T0193040

The Veterinary Book
for
Sheep Farmers

The Veterinary Book for Sheep Farmers

David C. Henderson

First published 1990
Reprinted 1991, 1994, 1995, 1997, 1999, 2000, 2002, 2006, 2010, 2020

Copyright © 1990 David C. Henderson

Published by Old Pond Publishing

Reprinted 2021 by
5m Books Ltd
Lings, Great Easton, Essex CM6 2HH, UK
www.5mbooks.com

A catalogue record for this book is avilable from the British Library

ISBN 978-1-903366-30-1

Cover design by Andrew Thistlethwaite
Phototypeset by Galleon Photosetting, Ipswich
Printed in Great Britain by Bell and Bain Ltd, Glasgow

CONTENTS

Appendices

Index

ACKNOWLEDGEMENTS

I would like to thank my many friends and colleagues who have helped during the prolonged gestation of this book. I have badgered them to supply information and photographs and to check the manuscript for me. They are Ken Angus, David Blewett, David Buxton, Bob Coop, Neil Gilmour, Alastair Greig, Hugh Reid, Mike Sharp, John Spence and Neville Suttle.

I have also borrowed photographs from Alex Donaldson, David Doxey, John Egerton, Mike Geary, Lorna Hay, Gareth Jones, John King, Francis David Kirby, Bill McKelvey, David Mellor, Elspeth Milne, Hugh Reed, John Robinson, Angus Russell, Barti Synge, Jill Thomson, Ian Wilmut Eddy Winkler, Coopers Pitman-Moore, the Central Veterinary Laboratory, John Deere (The Furrow), Medata Ltd and the Upjohn Company. The Agricultural Training Board kindly allowed me to reproduce their training material on sheep dipping.

Both Brian Easter and Alan Inglis have taken photographs for me and have developed and printed my own efforts—the best black and whites are theirs. Eddy Gray and Leslie Inglis took the excellent electron microscope pictures throughout. I thank all these people and the organisations to which they belong for their help.

The illustrations throughout are by Alice Helen Henderson, BVM&S, MRCVS.

Mary Martin warrants special mention for her skilful word-processing of the manuscript and for her cheerful fortitude throughout. So too does John Spence for his invaluable and unstinting help and advice. Dr Ian Aitken, the Director of the Moredun Research Institute, kindly allowed me to use the facilities of the Institute and I thank him and the Animal Diseases Research Association for their support.

Roger Smith and Julanne Arnold of Farming Press Books have been constructive and helpful throughout and I have valued their forbearance.

Since this book has been written at home during the early hours of the morning, the evenings, the middle of the night, weekends and holidays, my apologies go to my family, who have had to endure considerable disruption to their lives. My special thanks to my wife Alice, for her encouragement and gentle cajoling, and to my sons John and Roy, who have trouped through with innumerable cups of tea, coffee and helpful remarks!

To the memory of
Catherine Louise Henderson
who died in December, 1970

PREFACE

It is our duty to ensure the welfare of the flocks in our charge by maintaining the very highest standards of husbandry and health care through skilled and diligent shepherding. I hope that this book will be of some assistance in this regard since it has been written primarily for the guidance of sheep farmers and shepherds. However, I believe it will also be of benefit to agricultural advisers, to students of both agriculture and veterinary medicine, to veterinary surgeons who deal with sheep only on an infrequent basis and, indeed, to anyone who keeps a few sheep or has an interest in them.

The success of any sheep breeding enterprise depends upon a high level of reproductive efficiency. To that end I have included an account of the reproductive management necessary to achieve optimum results, beginning at weaning with the preparation for mating and, working on a calendar basis, through pregnancy to lambing, lactation and back to weaning. Many diseases and disorders associated with reproduction afflict sheep at specific stages of the cycle and I have slotted them in accordingly. Other diseases occur on a seasonal basis or may affect a particular age group. Others again do not fit any particular pattern and may arise at any time. These I have fitted in where it seemed most appropriate.

The idea of this calendrical approach was to encourage the reader to peruse a section of the book in advance of the event. For example, for a spring lambing flock, the chapters dealing with the care, welfare and diseases of the newborn lamb can be read early in the new year, so that the reminders contained therein will prompt the flockmaster and shepherd to make preparations in good time. I also hope that the husbandry and health programme set out in Appendix 1 will guide the reader in planning a regime for his or her own flock.

I make no apology for mentioning the role of the veterinary surgeon on numerous occasions. Too many sheep farmers call on their veterinary practice only for emergencies, usually around lambing time. It would be more cost-effective to use the veterinary surgeon's expertise in preventing and controlling disease. After all, a sick animal is frequently an indication of a failure to foresee problems and take avoiding action. This is discussed fully in Appendix 2.

It has been my aim to come to the aid of flockmasters in their constant battle to thwart the sheep in its desire to die for no apparent reason and in so doing to improve the wellbeing of this appealing species.

DCH
Broughton, Peebleshire
Scotland 1990

A NOTE ABOUT RECENT DEVELOPMENTS

Since the preparation of the first edition of this book there have been a number of developments to which I would draw your attention.

The advice given to farmers concerning the control of internal parasites has changed significantly because anthelmintic resistance has become a matter for considerable concern in the UK. The reader is referred to a document entitled *'Sustainable Control of Parasites in Sheep'* (SCOPS) which can be viewed on the National Sheep Association (NSA) website at www.nationalsheep.org.uk. It is important to appreciate that while the advice given is based on sound science, it has yet to be verified and flock owners are advised not to make significant changes to their present control measures without consulting their veterinary surgeon.

It is expected that a similar revision will shortly be made to the advice concerning the control of ectoparasites. Sheep scab is no longer a notifiable disease and has subsequently spread to all areas of the UK, seriously compromising sheep welfare. The *National Scrapie Plan* is a long-term, extensive genetic experiment with the aim of reducing the incidence of the disease in the national flock. Caseous lymphadenitis has moved from pedigree into commercial flocks and is likely to progress unless strenuous controls are implemented. A new and severe lameness now affects some flocks – contagious ovine digital dermatitis (CODD) – as if footrot were not enough to contend with!

Since the devastating outbreak of foot & mouth disease in the UK in 2001, the need for flock biosecurity has never been greater. The agriculture departments of all the devolved administrations in the UK provide information on how to protect animals from infectious disease, but Northern Ireland has a particularly helpful website at www.dardni.gov.uk – go to *'Biosecurity for Northern Ireland Farms'*. Whilst the advice given is equally applicable to all areas of the country, it is strongly advised that local veterinary advice is sought in devising tailor-made biosecurity measures which should be incorporated into the flock health plan.

DCH
Broughton, Peebleshire, Scotland, 2006

1

HEALTH AND DISEASE

Good health implies a soundness of body with all the organs, the muscles and the skeleton functioning normally. Fortunately, most animals are healthy, or reasonably so, for most of the time. Disease, on the other hand, is a state of ill health, which implies that some parts of the body are not functioning as they should. Disease may be due to one or more of a number of direct causes—sometimes referred to as the **exciting causes** of disease, although they are unlikely to be considered exciting to the animals concerned! The bacterium *Pasteurella haemolytica* is the exciting cause of one form of pneumonia in sheep. Copper deficiency in the diet of pregnant ewes may be the exciting cause of swayback in their lambs.

Apart from the direct causes of disease, there are numerous other factors which, although not able to cause disease themselves, may influence

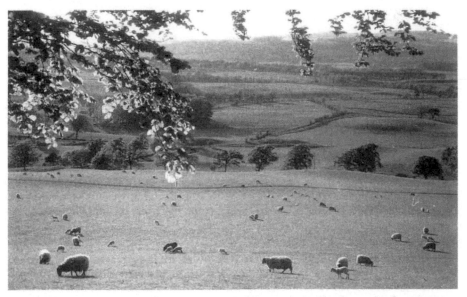

Plate 1.1 A group of healthy ewes and lambs on a productive upland pasture.

1

whether or not an animal will become ill or sustain an injury. These are known as the contributory or **predisposing factors**. It is known that the bacteria which cause pasteurella pneumonia can live in the upper respiratory tract of normal, healthy sheep without causing disease. However, should the sheep become stressed in some way, perhaps by being overcrowded in a poorly ventilated shed, then the bacteria may find their way into the deep recesses of the lung, multiply rapidly and cause pneumonia. In this example, the overcrowding and inadequate ventilation would be two of the contributory or predisposing factors.

Some of the more important exciting and predisposing causes of disease are discussed below.

EXCITING CAUSES OF DISEASE

Living organisms

When most people think of disease they think first of infectious disease. Strictly speaking, all living organisms capable of causing disease are parasites, but by tradition this term has been reserved for two important categories of relatively large living organisms, namely the **external parasites** which include ticks, mites, lice, keds and flies, and the **internal parasites**, which comprise roundworms, tapeworms and liver fluke. The other major category is that of the **microorganisms** which include viruses, bacteria and fungi, and these are discussed in more detail later in this chapter.

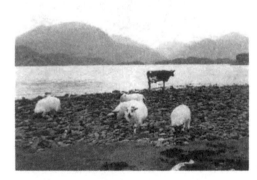

Plate 1.2 Lambs in the Scottish Highlands. Radioactive fallout from Chernobyl in 1986 has compromised the livelihood of many sheep farmers in the hill areas of the UK.

Physical and chemical agents

The definition of disease given earlier must include states which would normally be thought of as injury rather than disease. However, a lamb with a fractured leg is diseased, as is one which has been chemically burnt through the use of an inappropriate product, such as neat lysol applied to an area of flystrike. Radioactivity would also come under this heading and whilst clinical disease in sheep following the Chernobyl incident has not been recorded, nevertheless, heavily exposed sheep have been declared unfit for consumption in order to protect the human population against the possibility of disease (see Chapter 16). There must also remain the possibility of damage to the germ cells—the precursors of ova or sperm—which could result in the birth of genetically deformed lambs at some future date.

Genetic abnormalities

Occasionally lambs are born with some physical deformity, such as entropion (an inturning of the lower eyelid), an unperforate anus (where there is no connection from the gut to the exterior) or some functional abnormality of an organ. This may occur as a result of the mix of genes of the dam and sire. In these instances the genes donated to the affected lambs by their parents are the direct cause of the disease condition (This should not be confused with genetic susceptibility or resistance to disease, which is a predisposing factor—see below.)

Nutrition and feeding

What animals eat may influence their health very considerably. First and foremost, they must be offered a sufficient amount of food which will provide them with adequate energy, protein, vitamins, minerals and trace elements for their needs. An animal's requirements change with age and status. A twin bearing ewe in late pregnancy requires not only a great deal more food than a store lamb, but also a different balance in the constituents of the diet. Deciding what an animal's requirements are at any stage of its life is the science of nutrition. Providing those requirements is the art of feeding.

Most diseases caused directly through inadequate feeding are due to deficiencies, excesses or imbalances between individual nutrients and in particular of minerals, trace elements and vitamins. Magnesium deficiency in lush spring swards may cause hypomagnesaemia in lactating ewes. Copper deficiency in the diet of pregnant ewes may lead to abnormal development of the nervous system of the foetuses and the birth of swayback lambs. Similarly, a deficiency of vitamin E in the pregnancy ration may lead to white muscle disease and the sudden death of young lambs.

On the other hand, an excess of copper in the diet of housed sheep—for example, by feeding an inappropriate mineral supplement formulated for cattle—may precipitate cases of sudden death through copper poisoning. Free access minerals rich in iron, offered to sheep grazing swards with a perfectly adequate copper content, may be the cause of copper deficiency, since iron 'locks up' this element, making it unavailable to the animal. The excessive ingestion of soil—such as may occur when sheep graze turnips very close to the ground or badly poached leys in wet, muddy weather— may also cause copper deficiency because of its high iron content. Soil often contains the bacterium responsible for causing listeriosis. If silage is spoiled

3

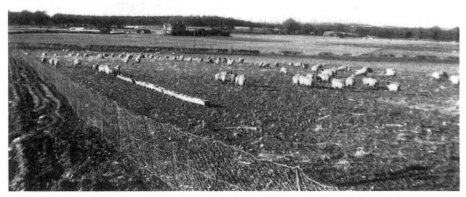

Plate 1.3 Lambs on a root break. Ingestion of soil (which has a high iron content) may make copper unavailable to the animal.

in the making and is also contaminated with soil, then the bacteria may multiply in the clamp or big bales and cause disease in sheep eating it. Certain plants may cause disease at a particular stage of growth, or if taken in excess. Too much clover may cause frothy bloat and an excessive intake of kale may lead to goitre in young sheep because of a deficiency of iodine. Under certain adverse conditions sheep may graze poisonous plants which they might not normally eat. Prolonged bracken intake may lead to bright blindness and sheep nibbling at yew trees for only a short time will surely die.

PREDISPOSING FACTORS OF DISEASE

Management and husbandry

Policy decisions taken by sheep farmers or shepherds can have a profound effect on the health of the flock. One particularly crucial decision is whether to keep a **closed** flock—where breeding replacements are home bred—or an **open** flock, where they are purchased. In the closed flock, it should only be necessary to purchase rams. This considerably reduces the risk of introducing infection, especially if they are purchased from a source with a high health status, are carefully examined before being brought onto the farm and are kept in quarantine for a period before mixing with the rest of the rams or joining the ewes. Even so, they may still bring in infection, for example, border disease, or they may contribute genes which make their offspring more (or less) susceptible to certain diseases, such as scrapie.

In the open flock, the risk of introducing infection is increased very substantially. Large numbers of animals are purchased and they may come from a number of different sources. The period of greatest risk is during late pregnancy and at lambing, when ewes may abort from one or more of a long list of highly infectious agents. The risk is not only to the home flock, but also to the newcomers, since they may become exposed to an infection which is under a degree of control in the home flock, but to which they are highly susceptible. Enzootic abortion is one of the most serious problems in the United Kingdom. It has long been of major importance, but it appears to be spreading further afield, due mainly to the considerable traffic in breeding females and the increase in intensification.

The provision of **parasite-free** or 'clean' **grazing** for lambs will ensure that they fatten more quickly and efficiently and will also reduce the need for frequent dosing with anthelmintics. However, the **strategic use of anthelmintics** to control worms or liver fluke disease on farms where other methods of control are impractical or uneconomic is an essential husbandry operation, not only because of the increased productivity it will bring, but also because it will improve the well-being of the flock.

A number of diseases are an ever-present risk on most, if not all, sheep farms. Some, such as the clostridial diseases and pasteurella pneumonia, are life threatening. Others, such as footrot, may be crippling, both to the sheep and to the profitability of the flock. Others, such as enzootic abortion and orf, may be a risk only in certain flocks. In all of the above examples, **vaccination** is an option for prevention or control. If a vaccine is not available, **routine medication** may be an alternative—for example, the use of monensin-medicated feed to reduce the impact of toxoplasmosis where abortions are expected.

The provision of an adequate standard of **housing** may significantly influence the health of the flock. If buildings are wrongly sited and badly designed and stock are overcrowded in them, then certain diseases may flourish. Atypical pneumonia may severely limit the productivity of animals in overstocked, poorly ventilated accommodation. Poor **hygiene** standards in buildings will increase the risk of infection. When an outbreak of diarrhoea occurs during lambing, almost every lamb born is likely to become infected because of the enormous build-up of infection in the pens, unless they are thoroughly cleaned out, disinfected and amply bedded down.

Whilst imbalances in the diet may be a direct cause of disease (see above), improper feeding may also predispose to disease. The provision of inadequate trough space for housed ewes in late pregnancy may lead to bullying. Some ewes may not receive their full ration of concentrates and the resulting energy deficit may precipitate cases of twin lamb disease (pregnancy toxaemia). A similar situation may occur in single bearing hill ewes, when the already meagre grazings are covered with snow and no supplementary feeding is on offer.

Inadequate feeding in mid pregnancy (or overfeeding in early pregnancy) may mean that the placenta or afterbirth (which transfers nutrients to the lamb from the ewe) does not grow to an adequate size. This will lead to the birth of small lambs, a reduction in the yield of colostrum and milk and poor mothering instinct in the ewe—all of which will increase the incidence

5

of lamb mortality and slow the growth rate of the surviving lambs.

Deficiencies of energy and protein in the diet may mean that the sheep is unable to mount a proper response to infection (see below), and recent research has shown that sub-clinical copper deficiency in lambs may make them much more prone to many of the diseases of early life.

Weather

Adverse or extreme weather conditions may have both direct and indirect influences on disease within a flock. Harsh weather at lambing time on the hill may increase lamb mortality substantially. Several seasons of wet summers are likely to increase the incidence of liver fluke on affected farms and conversely, several dry summers will reduce the risk because of the effect on the intermediate host snail population. As the weather warms during the summer, so the development of infective worm larvae on pasture speeds up, so that by mid-summer, the challenge to grazing lambs may be overwhelming. Footrot infection is not able to spread from sheep to sheep via the pasture unless weather conditions are suitable. The ground must be constantly wet for a prolonged period and the mean daily temperature must exceed 10°C.

Age and status

As a generalisation—to which there are always exceptions—younger and older animals are more prone to disease and injury than the middle-aged. The young may not have acquired immunity to particular diseases and the older animals' defences against infection may be compromised to a degree. The physiological status of an animal is obviously important. Mastitis is more likely in the lactating ewe and twin lamb disease only in the pregnant ewe. Around lambing and during lactation, ewes are less able to keep worm infestations under control due to changes in their hormone status. These changes allow the female worms to begin egg laying, so that the ewes then begin to add significantly to the pasture contamination which will challenge their lambs.

Stress

Stress is a very difficult concept to explain satisfactorily, but there is no doubt that animals, including humans, do undergo detrimental physical and physiological changes as a result of adverse factors in their environment. In some instances, it is possible to measure hormonal and other changes in blood which indicate that an animal may be in pain or distress. For example, cortisol levels in the blood of lambs rise after they have been rubber-ring castrated, indicating that they are feeling pain, and some lambs may demonstrate in their behaviour—by rolling about on the ground, for example—that they are suffering. This painful stress may prevent them from sucking colostrum if they are ringed during the first day of life. This in turn may predispose them to hypothermia or to infections such as watery mouth.

Stress may come in many forms and often several factors may act together to compromise the animal severely. For example, during hot humid weather, unsheared fattening lambs, overcrowded in an inadequately ventilated barn, are almost inevitably going to experience an outbreak of pneumonia, since the microorganisms responsible are very likely to be present in a proportion of the population.

Intercurrent disease

Animals already suffering from one or more diseases may become much more susceptible to others. Lambs with a sub-clinical copper deficiency have been shown to be considerably more likely to succumb to the diseases to which lambs are prone during the early weeks of life. Sheep afflicted by the virus-induced lung tumour jaagsiekte are known to be much more susceptible to pasteurella pneumonia, and often it is this infection which kills them before the tumour does.

Genetic susceptibility or resistance to disease

It is commonly acknowledged that some infectious diseases affect some species and not others. For example, foot and mouth disease does not normally infect humans—although there are a handful of recorded cases! Similarly, sheep do not suffer from mumps or whooping cough—they are said to be innately resistant by virtue of their genetic make-up. However, amongst closely related species, such as the ruminants, there are many shared diseases. Cattle and sheep both suffer from pasteurella pneumonia, liver fluke, Johnes disease, some of the clostridial diseases and many more. There are also infections which cause disease across many mammalian species, including man, such as salmonellosis, tuberculosis, toxoplasmosis and ringworm, although the symptoms and severity may differ and the strains of microorganism may vary between species of host.

The genetic make-up of an individual of a particular breed may make it more or less susceptible or resistant to particular disease conditions. For instance, the Texel breed is particularly susceptible to copper poisoning but more resistant to copper deficiency. This is in contrast to the Scottish Blackface which is more prone to deficiency and less prone to poisoning. Individual animals in a flock may be more or less susceptible to footrot, and there is some recent evidence that certain families of sheep within a breed may be more susceptible to broken mouth than others. Strains of sheep within a breed may be more resistant to a particular strain of the scrapie agent than others. Resistant sheep which become infected may die at a ripe old age from some other cause before the scrapie agent has time to cause clinical disease, whilst less resistant sheep which become infected may develop clinical signs in middle age and die.

Microorganisms

Microorganism is the collective term used throughout this book to describe a variety of extremely small living agents, a number of which are capable of infecting and sometimes of causing disease in animals and humans. It is these latter—the **pathogens**—which we are concerned with in this book. The main groupings are the bacteria, the fungi and the viruses, although there are a number of others—for example, the mycoplasma and the rickettsia.

Microorganisms are so small that it is difficult to imagine just how small, particularly in the case of viruses. The parasite worms of sheep are gigantic in relation to the largest microorganism and even they can be seen only with difficulty by the naked eye, being only the thickness of a hair and about half a centimetre long. (*Haemonchus contortus*, the barber's pole worm, is much larger than all the other worms and is clearly visible to the naked eye.) Bacteria can only be seen when magnified hundreds of times under the light microscope and only then when they are stained with special dyes. Viruses are so small that with very few exceptions they cannot be seen even under the highest power of the light microscope. However, they can be 'seen' indirectly using an electron microscope, which magnifies them many thousands of times.

Despite their extremely small size, microorganisms are capable of causing varying degrees of damage in their hosts, from a mild insult, such as a discrete local abscess, to severe injury or death in the case of acute mastitis or listeriosis.

VIRUSES

Viruses grow and multiply only inside the cells of their host animal. This they do by taking over the host cells and 'instructing' them to manufacture virus particles rather than do the job they normally perform. Consequently, the infected host cells fill up with enormous numbers of virus particles and then burst, releasing the new viruses which then infect neighbouring cells. The consequence of this is the destruction of host cells, often on a massive scale, especially if virus particles travel in blood and so reach all parts of the body (viraemia). The symptoms in the animal will depend on the type of cells which are destroyed and the degree of destruction. For example, the louping ill virus attacks cells in the central nervous system and so the symptoms are nervous in character and will eventually cause the death of the animal. The orf virus, on the other hand, attacks only cells in the skin and mucous membranes, and whilst this can cause considerable damage, it is rarely life threatening. Some viruses may cause tumours (cancer) and the retrovirus responsible for jaagsiekte is an example.

Viruses can survive for only a limited period outside the host, and then

8

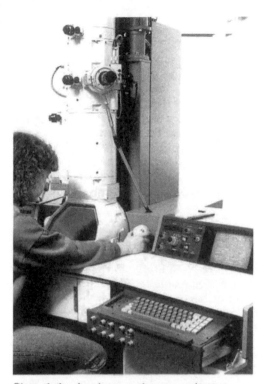

Plate 1.4 A microscopist at work at a transmission electron microscope. This machine can magnify up to one million times.

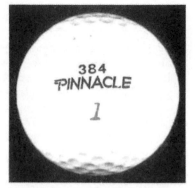

The three microorganisms photographed below have been magnified to the size of a golf ball. If the golf ball above were magnified to the same extent —

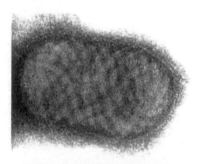

as the orf virus it would have a diameter of 6,060 metres or 4½ miles.

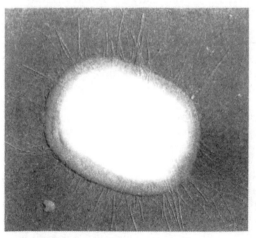

as *E. coli* it would have a diameter of 1,350 metres or 9/10 of a mile.

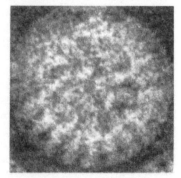

as rotavirus it would have a diameter of 24,960 metres or 16½ miles.

only if they are adequately protected from the environment. They cannot multiply outside the host, so if scientists wish to observe their effects on cells or need to grow them in the laboratory, they have to grow single layers of animal cells in glass vessels and infect them with the virus. They can then observe the effects on the cells using a light microscope, or the virus can be 'harvested' from these cell cultures. To confirm the diagnosis of a virus disease it is often necessary to set up a series of tests on blood to detect antibodies against the suspect virus (see below). Diagnosis can sometimes be confirmed by identifying the virus directly using the electron microscope, as in the case of diarrhoea in lambs caused by rotavirus.

BACTERIA

Unlike the viruses, many bacteria are able to multiply in the environment as well as in the animal's body. Listeria, for example, are able to multiply in silage under certain conditions. Many bacteria are also able to survive for long periods away from a host, such as the bacterium causing lamb dysentery, whereas others like the footrot bacterium *Bacteroides nodosus* may survive for only a few days.

Bacteria such as anthrax and pasteurella possess characteristics which allow them to invade further and further into the animal's body rapidly and effectively, and this allows them to do a lot of widespread damage very quickly. Others cannot easily invade the tissues and grow and multiply more slowly and only locally. They may, however, be even more devastating than the invasive bacteria, since they may produce poisons known as **toxins**, some of which are extremely potent. *Clostridium botulinum* toxin is the most poisonous substance known: substantially less than a kilogram would be all that was necessary to kill the entire human population of the world. *Clostridium tetani*, the cause of tetanus or lockjaw, multiplies in deep wounds or in tissues deprived of oxygen, such as those immediately under the rubber rings used for the castration and tailing of baby lambs. Here it produces a very powerful toxin called tetanospasmin, which affects nerve cells and produces the classical nervous symptoms of the disease.

Bacteria are generally much easier to handle than viruses. They can usually be grown in the laboratory—from blood, faeces, urine or a variety of post-mortem tissues—on special media which contain the sort of food bacteria require, such as blood. They may then be identified using a variety of laboratory techniques.

Where it is difficult or impossible to grow bacteria in the laboratory, evidence in the form of antibodies in blood may be looked for, as in the case of virus infections. Laboratory diagnosis, to confirm or dispute a diagnosis based on clinical signs and a history of the case or outbreak, is a vital step in the treatment and control of a disease.

A large number of species of harmless bacteria (and protozoa) inhabit the rumen. They are essential to the function of that organ and therefore to the digestion and well-being of the ruminant.

FUNGI

Fungi are lowly members of the plant kingdom that are closely related to bacteria. The only common fungal infection in sheep in the UK is lumpy wool (mycotic dermatitis), the development of which is more related to factors such as the weather conditions than to animal to animal transmission. Ringworm is another fungal disease but it is uncommon in sheep in the UK.

SOURCES OF MICROORGANISMS

Some microorganisms which cause disease in animals are found very widely in the environment, especially in the areas where animals are kept. The bacterium *E. coli* and the virus rotavirus (both of which cause diarrhoea in young animals) can be found as contaminants of bedding, food and water supplies, vehicle tyres, shepherds' hands, clothes, boots and lambing equipment. Indeed, where there has been an outbreak of scour it would be difficult to find any object in the vicinity which was not contaminated. The clostridial bacteria—different members of which cause diseases such as lamb dysentery, pulpy kidney and tetanus—are also common contaminants of sheep surroundings. This group of bacteria is capable of forming highly resistant forms, called **spores**, which can survive in soil and elsewhere for very many years, so that they are a constant threat to any livestock enterprise. Vaccination is therefore essential against this group of bacteria.

Other bacteria have a much more restricted distribution. When an animal dies from anthrax, the blood contains countless millions of the bacteria responsible. Immediately any blood is exposed to the air—through oozing from the various orifices or by the carcass being cut open—the anthrax bacilli form very resistant spores. These will contaminate the soil and herbage wherever the blood is spilt, and as the spores can probably survive for 50 years or more, this area can be considered a permanent risk. Anthrax is now a rare disease in the UK, and so the areas of contamination are relatively few, especially since it is a notifiable disease and every effort is made to reduce contamination by careful disposal of the dead animal and treatment of the surrounding area. The main risk from anthrax in the past was from uncooked meat products imported from countries where the disease is endemic, but this trade has long been prohibited.

Foot and mouth disease virus is the most infectious microorganism known, in either animal or human medicine. The UK operates a slaughter policy to eradicate the disease on the relatively rare occasions that it is imported into the country. In consequence, the virus is not found in the UK except during an epidemic. Since it is not able to survive for long outside its animal hosts, the virus is destroyed along with the slaughtered animals.

Some animals infected with a microorganism may either not become

11

diseased or else recover, but not succeed in eliminating the microorganism from their bodies. These carrier animals, whilst appearing normal, or relatively so, will continue to excrete the bacteria or virus and thus remain a source of infection for their flock mates for considerable periods, or even for the rest of their lives. This state of affairs occurs in the virus infection known as border disease and also in some cases of salmonellosis.

THE TRANSMISSION OF INFECTION

Microorganisms employ a number of different methods of transmission. In respiratory diseases such as pasteurella pneumonia, the bacteria are coughed, sneezed or simply breathed out on minute droplets of water (aerosol) which float around in the atmosphere to be breathed in by other sheep in close proximity. Obviously, stocking rate will influence the degree of spread, as will the efficiency of ventilation and the prevailing weather conditions.

Bacteria and viruses responsible for causing diarrhoea in newborn lambs depend upon thorough contamination of the lambing area, so that each new lamb will inevitably become infected by mouth as soon as it is born. The important causes of abortion in ewes are also transmitted by mouth. When a ewe aborts in the lambing area, other ewes nose around the dead foetus, afterbirth and fluids and so may become infected themselves. Other microorganisms which contaminate the lambing area, such as one of the bacteria which causes footrot (*Fusobacterium necrophorum*), infect lambs via the wet navel cord.

The 'friendly' bacteria and protozoons which keep the rumen functional are also transmitted by mouth from ewes to lambs, so that when the lambs become ruminants these microorganisms are already present in the gut and take over that part of the digestive function.

Some microorganisms are transmitted by an intermediary. Louping ill virus, the organism causing tickborne fever and probably the bacteria responsible for tick pyaemia are all transmitted via the bite of the sheep tick. Spread of infection at mating (venereal) is not an important method of transmission of infection in sheep in the UK, although in other species of animal and on a world-wide basis it is very significant.

Just because an animal comes into contact with an infectious microorganism does not mean that the animal will become diseased. Animals have a number of defence mechanisms at their disposal to ward off infection or to prevent disease becoming established and these are discussed in the following pages.

Protection Against Infection

All animals are continually being invaded by microorganisms from birth to death. Whilst most of them are completely harmless, a number are potentially or downright dangerous. However, most animals are healthy for most of the time providing that they are well fed and husbanded and are not exposed to overwhelming infection. This is not an accidental situation, but rather the result of an extremely sophisticated defence system which has developed over time.

PHYSICAL BARRIERS TO INFECTION

The body's first line of defence against infection consists of a series of physical barriers which prevent microorganisms from getting into the body tissues.

Respiratory tract

Many thousands of bacteria are breathed in through the nose and mouth daily, but few, if any, ever get into the deepest recesses of the lung. As the air passes through the nostrils, larger particulate matter—including dust and the minute droplets of moisture which transport bacteria and viruses—are trapped on the hairs and in the sticky **mucus** on the inner surface of the nostrils. Those that escape these defences are trapped in the mucus which lines the air passages. The cells on the surface layer of the air passages, which make up the **mucous membrane**, are also armed with hair-like structures called **cilia**, which waft the mucus and the entrapped microorganisms upwards and outwards. The mucus will eventually be coughed up and swallowed, together with any microorganisms it may have trapped.

Gut

Microorganisms which are ingested and swallowed by ruminants will be mixed into the huge volume of rumen contents. Many will perish here because the conditions in this 'fermentation vat' will be unsuitable for their growth and multiplication. Some will survive, however, and will move into the stomach or abomasum which contains hydrochloric acid at a concentration which will kill many microorganisms that survive the rumen. Any remaining survivors must then run the gauntlet of the intestine with its very different conditions, such as the alkaline environment of the small intestine.

Skin

Many bacteria land on, or adhere to, the skin. Healthy skin secretes a host of different chemicals on its surface which actively kill bacteria or prevent them from multiplying and establishing colonies. Some 'friendly' bacteria (commensals) are able to survive on the skin and help keep the potentially dangerous ones at bay through competition.

Reproductive tract

Microorganisms may enter the reproductive tract on the penis or in the semen of the ram at the time of mating. The slightly acidic conditions of the vagina may destroy some microorganisms and the flushing action of urination will get rid of others. A number of 'friendly' bacteria may establish in the lower reproductive tract (vagina) and some of these may help to ward off infection by other disease-producing bacteria.

Eyes

Eyelashes and eyelids protect the eye from damage by large particles. Tiny moisture particles containing bacteria and viruses, which land on the eyeball or its surrounding tissues, stick to the thin film of moisture flowing over the surface. This moisture is continually flushed away into the back of the throat via a narrow tube from the corner of the eye and replaced with fresh from the tear glands. When the eye is physically or chemically damaged or infected by microorganisms, the tears flow much more freely in an attempt to flush away the damaging agent. If an infection becomes established, blood vessels may grow across the surface of the eyeball (cornea) and transport white blood cells to the damaged area (see below). This interferes with vision temporarily or, if the damage is severe, sometimes permanently.

Inner body surfaces

All the above examples are of 'surface' defences. Whilst it will be obvious to the reader that the skin is on the surface of the body, it may be more difficult to accept that the inner lining of the gut, the air passages and all of the other orifices of the body are also surface structures, but this is nevertheless the case. The skin is a tough, relatively dry outer surface layer, whilst the inner surfaces are lined by a much more delicate covering, the mucous membrane. As the name implies, this layer is covered by mucus, secreted by special cells in the membrane. Mucus itself is a very important barrier to infection. It is only in relatively recent times that researchers have begun to appreciate just how important this sticky liquid is in the defence against infection. Apart from forming a physical barrier on the surface of the gut or respiratory tract, it also contains antibodies and other protective substances.

SECOND LINE DEFENCES

Microorganisms may breach the first lines of defence described above in a number of ways. For example, a scratch in the skin may allow the orf virus to enter the tissues and establish an infection, or the bite of the sheep tick may introduce the virus which causes louping ill. Warm, wet conditions underfoot may denature the skin between the cleats of the sheep's foot and allow the bacteria responsible for footrot to establish an infection. The flagella-like structures (pili) on the surface of disease-producing *E. coli* allow them to attach to the gut wall and so establish themselves. Poor ventilation in a building may lead to inefficient air flow, not only in the sheep shed, but also in the air passages of the sheep. This will reduce the efficiency of the cilia and allow the establishment of infection by either bacteria or viruses.

INFLAMMATION

As soon as an infectious microorganism—or, indeed, foreign material of any kind—breaches the first lines of defence and gains access to the tissues underneath, a truly remarkable series of events is set in train.

Damage to tissues—such as would occur following physical damage to the skin, or infection in some part of the gut—stimulates the release of chemicals which 'sound the alarm'. The blood vessels in the damaged area increase in diameter and so allow more blood to flow through them. They also become more permeable, so as to allow some of the components of blood to 'leak' out. These include white blood cells, which are needed to deal with any foreign intruders, and blood plasma, which helps to dilute the invaders or any toxins they may produce. A substance called fibrin also leaks out of the blood vessels and forms a 'web' in an attempt to trap microorganisms and so give the body's other defences a better chance to deal with them.

This process, which is called **inflammation**, causes the area concerned to become swollen, red and hot, due to the increased blood flow and its consequential events. This causes pain to a varying degree depending upon the extent of the damage and the number of nerve endings present in the affected area. The inflammatory process can easily be seen on the skin surface, but the same series of events will occur in any part of the body to a greater or lesser degree. This response to injury can sometimes be most inconvenient to the animal—for example, by stiffening up an injured limb, so making walking difficult—but it is a vital process on the road to recovery, since it focuses all the second line defence mechanisms on the injured or infected area. Inflammation reflects the 'heat of battle' which is the body's reaction to damage or infection.

The battle is a ferocious one, with no holds barred. It takes place between the invader and a series of specialised cells from various parts of the body which launch a coordinated attack. A short and much simplified description of the battle is given below, not only for the interest of readers, but also to provide a better understanding of the use of vaccines and antisera, and of the value of colostrum.

CELLULAR DEFENSES

When an animal becomes infected initially, the tissues of the body are invaded by relatively few microorganisms. However, once they begin to multiply, their numbers increase very rapidly and their presence in the body becomes 'noticed' by specialist cells whose job it is to defend the animal against invasion. There are a number of different types of cell which all have specific jobs to do and which cooperate with each other

15

in a remarkable way to mount a most effective, coordinated and usually successful defense against infection.

Apart from the red blood cells, which combine with oxygen in the lungs and yield it up to the tissues, there are a number of other types of cell in blood and these are known collectively as **white blood cells**. These are produced in the bone marrow and are vitally important in defending the body against invasion by infectious microorganisms.

PHAGOCYTES

One series of white blood cells is called **phagocytes** or 'feeder' cells. These are able to recognise any kind of 'foreign' material—be it a virus, a bacterium or a speck of coal dust—which gets past the body's first line of defences and into the tissues. Phagocytosis is a process whereby the cell

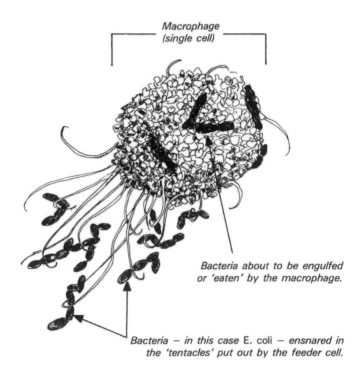

Macrophage
(single cell)

Bacteria about to be engulfed or 'eaten' by the macrophage.

Bacteria – in this case E. coli – ensnared in the 'tentacles' put out by the feeder cell.

Drawing based on a scanning electron microscope photograph which shows a feeder cell, or macrophage, at several thousand times magnification. Macrophages are one of the body's defences against invasion by microorganisms. One is shown here feeding on bacteria coated with substances (opsonins) which make them 'tastier' to the feeder cell.

Figure 1.1 A macrophage or feeder cell ensnaring and engulfing bacteria.

pushes out long pseudopodia or false feet from its surface. These catch hold of the intruding microorganisms and draw them towards the cell, which then engulfs or surrounds them, just as an amoeba does with its food. Once the microbe is inside the cell, it is covered with enzymes which enable the cell to kill and digest it. Sometimes the feeder cell is itself killed by the bacteria it ingests during this process. Indeed, some infectious agents have developed techniques which enable them to survive this attack. The accumulation of dead bacteria and phagocytic cells at the site of a wound is known as **pus**.

Phagocytic cells can recognise normal body cells as 'self' and so leave them alone, unless they become damaged (by a virus for example) or are abnormal in some way (such as cancer cells), in which case they destroy them. Viruses, bacteria and other microorganisms are recognised as foreign because they have a different arrangement of proteins on their surface from the body's own cells, which sets them apart. These proteins are called **antigens**. When microbes have been engulfed by phagocytes, they, or their dismembered parts, are carried in the lymph or blood to lymph nodes or to other lymph tissue about the body. Here they are 'presented' or 'displayed' to other specialised cells which learn to 'recognise' them.

One series of special cells—the **B cells**—have on their surface perhaps as many as one hundred thousand or more different receptors, each capable of locking onto a specific antigen on a particular microorganism. As there are literally millions of these cells in the body there is likely to be a receptor site to fit almost any foreign antigen which invades the body for the first time. As soon as a B cell comes across an antigen for which it has a receptor, it locks onto it. This reaction stimulates the B cell to divide rapidly, so producing huge numbers of cells all identical to each other and to the parent cell, called **clones**. Some of these clones remain in the body for life as **memory cells**. An identikit picture of each new invader is produced in this way, so that a 'rogues' gallery' is steadily built up over the years. In the event of a second or subsequent attack by the same microorganism, the body can recognise it immediately and act more rapidly and effectively as a consequence.

ANTIBODIES

Following rapid cell division, the B cells change into another type of cell, called a **plasma cell**. These are of great importance because they manufacture **antibodies**, which are special proteins sometimes referred to as **immunoglobulins**. They are manufactured in plasma cells to a precise configuration which fits exactly a specific antigen on the surface of a microorganism, or a toxin (poison) produced by a microorganism. An antibody can only combine with its specific antigenic counterpart. Antibodies produced against antigens on the surface of the bacterium which causes lamb dysentery, for example, are not able to bind with antigens of the bacterium causing pasteurella pneumonia or vice versa. Antibody production takes

17

place mainly in the spleen, the lymph nodes and lymph tissue in the gut and respiratory tract. When an animal becomes infected in the normal course of events and responds by producing antibodies, this is said to be a **naturally acquired active immunity** and is usually of reasonably long duration.

Antibodies in the diagnosis of disease

Following invasion by a microorganism for the first time, antibody production takes some days to get into gear and it is usually a week before antibodies specific to a particular disease can be detected in blood serum taken from the infected animal. Blood sampling for a particular antibody is an important technique used in the diagnosis of disease. For example, if toxoplasma abortion is suspected in a flock, then blood samples from aborted ewes can be taken and tests set up to look for the tell-tale antibodies which will provide evidence of infection with toxoplasma organisms at some time during the ewe's life. A positive result does not always mean that toxoplasma was the cause of the current abortion, however, since the ewe may have been infected the previous year and still retain some antibody in the blood. A second blood sample, two or three weeks after the first, may show a higher or lower level—or **titre**—of toxoplasma antibody. If the titre is higher, it probably means that the ewe is currently infected with the toxoplasma organism and is building up her antibody defences. If the titre is lower then it is probable that the ewe was infected at some earlier time of her life. This in itself is useful information, since it means that the search must be widened to look for antibodies to some other infectious abortion agent. What would happen in practice is that sufficient blood would be taken so that several tests could be undertaken to look for a whole range of antibodies against the long list of microorganisms which may cause abortion in ewes.

Because of the 'memory cells' stored in the body's immune system, should infection with the same microorganism occur a second or subsequent time (reinfection), then the system can get into gear very quickly, because the template for the particular antibody is already present and can be copied without delay. Animals may be vaguely unwell for a couple of days after reinfection, but once antibody production and the other antimicrobial defences get into full swing, the invaders are soon squashed.

ANTISERUM PRODUCTION

Reinfection usually produces high levels of antibody in blood and these antibodies can be harvested in blood serum and given to other animals who may be at particular risk from a dangerous infection. For example, if a horse—which has a large blood volume—is given a small, sensitising dose of lamb dysentery toxin (an antigen), it will produce antibodies against the toxin, which are called **antitoxins**—but only in relatively small amounts. However, if the horse is rechallenged with toxin it will produce very much larger amounts of antitoxin. A quantity of blood can then be taken from

Vaccines contain specific antigens which stimulate the animal to produce its own antibodies.

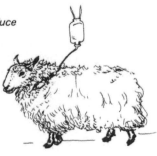

Ewes vaccinated annually during late pregnancy will transfer large quantities of antibodies into their colostrum in the days immediately before lambing, to protect their lambs, which are born without any antibody protection.

Lambs which suck colostrum in adequate amounts soon after birth will be protected (for a finite time) against the diseases to which the ewe is naturally immune, or against which she has been purposely vaccinated. Unvaccinated ewes transfer very limited disease protection to their lambs. The lambs must therefore be given 'ready-made' antibodies against the killer diseases of early life, such as lamb dysentery and pasteurella pneumonia.

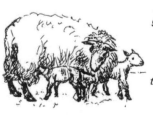

As lambs grow, they gradually use up their supply of colostral antibodies, and must therefore be vaccinated themselves, especially when they are to be retained as breeding replacements.

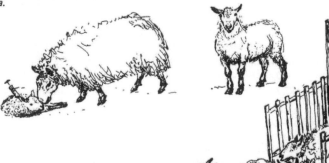

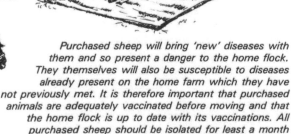

These antibodies are usually prepared by vaccinating horses, collecting blood from them and separating the serum which contains the antibodies (antiserum). This can then be injected into lambs at birth to provide them with instant protection.

Purchased sheep will bring 'new' diseases with them and so present a danger to the home flock. They themselves will also be susceptible to diseases already present on the home farm which they have not previously met. It is therefore important that purchased animals are adequately vaccinated before moving and that the home flock is up to date with its vaccinations. All purchased sheep should be isolated for least a month immediately on arrival.

Figure 1.2   Protective antibodies.

19

the horse, the red cells removed, and the remaining serum will be rich in lamb dysentery antitoxins. If newborn lambs are at particular risk from this disease—perhaps because their dams were not vaccinated against it, or because they did not get sufficient colostrum for one reason or another—they can be given antitoxin to provide immediate protection (see Chapter 9). This is known as **artificially acquired passive protection.**

The horse can be treated on a number of occasions in this way and several harvests of blood taken. The horse is chosen partly for its large blood volume and also because, although it recognises the toxin of lamb dysentery as an antigen and reacts by producing antibody against it, it is unaffected by the disease. It is said to be genetically or inherently resistant.

HOW ANTIBODIES PROTECT AGAINST DISEASE

When antibodies attach to antigens on the surface of a bacterium or virus, they may inconvenience or kill the microorganisms in a number of ways. They may prevent them from attaching to the surface of the gut so that they are unable to 'hang on' and cause damage. If a bacterium is motile—that is, capable of propelling itself along—antibodies may disable it, so that it cannot invade the body tissues. Antibodies may prevent microorganisms from growing or multiplying. They may have the ability to cause the invading microorganisms to stick to each other (agglutinate), which makes them more accessible to the cells which 'eat' or phagocytose foreign invaders. Antibodies or antitoxins may combine with the poisonous products of microorganisms (toxins), so neutralising them and rendering them harmless.

There are about nine special proteins in blood called **complement factors.** When antigens and antibodies combine, the chemical reaction attracts complement to the site of attachment. When all nine factors are present, complement is then able to penetrate the bacterial cell wall. This lets fluids into the bacterium which then swells up, bursts (lyses) and dies. The presence of antibodies on the surface of a microorganism also attracts **killer cells** to the site, which then destroy them. The combined effect of the above actions of antibody is to bring on the inflammatory response (see above), which, by increasing blood flow, brings ever-increasing numbers of feeder cells, killer cells and antibodies to the site of infection.

Vaccines and Vaccination

In 1774 in the village of Yetminster in Dorset, a farmer called Benjamin Jesty inoculated his wife and children with fluid from the blisters on the teats of cows affected with cowpox, from the neighbouring village of Chetnole. This was the first recorded case of deliberate vaccination. Indeed, the word **vaccination** is derived from the Latin for a cow—*vacca.*

Jesty, of course, did not know that he was inoculating his family with a live virus, but he was aware—like most country folk of the time—that milkmaids who caught the relatively mild, although disfiguring, disease of cowpox were apparently protected from the fatal or blinding disease of smallpox. In Gloucestershire in 1796, Dr Edward Jenner inoculated a boy called James Phipps with cowpox material taken from a human case of the disease. Subsequently, Jenner challenged the boy by inoculating him with smallpox and showed him to be immune to the infection. A brave boy and an even braver doctor!

From these humble country beginnings sprang one of the most important medical techniques in the fight against disease and one which has hardly scratched the surface of its true potential even today. In the case of smallpox, the combination of more sophisticated vaccines than those used by either Jesty or Jenner, together with some remarkable organisation and education, finally eradicated this dreadful scourge from the face of the earth more than 200 years later. Cowpox and smallpox are from the same family of pox viruses and have a very similar structure. When Jenner inoculated James Phipps with cowpox, the virus antigens would stimulate the boy's defense system to produce specific antibodies against those antigens. When he was subsequently challenged with the dangerous smallpox virus the cowpox antigens would be sufficiently similar to lock onto the smallpox and prevent it causing disease. The same principles are used today when preparing vaccines, although there is not always a convenient, closely related and naturally mild disease from which to prepare a safe vaccine.

It was another brilliant scientist, Louis Pasteur, who, in 1897, discovered a different method of safe vaccination quite by accident, whilst working with the poultry disease known as fowl cholera, caused by a bacterium named after him—*Pasteurella multocida*. Pasteur had left some bacteria on his laboratory bench when he went off on his holidays. On his return he noted that the normally potent disease-producing bacteria were not making birds sick and that some birds which he had inoculated with the old bacteria left on the bench could not then be infected by inoculation with fresh, potent bacteria. The prolonged growth over the holiday had weakened or '**attenuated**' the pasteurellae so that they could no longer cause serious disease, but would still stimulate an immune response and the production of protective antibodies. Pasteur subsequently grew his bacteria in the absence of oxygen to attenuate them and to make them safe enough to use in a vaccine.

LIVE VACCINES

Pasteur's type of vaccine is known as a **live attenuated vaccine**. Generally only one dose of such a vaccine is required to provide protection, since the attenuated bacteria or virus in the vaccine will be able to multiply to a limited extent in the animal. This increases the amount of antigen presented to the animal very considerably, so mimicking a natural infection. The animal responds by recognising the antigen and then by producing ever-increasing amounts of antibody (as described above) until it is able to overwhelm the deliberate infection. By this time the animal will have manufactured large amounts of antibody which will be only slowly destroyed. This will protect it against infection by the naturally occurring and dangerous microorganism. This is known as an **artificially acquired active immunity** and it generally provides protection against infection for a prolonged period of months, years or even a lifetime in some cases. It should be appreciated that whilst such vaccines are not able to produce the disease they are given to protect against, nevertheless, the animal may appear a little unwell and may run a fever for a short while after vaccination. They should therefore be treated with care during this period and not be unduly stressed, especially when vaccination is performed during pregnancy.

DEAD VACCINES

Vaccines can be made from killed bacteria or from toxins produced by bacteria. In this case at least two doses are required, separated by a few weeks, because the material injected is unable to multiply in the animal so that only a very small amount of antigen is presented to the animal. This is 'recognised' after the first injection and the information is stored in the memory cells. When a second dose of dead vaccine is inoculated into the animal some weeks later, the body immediately recognises the antigen and produces large amounts of antibody against it. However, the amount of antibody produced is usually significantly less than that following a live vaccination. The duration of protection is therefore shorter and so regular booster doses of dead vaccines are required to top up the level of immunity to a satisfactory protective level. The clostridial bacterial vaccines (e.g. '7 in 1') are dead vaccines, hence the requirement to boost ewes once or twice a year depending upon the level of risk.

Colostrum

Antibodies circulating in the blood of a ewe—as the result of natural infection or vaccination—are transferred in large quantities to the **colostrum** ('first milk') she produces in the days immediately before lambing. Since lambs become infected with microorganisms even during the birth process itself, it is vital that they suck colostrum from their mothers **immediately after birth and in sufficient quantity** to provide them with protection against infection if they are to survive and thrive. This type of protection is called **naturally acquired passive immunity**. The length of time a lamb will be protected will depend upon the particular antibody. For example, pasteurella antibodies present in colostrum will only protect the lamb for about three weeks after birth, whereas clostridial antibodies against diseases such as lamb dysentery, pulpy kidney and tetanus will protect for about three months. It is best if a lamb receives antibodies from its own dam, but it must derive them from somewhere and the alternatives are discussed in Chapter 8.

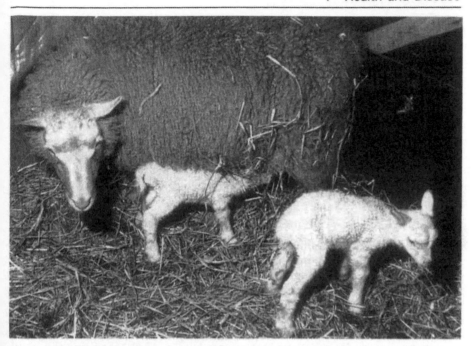

Plate 1.5 Finnish Landrace ewe suckling her lamb. Colostrum contains vital antibodies essential for lamb survival.

WHY VACCINATE?

It is obviously not possible, nor indeed necessary, to vaccinate animals against every microorganism they may come into contact with during the course of their lives. The farmer and the veterinary surgeon have to decide on the degree of risk to the flock and the level of protection required to make the sheep enterprise a profitable one, with due regard to the welfare of the sheep. Diseases such as the clostridial diseases are so common and so life threatening that it is essential to vaccinate all animals in the flock. In the case of the ewe, this will protect her and, in addition, it will provide protection for her lambs via colostrum.

Other diseases may be less than life threatening and the decision whether to vaccinate will depend upon the perceived degree of risk or the level of infection in the flock. For example, if the level of footrot in a flock is low and regular footbathing is sufficient to control the infection, then vaccination may be thought unnecessary. However, if lameness due to footrot is rife in the flock, then vaccination may be most helpful in reducing the level of infection when combined with the other methods of control.

The risk of infection with particular diseases will vary from farm to farm depending upon the terrain, climate and system of management. For

23

example, louping ill will only present a problem on tick-infested farms and then only if the tick population is itself infected with louping ill. Where this is the case, then vaccination of the flock is essential; otherwise sheep farming would be untenable, as it was on many farms in the north of England and Scotland in the days before a vaccine was available.

Where sheep have been farmed for many years, the particular risks will largely have been identified and a vaccination policy evolved to suit the farm. That is not to say that it will not need to be revised if the management of the flock changes. Where sheep are kept for the first time, local veterinary advice will be helpful in deciding on the essential and the optional vaccinations.

IMPROVING THE RESPONSE TO VACCINATION

In order to get an optimal response to vaccination—especially with dead vaccines—other components are added to the antigen to increase the immune response. Such substances, known as **adjuvants**, are more or less irritant to the body tissue, so that quite often a lump will appear at the site of the inoculation. With some vaccines the reaction will be hardly noticeable, but with others a large unsightly swelling will develop which may be painful.

In times past all sorts of strange substances were used as adjuvants, such as tapioca, starch or even breadcrumbs! Today, substances such as aluminium hydroxide or light mineral oils are used, but whilst reasonably effective they are far from satisfactory. A new generation of adjuvants which stimulate a strong immunity but do not provoke a reaction at the vaccination site is urgently required. It should be noted that a lump at the inoculation site does not mean the vaccine has not been effective, but rather the reverse. Oily adjuvants in particular will cause a nasty reaction in humans if vaccine is accidentally inoculated into, or scratched onto, the skin, and medical attention should be sought immediately.

Live vaccines—such as that against orf—depend upon the micro-organisms multiplying in the tissues and so the vaccine is introduced into the skin via a deliberate scratch made by a special applicator dipped in the vaccine. It is essential that the virus is not killed through the use of spirits, disinfectants, dips or pour-ons; otherwise the vaccine will not 'take'. If a scab does not form at the site of an orf vaccination within a few days, then the animal must be revaccinated.

It is essential always to read the vaccine manufacturer's instructions and to follow them strictly. Needles and syringes should be changed as instructed and empty vaccine containers disposed of safely. Never vaccinate sheep in bad weather or when they are sick, wet or dirty. Sick animals should be marked so that they can be done when they have properly recovered. Never mix vaccines or administer another vaccine or any other treatment at the same time, unless the manufacturer or your veterinary surgeon advises that it is safe to do so. **Particular care should be taken in the case of pregnant animals.**

Antimicrobial Drugs

Whilst the body has a very sophisticated defence system to defend itself against infection, there are occasions when the invading microorganisms gain the upper hand and the animal becomes so sick that its life may be threatened. Under these circumstances the animal will often benefit by being treated with drugs which kill or inhibit the growth of the invading microorganisms. These drugs, collectively known as antimicrobials, consist of two main groups. The first are chemicals synthesised by man—the **chemotherapeutics**—and the second are naturally occurring substances produced either by bacteria or fungi—the **antibiotics**. The sulphonamides are examples of chemotherapeutic agents, whilst penicillin and tetracycline are examples of antibiotics. It has been possible to determine the chemical structure of some of the antibiotics and to synthesise them in the laboratory. For the purpose of simplifying the following discussion all antimicrobial drugs will be referred to as antibiotics.

Numerous chemical substances are capable of killing microorganisms, but relatively few can do so without also killing or damaging the animal's own cells. Some of the more toxic chemicals which are unsuitable for animal treatment can be used as **disinfectants** for sterilising buildings and some less toxic substances as **antiseptics** for the sterilisation of the skin prior to surgery or the injection of an antibiotic.

Antibiotics are principally used to treat infections caused by bacteria or fungi, as very few have any effect upon viruses. When they are used in viral infections, such as orf, it is usually to control opportunist bacterial infection of the tissues which have been damaged by the virus.

Bacterial cells are similar to body cells, but they differ in a number of important ways. Also, the various types of bacteria have different characteristics. The problem facing scientists attempting to discover or develop new antibiotics is to identify these differences and to find compounds which can selectively attack without damaging the host animal. Penicillin, which was discovered by Sir Alexander Fleming in 1929, is still one of the most widely used antibiotics. Its interference with the formation of the bacterial cell wall causes a leak that results in the death of the bacteria. Antibiotics like penicillin which kill bacteria are known as **bacteriocides**. Penicillin is effective against a restricted, although important, group of bacteria (known as the gram positives) and is therefore said to be a narrow spectrum antibiotic. The tetracyclines interfere with the protein production of a wide range of bacteria (both gram positive and negative) and are classed as broad spectrum antibiotics. At the dose rates which can be safely administered, the tetracyclines do not kill bacteria, but disable them sufficiently for the body's own defence system to finish them off. They are therefore known as **bacteriostats.**

It is important to appreciate that **antibiotics are used to assist the body to overcome infection.** If the body's defence system is compromised—for example, through the administration of steroid drugs—then the animal is less likely to be able to overcome the infection despite help from antibiotic treatment.

USES OF ANTIBIOTICS

These drugs may be used to treat sick animals based on your veterinary surgeon's diagnosis of the disease. The choice of antibiotic will depend upon a number of factors, such as the species of animal, the suspected or confirmed bacteria responsible, the site of infection in the animal's body, the method of action of the antibiotic and the cost of medication. Treatment will hopefully ensure survival of the sick animal and speed up its recovery, so reducing the degree of pain and suffering. It will also reduce the contamination of the environment with infectious bacteria and therefore reduce the risk to in-contact animals. Indeed, in-contact animals may be treated even though they are showing no symptoms, on the assumption that they are likely to become infected. This is known as **preventive therapy** and can be justified under specific circumstances. It is less easily justified if used in place of good husbandry. Certain antibiotics which are not prescribed in human medicine are permitted as animal growth promotors, although these are rarely, if ever, used in sheep production in the UK.

ANTIBIOTIC RESISTANCE

There is no conclusive evidence that low level use, or indeed high level use, of antibiotics in animals presents any hazard to man in terms of bacterial drug resistance or antibiotic residues, providing they are used in accordance with the label recommendations. Almost all problems of antibiotic resistance in humans arise from the misuse of these drugs in man and not through their veterinary use. Nevertheless, antibiotics are valuable drugs and should be used responsibly and always under prescription and on veterinary advice.

Resistance is said to occur when a bacterium is no longer susceptible to a particular antibiotic or group of antibiotics. It can occur in a number of ways but is generally not related to the frequent use of a particular antibiotic. In a rapidly multiplying population of bacteria there will always be a proportion of variants, or mutants, some of which may be resistant to a particular antibiotic. If the treatment wipes out all the susceptible bacteria, then the remaining population will be resistant to that antibiotic. Generally it is high level therapeutic use of antibiotics, for the treatment or prevention of disease, which exerts this type of selection pressure, rather than the low level rates used for growth promotion. This is contrary to popular belief.

Drug resistance problems are most commonly encountered in hospitals, where there are large populations of patients undergoing treatment with high doses of antibiotics.

SIDE EFFECTS OF ANTIBIOTICS

Most of the commonly used antibiotics have a wide margin of safety at the recommended dose rates. Generally, the bacteriocidal drugs are more likely to produce side effects, but these are rare. (It is well known that penicillin produces hypersensitivity in a small proportion of humans.) Occasionally there is a reaction at the site of injection of a drug. If the dose rate is exceeded, then toxic effects may occur—for example, liver damage—especially in animals already suffering from a liver complaint, or in old or very young animals. Extra care should always be taken with pregnant animals.

There is a 'friendly' resident flora of microorganisms in the gut of all animals, including man. Prolonged antibiotic treatment by mouth may wipe out or significantly alter this population and this may allow less desirable microorganisms—such as certain fungi—to colonise the gut and lead to digestive upsets. The adult sheep is a ruminant which depends totally upon the bacteria and protozoa in the rumen to perform the first stage in food digestion. Thus, antibiotics should never be given by mouth to older lambs or adult sheep, as they can seriously interfere with rumination.

Different groups of antibiotics act in different ways and are sometimes antagonistic to each other. For example, penicillin and the tetracyclines are incompatible. As a general rule, never administer any mixture of drugs or vaccines without first consulting your veterinary surgeon.

The animal's own defences against disease, with perhaps some help from antibiotics, can triumph over adversity only if the animal is given every chance through good nursing. The following section deals with this important aspect of husbandry.

The Care and Welfare of Sick and Injured Animals

It is the duty of sheep farmers, shepherds or anyone who has charge of sheep to identify sick or injured animals promptly and to give appropriate treatment immediately or obtain veterinary advice as soon as possible. It is a simple enough matter to spot a lame sheep or to decide that a sheep which constantly walks around in circles is unwell, but it takes considerable skill, experience and commitment to detect animals in the early stages of many diseases.

STOCKMANSHIP

Stockmanship—and both sexes are implied!—requires that the person has an empathy with, and a respect for, the animals in his or her care. It is often said that stockmen are born, not made, but many people with no experience of farms or livestock make excellent stockmen with training, providing they have the necessary qualities. If those qualities are missing, then an individual will never become a stockman and should not be given charge of animals.

Observation

An essential skill for any stockman is observation, since it is only by knowing what is the normal behaviour of a flock or an individual animal that the abnormal can be recognised early. The good stockman will act promptly and attempt to identify the problem—for example, by examining a slow, stumbling newborn lamb which may be starving and chilled, or by checking a ewe which is apparently losing condition whilst its flock mates thrive. If the problem can be identified and treated promptly, this will alleviate pain and suffering and also reduce the risk of the spread of any infectious disease.

Nursing and aftercare

A most important but often neglected aspect of the treatment of sick or injured animals is the monitoring of progress and appropriate nursing and aftercare. Many animals which receive good treatment initially either die or have to be destroyed eventually because of a lack of adequate nursing care. This is a time-consuming, highly skilled but vital aspect of treatment and is discussed in a number of places in this book in relation to specific disease conditions.

Checking the flock

Sheep are kept under a wide variety of husbandry conditions, from the most extensive hill flocks with ewes stocked at only one to five or even ten acres, to intensive flocks with a thousand or more ewes lambing under one roof. Obviously, the hill shepherd can observe only a very small proportion of the lambings of the single bearing ewes on the high ground, but may be able to attend most of the births of twin bearing ewes brought down into the in-bye fields. Time is limited—especially where shepherds are charged with looking after more and more sheep—and it makes sense to concentrate on those animals where problems are most likely to occur.

In lowland housed situations, there is much more pressure on the flock and much more that can go wrong. Therefore, sufficient skilled shepherding and semi-skilled assistance is vital if the flock is to be cared for adequately and the welfare of sheep safeguarded. A ewe flock which needs looking at once a day post-weaning may require attention 24 hours a day if ewes have been synchronised to lamb over a short period.

Attention to the flock is not sufficient in itself, since the shepherd must know what to look out for—for example, animals not eating at the trough, lying apart from the flock, grinding their teeth incessantly or losing their

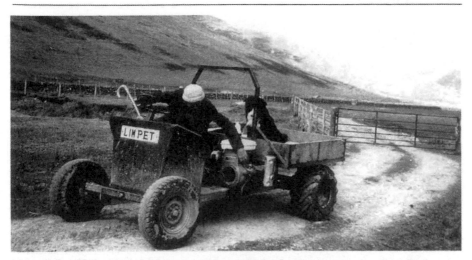

Plate 1.6 All-terrain vehicles can make hill shepherding more effective. Sick animals can be transported to shelter, and it also gives the dogs a chance to rest their legs and advise on engine tuning!

wool. The animal must be caught and examined as soon as possible and marked for ease of identification if necessary. The action required will depend upon a number of factors, and careful thought should be given as to what will stress it least.

It is never easy to catch an injured animal without causing it more pain. Fractures are particularly difficult, since further damage of a serious nature may be inflicted while catching the animal. Such cases should never be loaded into the back of a truck unattended and driven for miles. Transporting them a short distance back to the steading may be acceptable, providing someone can restrain them adequately in a suitable vehicle.

Hospital area

If it is possible to move an animal without causing it further pain or suffering, it should be taken indoors. This will protect it from the weather, from predators and from competition with the rest of the flock (at the feed trough for instance). It will also make good nursing a practical proposition.

On hill farms suitable pens can be located strategically about the hill, as these will be essential at lambing time. In lowland circumstances the hospital area should be situated away from the lambing area so that any infection can be contained. A disinfectant footbath should be provided, and separate boots and overalls used to avoid transfer of infection. Hand washing facilities should be provided, since personal hygiene is important because a number of diseases are transmissible to humans.

The accommodation should be bright, well lit and adequately ventilated

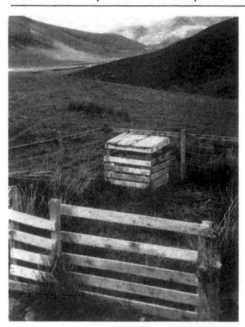

Plate 1.7 Enclosure and pen in isolated hill site for problem cases at lambing and other times.

Plate 1.8 (*Below*) If possible, buildings should be cleaned thoroughly immediately after use. Note that where a zoonotic disease has been present, power hosing as shown here will cause an aerosol, and the operator should wear a protective mask.

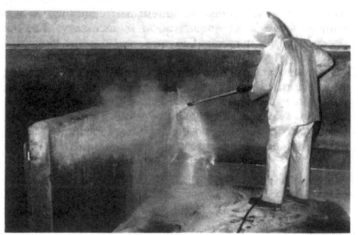

without draughts. The floor should be deeply bedded with clean, dry, mould-free straw. A layer of slaked lime under the straw will keep the floor drier and help kill any residual infection from previous occupants, especially if there is an earthen floor. Fresh bedding should be added frequently, both for comfort and to bury infected faeces, urine or other discharges. Straw bales make good pen divisions as they are solid, give good protection from draughts and can be burned along with the bedding after each

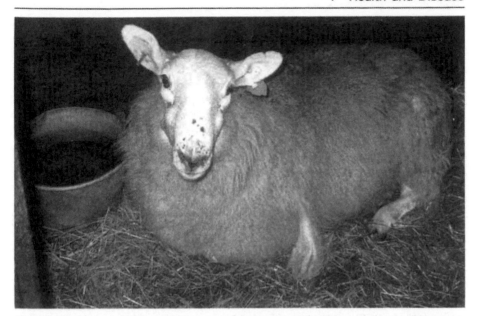

Plate 1.9 Fresh water must be accessible to sick animals at all times. (This ewe has jaagsiekte.)

occupant. The pen should be disinfected after each occupant where this is practical.

Food and water

It is surprising how often feeding and watering are neglected. Fresh clean water must be provided at all times. It must be accessible to the sick animal, which may not be able to rise or may be disinclined to move if it is in pain. The water container should be secured so that it cannot be tipped over. Fresh food should be offered in small quantities and any stale or wet material removed and discarded and not fed to other animals for risk of infection. Freshly cut greens from the garden are more likely to tempt a reluctant eater than some moderate to poor hay. Appropriate food should be chosen—for example, it would be sensible to offer good-quality roughage to an animal with a digestive upset from overeating on a concentrate ration. Sometimes it may be necessary to withdraw food altogether for 24 hours or more, but fresh water should always be available.

Inspection

Sick animals must be inspected several times each day, especially when they are unable to rise. **It is vitally important to prop up sheep which are unable to support themselves,** since they are ruminants and need to get rid of the gases which accumulate in the rumen or else they will suffocate.

Pneumonia is common in animals which are not adequately nursed in this way. Animals which cannot stand should be examined for bedsores and treated appropriately with soothing ointment and padding for protection if necessary.

It is all too easy to overlook slow deterioration in a long-term patient, so it is a good idea to handle the animal at hospitalisation and make a note of condition score and any other remarkable points on a board hung on the pen. This board can be used to record the diet, plus any medication which is prescribed. Consult your veterinary surgeon where an animal is failing or not responding to treatment. Where the case is hopeless the animal should be humanely destroyed to avoid further unnecessary suffering (see Appendix 3).

MEDICATION

New legislation in the UK—Animals and Fresh Meat (Examination for Residues) Regulations, 1988—requires farmers to record all treatments given to their animals and also all drugs stored on the premises. This includes medications mixed with feed on the farm, such as coccidiostats. Ask your veterinary surgeon how to record this information. Your local Animal Health Office of MAFF will supply details, and an organisation called NOAH, 12 Whitehall, London SW1A 2DY, can supply animal medicine record books which include a code of practice for the safe use of veterinary medicines on the farm. Only brief details will be given here.

All medicines must be kept locked away and out of the reach of children. It is most important to administer medicines strictly as prescribed and with care. Always follow your veterinary surgeon's instructions or those printed on the medicine pack or data sheet. Dose rates have been carefully computed and are usually related to body weight, so it is desirable to weigh animals accurately where the dose is by body weight. Weight is often estimated and the guess wildly wrong, especially with sick animals which may have lost considerable weight through not eating. Overdosing of a sick animal is dangerous and may hasten death. Special care should also be taken with pregnant animals.

Frequency and timing of treatments is also important. Do not continue medication for longer than prescribed, but ensure that the full course of medication is taken. Always pay heed to the withdrawal periods following treatment before animals can be sent for slaughter or before milk can be used for human consumption.

Never use out-of-date medicines and remember that half-used containers of certain products (particularly vaccines) may become heavily contaminated with bacteria. Such products will have warnings on the label.

Injections

Always use sterile needles and syringes for drugs given by injection. Disposables are reasonably priced and should be kept in their sterile wrappers in a clean place until needed. Choose a clean area of skin in the area of the body recommended by the manufacturer or your veterinary surgeon. Take care not to contaminate the needle before injecting the sheep. If bacteria are inoculated, an abscess may develop at the site which may result in serious complications. (Be sure not to inject yourself or your workmates. If you do so, seek medical attention immediately, taking the product or data sheet with you. Oil-based vaccines in particular can produce a serious and painful reaction.)

If a large injection has to be made, then more than one site may be used, but follow the instructions carefully with regard to the route of injection— that is, intramuscular or subcutaneous. Where there is a choice, always choose the subcutaneous route (under a fold of the skin) as this is often (although not always) less painful and the chance of reducing the value of the carcass is also reduced. A common fault with subcutaneous injection is to go through both sides of the fold of skin and inject the drug into the fleece! It is highly desirable to use the subcutaneous route in baby lambs wherever possible, since there is so little muscle and it is very easy to damage nerves or bone and to cause considerable pain.

No one should be allowed to inject sheep before receiving training in how to do the job correctly. The task is often done in a careless and irresponsible manner. The Agricultural Training Board can arrange courses locally.

Oral medication

Some medicines can be given by mouth, but great care should be taken because sick animals may have difficulty in swallowing. Liquids can be given by stomach tube where the animal can swallow a tube but might have difficulty swallowing a substantial quantity of liquid. Unconscious animals should never be given oral medication as they are unable to swallow.

Animals should be handled with a minimum of force and should be relaxed (not struggling) when they are drenched. Deliver the medicine into the side of the mouth slowly and in small amounts and allow the animal plenty of time to swallow. Keep the sheep's mouth shut until all the medicine is swallowed, but allow it to breathe through its nose.

PAIN

Whilst sheep are somewhat undemonstrative creatures, there is no doubt in the author's mind that they feel pain to a degree comparable to other animals and humans. Apart from the pain associated with physical injury, many disease conditions are also painful—for example, acute liver fluke or laminitis. If you think an animal is suffering, your veterinary surgeon can often provide relief with mild or powerful pain killers as appropriate, or with other drugs which can reduce the heat and swelling associated with inflammation. If an animal is suffering serious pain and is unlikely to recover, humane euthanasia should be considered.

CODES OF RECOMMENDATIONS FOR THE WELFARE OF LIVESTOCK: SHEEP

These codes for the UK are being reviewed for updating at the time of going to press, and they will be distributed in due course. They should be on every sheep farm and available to every shepherd. Should you not receive a copy write to MAFF in England and Wales, to DAFS in Scotland or to DANI in Northern Ireland.

2

PREPARATION FOR MATING

The Seasonality of Breeding

THE EFFECT OF DAY LENGTH ON THE BREEDING SEASON

The sheep is a seasonal breeder in the UK, and the main factor influencing when breeding will occur is the proportion of hours of daylight to dark—photoperiod.

At the base of the brain is the pineal gland, which starts producing the hormone called melatonin as soon as it gets dark, and ceases production when dawn breaks. When the days get shorter in the autumn, sufficient melatonin is produced to initiate the start of breeding cycles in the ewe. As the days begin to lengthen once more in the spring, there is insufficient production of melatonin and the breeding season peters out until the following autumn.

It is not simply the day length which is important, but also whether the day length is steadily declining or increasing. Increasing day length is more inhibitory to breeding and this accounts for the fact that it is more difficult to bring ewes into heat in spring and early summer, rather than after the longest day (21 June) has passed.

In the tropics where day and night are of roughly equal length, the native sheep breeds have no breeding and non-breeding seasons as in northern or southern regions of the world, so that ewes may breed all year round. However, there are still some periods of the year when breeding is more successful than at others. Sheep moved from the northern to the southern hemisphere, or vice versa, will eventually adjust and breed at the same period as the native sheep, although it may take them a year or two to settle down.

Other factors have an effect on the onset of the breeding season, but in the fine tuning rather than in its overall control. Shepherds will be aware that a cold spell of weather in autumn may 'bring ewes on' sooner than when the weather is warmer. Sheep at high altitudes may be slower to start breeding, but it is difficult to separate this from the poorer level of nutrition associated with hill sheep which also has an inhibitory effect. Ewes in very poor body condition are likely to be slower in coming to the ram, to have a poorer conception rate and a higher barren rate and to produce fewer lambs, than ewes in average to good body condition. Disease may also affect the body condition of ewes and rams and thus exert an indirect effect upon fertility.

LENGTH OF THE BREEDING SEASON

Breeds vary considerably in the length of their breeding season. The shortest day (21 December) is the mid point of sexual activity for most breeds, but the peak of activity is generally in October or November, and that is when they are usually most fertile. The mountain breeds such as the Scottish Blackface, Swaledale, Cheviot and Welsh Mountain have a short breeding season of about three to four months—time to fit in five to seven cycles of around 17 days each. Crossbreds such as the Mule, Masham, Greyface and Scottish Halfbred have an intermediate breeding season of around five months in length, whilst Suffolks and Suffolk crosses may fit in 10 or 11 cycles in a period of around six months.

Unique among British breeds is the Dorset Horn, which has a very long sexual cycle of around eight months. The peak of its breeding activity tends to be several weeks earlier in the year than for other breeds. In flocks where rams are run with the ewes all year round (an ill-advised thing to do) a few Dorset Horn lambs may be dropped during every month of the year. This feature of the breed is often made use of in early, or out-of-season, breeding flocks. Crossing the Dorset Horn with a breed of high fecundity, such as the Finnish Landrace, produces female progeny with intermediate fertility and intermediate length of breeding season which can be used to advantage in these systems.

Crossing any two breeds with different lengths of breeding season will produce female progeny with an intermediate breeding season. In general, breeds with a short breeding season start their sexual activity later in the autumn and finish earlier in the spring.

Apart from the major differences between breeds, there is also considerable variation between individuals of the same breed and this fact has practical significance. In flocks with a mixture of breeds, the variation may be even greater. In the absence of the ram, ewes tend to trickle into sexual activity and there may be several weeks between the time when the first ewe and the last ewe have their first heats. These events will be detected only by the ram of course.

Generally speaking, it is best to mate a particular breed at the time of year when the fertility will be optimal, rather than to attempt ambitious early breeding schemes with an unsuitable breed. Also, changing breed is not always acceptable, and so the ewes may be manipulated in one way or another to persuade them to breed when they would not normally do so, hopefully without compromising fertility too greatly. However, the further away from the peak of breeding activity that mating takes place, the lower will be the conception rate, the higher the barren rate, the smaller the lamb crop and the more protracted the lambing period.

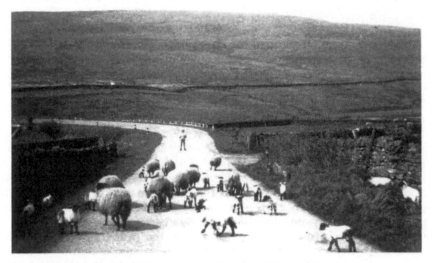

Plate 2.1 The Swaledale and other mountain breeds have a very restricted breeding season.

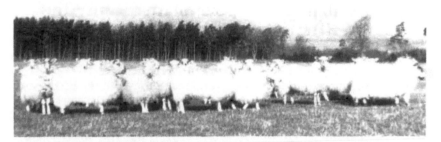

Plate 2.2 Scottish Greyface (*above*) and Scottish Halfbreds (*below*) have a breeding season of intermediate length.

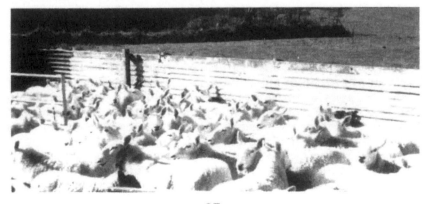

THE BREEDING SEASON IN RAMS

It is not often appreciated that rams also have a breeding season. It is true that rams of most breeds are capable of working all year round, but it is perhaps not so widely appreciated that their performance—in terms of both sexual drive and the fertilising capacity of their semen—may decline during the period of the year when ewes are not sexually active. This is due to the same factors as in the ewe, since day length affects the hormone levels of both sexes. This has important implications for early and out-of-season breeding programmes. The factors affecting ram performance are discussed in detail in the following pages.

A successful lambing is dependent upon planning which begins at least seven or eight months earlier, with the selection and preparation of both ewes and rams for the forthcoming mating season. It will be assumed here that the flock is a spring lambing one. Flocks attempting early lamb production or frequent breeding have some special preparatory requirements which will be described in the chapter on the manipulation of breeding.

RAM MANAGEMENT

Deciding on the Size of the Ram Stud

Once the size of the ewe flock is decided, it is important to determine how many rams will be required to serve the ewes effectively and of what breed and age group they should be. This should be done as early as possible, so that newly purchased rams can be examined along with the established ram stud six to eight weeks before mating is programmed to start.

It is always wise to err on the generous side to allow for contingencies. If the purchase price and maintenance costs of a good-quality commercial ram are costed out over the total number of lambs he will sire throughout his working life, it will be a very reasonable sum indeed. As the ram plays such a crucial role in the overall breeding performance and therefore profitability of a flock, it is unwise to buy poor-quality rams because they appear cheap or to purchase fewer rams than are necessary to perform a satisfactory job.

Leaving aside the genetic merit of the ram and considering only his breeding ability, a sound and fertile ram is capable of getting a lot of ewes pregnant. Consider the fact that the majority of lowland ewes and a significant proportion of hill and upland ewes will produce more than one egg and that ewes will become pregnant even if only one egg is fertilised. However, if two or more eggs are shed but only one is fertilised—perhaps because the ram is overworked or sub-fertile—this represents a considerable loss of breeding potential and hence profitability.

The problems do not stop there, however, since losses of embryos inevitably occur in early pregnancy. If only one egg out of two is fertilised and is subsequently lost, then the ewe either returns to service (repeats) when the rams are still with the ewes, in which case she has a second chance, or else she does not return until after the rams have been pulled out, in which case she becomes a barrener.

THE WORKLOAD ON RAMS

Rams have very considerable powers of sexual recuperation. However, if they are overworked by having too many ewes to serve, then the quantity of semen ejaculated will be reduced. Also, the quality of the semen, as judged by the number of sperm per unit volume of semen, will also deteriorate and the proportion of immature sperm, which are incapable of fertilisation, will increase. Therefore the effectiveness of the semen deposited in each ewe served will be significantly reduced. Fewer ewes will 'hold' to matings and fewer eggs per ewe will be fertilised. The overall consequences are that the lambing period will be extended, the lamb crop lower and the number of barren ewes increased. The workload assigned to each experienced ram is therefore important and this will vary to some extent with breed and the terrain where mating is to take place.

On extensive hill grazings rams have to seek out the ewes on heat, as well as ewes on heat seeking out the ram. This involves travelling considerable distances, often in difficult weather conditions in late November, December and early January. It is therefore most important that hill rams are physically sound and sexually active and that at least three experienced rams are run with every 100 ewes. If hill ewes are brought down off the high tops

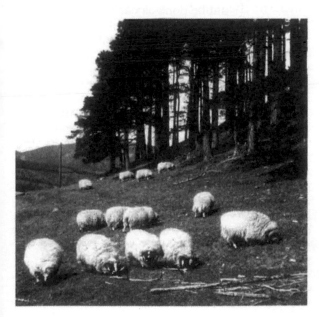

Plate 2.3 A group of fit and healthy Scottish Blackface rams immediately before the start of the breeding season in November on a Borders hill farm.

39

on to areas of enclosed hill for tupping, then less travel is involved. The number of rams can therefore be reduced and one experienced ram to 50 or 60 ewes is considered acceptable. On hill farms which have improved ground on which to flush ewes and the facilities to lamb ewes on the lower ground where they can be more closely shepherded, the expectation is that there will be a reasonable proportion of twins. It does not, therefore, make sense to reduce the ram power to a level which fails to take full advantage of the benefits of flushing the ewes. One ram to 40 or 50 ewes would be a better ratio under these circumstances.

In lowland flocks the above argument is also valid, and similar ram to ewe ratios of one to 40 or 50 are recommended.

With prolific breeds such as the Finnish Landrace, the average ram is generally very active and can serve more ewes and more frequently than the average ram of the less prolific breeds. However, one of the reasons why the ewes of these breeds are more prolific is that not only do they shed more eggs, but the rams are sufficiently potent to fertilise a high proportion of the eggs. If rams are overworked by being given too many ewes to service, some prolificacy will be sacrificed.

Ram power in synchronised flocks

Where rams are introduced early in the breeding season, following the use of teasers, a higher proportion of rams should be used to take account of the short period of intense activity—for example, one ram to 20 or 30 ewes. Where flocks have been synchronised in heat by the use of sponges, then the intensity of mating is extreme, with a group of ewes all coming into heat within hours of each other and the rams having to cope with an intense period of activity. In these circumstances very high ram to ewe ratios of at least one ram to 10 ewes are required, although only for a short period of two to three days (see Chapter 3).

INEXPERIENCED RAMS

The ram power suggestions above apply only to mature and experienced rams. Ram lambs and inexperienced shearlings must be given much less responsibility. Ram lambs start to produce sperm at around two to three months of age, but usually cannot mount and ejaculate until they are around four or five months old. By the time they weigh around two-thirds of the mature weight for the breed—at around six months of age—they will be capable of producing a reasonable semen sample, containing mature sperm capable of fertilisation. There is, however, a tremendous range of activity, and care should be taken to see that precocious ram lambs do not serve their ewe lamb flock mates, or that too much reliance is not placed on less forward animals.

Ram lambs are often reared in all-male (bachelor) groups after weaning, with no contact with females during their early sexual life, so that homosexual tendencies are therefore not uncommon. When such rams

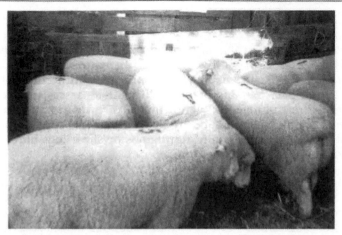

Plate 2.4   Polled Dorset ram lambs at a Dorchester sale
in May. Young, inexperienced rams should not be
overworked.

are joined with ewes they tend to sniff under the belly (having been used
to sniffing around the sheath and testicles of other rams) and may fail to
find the vulva, or may serve into the ewe's rectum. Others will mount the
ewe's head end and those that do find the correct way to go about it may
be so used to males moving forward, away from their advances, that they
may fall backwards off the ewe when she stands still! Most rams adjust in
time, but perhaps not before seriously disrupting the breeding programme.

Ram lambs should therefore be run with around 20 to 25 experienced
mature ewes at most in their first year. Lambs which are overworked in
their first season may not perform so well subsequently. Mature rams
can be run alongside ram lambs as a backup, but if they are working in
relatively small fields, the older rams may inhibit the ram lambs or even
bully them. Thus, one reason why ram lambs do not work well the following
season may be that they are sexually inhibited.

Ram lambs should not be run with groups of synchronised (sponged
or teased) ewes, nor should they be used on ewe lambs or gimmers which
have not been mated before. Such 'maiden' females are also sexually
inexperienced and tend not to seek out the ram like mature ewes. (A mature
ram should always be used on maiden ewes, but not so heavy a specimen
that they collapse under his weight!) Ram lambs should be test mated with
a small group of ewes to see that they know how to go about sniffing out
ewes in heat, mounting and thrusting, before letting them loose in the
flock. The ability to thrust and to ejaculate forcefully and dexterously is
genetically inherited. Rams which are good in this department are likely to
be more potent and their female offspring are also likely to be more fertile.

AGE OF THE RAM STUD

The age of the ram stud should be reviewed. Rams tend to be most fertile between the ages of two and five years and thereafter decline in both libido and potency. Individual rams may, of course, remain fertile for longer or for shorter periods, but this may be difficult to assess in flocks where several rams are run together with a bunch of ewes (multi-sire matings). Older rams should therefore be treated with some suspicion and there should always be a proportion of ram lambs or shearlings introduced each year to maintain a balanced age range.

EFFECTS OF INFERTILE RAMS ON FLOCK PERFORMANCE

Around 10% of rams examined by veterinary surgeons are considered unfit for use, because of sterility (an absolute and permanent inability to fertilise), infertility (a temporary inability to fertilise) or sub-fertility (a degree of reduced fertility). This may sound a small proportion of rams and hardly worth the effort and expense of ram examination. However, consider the situation where a sub-fertile ram is running singly with a group of ewes. Since most of these rams will be able to serve ewes, then where the ram is wearing a raddle harness the first inkling that a problem exists will be

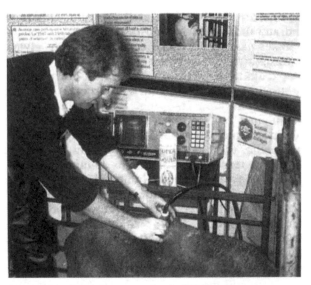

Plate 2.5 Suffolk ram project, Edinburgh University, measuring muscle and fat depth in the live ram lamb. Rams are given an index based on these measurements plus live weight. Rams with a high index should improve flock performance.

some days after the first change of raddle colour, when more ewes than expected begin returning to service. If rams are not raddled, the problem may be discovered only at scanning for pregnancy diagnosis, or worse still at lambing time.

Where rams are run in groups with the ewes, then one dud ram in a group of three or four may appear to make little difference, provided of course that the other three are sound, capable rams. However, if the problem ram is aggressive and dominant, he may prevent the others from serving all but a few ewes. This may lead to a very high return rate and in consequence a spread of lambing, a lower lamb drop and an increase in barren rate. This effect is well illustrated by some trials carried out by Australian workers. One group of around 100 ewes was run with three fertile rams and the return rate to the first service was 18%. In two similar groups of ewes, each run with two fertile rams and two sterile (vasectomised or teaser) rams, the return rates were 46 and 37%.

It therefore makes good sense to weed out unsuitable rams or, better still, not to purchase or retain them in the first place, as much because of the damage they can do as for what they cannot do. Also, since the remaining rams do not have to cover for infertile rams, there should be more ram fertilising-power per ewe in the flock, which should improve breeding performance all round (see below).

PURCHASING A RAM

In closed flocks the purchase of a new flock ram represents the only opportunity to introduce fresh genetic material. Therefore the choice of ram may have a profound effect upon the profitability of a flock, not only because of his sexual ability in getting ewes into lamb, but also because of his effect upon the genetic quality of the offspring. Yet despite this, the purchase of a ram is often a hit or miss affair, with little or no attention paid to its genetic potential, its likely physical performance, its health, or the disease status of the flock from which it is purchased. It is unthinkable that a dairy farmer would buy a cow without examining its udder and yet the majority of rams are purchased with only the most superficial examination of their vital equipment.

When purchasing a ram it is best to do so as early as possible and preferably six or eight weeks before it is required to join the ewes. Rams take time to settle down to a new farm and need time to adjust before being expected to perform. They must also be fed appropriately—the equivalent of flushing for ewes—so that they are in good body condition and capable of producing plenty of good-quality semen. Ram sales in the UK are timetabled largely to suit the vendors who wish their rams, and ram lambs in particular, to be well grown at the time of sale. From the purchaser's point of view the sales are at least two months too late.

One of the prime objectives in buying a ram should be to select one that will improve the flock. It is preferable, therefore, to buy from a reputable

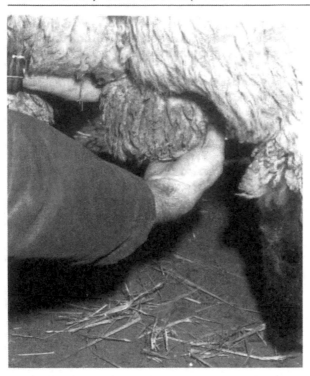

Plate 2.6 Even at a public sale it is possible to examine the scrotum of a ram. This animal would be rejected by virtue of the small size of the testicles, as testicular hypoplasia is an inherited condition and affected rams should not be used for breeding.

breeder who has a recorded flock. In the UK the Meat and Livestock Commission operates a Sheep Improvement Service and publishes a register of breeders whose flocks are recorded and in which purchasers can examine both rams and records. Wherever possible, have a look at the progeny of a ram you are considering buying (if he has worked in the past) and also at his siblings and parents.

One important feature of a ram which affects not only the fertility of the ram itself, but also that of his female progeny, is the size of the testicles. Workers in Edinburgh have shown that the female offspring of rams with large testicles are themselves more fecund than females descended from rams with small testicles. (The New Zealanders refer to this as the 'big balls syndrome'!) Apart from the effect upon the female line, there is a much more direct effect—namely that upon the ram's own fertility. The larger the testicles, the greater the sperm-producing capacity. Therefore always purchase a well-endowed ram and make sure he has two testicles of roughly equal size. Whilst single-testicle rams are often fertile, they can hardly produce as much sperm as even a moderately endowed ram with a full set. Whilst it may be impractical or unacceptable to tip a ram up onto his rear end at a public sale, it should still be possible to crouch down and examine the testicles and go through a shortened version of the detailed examination described later in this section.

Health

Enquire about the health status of the flock, particularly in relation to important diseases such as scrapie, which, if imported into the flock, may have little effect in the short term, but may cause considerable financial loss in the long term. (The newly introduced Sheep and Goat Health Scheme operated by ADAS, and the Premium Sheep Health Scheme operated by the Scottish Veterinary Investigation Service should help in identifying flocks of a given health status.) It is often helpful if other farmers you know have had rams from the same source and have information regarding their health and performance.

Whilst the purchaser has to rely on the word of the vendor as regards the general health status of his flock, the purchaser can at least cast an experienced eye over the ram itself and look for signs of the common problems which affect rams. First of all, the ram should be in good body condition—if not, then the question should be asked why not? Is it because some underlying disease is pulling the ram down in condition? If there is no plausible explanation, then reject the ram, however tempting his other assets may be. Rams should look alert and healthy and preferably be aggressive in character rather than 'soft and cuddly'. Aggressive rams are more likely to have a stronger sexual drive and to be more fertile.

Examine the ram for signs of all the common diseases which affect rams in particular (see below) and ask yourself whether any disease is going to compromise the working ability of the ram (e.g. footrot) or spread infection to the rest of the flock (e.g. orf), or both. If in any doubt, reject the ram. Enquire also regarding the routine health care measures which have been applied to the ram. However, even if the vendor assures you that the ram is vaccinated and wormed, you have no guarantee that these or other measures have been carried out effectively. If the vendor does not vaccinate his flock with the combined clostridial vaccines, this would suggest that the health care generally is likely to be suspect. For peace of mind, therefore, it is safer to assume that a ram is unprotected and to fit him into your own flock preventive health programme as soon as he has settled down in his new surroundings.

Care should be taken with certain long-acting products, such as copper preparations, since giving a repeat dose to an already treated ram could poison him. If in doubt ask your veterinary surgeon to blood sample him before administering any treatment.

Conditions of sale

If a cursory examination gives no cause for concern and everything else appears in order, then the ram can be purchased, preferably with a written and signed condition (not just a warranty) that the vendor will accept him back if he proves infertile or unfit for work for any other reason and will refund the money and all expenses incurred. In the case of a ram bought at the ram sales, the auctioneer's rules should be read carefully, as there is likely to be a deadline for reporting complaints.

Once home, the ram should be kept well away from the ewe flock and initially from the other flock rams also. Once he has settled down after the journey—say the next day—he should be given a more thorough examination. If there is any doubt about his soundness, then contact your veterinary surgeon without delay and ask him to examine the ram and complete and sign a suitable document. Report any complaint to the vendor or auctioneer as soon as possible. If there is any doubt about his breeding ability, act promptly. Whatever you do, do not wait until mating time to see if the ram is working satisfactorily. Not only will you jeopardise your chances of a replacement or a refund, but you will not have time to purchase another ram and give him a fair chance to settle in and work well in the flock. Many ram breeders will offer to replace a returned ram with another. This is often done late in the day and purchasers should beware, since many replacement rams are no better or may be even worse than the original.

Physical Examination of the Ram

Preparation of rams for the breeding season should begin at least six to eight weeks before they are to join the ewes. The first task is to give each ram a thorough examination. This allows time for replacement rams to be purchased to take the place of any which fail to come up to standard, or which for one reason or another were overlooked after the end of the previous breeding season.

This early examination will also identify rams which are in only moderate or poor body condition in time for extra feeding and other measures to help correct the situation. Examination of the reproductive organs in detail will reveal any obvious abnormalities which may make the animal unsuitable for breeding. A health check will identify any conditions which may affect the ram's performance or pose a risk to the ewe flock. There should be sufficient time to treat any disease and to effect a cure, so that by two to three weeks before mating is due to start, rams are in good health and first-rate physical condition.

Instruction in ram examination

Although ram examination is a relatively straightforward procedure, it takes considerable experience and clinical judgement to decide upon what is normal or abnormal and, in the case of the abnormal, upon what is significant in terms of breeding ability and what action should be taken. It is therefore strongly recommended that a veterinary surgeon carry out these pre-mating examinations. Nevertheless, some shepherds and farmers may wish to carry out the preliminary examination themselves, at least to the point where they come across some abnormality. To get the most out of this, they should

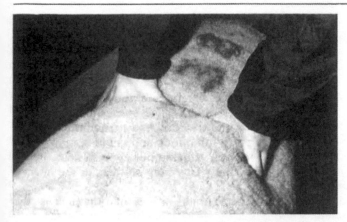

Plate 2.7   Rams must be in prime body condition (CS 4) before mating. It is important to have good body length from withers to tail-head. This ram at CS 3.5 would require three weeks of good feeding to achieve CS 4.

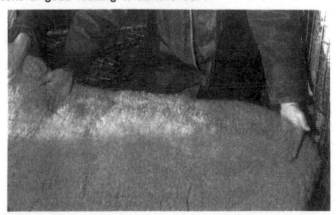

receive practical instruction from their veterinary surgeon during one of these examinations, as there is no substitute for 'hands-on' experience. In the UK, the Agricultural Training Board will organise courses where there is a sufficient demand. The description which follows is intended to give some guidance on how to proceed with such an examination.

OVERALL APPRAISAL OF THE RAM

The examination begins with an overall appraisal of the animal. Is he a good specimen of the breed and well grown for his age? Factors such as good body length, overall conformation and large testicles are much more important than pernickety points about face markings and the shape of horns, beloved of ram breeders and purchasers alike. A detailed

47

physical examination then follows, starting at the head and working back, finishing with the ram sitting up on his rear end for an examination of the reproductive organs, and finally of the feet.

Head

The head should be alert and the face bright and there should be no discharge from the eyes, ears, nose or mouth. The eyes should be clear and bright and any disorder diagnosed and treated. Apart from affecting the ram's eyesight, eye conditions are often infectious and could spread to the ewe flock when the ram is nosing around, sniffing out ewes in heat. Be on the look out for headfly damage, especially in young animals of the horned breeds, and treat appropriately.

Occasionally, and especially in fine skinned breeds of ram such as the Milksheep, Friesland or Finn, a crusty, crumbly, horn-like growth may occur on the top of the head, often following fighting. Affected rams should be isolated until your vet has investigated the lesion, since some of these horny growths have been shown to contain the orf virus. Avoid handling the affected area if possible and wash your hands immediately after accidental contact, since the infection can spread to humans.

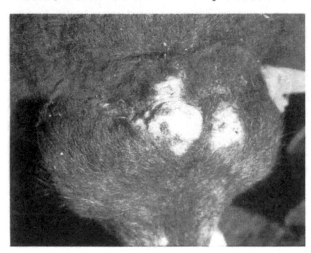

Plate 2.8 Some lesions, like this on the top of the head, may be due to orf. Such rams can introduce the disease to a clean flock.

Teeth

The condition of the mouth and teeth are important since any problem which makes eating difficult could affect body condition. Many abnormal conditions of the shape of the mouth, such as undershot or overshot jaw, are genetically inherited, and it is important not to breed such traits into the flock. Be quite ruthless in weeding out affected rams and preferably avoid purchasing them in the first place.

The incisor teeth—that is, the eight at the front in the lower jaw only—

should meet the hard ridge of toothless gum on the upper jaw called the dental pad. This allows the animal to graze effectively. Any tendency for the lower incisor teeth to project forward of the dental pad should be avoided—Leicesters and Border Leicesters appear to be particularly prone to defects of this type. Beware too of broken mouth since this will shorten the effective life of the ram, and it is also possible that there may be some genetic susceptibility to the condition.

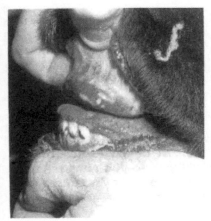

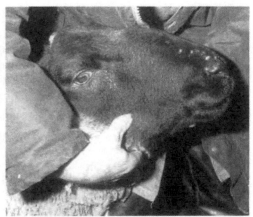

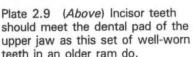

Plate 2.9 (*Above*) Incisor teeth should meet the dental pad of the upper jaw as this set of well-worn teeth in an older ram do.

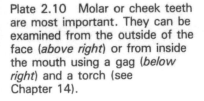

Plate 2.10 Molar or cheek teeth are most important. They can be examined from the outside of the face (*above right*) or from inside the mouth using a gag (*below right*) and a torch (see Chapter 14).

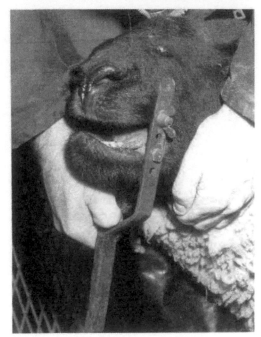

49

Molar teeth—those at the side of the mouth—cause at least as much trouble as incisors. It is quite easy to lose the tip of a finger in trying to examine them, so it is best to use a gag or to run your fingers along the outside of the face. Uneven wear of upper and lower sets of molars may leave a sharp ridge on the outside edge of the upper molars which can easily be felt through the cheeks. The sharp points can damage the cheeks and set up infection in the mouth, and food may lodge between the teeth and the cheeks. Avoid such rams since these problems are likely to recur time and again.

Feel the shape of the face and jaws and compare with other rams in the group. Any lumps and bumps should be investigated. Healed fractures of the jaw—through injury or fighting—may leave a hard lump, but so too may certain infections, perhaps via an infected tooth root. Serious infections of the jaw, tongue or cheeks may interfere with eating and can lead to poor body condition.

Brisket sores

Ill-fitting or inadequately adjusted raddle harnesses can cause brisket sores which, if not treated properly at the end of the mating season, become badly infected. This may be very painful, so that rams refuse to work, especially when harnessed. If brisket sores are not discovered until the pre-mating examination, then they should be treated immediately since

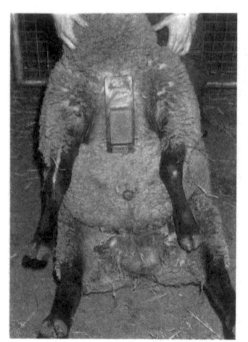

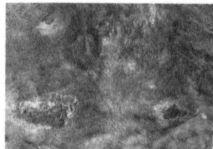

Plate 2.11 Ill-fitting harnesses may cause brisket sores which can put rams off their work. The sores in the plate to the right are scabbed over and in the process of healing, but some will require treatment.

they are often more difficult to cure at this advanced stage. Indeed, some may prove impossible to cure in time for mating and this may mean that an otherwise sound ram is unsuitable or unable to work, with or without a harness. Your veterinary surgeon will advise you on the best treatment, which often involves cleaning up the wounds and treating with antibiotics, both by injection and with local creams or ointments.

Feet and legs

Rams need to be very active for a relatively short period of the year and it is vital that they can perform their duties without let or hindrance. It is therefore of the utmost importance that they are not lame, either through limb or joint abnormalities, or through foot infections since any pain or discomfort can put them off their work very readily. A ram with footrot, especially in the hind limbs which have to carry his weight and thrust when mounting, will either perform inadequately or not at all.

Rams with abnormalities of the limbs, such as excessively sloping pasterns, splay feet or corkscrew toes, should never have been purchased or retained for use in the first instance, since all these conditions are thought to be genetically inherited. Any ram lamb with a joint infection via a navel infection should not be retained for breeding.

Strict precautions should be taken at dipping to see that uncontaminated dip is used, since an episode of post-dipping lameness in the ram stud shortly before mating would have a disastrous effect on the breeding programme.

Foot problems are the most common reason for lameness and these are dealt with in detail in Chapter 15. Some breeds of ram—the Suffolk, for example—appear to be prone to growths which occur between the digits, called interdigital fibromas. These can often be treated or removed surgically under local anaesthetic by a veterinary surgeon. Any such treatment

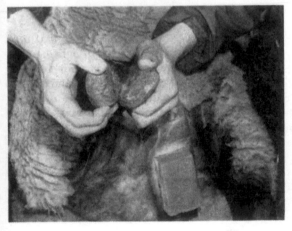

Plate 2.12 It is crucial that rams' feet—fore and hind— are in excellent shape well before tupping time (see also Colour plates 72–74).

51

must be carried out well ahead of the breeding season, since healing will take several weeks. As there is probably some relationship between this condition and the poor anatomy (shape) of the foot, it may not be wise to continue using affected rams, especially in pedigree flocks producing rams for sale.

Wool

The fleece should be examined to reveal any external parasite problems or the presence of lumpy wool, and these should be treated accordingly. Matted or urine-stained wool around the sheath should be very carefully clipped away to prevent any obstruction to the act of mating.

As will be explained later, the production of fertile sperm from the testicles depends upon their being at a lower temperature than the body. When rams are to be used early in the breeding season—for example, in August in the UK—it is as well to clip the wool off the scrotum in those breeds which have a significant amount of growth. This should be done well in advance of mating, such as at the time of ram examination.

EXAMINATION OF THE REPRODUCTIVE ORGANS

Examination of the genital organs of the ram should precede inspection of the feet (when the hands are clean) and be done whilst the ram is sitting up on his tail end. It will include an examination of the sheath, penis, scrotum and testicles. It may be necessary for your veterinary surgeon to collect and examine a sample of semen from any rams about which there is some doubt.

On first tipping the ram up, the colour of the inside of the thighs should be noted. In the weeks leading up to mating these should become progressively more reddened ('flushed') and greasy. At the early examination this may not be very obvious, but at the examination two or three weeks before mating all rams should be well coloured up.

Scrotum and testicles

The scrotum is the sack or 'purse' which contains the testicles and also the storage vessels for sperm, the epididymides, which are attached to the testicles. Before any detailed examination of the testicles is undertaken it should be stressed that they are very delicate, sensitive organs and should therefore be handled with care to avoid both pain and possible damage. Handle them as you would ripe tomatoes! The reader will notice the use the plural, because it is unwise to purchase or select for breeding, any ram—however good he may appear in other ways—which has only one testicle.

The scrotum should feel heavy when lifted up and should be covered in soft, clean skin. There should be no evidence of injury or disease (such as dermatitis), which might be painful or uncomfortable and perhaps discourage rams from working. The skin should be supple and should slide freely

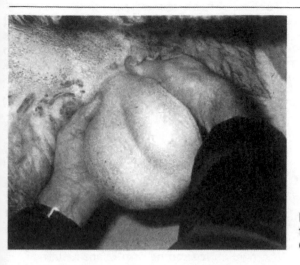

Plate 2.13 Handle the testicles with care when examining them.

over the testicles, which themselves should feel firm, plump and springy with no suggestion of excessive hardness or softness. Any restriction of movement may indicate that there has been some injury or infection which has healed, leaving scar tissue which tends to bind the testicles to the scrotum. This is a bad sign, because any damage which causes an orchitis (an inflammation of the testicles) or an epididymitis (an inflammation of the semen storage organ) almost inevitably leads to sterility, infertility or an unacceptable degree of sub-fertility.

SIZE AND MEASUREMENT OF THE TESTICLES   In a normal, healthy, fertile ram the scrotum and therefore the testicles within it should be large. During late winter, spring and early summer in the UK, the testicles are considerably smaller in most breeds and individuals. Once the longest day has passed, the testicles begin to increase in size so that they are at their largest when the rams—and the ewes—are at the peak of their fertility in the autumn and early winter.

As a general rule, rams of the more prolific breeds, such as the Finnish Landrace, have larger testicles in relation to body size than those of the less prolific breeds, such as the Dorset Horn. The larger the testicles, the more sperm and the more male hormone will be produced. Both of these factors affect the fertility of a ram as measured by his capacity to mate a large number of ewes in a short time and to fertilise a high proportion of the eggs shed by the ewes, so maximising the lamb crop. Much emphasis is placed on achieving a high ovulation rate (number of eggs shed at oestrus) by the ewe flock. In contrast, far too little emphasis is placed on ensuring, as far as is possible, that the rams are adequately fertile. It is not simply a matter of the ram depositing semen inside the female, but of the quality and quantity of the semen—and of sperm in particular—which is important.

A tape measure is handy to measure the circumference of the scrotum at its widest point. Obviously size will vary with breed, age and time of

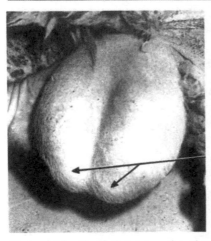 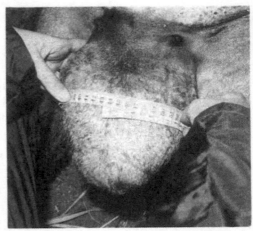

Plate 2.14 *(Left)* Scrotum of a shearling Suffolk ram at start of the breeding season. The testicles should be large, evenly sized and free from any hard lumps or other abnormalities. Note the clean-skinned appearance. The epididymides are at the bottom of the scrotum attached to the testicles (arrowed), and at the peak of the breeding season they may contain as many as 80 thousand million sperm.

Plate 2.15 *(Right)* The vital statistic of this mature Suffolk ram is a scrotal circumference of 43 cm. Testicle size is correlated to fertility.

year, but as a general guide, mature downland or longwool rams (such as the Suffolk or Border Leicester) should measure around 36 to 38 cm in circumference within two or three weeks of mating. Some allowance should be made when measurements are taken two months before mating. Mountain breeds, such as the Scottish Blackface, are generally slightly smaller at around 34 to 36 cm, and there is often a greater difference in size between the breeding season and the non-breeding season than there is in downland rams.

Ram lambs will obviously be smaller and size will be influenced by both physical maturity (body size) and the season of the year. Again, as a guide only, ram lambs of the downland and longwool breeds should measure around 30 cm and hill breeds 28 cm in their first autumn, at around 7 to 9 months of age. For shearlings, at around 18 months of age, the measurements should be within 3 or 4 cm of the mature size for the breed.

ORCHITIS Examination of the testicles may reveal that they are small and shrunken or contain hard lumps. If the insult has been recent, the testicles may be hard, swollen and painful (see Plate 2.16). Even if the initial damage involves only one testicle, the other inevitably suffers also. This is because of pressure due to swelling and because of the higher temperature due to the inflammation. The examination of a semen sample from such a ram would confirm that it was unsatisfactory due to the presence of small numbers of sperm and a high proportion of abnormal sperm.

Treatment of cases of orchitis, from whatever cause, is unsatisfactory and is unlikely to restore fertility to any useful degree. It is therefore unwise to use affected rams during the current breeding season and, indeed, the majority should be culled without delay. If any such rams are retained, they should be clearly identified for re-examination before the following year's breeding season, but it is unlikely that they will prove satisfactorily fertile.

In areas of the world other than the UK, specific infections such as brucellosis (*Brucella ovis*) may cause orchitis. Damage to the testicles is severe and rams may spread infection throughout the flock and should be culled immediately they are diagnosed. Fortunately, this organism does not occur in the UK.

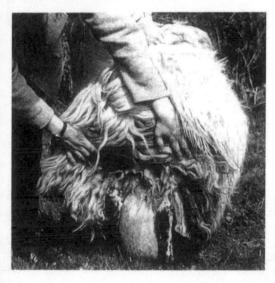

Plate 2.16   Orchitis (inflammation of the testicle) in a Scottish Blackface ram. The scrotum is dragging on the ground in this severe and painful case. Despite treatment this animal would never again be fit for breeding.

RIG   There are a number of defects of the testicle which have a genetically inherited basis. The first of these is the rig or cryptorchid. In this condition, either one or both testicles are either undescended or only partially descended from the abdominal cavity (where they originally develop) into the scrotum. It is important that the testicles lie in the scrotum, because there they are maintained at a lower temperature than in the abdominal cavity. This is essential for the production of sperm (spermatogenesis). Therefore a double-rig—a ram with both testicles retained in the abdominal cavity and an empty scrotum—will usually be sterile. A ram with only one descended testicle will probably be capable of getting ewes in lamb, but because the total weight of functional testicle is only half that of a normal ram, such a ram would have to be considered sub-fertile.

Ram lambs with partially descended testicles—that is, which lie somewhere in the canal between the body cavity and the scrotum or in some other abnormal position, such as alongside the penis—should also be rejected.

It is sometimes suggested that double-rigs be used as teasers. This is not recommended, since there is just the possibility that some viable sperm may be produced and this could cause havoc in a breeding programme.

TESTICULAR HYPOPLASIA The second inherited condition is called testicular hypoplasia, which simply means small testicles. The condition may affect one or both testicles but, as discussed above, either situation is equally unsatisfactory. Where one testicle is obviously small, there is no difficulty in detecting the problem. If both appear small, then measure the circumference of the scrotum and if the size is significantly below that expected for a particular breed or age of ram, the ram should be rejected. If in doubt, your veterinary surgeon can examine the ram and collect semen from him. Affected rams usually produce an unsatisfactory sample.

HERNIAS AND RUPTURES The third genetically inherited abnormality is inguinal hernia or rupture. This involves a loop of bowel becoming trapped in the scrotum alongside the testicle, having escaped from the abdominal cavity via the narrow inguinal canal between the abdomen and the scrotum (it is down this canal that the testicles travel around the time of birth). Normally, hernias are only one-sided (see Plate 2.18). The presence of bowel in the

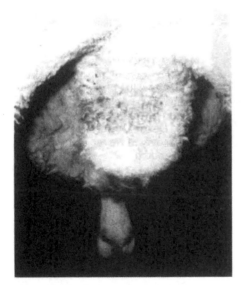

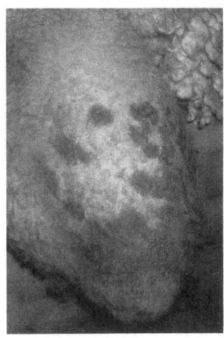

Plate 2.17 Cryptorchidism in a Perendale ram. Neither testicle has descended into the scrotum and the ram is unsuitable for breeding.

Plate 2.18 (*Above right*) Inguinal hernia in a Perendale ram. A loop of gut has descended into the scrotum and is lying alongside the right testicle.

inguinal canal interferes with the blood supply to the testicle and causes it to swell up. At this stage it is painful and the shepherd may observe an affected ram as somewhat stiff or apparently lame. The affected testicle then tends to shrink and shrivel up due to the lack of a blood supply. Your veterinary surgeon can confirm the diagnosis.

Strictly speaking, hernias are present at birth (congenital), whereas ruptures are acquired after birth. Hernias are genetically linked and ram lambs showing this defect should not be retained for breeding; neither should they be castrated for fear of the loops of bowel cascading onto the ground, in the case of surgical castration, or of bowel being pinched in the rubber ring or Burdizzo, in the case of the bloodless castration methods. If it is necessary to castrate such an animal, a veterinary surgeon **must** carry out the operation.

Rupture of bowel into the scrotum of rams is rare, although it is occasionally reported after rams have been fighting, especially in the Scottish Blackface breed. The theory is that some Blackie rams have a genetically inherited weakness of the inguinal canal and that the tremendous abdominal pressure which is built up at the moment of impact during head fighting forces gut through the canal into the scrotum.

However, whether it is a hernia or a rupture, affected rams should be rejected for breeding purposes.

SPERM PRODUCTION IN THE TESTICLES The testicles produce both sperm and the sex hormones which give rams their maleness and sexual drive. Sperm production starts in the ram with the onset of puberty and continues non-stop for the whole of the ram's life, unless disease or injury intervene. The numbers of sperm which a ram can produce are quite staggering. It is estimated that a fit and fertile ram at the peak of the breeding season will be producing around 20 million sperm from each gram of testicle every day! The sperm leave the testicle suspended in a fluid which transports them to the epididymis, which lies attached to the surface of the testicle and therefore also within the scrotum.

SPERM STORAGE IN THE EPIDIDYMIDES The two epididymides (see Colour plate 2) consist of many yards of coiled tube, and as the sperm are carried through this long tube they continue to mature and develop the power to swim of their own accord and to fertilise an egg. Without this period of development in the epididymides the sperm are useless. The fully mature sperm are stored in the 'tail' of the epididymis, which can easily be felt through the scrotum, attached to the bottom of the testicle. At any one time, there may be in the region of 40 thousand million sperm stored and maturing in the tail of each epididymis.

Rams, which have to serve many ewes over a short period, require a large reservoir in which to store mature sperm ready for action. Therefore the epididymides are very important organs and any damage or infection will have serious consequences upon fertility. Disease or injury to the testicles, such as orchitis, will also damage the epididymides, and there are also a number of conditions which affect the epididymides only. So during the

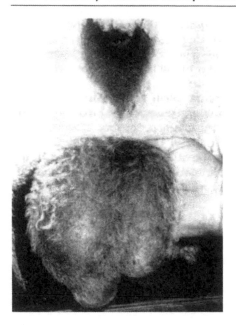

Plate 2.19 Epididymitis in a Suffolk ram—an inflammation of the sperm storage organ, situated at the bottom of the testicle.

course of a ram examination your veterinary surgeon will examine these important organs carefully. There should be no hard lumps or other abnormalities and the 'tails' of the epididymides should be easily distinguishable at the bottom of the testicles. In a mature ram the epididymis should be about the size of a walnut—only much less hard! In the event of any abnormality, a semen examination will be required. Treatment is unlikely to bring about a return to fertility and affected rams should be culled.

ACCESSORY SEX GLANDS There are a number of other organs in the male—called the accessory sex glands—which produce a variety of fluids that mix with the sperm immediately prior to ejaculation to produce semen. These organs lie within the body cavity and so cannot be examined directly (see Colour plate 1). Infections do occur in these glands on occasion but will probably go unnoticed unless a semen sample is examined.

Where a ram is not thought to be performing adequately and a clinical examination has revealed no obvious problem, then a semen sample may show that the sperm are very sluggish in their movements or that there is infection somewhere along the reproductive tract. This may be the first clue that a problem exists in the accessory sex glands. In some cases these infections clear up on their own or following treatment and fertility may be restored. In other cases the damage may be permanent with resultant infertility.

Prepuce and penis

The prepuce or sheath protects that part of the penis which is extruded momentarily during the act of mating. The delicate inner lining of the sheath is continuous with the equally delicate outer covering of the free end of the penis.

There are a number of abnormalities of the penis and sheath which may prevent a ram from erecting or introducing the penis into the vagina of the ewe, or from ejaculating in a forwards direction. Some of these deformities may be obvious to the experienced eye at an examination of the genitalia, but many may only become apparent at mating time. Indeed, some may go unnoticed altogether as rams may mount perfectly satisfactorily but may not be introducing the penis into the vagina and ejaculating. Suspicions may not be raised until an unacceptable proportion of ewes are marked with the new raddle colour at first return. This emphasises the need for careful observation of rams during the mating period.

Great care should be taken at shearing to avoid damaging the sheath, and any wounds must be treated appropriately and immediately if they do occur. If there are likely to be flies around at this time, a suitable fly repellent cream (**not dip**) should be applied. Even if injuries are treated successfully, the healing process may cause quite extensive scarring in this delicate area which may prevent erection of the penis and successful mating. It is important, therefore, to get practical instruction from your veterinary

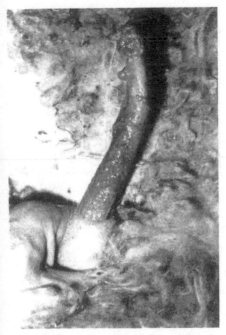

Plate 2.20   Extrusion of the penis of the ram. Any defect, injury or disease which prevents erection may prohibit successful mating.

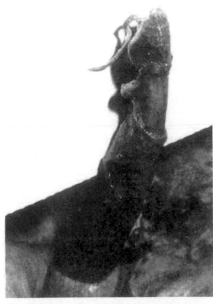

Plate 2.21   Vermiform appendage ('worm') on the tip of a ram's penis. This sprays sperm onto the cervix by a twirling action at ejaculation.

surgeon on how to extrude the penis so that it can be carefully examined (easy if you know how, almost impossible if you don't). Note how easily, or otherwise, the penis can be protruded from the sheath and look for any signs of injury or infection, such as the presence of inflammation (redness) or any abscessation (pus).

There should be a small worm-like process on the end of the penis called the **vermiform appendage**. The function of this 'worm' is to spray the semen onto the cervix (opening of the womb) by a twirling action during ejaculation. Sometimes this 'worm' is lost through injury (e.g. at shearing) or infection, but this does not necessarily affect the fertility of a ram, provided that the orifice at the end of the 'worm' is patent so that sperm can escape. Rams should not be rejected just because the worm is partially or totally lost, but it is there for a purpose.

GENITAL ORF There are a number of infections which affect the sheath and/or penis. The orf virus may cause infection on the sheath and occasionally on the penis. If small growths or pustules form at the opening of the sheath, orf should always be suspected and the ram isolated from other rams. If the diagnosis is confirmed then any affected rams should on no account be used for breeding, since the infection will spread rapidly throughout the ewe flock and therefore to other rams also running alongside the affected ram. Occasionally the orf infection may be so severe that the rams refuse to work because of the pain involved at mating, with resultant disruption to the breeding programme.

If rams are not examined before mating, the problem may only become apparent shortly after the rams are joined with the ewes. Under these circumstances, affected ewes and rams should be isolated from 'clean' ewes and any new cases removed to the infected group. This should help to limit the spread of the disease in small flocks, but it may be totally impractical in large flocks.

Interestingly, despite the very infectious nature of the orf virus, an outbreak around mating time which affects the genital organs of both ewes and rams does not necessarily persist in the flock to cause disease in lambs or on ewes' udders. Vaccination should **not** be used in flocks where only the genital infection is present.

If orf is suspected when examining rams before mating, then the examiner's hands should be washed before handling the next ram to prevent spreading infection and to protect the operator.

ULCERATIVE BALANITIS Another condition, which occurs a few weeks after the rams have been turned out and which may be confused with orf, is called balanoposthitis or ulcerative balanitis and vulvitis. It may cause very severe damage to the penis of rams. The first sign of an outbreak is that the wool around the vulva of ewes is blood-stained. Closer examination of the flock reveals that affected ewes have raw, bleeding patches (ulcers) on the vulva, which is also very swollen. Rams have a similar swelling and ulcers on the sheath, especially at the tip (glans) of the penis, and these may bleed profusely at mating. It is mainly this blood which stains the ewes' wool.

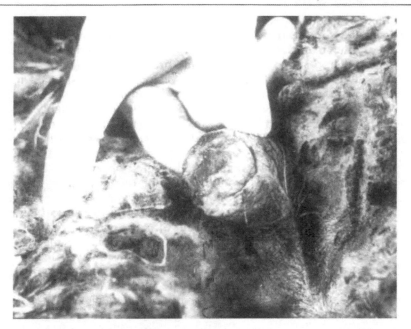

Plate 2.22   Ulcerative balanitis on the penis of a ram (*above*) and on the vulva of a ewe (*below*). Note the bloodstained short wool on the ewe. The veterinary surgeon is wearing gloves, as lesions like this on the penis and vulva may be caused by orf.

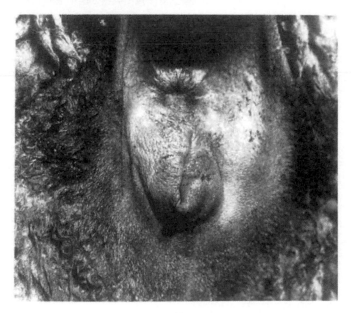

The ulcers in both ewes and rams are painful. Ewes may hold the tail away from the sores and whilst very badly affected rams may refuse to serve ewes, the majority will continue to do so. Surprisingly, there is usually little disruption to mating and the breeding programme.

Usually all the rams in with a group of ewes will become affected and it is difficult to know what action to take. Rams should preferably be withdrawn and given antibiotic treatment by injection and by using a suitably soothing and healing cream squeezed into the sheath and around the tip of the penis. The hope is to minimise the damage and subsequent scarring which accompanies healing, since this may mean that the ram could be unfit for work in the following season. However, if the breeding programme is not to be severely disrupted, fresh rams would need to be found to cover the second half of the mating period. This is not necessarily very easy nor desirable, especially when it is known that the replacement rams are almost certain to become affected from sexual contact with affected ewes.

Up to one-third of the ewe flock may be affected but the majority heal satisfactorily without treatment. However, any seriously affected cases should be treated by your veterinary surgeon. It is most important that the drugs used are kind to the very delicate membranes of the vulva and penis; otherwise further damage may be done. As the cause of the disease is unknown, treatment is aimed at reducing the risk of secondary infection. If there are still flies about when outbreaks occur, fly strike is a risk. (Dip should **not** be applied to the wounds as it is very damaging to the delicate tissues.)

It is probable that infection is introduced into the flock by either bought-in ewes or rams. All purchased rams should be isolated for a month and carefully examined before mixing with the ram stud or joining the ewes. There may also be some ram to ram spread before mating due to homosexual activity.

PIZZLE-ROT In Australia and New Zealand there is a disease, known locally as pizzle-rot, which has the same scientific name as ulcerative balanitis (balanoposthitis) and similar symptoms but a very different cause. This is thought to be due to grazing on lush protein-rich pastures and mainly affects wether (castrated) lambs. Affected lambs may lose condition and some die. Damage to the sheath and penis may lead to urine-staining of the fleece and subsequent fly strike. Treatment and prevention consist of implants of the male hormone, testosterone, removal from the offending pastures and supportive treatment, such as the prevention of fly strike. Surgery may be necessary in some cases. The condition does not occur in the UK.

Semen Collection and Examination

If there is some doubt about the breeding ability of the ram—for example, if the testicles appear to be abnormal or small for age or breed—consult your veterinary surgeon, who may consider it necessary to collect and examine a sample of semen. The technique—known as electroejaculation—should only be carried out by a qualified veterinary surgeon who should make the decision as to whether it is necessary. It should not normally be undertaken as a routine on all rams in the stud as it is an uncomfortable procedure. Exceptions to this rule may be necessary occasionally, for example, where rams are run singly with a group of ewes.

ELECTROEJACULATION TECHNIQUE

The ram is either left standing or may be laid on his side. A battery operated probe, which is capable of delivering a low voltage current, is inserted gently into the rectum with the aid of a lubricant. A container suitable for collecting semen is held at the opening of the sheath and the current in the probe is switched on for three or four seconds. This may need to be repeated two or three times, with a rest of a few seconds between each electrical shock. Ejaculation (usually without erection) generally takes place in the rest phases between stimulations and it may be necessary to 'milk' the sheath to retrieve the sample.

Even a skilled operator may not always be able to collect a sample at the first attempt. If so, the ram may be rested whilst the remainder of the ram stud are examined and then a second attempt made. If this is unsuccessful, any further attempt should be left to a later date. Collection using the electroejaculator does not give as good a sample as does the artificial vagina

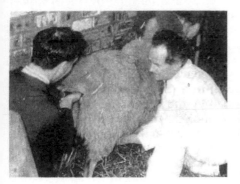

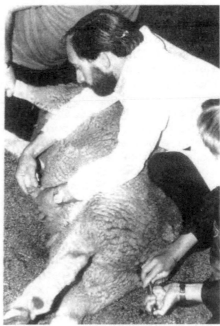

Plate 2.23 Electroejaculation in the ram in the standing or prone position. This procedure should be carried out by a veterinary surgeon and only when absolutely necessary, as it is an unpleasant procedure for the ram.

(AV) which is used when collecting semen for artificial insemination, but the latter method requires the use of teaser ewes and rams require training in order to produce a good sample. Therefore the AV is not always a suitable technique for on-the-farm ram semen collection.

If collection is attempted outside the breeding season, then with British breeds at least, semen production may be reduced in both quantity and quality. Where the rams have been kept well separated from the ewe flock—as they certainly should be in the period leading up to mating—then it is possible to 'ginger-up' the rams by running them in a paddock adjacent to a small group of ewes which need not be sexually active.

Where a ram has already been running with the ewe flock and for some reason requires testing—perhaps because ewes have not been 'holding' to him—then the ram should be withdrawn from the flock and rested for two or three days before semen collection is attempted. Otherwise, any sample is likely to be unrepresentative if the ram has been serving ewes and has depleted his semen reserves. In any case, rams should not be condemned because it is not possible to collect a sample.

EXAMINATION OF THE SEMEN SAMPLE

The veterinary surgeon carrying out such an examination will be looking for a number of characteristics. Sperm need to be very active in order to swim the relatively huge distance from where they are deposited in the vagina, through the cervix, across the uterus and into the oviduct to meet the egg and accomplish fertilisation. Therefore the motility of the sperm is most important.

This is estimated by placing a small drop of semen onto a warm glass slide and placing it on a microscope with a heated stage to keep the sample warm, as any cooling will immediately reduce the activity of the sperm. The sample will be scored from 0 (dead) to 5 (highly active) as adjudged by the wave motion (or lack of it) caused by the swimming movements of the sperm. The wave motion will depend upon the number of sperm per unit volume of semen, the proportion of them which can swim normally and the speed at which they swim. Providing a reasonable sample has been obtained and it has been kept warm during the examination, then the estimated score does relate quite well to the fertility of the ram, other things being equal—such as his willingness to serve. Scores of 2 or less are normally considered below standard and would warrant a closer examination of the sample.

By increasing the microscope magnification to 400 times and diluting the semen sample one hundredfold, it is possible to observe individual sperm. Providing the sample has been kept properly warm, the swimming movements of individual sperm can be seen. Providing at least half of them show normal forward movements, the semen sample would be classed as satisfactory as far as the motion of the sperm is concerned.

Special staining techniques can be used to determine the proportion of live to dead sperm in a sample of semen and also to identify the type and proportion of any abnormalities. Some abnormalities may explain why sperm cannot swim—for example, if the head and tail of the sperm have become detached. The presence of immature forms of sperm may indicate that a ram is being overworked.

Staining may also bring to light the presence of certain cells which should not normally be present in the semen. White blood cells, for example, would indicate damage or infection in some part of the reproductive tract, such as the testicles. This would usually mean that the ram was unsuitable for breeding.

Sperm numbers in the ejaculate

The volume of semen a ram ejaculates and the concentration of sperm in the sample determine the total number of sperm deposited in a ewe. It is important that very large numbers of sperm are deposited at mating because very few of them actually reach the oviduct where the eggs are waiting to be fertilised. The average ejaculate of a mature ram during the breeding season is around one millilitre and this quantity will contain around three to four thousand million sperm! Such a semen sample would have a thick, creamy consistency, good motility and a low proportion of abnormal sperm. High-quality semen has been shown to equate with an above-average proportion of multiple births in the ewe flock.

A subnormal ram may produce a sample which looks like cloudy water or thin milk and is only likely to contain around 100,000 to a quarter of a million sperm in one millilitre. These numbers are quite useless as far as fertilising ability is concerned.

Any assessment of the fertility of a ram is judged on a full examination, including all the tests mentioned above, plus others which may occasionally

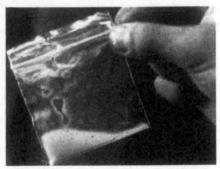
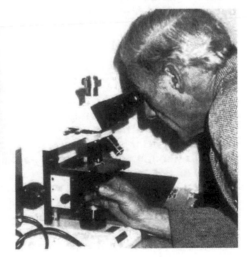

Plate 2.24 (*Above*) A good creamy semen sample collected in a plastic bag. Such a sample should contain large numbers of highly mobile sperm when examined under the microscope (*right*).

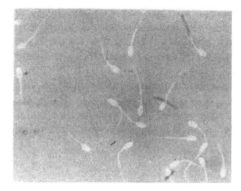

Plate 2.25 A normal sample of ram semen under the miscroscope at low (*left*) and at high (*below*) power. One sperm in the lower picture has a bent tail which will prevent it from swimming effectively.

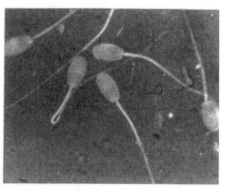

be necessary, such as biochemical tests. It should then be possible for your veterinary surgeon to give you an objective judgement of the ram's likely breeding fitness at the time of the examination. The final test, of course, is how the ram actually performs amongst the ewes, both in terms of mating and ejaculating ability and in his capacity to fertilise.

TESTING FOR LIBIDO

All being well, there is every chance that if a ram is fit and healthy and has passed a ram examination, then he will be capable of producing good-quality semen. However, a further crucial test remains—that of his ability to seek out ewes in heat and to mount and serve them satisfactorily. It is only when a ram is put to work that his libido is tested. It is possible to check this prior to his joining the ewes by means of a short test of sexual ability, although some concerns have been expressed over the welfare aspects of this technique.

The ram is put in a pen or small paddock with three or four ewes which are in heat either naturally or by using a synchronisation technique (see Chapter 3). He is given 12 minutes to see how many ewes he can serve, and during this time a good ram should be able to mount and ejaculate up to four times. He can also be given a score for his dexterity at mating. For example, a ram would be given a very poor score if he failed to ejaculate despite frequent intromission.

Generally speaking there should be little problem with fit, healthy, mature rams, but problems may arise with 'virgin' rams or inexperienced shearlings, or with ram lambs that have been run only with other males and thus are accustomed only to homosexual experiences. Rams which show little interest—poor libido—are quite likely to remain that way for life. On the other hand, a keen, active ram lamb will generally achieve a competent level of dexterity by dint of experience, providing he is not overworked in his first season. Approximately four out of five rams will pass a libido test satisfactorily.

Management of Rams Before and During Mating

FEEDING

The sperm produced in the testicles of a ram today will not be mature and capable of fertilisation for at least two months, as development takes around six or seven weeks in the testicle itself and the maturing and storage time in the epididymis takes another fortnight. Feeding plays an important role in this process and the most sensible approach is to attempt to maintain rams in good body condition all year round rather than to make a last ditch attempt to feed up a thin ram in the last fortnight before tupping. As it takes roughly six weeks of good feeding to put one condition score onto a sheep,

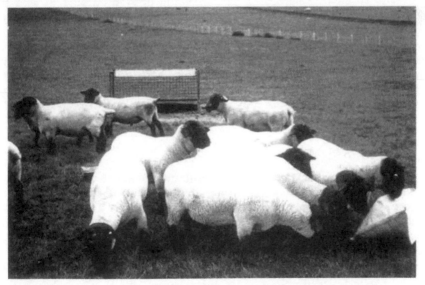

Plate 2.26 Rams need a high protein diet to flush them for mating. These are rams on the University of Edinburgh Suffolk breeding project.

it is important to check the rams early enough so as to do something for the thinner ones.

During the two months leading up to mating rams should be fed to improve steadily in body condition so that they are around condition score 3.5 to 4 a fortnight before they join the ewes. This is somewhat higher than advised for ewes at mating, as it must allow for the inevitable weight loss which occurs during the mating period.

The energy portion of the diet is especially important for ewes during the flushing period and whilst this is also true for rams, it is protein that is particularly important for the growth of the testicles and therefore for sperm production. (The testicles grow very appreciably in size once the longest day has passed.) Therefore, late summer and autumn grazing should be supplemented as necessary with a high energy concentrate containing around 16% protein and with a proportion in a non-degradable form such as fishmeal. A simple way of adjusting the protein content is to use a lamb creep feed (e.g. 17% protein) and mix it with whole barley to give a final 16% protein concentrate. The vitamin, mineral and trace element status of the ration should be appropriate to the conditions on the farm (see Chapter 11).

As rams will need to be fed concentrate throughout the mating period, it is useful to train them to eat from the bucket or out of the trough in a temporarily fenced-off corner of the field, so that the ewes (who would not normally be fed concentrates at this time) cannot get at the food. During mating this technique can be a useful method for catching rams for checking them over, adjusting harnesses and changing crayon colours or swapping them over to a different group of ewes. Training should take place before the rams join the ewes.

Any rams in poorer condition should be given individual attention and extra feed. Where rams are fed as a group, some bullying may prevent the dominated rams from getting their fair share of feed. They should be condition scored again a month before mating to see if they are responding to feeding. If not, then there may be an underlying health problem, such as chronic liver fluke disease, which will have to be corrected.

HEALTH MEASURES

It is most important that rams should be included in the preventive medicine programme which is used on the farm. Rams already in the scheme will require only booster vaccinations, but rams recently purchased should be given primary and secondary vaccinations. Vaccination against the clostridial diseases and pasteurellosis should always be carried out, and footrot vaccination is strongly recommended for the ram stud.

On hill farms where louping ill is present, it is most important to keep newly purchased rams away from the tick-infested areas of the farm on arrival. Always assume they are unprotected, even if they are from another tick-infested farm. They should be vaccinated against louping ill as soon as they have settled down after arrival and at least a month before they are due to join the ewes on an infected hill. This is particularly important on farms where there is an autumn tick rise. Both tickborne fever and louping ill are serious diseases in unacclimatised animals of any age. The fever produced will drastically interfere with sperm production in the ram and if this occurs in autumn, before or during mating, the ram may be infertile for a prolonged period. If the disease progresses, then the ram may end up paralysed or dead.

Anthelmintics (wormers) for the control of parasitic gastro-enteritis (worms) should be administered as early as possible; do not leave dosing until the week before joining with the ewes. Chronic liver fluke will pull rams down in condition. If the disease has been overlooked during the previous winter and spring and there are thin rams about when food is plentiful, then samples of faeces should be examined by your veterinary surgeon for the presence of fluke eggs. If positive, then all the rams should be treated. (Obviously the ewe flock should be checked and treated if necessary.) Acute liver fluke commonly occurs in the period around mating, especially after a wet summer. On fluke-infested farms, treatments will need to be administered at appropriate intervals throughout the autumn, winter and spring.

Compulsory legislation for the control of sheep scab may require the flock to be dipped just before or during the mating period. It is sometimes

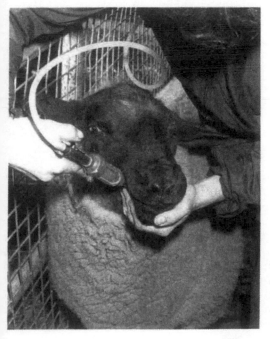

Plate 2.27 Ram being dosed for worms with an anthelmintic. Rams are often neglected as regards preventive medications.

69

said that rams are put off working by the smell of dip from the ewes, but if both sexes are dipped together this should not present a particular problem.

MIXING RAMS

Where possible, it is best to run the rams in the actual groups they will be in when they are to join the ewes. This is to allow time for a hierarchy to become established early, so that fighting and bullying is minimised after joining, allowing rams to concentrate on serving ewes. Generally speaking the most aggressively male rams—which are often also the largest—will tend to be dominant. Hopefully these will also be the most fertile and potent, but this is not always the case.

Newly purchased rams, once they have finished their quarantine period, should be introduced to the other rams they are to work with. This should be done close to the farmstead so they can be observed closely, since fighting—occasionally to the death—may break out.

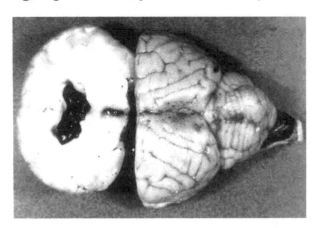

Plate 2.28 Brain haemorrhage. Note the blood clot in the cerebrum (left). Such damage can occur when rams head-butt.

PREPARATION OF RAMS FOR OUT-OF-SEASON BREEDING

In early lambing or out-of-season breeding flocks, rams are expected to perform at a time of year when they are likely to be less fertile. Similar treatment to that described earlier for ram lambs will help to stimulate both semen production and sex drive and therefore overall fertility. In the case of mature rams, where it is not desirable to have teaser ewes actually mated, a similar result may be obtained by running a small group of ewes in a secure paddock adjacent to the rams. Otherwise, teaser ewes should only be left in with the rams for long enough to allow each ram to mount and ejaculate once. This may only take a short while and should be repeated twice daily for two or three days.

Another alternative is to subject rams to artificial autumn conditions by housing them and blacking out any daylight, so that they have 16 hours of darkness and only eight hours of daylight when they are turned out to graze. This stimulates hormonal activity (via melatonin from the pineal gland), thereby increasing both testicle size and sperm production. This method takes some time to take effect and so must be operated for two to three months before the rams are required to work. Artificial lighting regimes are costly and cumbersome and mean that animals have to be housed at a time when there is ample grass outside. Nevertheless, it may be feasible for a small group of rams if a suitable shed is available providing an efficient mechanical ventilation system is in place. Synthetic melatonin can be used for this but is unavailable commercially in the UK at present.

Keeping rams separate from the ewe flock

It is most important to keep rams well away from the main ewe flock in the months leading up to mating. By 'well away' is meant out of sight, sound and particularly smell. Chemicals given off by rams at this time—the pheromones—are very potent and will sexually stimulate the ewes initially. However if rams remain in close proximity with the ewes, but are not joined with them for mating, then the pheromone effect will diminish. This will tend to delay the mating period when the rams are eventually introduced and will lead to a more protracted lambing—exactly the opposite to what is desirable. (Billy goats will also stimulate ewes in a similar fashion, so they too should be kept away from the ewe flock, as well as the doe herd.)

TIMING THE INTRODUCTION OF RAMS

In many flocks, mating goes on for far longer than is necessary or desirable. However, it is possible to shorten the time the rams run with the ewes and yet to achieve lambing results as good as or frequently better than in flocks with a lambing period twice as long, without resorting to the use of teasers or artificial methods.

One of the most important decisions to be taken is when to lamb the flock. It is therefore important to know the extent of the breeding season of the breed of ewe involved. This is because the compactness of mating will depend to a large extent upon the response of the ewes to the introduction of the rams. In a flock consisting of ewes of one breed, not all of the ewes will begin their sexual activity at the same time. Many will take weeks to do so, but eventually, the majority of fit, healthy ewes in a flock will come into season. They will all be at slightly different stages of their oestrous cycle, but over a period of 17 days—the length of an average oestrous cycle—around 98% of the ewes should exhibit heat and ovulate.

Therefore, if the rams are introduced at this stage of the proceedings, they will have a nice steady supply of ewes coming into heat each day. If the rams are fertile and in plentiful supply, then a high proportion of the ewes (75% plus) should become pregnant to that first service period, at a time of year when they should be approaching peak fertility. This situation would apply to Suffolks in late September and to Mules in late October.

However, if rams are introduced into a flock where only a small proportion of the ewe flock could be expected to be sexually active—for example, Suffolks in early July or Mules in early August—then the situation will be very different. The presence of the rams will have a stimulatory effect on the ewes which have not yet begun sexual activity because of the 'ram effect'. This will bring most of these ewes into heat over roughly a ten day period, beginning two to three weeks after the rams are introduced. The rams will serve the small number of ewes which were already oestrous cycling around the time they were joined. There will then be a delay before the majority of the flock come into heat. This will tax the rams' performance severely and may result in a high 'return' rate to first service. In consequence there will be a prolonged lambing, with the probability of fewer lambs born and a higher barren rate amongst ewes. Therefore, fertile rams should not be introduced until the majority of the ewes are sexually active. If it is required to mate and lamb a flock earlier than is natural for the breed, teaser rams or sponges should be used (see Chapter 3).

RAM GROUP NUMBERS

Unless it is necessary for pedigree purposes for rams to work singly with a group of ewes, then they generally work better and produce better results if they are run as a group. Two rams together tend to disagree and may exhibit homosexual tendencies, whereas in groups of three or more there are generally fewer problems. For example, under lowland conditions at the peak of the breeding season, where three rams are running with a group of around 150 ewes, there will be approximately nine ewes on heat each day. The three rams together will tend to serve and ejaculate into these nine ewes on two or three occasions each day, although they may mount ewes without ejaculating more frequently than this. The load will not be spread equally, of course. Some rams may serve all nine ewes, whilst others may be less amorous or may be prevented from serving by other dominant rams.

Competition between rams is good because it is better if ewes are served on several occasions during the time they are on heat, preferably by more than one ram. These multi-sire matings generally result in a higher lamb crop, a lower barren rate and a shorter lambing than do single-sire matings at the same ram to ewe ratio. Part of the reason for this is that the competition between rams means that they serve ewes more frequently, so that each ewe receives a larger dose of semen.

Small mating paddocks are best where practicable, so that rams can get around to sniff-out the ewes in season with a minimum of effort. Where mating has to take place indoors, the space allowance should be generous and feeding appropriate. The floor surface should be non-slip, so as not to discourage rams from mounting. Footrot should be tightly controlled, since it usually spreads rapidly under housed conditions and could seriously affect the willingness of rams to work. Because rams are working in close proximity, dominant rams may prevent subordinate rams from working. This may also occur in very small fields, whereas in larger areas the subordinate rams can nip in quickly and serve a ewe in just a few seconds!

HARNESSING OR RADDLING RAMS

As a general rule, rams should be harnessed or raddled for a number of reasons. Most immediately, it enables the shepherd to tell if a ram is mounting ewes. Some skill is necessary to decide what the marks left on ewes actually mean. Whilst a heavily marked ewe may suggest that she has been properly serviced, it may also mean that she has been mounted on numerous occasions by a particularly inept ram who has never ejaculated into her. (One group of New Zealand workers recorded a ram which mounted 80 times before finally ejaculating!)

On the other hand, a faintly marked ewe may well have been mounted by an experienced and dexterous ram who ejaculated at the first attempt. It is important that rams are closely observed to see if they are performing satisfactorily from the point of view of seeking out oestrous ewes, mounting and ejaculating. If not, or if there is any doubt, then they should be replaced by another fit 'standby' ram immediately.

Crayon marks also provide information on how the ewes themselves are performing. It is useful for the shepherd to record the number of ewes marked each day so that the pattern of oestrus in the flock can be determined. Crayon colours should be changed around 14 days after ram introduction, that is, a few days before the first ewes served are likely to repeat should they not hold to first service. A change of raddle colour is the only way the shepherd has of knowing whether the rams are getting an acceptable proportion of ewes to conceive. The lighter raddle colours should be used first and the sequence chosen so that it is possible to distinguish the fresh colour on top of the old.

If a high percentage of ewes return to a second, third or fourth colour, then providing the ewes are in good body condition and within their normal breeding season, this would suggest that the rams were most likely at fault. Even though there are several rams in with a group of ewes, it is possible that more than one is at fault, or that one dominant ram is subfertile or infertile and is preventing less aggressive fertile rams from serving ewes. There is often a long delay of perhaps a cycle and a half (three to four weeks) before some problems come to light. Even if rams are replaced immediately, there will inevitably be a considerable delay and prolongation of lambing. Hence the importance of a pre-mating ram examination.

Harnesses should be fitted a week before the rams are due to join the flock and a crayon chosen to suit the weather conditions during the mating period. 'Hot' and 'cold' crayons in several colours are available, for use in hot and cold weather respectively.

73

REMOVAL OF THE RAMS

Rams should be withdrawn from the flock after five or six weeks at most; otherwise lambing will be unduly prolonged because of a small number of stragglers. Therefore some ewes will have three opportunities to mate during this period and others only two. The rams' semen reserves will become more and more depleted as mating progresses so that unless fresh rams are substituted, ewes served at the end will have less chance of holding to service.

Ewes should be permanently marked to identify those lambing to the first, second and third services. The flock can be divided into early and late lambing groups so that feeding during the last third of pregnancy can be rationed appropriately. Some shepherds may wish to change raddle colours on a more frequent basis, so as to identify weekly lambing groups. The only problem that arises here is to find a sufficient number of strong colours to overmark ewes.

Once the rams have been removed, a teaser ram can be harnessed and joined with the ewes for a three week period, to colour mark ewes which are barren. These ewes can then be marked and managed accordingly. The use of the teaser in this way may be thought unnecessary in flocks which use ultrasound scanning to detect pregnancy. It is very unusual for ewes to exhibit oestrus when pregnant, as a small percentage of cows do. Nevertheless, an occasional pregnant ewe may be marked by the teaser ram who sneaked up on her unannounced. Where scanning is used, the barren ewes should be checked for pregnancy prior to disposal.

MATING

The act of courtship and mating in sheep is a rather hurried affair. The ram moves amongst the flock, sniffing the air and the rear ends of ewes as he does so. Ewes in oestrus give off chemicals which the ram can detect and which signal their sexual state, and they frequently urinate following any initial attention from the ram. The ram may stick his nose in the stream of urine or sniff at the urine on the ground. He then throws his head back, curls his upper lip and takes a long intake of breath, drawing the odour over some very sensitive glands which detect the chemicals signalling that the ewe is ready to be served. This is known as the Flehmen reaction.

If the ewe is in oestrus and ready to accept the ram, she will show an interest in him and may nuzzle his scrotum, present herself to him and stand still for him to mount. A dexterous ram will mount the ewe, introduce the penis into the vagina and make vigorous thrusting movements leading to a final ejaculatory thrust, all within 10 to 20 seconds. He will then dismount immediately and either prepare to mount the same ewe again or move off to find another oestrous ewe. The act of ejaculation—rather than simply mounting and thrusting—is a very characteristic movement, and shepherds should be able to tell when a ram is ejaculating efficiently. The ability to

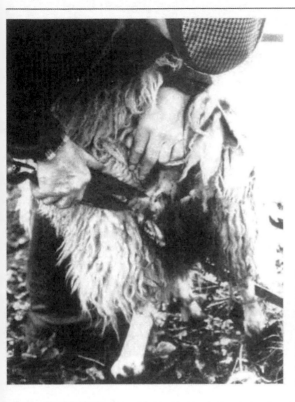

Plate 2.29 'Crutching' a ewe before mating. Removing excess wool around the vulva makes it easier for the ram to penetrate. Excess wool around the prepuce in the ram should likewise be removed.

thrust and ejaculate satisfactorily is an inherited characteristic. Rams which are good performers are likely to leave more semen high up in the vagina, close to the cervix, in a position that enhances the prospects of fertilisation.

Mating ability of rams

There is a wide variation in the ability of rams to mate effectively. A good ram is quite capable of mating 50 times in a week and some rams have been observed to mount up to 40 ewes in a day. Where good rams have access to a large number of oestrous ewes, for example, in a synchronised flock, they may mate with around 10 different ewes in 24 hours and mount each ewe three or four times. In one group of synchronised ewes, the author observed one Greyface ewe in heat race to the bottom of the paddock to greet the fresh rams. Within the space of just four minutes the ewe was properly mated by three Finn-Dorset rams a total of nine times!

The best rams will be capable of ejaculating every time they mount, or every other time. Average rams ejaculate every three or four mounts. Poor rams may perform much less effectively than this, or they may not be capable of ejaculating at all whilst giving the impression of being very busy. Good performances are not guaranteed to produce high conception and lambing rates. However, aggressive rams with a strong sexual drive

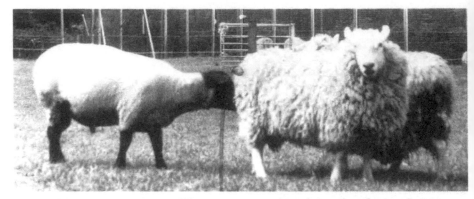

Plate 2.30 and 2.31 Ram sniffing an oestrous ewe (*above*) and preparing to mount (*below*). Sheep generally prefer to mate with their own breed or face colour if given the choice.

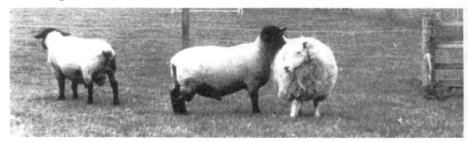

Plate 2.32 Dorset Horn shearling ram serving a Greyface ewe. The ram takes only a few seconds to ejaculate following mounting.

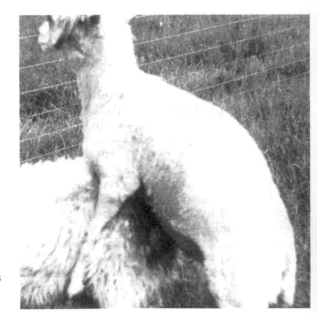

and high degree of dexterity are more likely to give satisfactory results than timid rams with poor sexual agility.

There is ample experimental evidence that rams have a highly significant effect upon litter size but the best rams may be difficult to identify in flocks where multi-sire matings of the same breed are the practice. The influence of the ram may be due to the better fertilising capacity of his sperm or to the better survival of embryos and foetal lambs during pregnancy, or indeed to a combination of both. Good performing rams tend to produce daughters of above-average fertility and rams bred from ewes of high fertility tend to be more fertile themselves.

The failure of a ram to mate satisfactorily may be due to a number of different factors, some of which have been alluded to already, such as the psychological factors associated with rams reared in bachelor groups or bullying by dominant rams, especially in very small paddocks. Ram lambs which have been overworked in their first season or have had their first sexual experiences with a group of synchronised ewes may be less than willing to work the following season. Also, ram lambs or shearlings which have been overfed, so that they are well grown for the ram sales (very close to tupping), are less likely to perform satisfactorily because of a reduced sex drive.

Sexual preferences

Carefully controlled trial work has shown that rams and ewes will mate with their own breed as a first preference—a form of racial prejudice! As an alternative, ewes would generally prefer to mate with a ram with a similar profile to their own breed. Head shape and colour would appear to be important. Where there is no alternative, ewes will mate with almost any breed of ram, but instances are recorded where ewes have resisted the advances of particular rams even when they were in heat.

Rams also have preferences—for example, they will usually go for the older and more experienced ewe. They also prefer ewes which are freshly in heat rather than those which have been served repeatedly already or are going out of oestrus. Older ewes tend to form 'harems' around a particular dominant ram who nevertheless may not be the most fertile. The lesson here is that virgin ewe lambs and gimmers should be run as a separate group with mature rams; otherwise they may be neglected. A ram of medium size should be used, so that ewe lambs do not move forward or collapse under his weight, in which case the ram may be unable to introduce the penis or to ejaculate. Careful observation should identify any problems associated with ram or ewe preferences, so that rams can be swapped around or groups adjusted in some way.

Effects of weather

Bad weather may affect the way rams work. During cold, wet conditions rams are more reluctant to serve. This may prove costly if a large number of ewes are in oestrus during bad weather. In early lambing or out-of-season

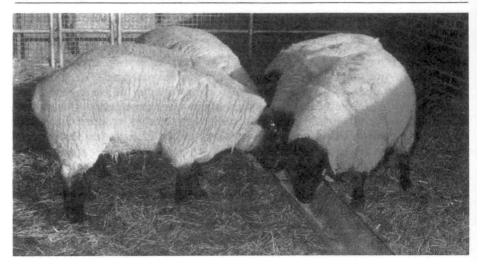

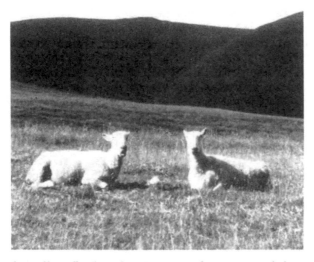

Plate 2.33 (*Above*) Trough feeding rams between matings. These rams have had two days of intensive mating amongst synchronised ewes and will be put back to work in two weeks' time to mate the repeats, so they must be kept in good condition. (The harnesses have been removed for the moment but the marks in the fleece can be seen.)

Plate 2.34 (*Left*) Bluefaced or Hexham Leicester rams. This breed and certain others may need shelter in severe winter weather, as they are not particularly hardy.

breeding flocks, the rams may have to work in very hot weather. The ewes will probably have been synchronised and it is vital that the rams work well for the critical two days of the induced oestrus. Some form of shelter from the sun may be provided where rams can retire for a brief period of rest. Alternatively rams can be housed in a cool shed during the hottest part of the day—say 10 am to 4 pm—and allowed to mate during the remaining 18 hours.

There are two adverse effects of hot weather. The first is an unwillingness to hunt out and serve ewes because of heat exhaustion. The second is that the effect of heat on the testicles, both directly and via a rise in body temperature, may damage sperm. All rams which have a woolly scrotum should have the wool clipped off well in advance of mating.

Ram care after mating

As soon as the rams have been withdrawn from the ewe flock they should be checked over for any signs of injury or disease, such as brisket sores or footrot, and any necessary treatment implemented immediately. Any rams which did not perform satisfactorily should be rigorously culled there and then, so that they are not forgotten and used again the following season.

Rams lose a considerable amount of weight during mating, even if they have been trough fed. They should continue to be hand fed until they are back into good body condition and should be maintained well throughout the year and given any preventive medicines, such as fluke drenches and vaccinations, at appropriate times along with the ewe flock.

Certain ram breeds, with fine skin and wool, such as the Bluefaced (Hexham) Leicester, may suffer somewhat during the worst of the winter weather. They should be housed overwinter unless a well-drained and sheltered grazing area is available. If kept outdoors, they should be properly fed to provide sufficient energy both to maintain body condition and to keep out the cold. Some breeders even provide waterproof overcoats for particularly delicate specimens!

Such care at the end of tupping will help considerably when it comes to preparing the ram stud for work again the following season.

EWE MANAGEMENT
Weaning to Mating

If there is a starting point for the preparation of ewes for the breeding season, then it is probably at weaning. At least two months should be allowed between weaning and mating, so that ewes have time to recover from the rigours of pregnancy and lactation. This is particularly pertinent to ewes suckling twins or triplets, when it may be tempting to allow lambs to continue sucking if ewes are still milking well. This temptation should be strongly resisted, since these ewes will have lost considerable body condition and need adequate time to make it up again before mating. If they are not given sufficient time to do so, then there may be a delay in the onset of sexual activity in autumn, a reduction in the number of eggs shed during oestrus and consequently a poor lamb drop.

The lumbar vertebrae in the loin region (behind the ribs) should be used to assess condition score (CS) in the sheep since this is the area where condition is last to be laid down but first to be lost.

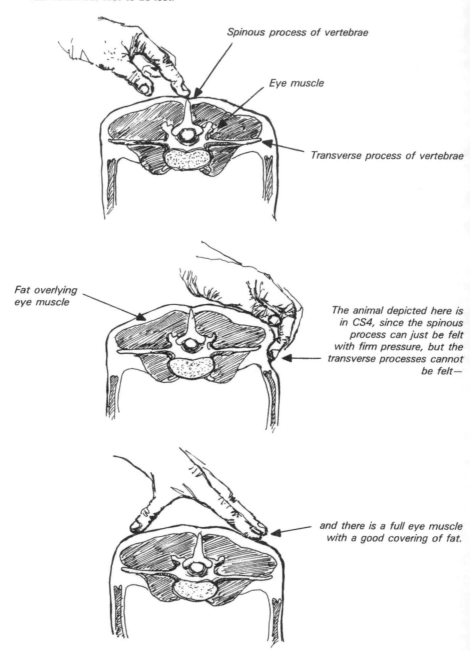

Spinous process of vertebrae

Eye muscle

Transverse process of vertebrae

Fat overlying eye muscle

The animal depicted here is in CS4, since the spinous process can just be felt with firm pressure, but the transverse processes cannot be felt—

and there is a full eye muscle with a good covering of fat.

Figure 2.1   The handling points for the condition scoring of sheep.

80

CONDITION SCORE TARGETS FOR MATING

Ewes should therefore be condition scored (CS) at weaning and managed accordingly to achieve the aim of CS 3 to 3.5 (or 2.5 to 3 on the hill) by two weeks before mating. Fat ewes in CS 4 to 5 are likely to have reared only singles, assuming that barren ewes were culled. They should be kept on bare grazing or at an increased stocking rate until they are down to around CS 3 to 3.5, at which they should be maintained. Ewes in CS 3 to 4 at weaning should be maintained at this condition on good grazing. Improved grazing and a reduced stocking rate will be necessary for ewes of CS 2 to 2.5, since they will need to put on a whole CS or more, which will take at least six weeks of good feeding. Thin ewes with a CS below 2 are likely to have reared multiples and will require some cereals to supplement good grazing—for example, a pound per day of mineralised whole barley. These thin ewes should be examined three weeks or a month later and the feed adjusted if necessary.

The best strategy for feeding ewes before mating is to allow them to build up steadily or to maintain body condition, rather than keep them hungry and attempt to flush them in the last three weeks. Good body condition is necessary for optimum ovulation rate and also to build up body reserves which can be drawn on during pregnancy, when feeding is generally of poorer quality and more expensive. Overfeeding on the other hand can be counterproductive, since it may have a depressive effect upon ovulation rate. Healthy lightweight ewes which are flushed well will generally out-perform fat ewes.

Despite nitrogen applications, good-quality grazing may be in short supply in late summer and autumn in some years. It therefore makes sense to utilise suitable grazing whenever it is available and to adjust the stocking rate so that ewes in only moderate body condition have an ample supply of good-quality grass.

Breeds vary in their response to flushing, with those of lower prolificacy, such as the Scottish Blackface or Swaledale, responding considerably better than the more prolific breeds, such as the Mules, Greyfaces or Finns. Other breeds, such as the Cheviot, will respond to flushing only if they begin from a medium condition score. In general, however, ewes which are mated in good condition, at around CS 3, will produce the optimum number of eggs and fewer of them will be barren than either fatter or thinner ewes.

Hill ewes

Hill ewes should be brought down off the high tops onto improved ground or in-bye fields for flushing where possible. The extent of flushing will depend on the availability of good-quality grass late in the year (October and November) and also on the desirability or otherwise of twins. Where there is very limited in-bye ground suitable for supporting ewes with twins during pregnancy and lactation, it is pointless to flush ewes to obtain twin ovulations. The result may be ewes with insufficient milk and small lambs

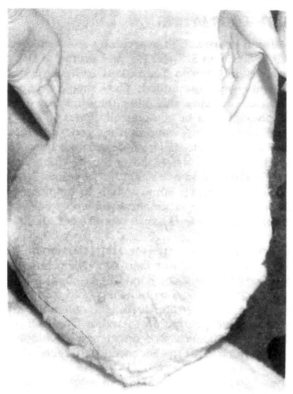

Plate 2.35 Condition scoring a ewe. (*Left*) The hands are positioned over the transverse processes of the lumber vertebrae (see Figure 2.1). This ewe at CS 2.5 needs a month of good-quality grazing to put on at least another half condition score before she goes to the ram.
(*Below*) This ewe is in condition CS 1.5: the bony spinous processes of the lumbar can be felt with the thumbs as a sharp ridge; there is very little eye muscle and no fat over the loin; the transverse processes are easily distinguished and the fingers can be pushed underneath.

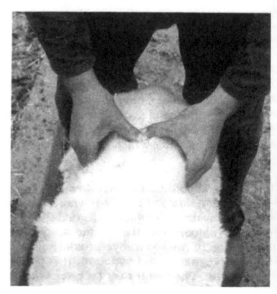

with a poor chance of survival. However, where there is sufficient grazing to support twins and especially where ultrasound scanning is practised to detect multiple births, then fields or fenced areas of improved hill can be cleared of sheep after weaning, fertilised and shut-up until required for flushing and early pregnancy grazing. After scanning, twin bearing ewes can be kept down on improved hill ground or in-bye fields. Single bearing ewes can be turned back onto the hill, except for those in poor condition, which should be held back and fed appropriately. Forage crops can also be used for flushing hill sheep.

It is important that hill gimmers are trained to eat concentrate feeds or feed blocks, as they will need supplementation at various times, such as in mid pregnancy. This should be done as early as possible after they return from the 'winterings' as ewe hoggs in April. Before turning them out onto the hill is a good time to start. Training is never 100% successful, but the majority learn and the benefits can be considerable in extra lambs sold off the farm.

It is most important on both hill and lowland farms that the improved feeding before mating is continued throughout mating and the early pregnancy period and even more important that sudden shortages of food are avoided during this period.

HEALTH

Weaning is an important time to check the health of ewes and to identify for culling any ewes with conditions which will make them unsuitable for breeding the following season. Around one-fifth of lowland ewes are culled annually, according to data collected by the Meat and Livestock Commission. Some of the diseases which may lead to culling are mastitis, lameness, broken mouth and liver fluke.

The majority of cases of mastitis occur during the first month after lambing. However, at weaning, ewes should be examined for the presence of any sores or injuries to the teats or udder and these should be treated to discourage contamination by bacteria and damage by flies. (Mastitis is dealt with in detail in Chapter 7.) Any ewes with hard or lumpy udders should be marked for culling. To discourage milk production, weaned ewes should be put onto sparse grazing and/or heavily stocked for four or five days, but under no circumstances should they be deprived of water for even a day.

Dry ewe therapy

Dry ewe therapy for the treatment of mastitis is a technique adapted from the practice of dry cow therapy. Since no special ewe preparations are available, each half of the udder is infused at weaning with half a syringe of a suitable dry cow intermammary antibiotic preparation. Although the most recent surveys suggest that post-weaning infections probably represent only a small proportion of all mastitis cases, the technique will be described here

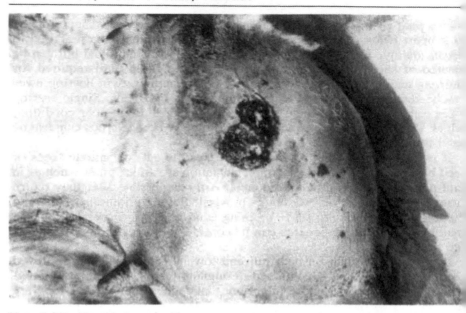

Plate 2.36 Mastitis is a significant cause of culling in the ewe flock. In this case the infection has burst to the exterior and is scabbing over.

for those who wish to consider its use. It is strongly recommended, however, that the pros and cons are discussed with your veterinary surgeon before proceeding. Dry ewe therapy works best where groups of lambs are all weaned together, since if one of twins is sold, the remaining lamb may suck the antibiotic out of the udder. The task should be carried out on a dry day with the most stringent hygiene precautions; otherwise it is pointless, since poor technique could actually introduce infection.

Two people are required to do the job properly. One tips up ewes and is therefore 'dirty' whilst another carries out the task and should keep 'clean' by not otherwise handling the ewes. The clean operator should preferably wear rubber gloves and wash them in a bucket of warm water containing a suitable disinfectant after treating each ewe. Paper towels, cotton wool, surgical spirit, intramammary tubes or syringes and an iodophor teat dip in a garden hand sprayer will be required. It is much easier if the clean operator works seated, with the ewe upturned in a cradle.

- All ewes should be treated.
- Any gross dirt should be washed from the teats and udder using a disposable paper towel soaked in disinfectant and then dried with another clean towel. If the udder and teats are clean and dry, they should not be washed.
- Each teat should be swabbed and the orifice gently rubbed for several seconds with cotton wool soaked in surgical spirit.

- Squirt a little milk from each teat to locate the orifice and to act as a lubricant.
- The nozzle of the intramammary tube or syringe should be very gently inserted into the teat orifice and approximately half the contents squeezed in and gently massaged up into the udder. Repeat for the other teat. (If

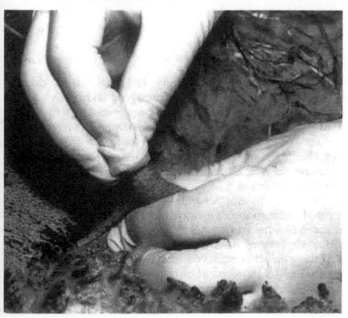

Plate 2.37 (*Above*) Swabbing the teat end with surgical spirit. It is essential that no infection is introduced: note the operator's rubber gloves which can be washed and dried between ewes.

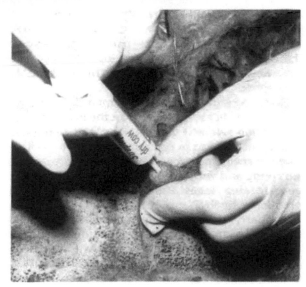

Plate 2.38   Infusing dry-cow penicillin/streptomycin into the teat orifice of a ewe. Providing strict hygiene is observed, there should be no objection to using half a tube in each half of the udder.

85

it proves difficult to insert the tube, do not persist, but gently 'fold' the end of the teat around the nozzle and squeeze the contents—sufficient should find its way into the teat.)

- Thoroughly spray the teats and surrounding udder with iodophor teat dip, or swab with cotton wool soaked in iodophor. (Do not apply any sticky ointments or Stockholm-tar, as dirt merely adheres to them, so increasing the risk of infection.)

FERTILITY OF EWES

Ewes which are well managed and adequately fed and which do not become affected by any disease which may, directly or indirectly, affect their ability to conceive are generally highly fertile when mated with fertile rams. Examination of eggs from ewes on embryo transfer programmes shows that, after one service, in excess of 90% of them are satisfactorily fertilised. Because of the death of a proportion of the early embryos the conception rate to a single service is generally around 75% in upland and lowland flocks of medium prolificacy.

Around 6 or 7% of ewes do not sustain a pregnancy, even though they may have conceived more than once during the breeding season. This is an average figure and will vary from year to year and from flock to flock depending on several other factors, many of which are managemental and not always the fault of the ewe. It is believed that only a very small proportion of these failures are due to anatomical abnormalities of the ewe which might prevent conception or development of an embryo.

Ewe lambs and gimmers are generally less fertile than mature ewes, in contrast to heifers which are generally significantly more fertile than mature cows. This is probably due to the fact that many ewe lambs are not sufficiently well grown and are often sexually immature at the time of mating. Gimmers, being sexually inexperienced, do not always encourage the attention of the rams and may not be mated at all when in heat, or may be mated too near the end of the heat, so reducing the chances of conception.

Body condition in ewes—which is usually under the control of the farmer and shepherd rather than the ewe—may have a profound effect upon conception rate and the maintenance of pregnancy. If body condition falls during mating and in early pregnancy, this will adversely affect the number of eggs shed, the proportion of eggs fertilised, the proportion of embryos surviving and will, in consequence, increase the number of barreners. With good feeding, many of these empty ewes would have been quite capable of producing lambs.

Similarly, where management during early pregnancy causes stress to ewes, for example, by dipping, dosing or gathering the flock unnecessarily, then a number of pregnancies will be terminated in these early weeks. Only a small proportion will be terminated because of genetic abnormalities of the embryo itself.

Giving ewes a second chance to breed

It is common practice in most flocks to give a second chance the following breeding season to ewe lambs or shearlings which fail to produce a lamb. It is also common practice in many flocks to cull mature ewes which are barren. However, from the above, it can be seen that a high proportion of these culled barreners would be perfectly capable of breeding subsequently if given the chance. Indeed, many are purchased by other farmers and successfully bred on their new farms. Because it is difficult or impossible to identify the small number which are unable to breed, there is a small risk in retaining such ewes. Nevertheless, with the high cost of replacements the risk may be considered worthwhile (except with the oldest ewes), providing they are sound in all other respects.

Infectious abortion, such as enzootic abortion, toxoplasmosis or salmonellosis, can result in considerable losses of lambs, especially in the first or second years of an outbreak. However, ewes which have aborted usually become immune to the specific microorganism involved for some years, even for life in some cases. As a general rule, therefore, aborted ewes should be retained in the flock. However, there are differences in the management of flocks according to the infectious agent or agents involved and the reader is referred to the section on abortion in Chapter 5 for details.

Damage at lambing time

Ewes which experience difficulties during lambing may be damaged internally whilst giving birth unaided, or through carelessness or ignorance when being given 'assistance'. Where rough handling has caused severe infection or tearing of the tissues—or even fractures of the bones of the pelvis—the healing process may result in a much-restricted exit for lambs at subsequent lambings. Where this is thought likely to give rise to difficult births in future, the ewe should be culled.

Ewes which prolapse the vagina before lambing or the uterus after lambing or which require a caesarean section because of some obstruction such as ringwomb should also be culled. Ewes with mastitis are unlikely to be able to feed lambs adequately, if at all, and should not be retained for breeding.

Selecting replacement ewes

It is wise to select female breeding replacements from among the offspring of ewes which have had troublefree lambings. Flock records should be consulted to avoid selecting replacements from ewes which have had any lambing difficulty. By pursuing a rigorous culling and selection policy on the lines indicated, it is possible to build up an 'easy-care' flock where assistance at lambing will only occasionally be required. This will depend to some extent on the ewe breed and to a lesser extent on the ram breed, since the ram generally has less influence on the size of the lambs born than does the ewe.

The Oestrous Cycle of the Ewe

The seasonality of sexual activity in ewes in temperate regions of the world as influenced by day length, breed, feeding and other factors has already been discussed. Once sexual activity has begun in a flock, the ewes tend to trickle into oestrus, so that individual members of the flock will all be at different stages of the oestrous cycle. Cycles normally continue on a regular basis, with ewes coming into heat roughly every 17 days and ewe lambs around a day less.

HORMONAL CONTROL OF OESTRUS

The oestrous cycle in the ewe is controlled by hormones. These are chemicals produced by various glands in the body which are released into the bloodstream to produce their effects on tissues or organs which may be a long way from where the hormones were produced. The word hormone derives from the Greek meaning 'I stir up', which is a particularly pertinent description for the sex hormones. In the ewe, the glands secreting the hormones which control the oestrous cycle are the **ovaries** (which number two, left and right), the womb or **uterus**, and a small gland at the base of the brain, called the **pituitary**, which provides overall control. The actions of the hormones are very complex and interrelated. They are also influenced by outside factors, such as day length and feeding. Only a very simplified explanation of events will be given here.

The 17 day cycle is, for simplicity's sake, divided into two phases. First is a period of around a day and a half when the ewe shows great interest in the ram and will allow him to mate with her. This is called **oestrus** or **heat**. The time a ewe is on heat depends upon a number of factors and is quite variable: the presence of the ram will hasten ovulation and shorten oestrus; prolific breeds tend to have a longer heat; oestrus is shorter in the middle of the breeding season and longer at the beginning and end; young females tend to have a shorter oestrus than mature ewes. For the rest of the cycle—some 15 days—the ewe is not interested in the ram and will not allow him to mate her. However, the ram will normally make little attempt to do so, since the ewe does not encourage him, nor does she give off any odours which tell him she is in heat.

The hormonal events around oestrus

A few days before oestrus, one or more fluid-filled, cyst-like structures called follicles (within one or both ovaries) rapidly increase in size. This comes about due to a hormone called **follicle stimulating hormone (FSH)**, which is secreted by the pituitary gland in the brain. These follicles also produce their own hormones, including a most important one called **oestrogen**.

Oestrogen is responsible for the behavioural changes in the ewe which

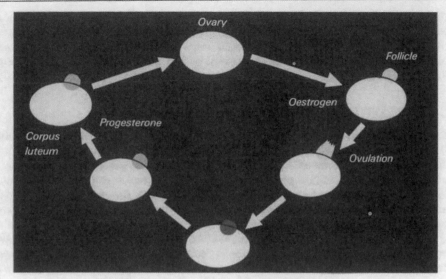

Figure 2.2 The ovarian cycle of the sheep.

make her attractive to the ram. Also, as the follicles increase in size and approach ripeness or maturity, so the quantity of oestrogen they secrete increases. Due to its action on the pituitary gland, oestrogen reduces the production of FSH and increases the secretion of another hormone called **luteinising hormone (LH)**.

It is LH which causes the final ripening and eventual rupture of the follicle, with the release of the ovum or egg in a relatively large quantity of fluid, in which it has been protected and nurtured during its development inside the follicle. The synchronisation of all these events is important, for it is essential that the eggs—which do not have a long life—are shed to coincide with mating, so that the chances of fertilisation are maximised.

Journey of the sperm

Oestrogen has at least one other important, although indirect, function: that of allowing another hormone—**oxytocin**—to bring about contractions of the muscular wall of the uterus. These movements aid the swimming movements of sperm, which have a very lengthy and hazardous journey considering their extremely small size. They must swim from the vagina (where they are deposited at ejaculation), through the cervix, across the uterus and up the oviducts to reach the eggs. In fact, very few sperm ever complete the journey. The majority fail to negotiate the cervix and are expelled from the vagina to the exterior. Those that manage to do so are looked upon by the ewe's body defences as 'foreign' material, with the result that many are destroyed by the white blood cells.

As the eggs are released from the follicle on the ovary they are caught in the funnel-shaped end of the **oviduct**—the tube leading from the ovary to

89

the uterus. The eggs must travel down the oviduct to be fertilised and thence on to the uterus where any fertilised eggs will develop. With the rupture of the follicles, oestrogen levels fall very low. Consequently, oestrous behaviour subsides and the contractions of the uterus cease, so protecting the tiny fertilised egg.

CORPUS LUTEUM AND PROGESTERONE

The gaping hole left on the surface of the ovary where the follicle once was fills up with blood and within a few days becomes a hard yellow structure called a **corpus luteum (CL)**, which begins to secrete yet another hormone, a very crucial one, called **progesterone**. This hormone prepares the uterus to receive the fertilised egg and later helps maintain the pregnancy. It also acts on the pituitary gland in the brain to turn off FSH and LH, so preventing the ewe from coming into oestrus in the meanwhile.

About 12 or 13 days after oestrus the ewe will 'know' whether or not she is pregnant. This comes about because the microscopically small embryo secretes chemical substances which alert the ewe to its presence. If the ewe is pregnant then the CL will persist on the ovary for several weeks, pumping out progesterone and so preventing the ewe from coming into oestrus, which could terminate the pregnancy.

If the ewe is not pregnant, either because she was not mated or because she failed to conceive, then after about 11 or 12 days the uterus secretes a hormone called **prostaglandin F2 alpha**, which causes the CL to shrivel up and progesterone levels to fall very low. This in turn means that FSH from the pituitary can again begin to stimulate more follicles to grow on the ovary and so the whole cycle begins all over again.

Oestrus signs in the ewe

Obviously, the whole point of oestrus or heat is to produce eggs and stimulate the ram to mate with the ewe so that sperm are introduced into the ewe's reproductive tract at the correct time to maximise the chances of fertilisation taking place. The signs of oestrus in the ewe are much less pronounced than in the cow and cannot be detected by the shepherd if rams are not running with the ewes. When rams are present, however, mature oestrus ewes will tend to remain near the ram and will stand still for him to mount. Sometimes they wag their tails vigorously ('flagging') to attract the ram's attention and some ewes may make half-hearted attempts to mount the ram and may nuzzle him under the belly and around the scrotum. Young females rarely exhibit any of these behavioural signs and where there is competition from older ewes they may go out of heat without being served.

Oestrus occurs when the follicles on the ovary are at their largest, almost fully ripe and on the point of rupturing to release the eggs. This timing is important because the ram will be stimulated to mount and deposit semen in the vagina so that sufficient sperm are present in the oviducts at the right time to meet the eggs on their journey from the ovary to the uterus and so maximise the chances of fertilisation. Where two or more follicles are present there is rarely more than a few hours' difference in time of their rupture.

Ovulation Rate

The number of eggs shed—the ovulation rate—is very variable both within flocks and between flocks and depends upon many factors such as the breed, the season of the year, body condition, the adequacy of feeding and the age and health status of the sheep. Ovulation rate sets the upper limit of the lamb drop in a flock. If the ovulation rate is low then the lamb drop will be low. If the ovulation rate is high then it is at least possible—although not inevitable—that the lamb drop will also be high. However, a high death rate amongst early embryos (see later) will lower the lamb drop and mask the fact that the ovulation rate may have been satisfactory. A low ovulation rate in an individual ewe means that there is less chance of her conceiving following mating, since, if only one egg is shed and it is not fertilised, the ewe will return to service 17 days later. This also increases the likelihood of a protracted lambing period. If two or more eggs are shed and one or more are fertilised, then the ewe becomes pregnant.

INFLUENCING OVULATION RATE

The farmer can influence ovulation rate and therefore lamb drop—for better or worse—in a number of ways. The important influences of condition score and of flushing have already been discussed. The choice of lambing date and therefore tupping date is very significant. At the beginning and the end of the breeding season, the ovulation rate for the flock as a whole is significantly less than in mid season (October and November in the UK) and this is reflected in the correspondingly higher lamb drops in March and April, whatever the breed involved.

The ovulation rate of individual breeds varies considerably, although it is lambing percentages which are usually quoted. (Ovulation rates are not usually measured, since this involves using a minor surgical procedure called laparoscopy, which actually allows the operator to view the ovaries and to count the number of ruptured follicles at oestrus.) Ovulation rates are generally about 30% higher than lambing rates, since approximately this proportion is 'lost' between fertilisation and lambing. So ewe breeds with 200% lambing or more, such as the Finn, Cambridge or Bluefaced Leicester, will produce around three or four eggs at each oestrus, whilst breeds with a lambing rate of below 150%, such as the Cheviot or Dorset Horn, will average around two ovulations.

The simplest way to increase ovulation rate through breeding is to cross low prolificacy ewes with high prolificacy rams. (Prolificacy is the number

91

of lambs born as a proportion of the number of ewes which lamb.) Mules and Greyfaces are examples of such, being the product of a Bluefaced Leicester ram over Swaledale or Scottish Blackface ewes respectively.

Where it is undesirable to change the breed, then selection within the breed by retaining replacement females from ewes producing multiple lambs is slow, because the heritability is low. Progress can be roughly doubled if, rather than selecting on lamb numbers, selection is made on ovulation rate using the laparoscope. This is unlikely to appeal to commercial farmers on grounds of cost and is only likely to benefit nucleus improver flocks. Even then, the welfare aspects of this technique give cause for some concern.

Fecundity genes

There are a small number of breeds worldwide in which a single gene has been identified which has a profound effect upon fecundity (the number of lambs born as a proportion of the number of ewes mated). The most familiar of these is the **Booroola** Merino gene which has been termed the **F gene**; others have been identified in Icelandic, D'man, Javanese and possibly the Cambridge breed. Merinos carrying the Booroola gene (which originated in a flock in New South Wales, Australia) have, on average, one extra ovulation at oestrus. Because, as a general rule, the more prolific a breed, the greater are the embryonic losses, this extra ovulation usually only results in 0.6 extra lambs, but this is of course a very large increase. As an example, a flock producing 140 lambs per 100 ewes to the tup before incorporation of the gene would produce $140 \times 0.6 = 84$ extra lambs, giving $140 + 84 = 224$ lambs per 100 ewes to the ram.

Where such a large number of extra lambs could prove embarrassing, a compromise can be arrived at in a flock by incorporating the F gene into only a proportion of the flock, say 50%. This would increase the lambs born per 100 ewes to the tup by $0.5 \times 0.6 = 0.3$ or 30%, so that in our example flock there would be an extra 42 lambs (0.5×84) giving 182 lambs per 100 ewes to the ram.

Because of the natural variation in ovulation rate between individual ewes in a flock, the effect of the F gene acts in the same way as any other method which increases ovulation rate. That is, the increase in lambs born is never spread evenly throughout the 'treated' ewes. Some will still give birth to singles, whilst others will have triplets or quads, which of course are smaller and more vulnerable and therefore need extra shepherding. Cross-fostering and other techniques will have to be employed to keep the extra lambs alive; otherwise the benefits could very easily turn into serious disadvantages.

Whilst this Merino F gene can be incorporated into other breeds, it is obvious that the Merino breed characteristics would not appeal to many British farmers. However, by backcrossing, the undesirable features can be diluted to an acceptable degree without losing the F gene. In other prolific breeds such as the Finn, the prolificacy is not carried on a single gene and therefore backcrossing to dilute the Finnish characteristics also dilutes the prolificacy proportionately.

Increasing ovulation rate through immunisation

Immunising techniques for increasing ovulation have only recently been introduced to the UK. They were initially used in the Antipodes, where they were primarily developed to improve both the prolificacy and consequently the fertility of extensively managed flocks of inherently low prolificacy, such as the Merino. However, they have not yet been adequately evaluated under a sufficiently diverse range of conditions for them to have found a niche in British sheep husbandry.

There are a number of naturally occurring compounds circulating in the ewe's bloodstream which have an inhibitory effect on the number of follicles which develop on the ovary. Some of these are male steroids or androgens—such as androstenedione. It is possible to produce compounds called immunogens which act like vaccines, so that when they are injected into the ewe they stimulate the production of antibodies which combine with and inactivate her natural steroids. This allows more follicles to develop in the ovaries and therefore more eggs to be released at oestrus.

The only commercially available compound in the UK at present is marketed as Fecundin (Coopers Pitman-Moore). Trials and commercial use have shown that it results in the production of around 25% extra lambs averaged over a number of different flocks, breeds and husbandry conditions. However, results have varied considerably, with some treated flocks producing no extra lambs or even rearing fewer lambs than untreated ewes, whilst other flocks have achieved in excess of 50% more lambs born. These large differences are due in part to the very wide range of management ability.

There is no doubt that this compound increases ovulation rate very substantially. The secret is to ensure that this translates into more lambs reared successfully. Any significant increase in the death rate of baby lambs from starvation, hypothermia and disease could hardly be justified on either welfare or economic grounds. It should be pointed out, however, that the problems are no different in practice from those which arise as a result of the incorporation of the Booroola gene into a flock.

Immunisation regime

The Fecundin treatment regime is very similar to that of many vaccination schemes, in that sheep which have not previously been immunised must be treated initially with two injections three to five weeks apart. The first injection should be given two months before the rams are to be introduced and the second at least a month before mating. It is most important that this second injection is not given less than a month before tupping, since this could reduce ovulation rate and hence lamb drop—the reverse of what is desired.

Ewes which have been immunised in previous years need only a single booster injection and this should be given at least a month before mating.

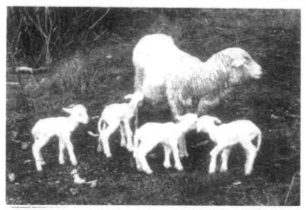

Plate 2.39 A Booroola Merino ewe with quadruplet lambs in Western Australia. The high prolificacy is due to a single F gene.

Plate 2.40 Scottish Blackface ewe with triplets as a result of immunisation with an anti-androstenedione (Fecundin). This flock is kept under lowland conditions. The technique would be contra-indicated in true hill flocks because of the probable high mortality amongst lambs.

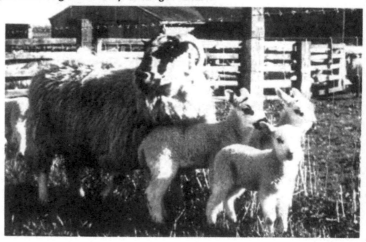

Gimmers joining the breeding flock will need two injections initially. After the second injection there is a rapid rise in the antibodies against the steroid which inhibits follicle development, reaching a peak between a week and a fortnight after the second injection. The higher the antibody level, the greater the increase in the number of eggs shed. Antibody levels then decline rapidly, so that three months after the second injection there is no effect upon ovulation rate. In between these extremes there will be a graded response. Where the second or booster injection is given much earlier than a month before tupping, then by the time ewes are mated, the effects of stimulation will be declining and there will be a poorer response or none at all.

Ewes must be sexually active when the rams are introduced. Where necessary, this can be manipulated by using either hormonal treatments or the ram effect to induce oestrus and ovulation without losing the effect of the immunisation. Ewes which are served early in the tupping period will receive the greatest stimulation although this may not necessarily be apparent, since ewes served later could be expected to produce more eggs as a result of being further into their breeding season.

To achieve an optimal response ewes must be in a good body condition (at least score 2.5), as ewes in poor condition may show no response to treatment. Adequate ram power at mating is crucial to maximise fertilisation rate and every effort should be made to reduce stress during early pregnancy since early embryonic death is generally higher in the more prolific ewes.

Husbandry in immunised flocks

Because of the natural variation in ovulation rate between ewes and because losses of embryos may occur during the early pregnancy period, there is no method, natural or artificial—nor is there ever likely to be—which will produce twins across the board. Therefore, where Fecundin or any other method is used to boost ovulation rate, it may be wise to scan ewes in mid pregnancy to identify those carrying twins and triplets. The flock can then be fed accordingly, so that the growth of the placenta—which governs the birth weight of lambs—is not compromised.

Good feeding during pregnancy also ensures that ewes have a good supply of the colostrum and milk which are so vital for lamb survival, especially in prolific flocks where lamb birth weights are inevitably lower and there is more competition at the teat. Failure to manage the flock as a prolific one may result in poor or even disastrous results.

On hill farms where ewes are confined to rough grazings on the open hill, it is unlikely that Fecundin will have any place, as ewes are unlikely to be able to rear the additional lambs born. Even if they could do so, it is doubtful whether the costs of treatment would be covered by the extra lambs sold. If hill farms have a high proportion of improved ground (say 20 or 25% of the total acreage) and ewes can be wintered during pregnancy on re-seeds, then the economics may just make sense. The management, and feeding in particular, would need to be stepped up to cope with the increased lambing percentage.

It is likely that this technique will prove most useful in lowland flocks with a usual lambing rate of about 120 to 160%, which could be raised to around 145 to 185% respectively. It is estimated that to cover the costs of the drug and the feed necessary for the extra number of ewes with multiple pregnancies, around 12 extra lambs need to be sold per 100 ewes to the tup. Each additional lamb sold thereafter would represent a profit. The costs need to be worked out over at least two or three years to take account of the higher cost of drugs in the first year. Flocks with a lambing percentage of around 175% could expect around 7 or 8% of ewes to produce triplets. However, after a successful Fecundin treatment (200% lambing), as many as 20% of ewes could produce triplets. Such flocks might therefore contemplate housing at lambing to help save lambs and make shepherding easier and this would add to the cost. In flocks which already have lambing percentages approaching 200%, the use of Fecundin may result in over 30% of ewes producing triplets and a significant proportion of quads. This requires an exceptionally high standard of shepherding and flock management with particular skills in artificial rearing and should not be undertaken lightly.

Immunising for more lambs in early breeding flocks

In early lambing flocks, profitability is highly dependent upon a good lambing percentage. However, the majority of ewes used on these systems are Suffolk cross types and the like, which start oestrous cycling relatively early but are of low prolificacy. (Overall national lambing percentages in early lambing flocks are only around 130%.) The use of Fecundin in flocks of low prolificacy is therefore tempting. Such flocks are generally sponged and treated with a follicle stimulating hormone (PMSG). If Fecundin is to be used, this sponging regime is essential, since all ewes must be oestrous cycling when the rams are introduced. Fecundin appears to have an additive effect to the PMSG and a lower dose of the latter may be used. However, whilst Fecundin raises the prolificacy of treated flocks, the fertility—that is, the proportion of ewes lambing in the flock—is reduced, so that there are a higher than expected number of barreners. The reasons for this are not clear, and until more trials have been carried out, this use of Fecundin should be carried out with caution.

PREGNANT MARE SERUM GONADOTROPHIN (PMSG)

Brief mention has been made of the use of the follicle stimulating hormone (PMSG), of which more will be said later (see Chapter 3). However, it should be pointed out here that PMSG is not a particularly suitable product for increasing ovulation rate in sheep. This is because ewes respond in a very unpredictable way to the drug: some produce few, if any, extra eggs whilst others produce excessive numbers. It would be very difficult to advise on a dose rate, since this would have to be adjusted according to breed, season and other circumstances and it would be easy to overdose and produce large litters. PMSG is essential for out-of-season breeding programmes in conjunction with the use of sponges and for the more precise timing of ovulation required for AI programmes. It should not be used to increase lambing percentage, especially when more precise methods are available.

Teasers

Teaser rams suddenly introduced to the flock just before the start of sexual activity in the ewes will induce oestrus earlier than intended. They also stimulate ovulation rate to a modest degree. This is discussed in Chapter 3.

Melatonin

Melatonin produces a mild superovulatory effect and its use is described in Chapter 3.

3
MANIPULATION OF BREEDING

Most sheep enterprises in the UK, with notable exceptions, are based on very traditional low input—low output systems. Apart from areas of Scotland and Wales, where sheep are the main enterprise on the farm, they are often run as a subsidiary, for example, as part of an arable rotation where they are used to consume arable by-products and to increase soil fertility, or as scavengers behind the dairy herd.

In dairy and pig herds there is often a high degree of control of the breeding programme, whereas in sheep flocks the rams are simply put in with the ewes at a traditional time of year for that area or farm. When the ewes actually start and finish breeding is usually left entirely to chance, with the result that lambing is not timetabled and is often unduly prolonged. Yet the means are available—often at very little extra cost—to organise the whole procedure so that lambing can be completed within less than a month and at a predetermined time to fit in with the other enterprises on the farm.

The benefits of being able to make better use of labour, buildings and feedstuffs and to finish lambs in even batches aimed at a particular market are obvious. Lamb deaths during early life—a very serious welfare problem, as well as a drain on the profitability of the flock—can often be minimised by using techniques which shorten lambing and allow for very close shepherding over a more manageable period.

Every flock will have its own particular aims and special circumstances and all the techniques to be described here will not be applicable to every farm. However, it is unlikely that there are many flocks which could not benefit in some way by using one or more of these techniques.

MANIPULATIVE TECHNIQUES AVAILABLE

It is possible to:

- synchronise oestrus and ovulation during the normal breeding season and thereby shorten the lambing period
- persuade ewes to begin breeding slightly earlier in the year than they would normally do
- breed ewes well outside their normal breeding season and also to produce more than one crop of lambs per year

- encourage ewes to produce more lambs than they would normally do by stimulating an increase in ovulation rate
- persuade all the ewes in a flock to lamb on a predetermined day of the year
- artificially inseminate ewes
- transfer embryos from one ewe to another
- produce identical twins
- produce transgenic animals

Transgenic animals are those which have had genetic material donated from another animal, not necessarily of the same species, incorporated into their own genetic material. Using this technique it may be possible in future to breed animals with the ability to grow faster and to produce leaner carcasses, to resist certain diseases without the need for vaccination and to produce a natural harvest of pharmacologically active substances. An example of the latter is already possible with ewes that can produce milk rich in one of the human blood-clotting factors required by haemophiliacs. This could replace the need to harvest it from human blood with all the attendant risks.

The Ram or Teaser Effect

This technique makes use of a powerful natural phenomenon, which is often poorly understood and improperly applied. It is a most effective method if used correctly and it is certainly underutilised.

PHEROMONES

Rams and teasers (vasectomised rams) secrete some very potent chemicals from their wool wax called **pheromones**. The smell of these substances produces an immediate and profound hormonal response in ewes, awakening them from sexual inactivity or **anoestrus**. Providing the ewes have been kept well away from the sight, sound and particularly the **smell** of rams for at least a month to six weeks, the presence of the males will produce an immediate and profound sexual response from the ewes. Within less than half an hour, the hormones which stimulate the start of oestrous activity will be circulating in the ewe's bloodstream in much-increased amounts. The effect of this is to stimulate almost every ewe in the flock to ovulate within a few days of introducing the males. The only exception will be ewes which have already begun oestrous cycles, which will be unaffected.

This ovulation—unlike the situation during the peak of the breeding season—is not accompanied by the behavioural signs of oestrus and so is called a **silent heat**. Since the ewes do not give off any odours or exhibit any of the usual behavioural signs of heat, the rams will not mate with the ewes at this time—except perhaps with a few which may already have been sexually active before the introduction of the rams.

Timing of teased heats

A proportion of the ewes in the flock will then come into a proper **behavioural oestrus** roughly 17 days (a full heat cycle) after this first early ovulation, that is, some three weeks after the males were first introduced. The rest of the flock will have a short oestrous cycle of only about a week in length, with ovulation occurring at a second silent heat. Again, these ewes will not be served by the rams. Usually the majority of these ewes will then go on to have a normal 17 day cycle followed by ovulation and accompanied by behavioural oestrus. On this occasion they will accept the ram for the first time, approximately four weeks after the males were first introduced.

This technique therefore results in two peaks of heat which occur roughly three and four weeks after the males are introduced. The teaser rams must not remain with the flock for more than two weeks at most. Indeed, a few days is all that is necessary to start the ewes off. Teasers must then be replaced with fertile rams, which will serve most of the ewes within a ten day period. The sequence of events is shown in Figure 3.1.

WHEN TO UTILISE THE TEASER EFFECT

The teaser effect can only be used satisfactorily in flocks where all, or at least the majority, of the ewes have not yet begun sexual activity, but who are within just a few weeks of their normal breeding season. Ewes already oestrous cycling are unaffected by the presence of the male in that their heat cycles will continue unaltered. Ewes which are in the middle of their non-breeding season (in deep anoestrus) are less likely to respond satisfactorily. Even if they do so, they will tend to lapse back into non-breeding mode when teasers are removed because of the inhibitory influence of long days on sexual activity.

The method can therefore be used to advance the breeding season of any flock, of whatever breed, by three or four weeks. If it is used much earlier than this, then the results may be disappointing, since the ovulation rate and therefore lambing percentage may be lower than is acceptable. The technique does not synchronise oestrus and ovulation as tightly as the sponge method and is therefore not suitable for artificial insemination programmes which use fixed-time insemination. However, where teasers are harnessed, ewes can be inseminated as they are marked. In this way the majority of ewes can be inseminated in less than a week, but the method is time-consuming.

Number of teasers required

Teaser rams should be introduced to the ewe flock at roughly the same ratio as fertile rams, that is around three per 100 ewes for the purpose of early breeding. (More may be needed for AI programmes, e.g. 5%.) When the

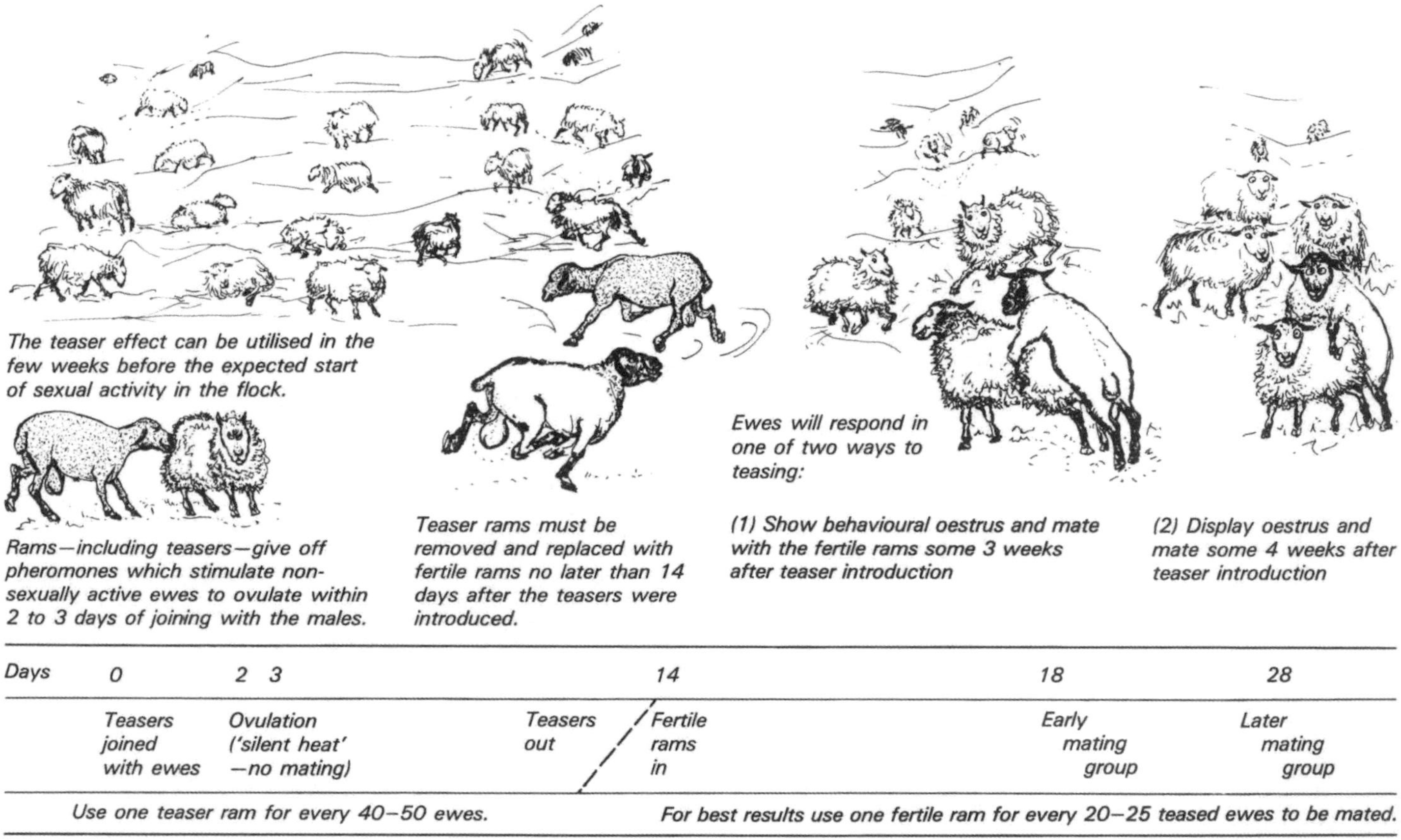

The teaser effect can be utilised in the few weeks before the expected start of sexual activity in the flock.

Rams—including teasers—give off pheromones which stimulate non-sexually active ewes to ovulate within 2 to 3 days of joining with the males.

Teaser rams must be removed and replaced with fertile rams no later than 14 days after the teasers were introduced.

Ewes will respond in one of two ways to teasing:

(1) Show behavioural oestrus and mate with the fertile rams some 3 weeks after teaser introduction

(2) Display oestrus and mate some 4 weeks after teaser introduction

Days	0	2	3		14		18	28
	Teasers joined with ewes	Ovulation ('silent heat' —no mating)			Teasers out	Fertile rams in	Early mating group	Later mating group

Use one teaser ram for every 40–50 ewes.   For best results use one fertile ram for every 20–25 teased ewes to be mated.

Figure 3.1 The ram or 'teaser' effect.

teasers are replaced by fertile males it should be remembered that because of the synchronising effect, the rams will be very busy and at least four rams per hundred ewes should be used and more if possible so as to achieve the highest fertilisation rate.

PREPARATION OF TEASER RAMS – VASECTOMY

Teasers can be prepared in a number of ways but the safest and most satisfactory way is to vasectomise a normal fertile ram. Any age of ram can be used, but young rams which have not worked are an unknown entity and old rams, on the other hand, will not have long to live. A ram which has worked before and which has a good sexual urge is the best type of candidate.

Your veterinary surgeon will carry out the operation for you either under general anaesthesia or under sedation with local anaesthesia. A length of the tubes leading from each testicle to the penis is removed. Sperm cannot then mix with the other fluids which make up semen, so that the ram cannot fertilise ewes. Since the testicles remain and continue to produce male hormone, the rams feel no different and are equally keen to mate

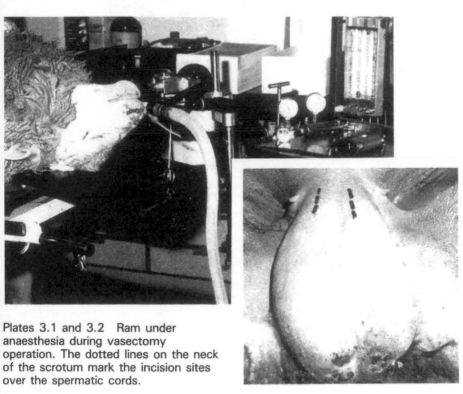

Plates 3.1 and 3.2   Ram under anaesthesia during vasectomy operation. The dotted lines on the neck of the scrotum mark the incision sites over the spermatic cords.

101

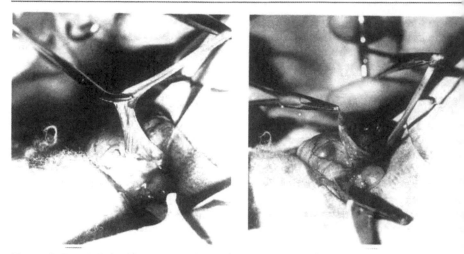

Plates 3.3 and 3.4 The spermatic cord is exposed (*left*) and a section about an inch long is removed (*right*). The operation is then repeated on the other side.

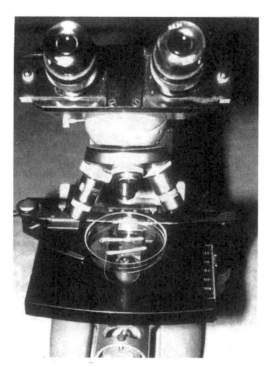

Plate 3.5 Microscopic examination of the excised cord helps your veterinary surgeon confirm that the correct 'tube' has been removed, since sperm may be present when the cord is squeezed onto the glass dish.

102

with ewes. The operation wounds heal quickly and rams are soon eager to work again, but should not be used as teasers for at least a month after the operation. This is because residual sperm in the tubes prior to the operation may survive for some little time and still be capable of fertilisation. Before use your veterinary surgeon can collect a sample of semen and check that no living sperm are present.

Vasectomised rams should be clearly and permanently identified in some way so that they are not used in error on the flock. They should be managed in exactly the same way as the other stud rams and should last for many years if well cared for.

Hormone treatment as an alternative to vasectomy

As an alternative to performing a vasectomy on an entire male it is possible to achieve comparable results by treating a castrated male with male hormones to make him feel and act like an entire ram once more. One such hormone is testosterone, which is administered by injection once a week for three weeks. After the third injection the teasers are ready to work, and for the purpose of teasing a flock early in the breeding season this treatment regime should be sufficient. Where the teaser is required to work for a prolonged period, for example in several sub-flocks or groups, additional injections will be needed at fortnightly intervals. Your veterinary surgeon will advise you and prescribe these hormones, which are the subject of debate in the European Community. At present it is permissible to use them to improve the reproductive performance of the flock.

Progesterone treatment of teased ewes

Where it is desired to persuade ewes to show a behavioural oestrus rather than just a 'silent heat' during the week following the introduction of teasers, they can be treated by injection with the hormone progesterone or with sponges containing one of the synthetic progestagens. If ewes are injected with progesterone immediately before the teasers are introduced or they are sponged a fortnight earlier than this and the sponges removed immediately before the teasers are introduced, then a high proportion of the ewes will show a normal heat with ovulation in the week following joining. Obviously, the teasers will have to be removed and the fertile rams introduced much earlier with this method. However, the use of sponges and a follicle stimulating hormone (PMSG) will achieve the same result and with a more satisfactory synchronisation.

Other tasks for teasers

Teasers fitted with raddle harnesses can be put to other useful purposes, namely:

- to identify ewes in heat for AI programmes
- to detect the proportion of ewes in heat at the beginning of the breeding season where sponges are to be used, so that a judgement can be made as to whether PMSG is necessary (see below)

- to identify barren ewes at the end of the breeding season once the fertile rams have been withdrawn from the flock

Sponges for the Induction and Synchronisation of Oestrus and Ovulation

It is possible to bring a whole flock of ewes into oestrus together at almost any time of the year by using hormonal treatments which mimic what happens naturally to ewes during their breeding season.

As explained in the section dealing with the oestrous cycle of the ewe, in Chapter 1, a yellow body or corpus luteum (CL) forms on the ovary at each of the points where an egg has been released. Each CL secretes the hormone progesterone which prevents the ewe coming into heat again immediately after ovulation. This allows the establishment of a pregnancy should mating and fertilisation take place. The CL remains on the ovary in non-pregnant ewes for just less than a fortnight. When it disappears, progesterone levels fall and only then can the ewe come into oestrus once more. Moreover, the ewe will only display a behavioural oestrus and become attractive to the ram if she has been under the influence of progesterone for about a fortnight.

It is possible to mimic the CL by using a safe and simple device called a pessary or **sponge**, which is impregnated with a synthetic progesterone compound, known as a **progestagen**. Sponges are made of polyurethane and are inserted carefully into the vagina of the ewe using a special applicator—a hollow plastic tube with a rod for pushing the sponge through the tube—as shown in Figure 3.2. The sponge slowly releases the progestagen, which is absorbed through the wall of the vagina and into the ewe's bloodstream. This prevents treated ewes from coming into heat for as long as the sponges remain in the vagina. Your veterinary surgeon will supply sponges and instruct you on their use and application in the first instance, since they are prescription-only medicines. They can be safely applied by any competent shepherd provided the procedure is not rushed and is carried out hygienically and with care (see later section on sponging ewe lambs).

Sponges are left in the ewes for approximately the same time as the CL is normally present on the ovary, namely 12 to 14 days. Providing they have been inserted correctly, less than one in a hundred sponges should be lost during this time. When the sponges are withdrawn from a group of ewes there is an immediate and rapid fall in the level of progesterone circulating in each ewe's bloodstream, closely mimicking what happens naturally in the ewe when the CL disappears. This 'takes the brakes off' and—providing the ewes were sponged during their normal breeding season—allows the other hormones which bring the ewes into oestrus to function.

The effect of simultaneous sponge removal in a flock is to bring all ewes into a fertile oestrus within a couple of days of each other. This allows the flockmaster a high degree of control over the timing and duration of lambing.

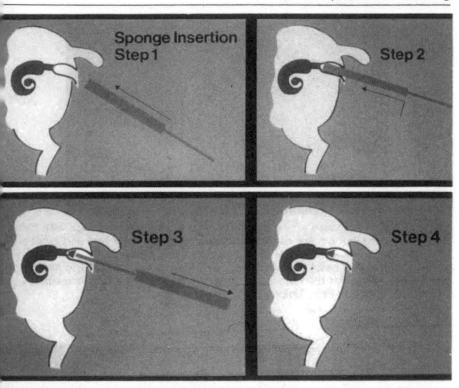

Figure 3.2   The applicator loaded with a sponge is inserted in an upwards and forwards direction into the ewe's vagina (step 1). The sponge is deposited up against the cervix (step 2). The rod holds the sponge in situ whilst the tube is removed (step 3). The nylon threads should be left hanging out of the vagina (step 4).

PREGNANT MARE SERUM (PMSG)

If ewes are to be persuaded to come into oestrus in a synchronised manner during the non-breeding season, the sponge alone will not be sufficient. A second hormone—**follicle stimulating hormone (FSH)**—must be given by injection at the time of sponge removal. This hormone is available as a product called **pregnant mare serum gonadotropin** or **PMSG**. PMSG is supplied as a freeze-dried powder, in which form it is relatively stable if kept cool. When required, it must be dissolved in the sterile water provided with it, but only **immediately before use**, since once in solution it deteriorates rapidly (within hours). It must not be used the following day, since its activity will have declined to a level where it is much less effective or totally ineffective. As it is a relatively expensive product, it should therefore be used in strict accordance with the manufacturer's instructions.

105

(*text continues on page 108*)

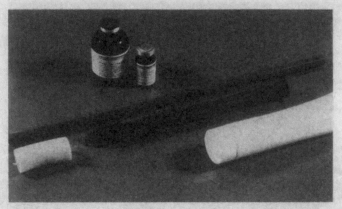

Plate 3.6 A progestagen impregnated intravaginal pessary or sponge with nylon strings attached (bottom left of picture), along with applicator (rod and tube) and lubricating antiseptic cream. The large bottle contains sterile water and the small bottle a freeze-dried pellet of PMS for use outside the normal breeding season. It is most important that the PMS is not made up as a solution until immediately before use. (Veramix Plus, Upjohn Ltd)

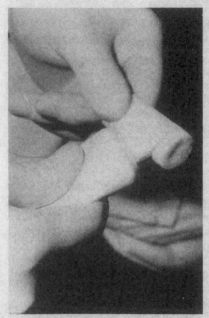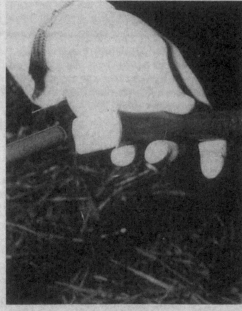

Plates 3.7 and 3.8 A small amount of antiseptic cream is applied to a sponge (*left*). This also acts as a lubricant. The sponge is then loaded into the applicator (*right*). Note that rubber gloves are being worn.

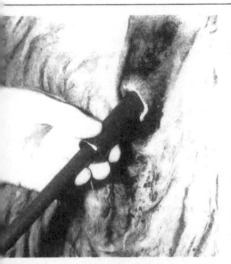

Plate 3.9   Applicator in the vagina of the ewe so that the sponge is located against the cervix.

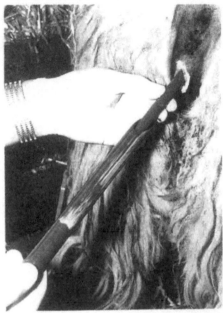

Plate 3.10   The rod holds the sponge in position whilst the sleeve (tube) is removed.

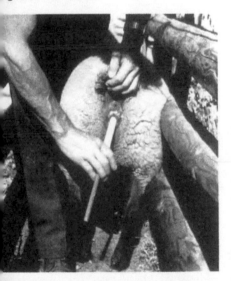

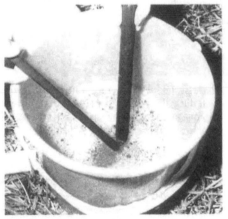

Plate 3.11   Providing ewes can be restrained adequately, sponging can be carried out singlehanded. It is important that ewes do not go into reverse gear, when there is a risk of damage to the vagina from the applicator. This Suffolk ewe is being sponged by a shepherd in South Devon.

Plate 3.12   Rod and tube being cleaned in mild soapy antiseptic solution. Cleanliness is vital to avoid vaginal infection. It is best to have several applicators in use so that some can remain in the antiseptic for a reasonable period.

107

The farmer and his veterinary surgeon have some tricky decisions to make as far as PMSG is concerned. The first is whether or not to use it at all and second, if it is to be used, at what dosage. If the only thing required is synchronisation of mating in a group of ewes, all of which are already oestrus cycling, then PMSG will not be necessary, since the sponge alone will do the trick. For example, Suffolk ewes would be oestrous cycling in the month of October, so that PMSG would not be required if the flock was to be synchronised with sponges. The one exception is where artificial insemination is to be used, in which case a small dose of PMSG will fine-tune the timing of ovulation, so that individual ewes can be inseminated at a predetermined hour (fixed-time AI).

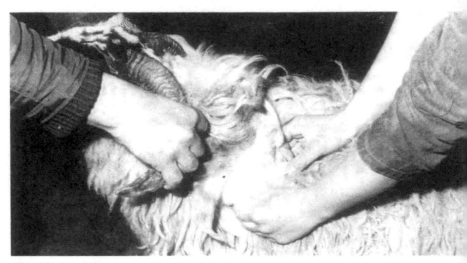

Plate 3.13   When pregnant mare serum is to be used for out-of-season breeding, it must be reconstituted and injected under the skin in the mid neck region at the time of sponge removal if natural mating is to be used. Different timings may be used for AI or ET.

Where it is desired to bring ewes into a fertile oestrus during their non-breeding season, then, since most or all of the ewes will not be oestrous cycling at that time, PMSG treatment will be needed for all ewes at sponge removal. The question of PMSG dosage then remains. This must be sufficient to initiate oestrous activity, but not so high as to produce too many multiple births. The further away ewes are from their normal breeding season, then the higher the dose of PMSG that will be required. It is generally unwise to be overambitious by attempting to breed too far outside the normal breeding season for the breed concerned, since the results may be disappointing.

The transitional period

In a flock of sheep, individual ewes will begin oestrous activity at different times. It will take several weeks before every ewe has come into heat for the first time and this is known as the transitional period. If sponges alone are used during this period, then only those ewes which are already sexually active will respond to the treatment. The main reason for using sponges is to synchronise *all* the ewes in the flock. PMSG must therefore be given to all ewes at the time of sponge removal, since the shepherd cannot identify which ewes are oestrous cycling and which are not.

The dose of PMSG used at this time will be lower than the dose needed in the depth of the non-breeding season. Since the different breeds and crosses of sheep have different breeding seasons it is sometimes difficult to decide on whether PMSG is needed. If in any doubt, take advice from your veterinary surgeon. The companies manufacturing sponges (Veramix from Upjohn and Chronogest from Intervet) have many years' experience of using their products in a variety of breeds, at different times of the year and under many different husbandry systems. They are always pleased to advise so that farmers can achieve the best results with their products.

Table 3.1   PMSG dosage guide in international units (iu) for a selection of breeds

	Dorset Horn, Finn × Dorset	Suffolk, Suffolk cross	Scottish Halfbred, Mule, Greyface
July	600–500	750–600	poor results
August	400–300	500–400	750–600
September	nil	300–nil	500–300
October	nil	nil	nil

Note: PMSG must be made up **immediately** before use from **in-date** material. Follow the manufacturer's instructions carefully. The higher dose given should be used at the beginning of the month and the lower dose at the end.

Sponge removal

Sponges are removed by pulling gently on the strings left hanging out of the vulva following application. If sponges do not come away easily, do not force them. Apply a little lambing lubricant to a clean finger and gently release the sponge if possible. Sometimes the strings will disappear, but they are usually to be found coiled up in the vagina. Strings may occasionally become detached from sponges, in which case the sponges should be removed by using the clean finger technique. Occasionally, your veterinary surgeon may have to remove them using forceps. (If sponges have been inserted carelessly and roughly, they may become lodged in the wall of the vagina, or, very occasionally, they may be pushed right through the vagina and into the body cavity, where they set up a peritonitis. These situations are very rare but serious and must be corrected by a veterinary surgeon.)

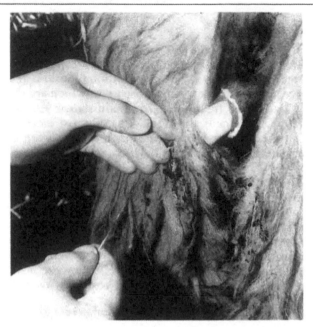

Plate 3.14 Sponges are left in the ewes for 12 to 14 days and are then removed by gently pulling on the nylon strings. It is normal for a small quantity of unpleasant smelling fluid to have accumulated in the vagina. Blood 'splashing' on the sponge is abnormal and is evidence of infection due to poor hygiene at application.

A small percentage of sponges may fall out of the vagina and how the ewe responds will depend on when the loss occurred. If the loss was soon after insertion, the ewe will not respond to treatment and will not be synchronised with the rest of the flock. If the loss occurs later, then she might have had sufficient progesterone to respond. However, it is usually impossible to say when the loss occurred and therefore best to assume that these ewes will not respond. If sponges are left in the ewe in error, she will not come into oestrus for as long as the sponge is in place.

When sponges are inserted into the vagina of the ewe, they are treated as 'foreign' material so that when they are withdrawn after two weeks there may be a small accumulation of unpleasant smelling fluid. This is an accumulation of mucus from the vagina and white cells from the blood. This will drain away quickly after sponge removal and should not interfere with conception. However, if sponging has been carried out in a slovenly and unhygienic way, so introducing infection with the sponge, there may be some blood-tingeing of the sponge as a result of inflammation in the vagina. This may damage sperm at mating, but fortunately is a relatively rare occurrence. In hot weather, the possibility of flystrike should be borne in mind. After removal, sponges should be burned, as such unsavoury items are a sheer delight to farm dogs and may cause them difficulty!

RAM INTRODUCTION AFTER SPONGE REMOVAL

After sponge removal, ewes should be left to their own devices for the next two days and kept well away from the rams. A few ewes will start to come into oestrus about 24 hours after sponge removal, and by 48 hours after sponge removal the vast majority will be in oestrus. **Rams should not be joined with the ewes until 36 to 48 hours after sponge removal**. If they are introduced earlier than this, then the conception rate—and therefore lambing rate—may be significantly reduced. Where rams are put in immediately after sponge removal, they will tend to serve the few ewes which come into heat early very frequently. The rams will deplete their valuable semen reserves so that when the majority of the ewes come into heat, they will not receive a high enough dose of sperm to ensure a high fertilisation rate.

At the start of oestrus, ewes which have been sponged tend to produce rather more mucus (a clear sticky fluid) than is normal. This tends to dilute the reservoir of sperm deposited at the cervix during ejaculation. This mucus has usually reduced significantly later in oestrus. The 'transport' of

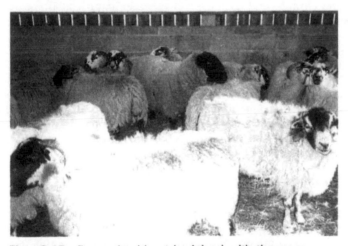

Plate 3.15   Rams should not be joined with the ewes until 36—48 hours after sponge removal, by which time most if not all of the treated ewes will be in heat.
Although these housed ewes have plenty of space, note how they crowd the ram, eager for his attentions. When rams have to work indoors it is essential that the floor is non-slip.

sperm up the ewe's reproductive tract is somewhat impaired immediately after sponge treatment, but this adverse effect is also reduced later in oestrus. These are other reasons for delaying the introduction of the rams.

It is equally important that rams are not joined with synchronised ewes too late; otherwise some eggs will have deteriorated before sperm can reach them in the oviducts.

RAM POWER IN SYNCHRONISED FLOCKS

Much has already been said about the fitness and fertility of rams, and in flocks which have been synchronised with sponges this is particularly important. Rams have evolved over thousands of years to cope with serving large numbers of ewes over a few weeks, but here they are being asked to service the whole flock—perhaps several times over—in only two days! Therefore, rams should be in prime condition and there must be an adequate number of them to share the heavy work load.

During the breeding season, at least 10% rams should be made available in synchronised flocks. If more rams are available, then they should be used. Outside the normal breeding season, when the rams' semen reserves and libido are lower, 20% (one ram to five ewes) should be the aim. In early lambing flocks or in out-of-season breeding or frequent breeding flocks, a respectable lambing percentage is vital for economic viability. It is therefore pointless going to the trouble and expense of synchronising the flock and then not supplying sufficient ram fertilising power. It is not just the proportion of ewes pregnant which counts, but the number of embryos conceived.

Rams used in synchronised flocks must be sexually mature. They must have worked previously and have a proven performance record. Ram lambs or shearlings which have not worked before are unsuitable. Mating time in a synchronised flock is a very different affair from in a conventionally mated flock. When rams are introduced to a flock where all the ewes are on heat simultaneously, it takes an experienced ram to cope. Ram lambs have been observed to turn tail and run away when surrounded by a bunch of mature ewes eager for attention!

Mating groups

There are a number of ways of organising mating in sponged flocks. The most commonly used and least disruptive is to run a bunch of around 50 ewes with five or more rams in a small paddock near the farmstead at a high stocking rate (50 to 60 per hectare). This ensures that rams can get round all the ewes without unnecessary travelling. The shepherd can observe the mating closely to see that all rams are working well and that bullying or other problems are averted. Early observations are crucial in order to pick out suspect rams, which must be replaced immediately.

It is not always necessary to harness rams for this first service period since 95 to 100% of the ewes should be served if they have been treated correctly. In fact, the great pressure of work may mean that the harnesses rub the rams sore, especially if not fitted carefully a week before joining and adjusted daily. This discomfort may make the rams less willing to work to full capacity. Rams must be harnessed for the repeat service to identify those in the later lambing group. If a harnessed teaser is put in with the ewes after the second service period, he will identify barreners.

Hand mating

An alternative to paddock mating, especially in flocks where rams are in short supply, is so-called hand mating. A harnessed teaser ram is run with the synchronised ewes from about 24 hours after sponge removal. Marked ewes are pulled out of the main flock, allowed to mate with a fertile ram and then kept in a separate paddock with other served ewes but no rams. They are then remated some 8 to 12 hours after their first service. Alternatively ewes can simply be taken out of the flock at random for mating at 48 hours after sponge removal without the aid of a teaser, since most ewes should be in heat by this time. Rams must be carefully observed to see that they actually ejaculate, rather than just mount ewes. Only one ejaculation should be allowed before the ewe is removed. Rams should be rested for a quarter of an hour between matings.

Ewes mated in the early morning can be re-mated in the evening and those mated in the afternoon remated early the following morning. Alternatively, ewes may be hand mated once only around 48 hours after sponge removal and then turned out with fresh rams in a paddock.

Hand mating regimes can work well but are labour intensive and time-consuming. Ewes unused to being handled indoors may find it stressful at a time when stress should be minimised. The results are unlikely to be any better than a paddock mating where a sufficient number of rams are available. It is claimed that one ram to 15 ewes is sufficient for hand mating systems, but where insufficient ram power is available in a flock, then it is probably wiser to abandon the idea of synchronisation programmes altogether, unless artificial insemination is a viable alternative (see later).

Obtaining extra ram power

It is often possible for individual farmers without sufficient rams for planned breeding programmes to borrow or hire extra rams. In some areas, groups of farmers sponging their flocks operate ram sharing schemes. All the rams are usually kept on one farm where they are prepared for tupping. The various flocks involved will usually stagger their sponging times so that the rams can move around the flocks in turn, with at least four or five days' rest between each flock. Whilst there is always a disease risk in moving stock from farm to farm, the risk is probably no more—and may be considerably less—than when buying rams at sales where the health status of the flocks from which the rams originate is rarely revealed.

Withdrawing rams and repeat mating

At the first mating, which begins 48 hours after sponge removal, the majority of ewes will be served in the 24 hours after the rams are introduced, that is, during the third day after sponge removal. The remainder are mated on the fourth day. After this time there are unlikely to be many, if any, ewes left in heat and the rams should be removed after their two days of intensive sexual activity. They should be rested for the next 10 or 12 days and fed well to make up some of the weight loss they will inevitably experience. Not all of the rams will be required for the 'repeat' mating, providing a good conception rate to first service of 65 to 85% is achieved. Less than a third of the ewes (15 to 35%) should return to service. The proportion returning will depend upon such factors as breed, time of year, feeding, ram fertility and libido and management generally. Even the weather may play a role, since a spell of wet, windy and cold weather over the two day tupping period may adversely affect the rams' desire to work.

For the repeat service, at least one ram to 30 ewes should be run with the flock for one week, beginning no later than 16 days after sponge removal, that is, 12 days after rams were withdrawn following the first service period. If all the rams used for the first service are still available, then use more than 3% to maximise the conception rate. The repeat service will also be synchronised, although not quite so tightly as the first because of the natural variation in ewe oestrous cycle length. Some flockmasters deliberately wait until this second service period before mating any ewes, to take advantage of the higher conception rate at this time. The same ram to ewe ratio will be required (10%) and the lambing will be a few days longer and, of course, two to three weeks later.

An important practical point when synchronising flocks in the **non-breeding season** is that sponge/PMSG treated ewes **will not return to service 17 days later**. Instead they will lapse back into sexual inactivity (anoestrus) because of the inhibitory effect of day length. Therefore **it is essential to mate ewes at the oestrus immediately after sponge removal and to try to achieve maximum conception rates at this time.** Remember that the costs of treatment for the whole flock have to be spread over the number of lambs sold from only the proportion of the ewes which conceive to the first and only service.

Where a short three week lambing is required, the rams are removed after the second service period and teasers introduced with a new raddle colour to identify barren ewes. In well-managed synchronised flocks the barren rate should be little different from that in a non-synchronised flock at the equivalent time of the breeding season.

LAMBING TIME IN SYNCHRONISED FLOCKS

Lambing time in a sponged flock is highly predictable. The ewes which conceived to the first two day service period will lamb down over

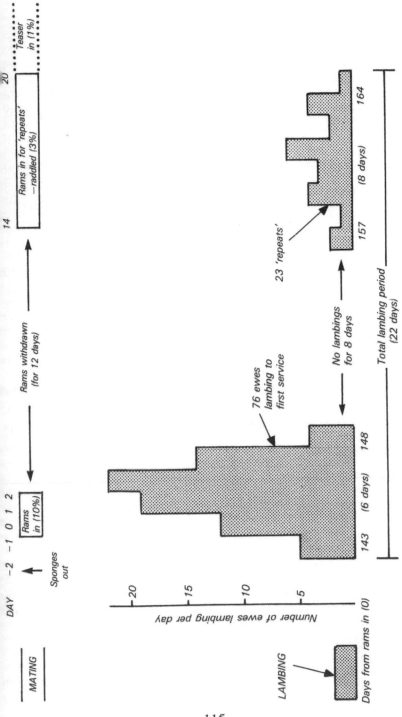

Figure 3.3 Mating and lambing in a synchronised (sponged) flock of 105 Greyface ewes within the breeding season (March lambing).

115

approximately a week. There then follows a week without any lambings followed by the ewes which held to the second (repeat) service which lamb down over roughly a 10 day period. The whole lambing is over in around three to three and a half weeks. The week when no lambings occur should be used to clean out the lambing area and bed down generously with fresh straw for the second group. This helps to break the chain of infection which inevitably builds up at lambing time.

Table 3.2 Sponging programme for a large flock of Suffolk cross Greyface ewes

Pre-mating management

June/July	Ewes weaned and condition scored
August 24th	Ram examination and teaser testing
September 1st	Teasers joined with flock of 800 ewes

Mating management

September 21st	Teasers removed and sponges* inserted into 300 oestrous cycling (marked) ewes
October 4th	Sponges removed after a 13 day insertion period
October 6th	Fertile rams joined at 1 ram to 10 ewes (10%)
October 8th	Rams removed after a 2 day mating period
October 20th	Harnessed teasers joined to mark 'empty' ewes

Lambing time (March)

257 ewes lambed to the two day mating period (86% of the 300 sponged)
449 lambs born to 257 ewes which lambed (175 lambs born per 100 ewes lambed)

170 ewes (66%) lambed over a 60 hour period (day 146 to 148 of pregnancy)
All 257 ewes lambed within 6 days. Extra skilled labour employed over lambing

*Veramix from Upjohn Ltd.

Sponging programmes should be tailor-made to suit particular flock requirements. Table 3.2 illustrates how the method was used in part of a large flock of 800 Suffolk cross Greyface ewes. The farmer wanted to reduce the number of ewes lambing in April and to have at least 200 ewes lambing during one week only in early March.

Teaser rams were run with the whole flock of 800 ewes to identify for sponging 300 ewes which were already oestrus cycling, so that PMSG would not be necessary. Instead of returning the fertile rams to the flock for the repeat service, harnessed teasers were joined to identify those ewes which had not held to the first service so that they could be mated in November with the April lambing flock. The excellent result of 86% of ewes lambing to the two day service period (October 6th to 8th) shows what can be achieved by attention to detail and top-class husbandry and management.

SPONGING EWE LAMBS

A number of sheep farmers use sponges for advancing the breeding season of ewe lambs and for synchronising their lambing, although neither of the sponge manufacturers recommends this. Nevertheless they can be used successfully, providing the limitations—of ewe lambs, rather than sponges—are appreciated.

It is generally accepted that to achieve reasonable reproductive performance, ewe lambs must be old enough, big enough and sufficiently sexually mature at the time of mating. They should be at least two-thirds of mature ewe weight and at least seven months of age. Even then there is no guarantee that they will have had their first oestrous cycle, even though it is in the midst of the breeding season for the particular breed concerned. Oestrus is generally shorter and less intense than in mature ewes and, as a rule, fewer eggs are shed. Conception rates are also lower than in ewes and embryo mortality higher. Lambing rates of around 60 to 80% are normal in naturally mated flocks and sponging will not necessarily improve that result.

Do not attempt to sponge ewe lambs unless you are experienced in doing the job in adult ewes. Sponges should be inserted with very great care and the job should never be rushed. The vagina is much less roomy than in the mature ewe, so that a small sponge is preferable. Also there may be strands of hymen tissue across the vagina of virgin sheep and if sponges are roughly applied the bleeding which occurs may 'heal over' the sponge and make it difficult (or even impossible in a few cases) to remove the sponge. Rather than using the special applicator provided, it is usually easier and safer, especially in small breeds, to use the clean finger technique to gently push the sponge into the vagina with a small amount of a suitable antiseptic cream (too much lubrication may mean sponges will slip out). If resistance is felt or the animal is obviously in discomfort, then give up and abandon the idea for that animal. Better results will be obtained and the welfare of animals safeguarded if ewe lambs are sponged selectively.

A small dose of PMSG should be used in ewe lambs, even within the breeding season, since it is not necessarily known if they are oestrous cycling, or even if they have reached puberty. A small dose of around 300 to 400 international units is sufficient, since it would be undesirable to stimulate any extra ovulations which might lead to multiple births. Better conception rates will usually be achieved if mating is left until the first repeat oestrus.

Mating management is important with ewe lambs and especially so in sponged animals. As the heat is generally of low intensity, they will not normally seek out the ram. They should be mated separately from the mature ewes and a higher ram to ewe ratio (e.g. one ram to seven or eight ewe lambs) employed. Rams should be of medium size, mature, sexually experienced and of a high libido so that they actively seek out ewe lambs in heat.

The benefits of sponging ewe lambs are largely associated with ease of

117

management. The costs per lamb born or reared are higher than for adu
ewes because of the lower lambing percentage and higher barren rat
This should be appreciated before embarking on a ewe lamb synchronisin
programme.

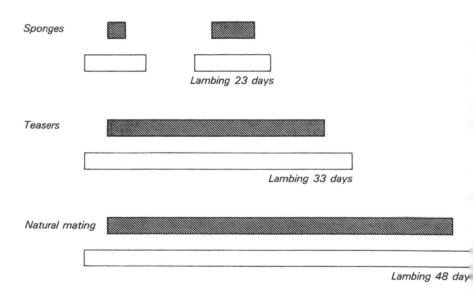

**Figure 3.4 Comparison of three mating systems applied during the
breeding season. Shaded area, mating; non-shaded area, lambing.**

ADVANTAGES OF SPONGE SYNCHRONISATION

There are a number of benefits from synchronisation with sponges, an
these will vary from flock to flock. Some examples are listed below:

- Forward planning is possible. Lambing can be timed to fit in with othe
  enterprises on the farm or to coincide with periods when skilled extr
  labour is available. In the UK, for example, early lambing Suffolk cros
  ewes could be sponged for the first group to lamb in the week befor
  Christmas, with no lambings over the Christmas holidays, and the second
  smaller group lambing during the first week in January. (Pedigre
  Suffolks would have to lamb immediately after January 1st, of course!
- The feeding of the flock can be more accurately apportioned whe
  precise mating dates are known and when all ewes are due to laml
  within a few days of each other in two distinct groups.
- Scanning can be carried out at the optimum time to suit both matin
  groups.

118

- Health measures can be timed with more precision to maximise benefit. For example, clostridial vaccination in late pregnancy given to ewes with a short and precise lambing period is likely to produce optimal protection for a greater proportion of lambs.
- Best use can be made of buildings and of labour. Almost half the labour costs of a sheep enterprise are incurred at lambing time. In a sponged flock with a short, precise three week lambing, a 24 hour watch can be provided during the first week and the last week when lambs will be coming thick and fast. Labour will be fully utilised, rather than incurring a great deal of overtime spread over a longer and less productive period.
- Buildings used for other purposes such as grain storage or cattle courts can often be utilised when the lambing dates are known accurately and can be timetabled in advance.
- **More newborn lambs can be saved**. This must be the first priority in any flock, but by housing at lambing and by drafting in extra skilled labour, it should be possible to save a very significant number of lambs which would otherwise perish in flocks with a more protracted lambing period.
- Fostering of lambs is considerably easier, especially in small flocks where the lambing often goes on even longer than in larger flocks. With ewes lambing very frequently, it is usually easier to pair up ewes and lambs. This is made more convenient still if the flock has been scanned for the number of lambs in each ewe. In some synchronised flocks all ewes are penned individually at lambing time, with single bearing ewes and triplet bearing ewes on opposite sides of the passageway so that cross-fostering is made even easier.
- Lambs born over a short period can be reared and weaned together in even batches for slaughter or sale.
- By using PMSG at the time of sponge removal, it is possible to synchronise not only oestrus but also ovulation, so that artificial insemination and embryo transfer can be utilised.
- Ewes can be persuaded to breed earlier than they would normally do, or even to breed during their non-breeding season.
- By synchronising mating and inducing lambing, ewes can be timetabled to lamb more frequently than once a year—for example, three times in two years (see later).

Flocks most suitable for sponging

In very large flocks, synchronisation may lose some of its benefits, but for medium-sized flocks of up to around 300 ewes and for small flocks, the management benefits can be considerable. Indeed, for small flocks and especially for part-time managed flocks, sponging is an ideal technique. Where PMSG is used for early or out-of-season lambing, it is essential to use suitable breeds with an extended natural breeding season and reasonable prolificacy, so that a respectable lambing percentage is achieved; otherwise the economics may not make good reading.

Before finally deciding to synchronise the flock, do discuss the technique thoroughly with your agricultural adviser and veterinary surgeon, because there are a number of disadvantages as well as all the advantages. For example there is a high requirement for fit and fertile rams, and housing is essential in a synchronised flock, since a spell of atrocious weather over the busy first week of lambing could be disastrous for the lambs and also for the gross margin.

Other Manipulative Techniques

There are a number of other methods of synchronising oestrus and ovulation or of encouraging ewes into sexual activity during their non-breeding season.

PROSTAGLANDINS

Prostaglandins are a group of natural or closely related synthetic compounds which can be used to synchronise groups of ewes, in much the same way as groups of heifers or cows. They also have the same restraints as they do in cattle, namely that they can be used only in animals which are already oestrous cycling and that means during the breeding season only.

It is the ewe's own natural prostaglandin, which is secreted from the uterus every 17 days, that causes the yellow body or corpus luteum (CL) on the ovary to fade away and so allow the ewe to come into oestrus once more. By injecting prostaglandin into ewes which have a CL, they can be induced to come into oestrus and to ovulate a few days later. In ewes with no CL on the ovary, such as anoestrus ewes or ewes just about to come into oestrus, the drug has no effect.

As it is not possible to determine which ewes are at which stage of their oestrous cycle, a system similar to that used for groups of heifers is

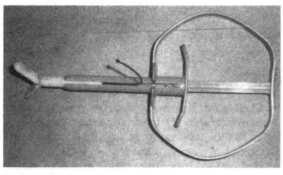

Plate 3.16 CIDR—a Silastic intravaginal device impregnated with natural progesterone (similar in concept to PRID for cattle)—is an alternative to sponges in New Zealand only, but at twice the cost. The CIDR is shown part-loaded in its applicator. When fully loaded, the wings (left) are folded away for insertion into the vagina. When the applicator is removed the wings spring open and hold the device in place in the vagina.

mployed, with two injections being given some nine to 14 days apart (there
s some debate over whether a shorter or a longer period between the two
ijections gives the best results). The majority of the ewes should come into
eat some two to three days after the second injection. They can then be
erved naturally by the rams, using the same ram to ewe ratio as for sponges
it least 10%), or they can be artificially inseminated.

Prostaglandins are potent drugs and pose a risk to pregnant women and
sthmatics and are therefore under veterinary control. They are also more
ostly and often less effective than sponges. These restrictions, together
ith the fact that prostaglandins can be used only within the breeding season,
ean they are unlikely to be widely used in sheep synchronisation.

MELATONIN

he small gland at the base of the ewe's brain called the pineal gland
esponds to the onset of darkness within only a few minutes by releasing a
ormone called melatonin into the ewe's bloodstream. At dawn, the produc-
on of melatonin ceases equally rapidly. During the long summer days little
elatonin is released, due to the relatively few hours of darkness, but as
e evenings draw in, a level is reached where there is sufficient melatonin
resent in the bloodstream to trigger off the start of sexual activity in the
we.

Synthetic melatonin is a safe and readily available product. (Originally
was extracted during the decaffeination of coffee beans.) If the hormone
administered to ewes—as a feed additive or an implant, or incorporated
to a soluble glass bolus which slowly releases the hormone as it dissolves—
is possible to make ewes think that autumn and the breeding season have
rrived. To date, melatonin has been used only in research and development
ials in the UK and is not yet available commercially. It has shown promise
r the purpose of inducing ewes to begin breeding several weeks earlier
an normal. If its early promise is fulfilled, it could become an alternative
the teaser ram or to sponges with PMSG for early lambing flocks. It has
o effect on ewes already oestrous cycling, nor does it always work sat-
factorily deep into the non-breeding season. It does not synchronise oestrus
ewes, but this could be arranged by using melatonin along with sponges
s a replacement for PMSG. Melatonin has only a modest superovulatory
ffect (inducing the shedding of a large number of eggs), which could be
n advantage in some flocks.

Since individual ewes in a melatonin treated flock all begin their sexual
ctivity at slightly different times, it could be expected that fewer rams would
e necessary than in a sponge synchronised flock. Fertility has varied widely
the trials to date. Work using the slow release soluble glass capsules has
iven good conception rates and respectable lambing percentages in ewes
ated some weeks earlier than normal for the breed. For example, in one
ial, Mule ewes treated in late June with a slow release capsule had a

conception rate approaching 90% when mated in late August and lamber down at 170 lambs per 100 ewes mated.

One significant problem with melatonin treatments is that there is a long lead-in period of some six to eight weeks between the start of treatment and the onset of sexual activity and the medication must continue throughout this long period. If treatment is applied later than this, there will be no advancement of sexual activity. Conversely, if ewes are started on a treatment regime too early they may not respond, since they apparently need a period of exposure to long days before they are able to do so. Recent trials in the North of Scotland have shown that where short-term melatonin treatments of about one month's duration are used, not only do they not work, but they may actually delay the time when a particular breed of ewe would be expected to begin oestrous activity naturally. Caution will therefore have to be exercised when these products become available commercially.

LIGHTING REGIMES

Various attempts have been made over the years to manipulate the breeding season of ewes (and rams) by using various **lighting regimes** to overcome the inhibitory effect of long days on sexual activity. Most of these regimes have been cumbersome, impractical and costly, requiring the confinement of sheep when there is ample grazing available and the lightproofing of buildings, with the attendant problems of artificial ventilation. Since the discovery in the last decade of the role of melatonin (see above), these lighting regimes, which attempt to reverse the seasons, would appear to be largely redundant and will not therefore be discussed here.

Artificial Insemination

Artificial insemination, or AI, is a method of breeding ewes without their having any direct contact with the ram. Semen is collected from the ram by training them to serve into an artificial vagina. The semen may then be used to inseminate ewes within 20 to 30 minutes of collection or it may be diluted, chilled and used to inseminate ewes within 10 hours of collection. Alternatively, the semen may be diluted, deep-frozen in straws or pellet and kept for an indefinite period. When required, it is thawed out and used immediately.

SEMEN FOR INSEMINATION

Semen is always examined under the microscope before it is used or frozen to determine the motility and the concentration of sperm, that is, the number of sperm per millilitre of semen. A mature ram during the breeding season should produce about 1 millilitre per ejaculate, and this should contain

ound 3,000 or 4,000 million sperm. A good sample may be divided into
▶ or even 20 individual doses of around 200 to 400 million sperm for each
ve.

Rams will generally produce more semen with a higher concentration
sperm during their normal breeding season. Therefore, where semen is
be deep-frozen, it makes sense to collect it at this time. Out-of-season
semination of ewes generally gives poorer results, and if the semen is also
llected out-of-season, then much more of it will be needed to achieve an
ceptable result. About 20 semen collections a week can be taken from
ram during the breeding season, but only four or five a week out of
ason.

PROGRAMMES

wes must obviously be in oestrus when they are inseminated. Oestrus
n be detected during the breeding season by running raddled teasers (one
50 ewes) with the flock, and ewes which have been coloured can be
awn out of the flock and inseminated. As the oestrous cycle of the ewe is
7 days long and since all ewes will be at slightly different stages of their

Table 3.3   Artificial insemination programme for ewes using a single fixed-time
insemination with fresh or chilled semen.

ay	Weekday	Time	Operation
16	Monday	any time	Insert sponges in ewes.
2	Monday	9 am	(i) Withdraw sponges.
			(ii) Inject PMSG: 350 to 500 iu* in breeding season or 500 to 1000 iu out of season.
	Wednesday	throughout the day	Collect semen from rams, examine, dilute and chill as necessary.
		4 pm	Inseminate ewes into cervix (55 hours after sponges removed) with at least 100 million sperm (200 million if available).
12	Monday	any time	EITHER introduce raddled teaser ram to mark returns for a repeat insemination, OR introduce raddled fertile rams (5%) to cover ewes which return to oestrus.

u = international units

OTES

wes must be in good body condition and should have been weaned at least two months before.
ose of PMSG varies, not only with the time of year, but with the breed of ewe.
ouble insemination with fresh semen is usually considered uneconomic unless by DIY AI.
ewes are inseminated well outside the breeding season, those that do not conceive will not
turn to oestrus 17 days later.

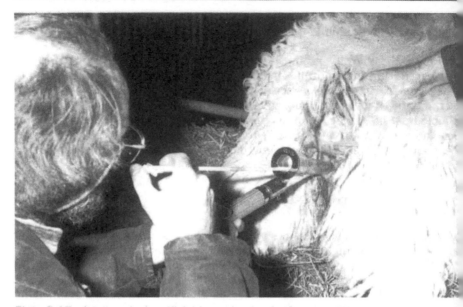

Plate 3.17 Intracervical artificial insemination in the ewe. With the ewe restrained over a rail and supported with bales, a speculum with a light source is inserted into the vagina to locate the cervix. The insemination pipette with the semen in its tip (out of sight) is inserted a short distance (a few millimetres) into the cervix. A syringe full of air (right hand) is used to eject the semen from the pipette.

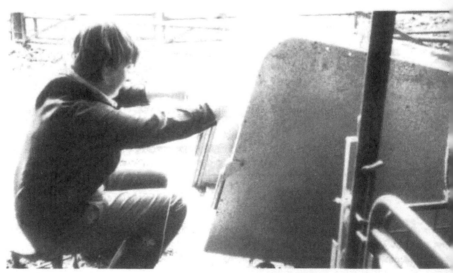

Plate 3.18 Ewes may be restrained in a tipping crate for artificial insemination.

heat cycle, only about six out of every hundred ewes will come on heat each day. It will therefore take at least 17 days to inseminate the flock. This is a cumbersome, time-consuming business. It is also stressful for the flock to be gathered so frequently and this can reduce conception rates and cause some embryonic loss. Rams also have to be collected from daily if fresh rather than frozen semen is to be used. Needless to say, this method is not popular in the UK, but in some parts of the world where very large flocks are run and labour is plentiful, the technique is commonly used. In the Soviet Union, for instance, it is estimated that some 50 million ewes are artificially inseminated each year.

In the UK, artificial insemination is invariably carried out on ewes which have been synchronised using sponges and PMSG (usually given by intra-muscular injection). The PMSG is always necessary where fixed-time AI is to be used, since it fine-tunes the synchrony of ovulation. Using this system, large numbers of ewes can be inseminated in a day.

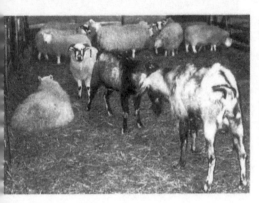

Plate 3.19 It is crucially important that rams are kept well away from synchronised ewes on an AI programme, especially after sponge removal; otherwise the timing of ovulation will be advanced and the results disappointing. Billy goats will exert the same effect and must also be kept clear.

A typical AI programme is shown in Table 3.3. Conception rates to AI using fresh semen in such a programme should be in the region of 60 to 70% except outside the breeding season, when they tend to be lower.

Semen can be deposited in a number of parts of the ewe's reproductive tract. The poorest results are obtained when it is left in the vagina close to the cervix—the so-called 'shot in the dark' method. Much-improved conception rates result from depositing semen about 1 cm into the folds of the cervix. (It is very difficult or impossible, as well as stressful for the ewe, to attempt to thread the catheter—the instrument used to deposit semen—through the full length of the cervix and into the uterus, as is done in the cow.)

INTRAUTERINE AI

A novel technique is now available whereby semen is deposited directly into the uterus—intrauterine AI. This method gives excellent conception rates, even using low doses of semen. The ewes are synchronised as

125

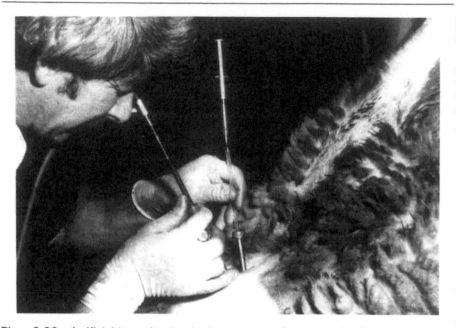

Plate 3.20 Artificial insemination by laparoscopy. By this method semen is deposited directly into the uterus, so bypassing the cervix. High conception rates can be achieved. The ewe is tranquillised and given a local anaesthetic at the place where the instruments are inserted into the abdomen. The insemination pipette is at right (in operator's left hand). The other instrument is a fibre optic laparoscope for grasping and visualising the uterus. A similar technique can be used for embryo transfer.

before, sedated and given a local anaesthetic into the abdominal wall where the instruments are to be inserted. The ewe is held in a cradle on a steep incline, while a fibre optic laparoscope is inserted through a small incision into the body cavity. This instrument allows the veterinary surgeon to see what he or she is doing, so that the uterus can be located. A second small incision is made into the abdomen and through this a syringe is introduced allowing the semen to be injected directly into the uterus. Despite being a more expensive technique, the results are so good that it is likely to be cost-effective where frozen semen of genetically superior rams is used in upgrading programmes, where frozen semen is imported or exported, or where high conception rates are essential in superovulated ewes on embryo transfer programmes.

There is, quite rightly, some concern about the welfare implications of performing this technique, despite the use of anaesthetics. These will have to be addressed before the method is used widely in commercial flocks.

126

However, at present the costs are likely to make it prohibitive in most commercial flocks.

ADVANTAGES OF AI

There are a number of reasons why AI might be advantageous to a particular farmer or in the national sheep flock:

- Where genetically superior rams have been identified, AI is the only feasible method of widely disseminating the genes. (If rams with poor genetic merit are used in AI programmes, the results would be conversely disastrous.) In a normal flock a ram may mate with around 50 ewes a season. With conventional AI (intracervical), a thousand ewes a season could be inseminated with fresh semen from one ram. Using intrauterine AI and frozen semen, as many as 25,000 ewes could be inseminated annually with semen from one highly fertile ram. Commercial flock owners could benefit from AI by using superior sires which would otherwise be too expensive to purchase (this is analogous to the situation in cattle AI).
- The deep-frozen semen of superior rams (including those in the process of being assessed) or of the rare breeds can be used long after their death.
- The health risk in purchasing, borrowing or hiring rams can be reduced by purchasing semen from ram studs with a veterinary monitored health status.
- Where oestrus synchronisation is employed, extra rams are required to mate the ewes over a very short period of two days, and AI can reduce this requirement. Since semen is evaluated before use, AI will also reduce the risk of using infertile rams and overcome such problems as dominance by a sub-fertile ram. In early and out-of-season breeding, the rams have to work out-of-season, when libido, semen quantity and quality may suffer. The predetermined dose of sperm used is calculated to maximise the chances of fertilisation. Semen can be collected and frozen during the ram's normal breeding season for use out-of-season.
- Intrauterine AI can be used to achieve high fertilisation rates in ewes which have been superovulated for embryo transfer purposes.

Embryo Transfer

Embryo transfer (ET) is a sophisticated technique whereby certain ewes (donors) are mated by natural service or are artificially inseminated. The fertilised embryos are recovered from the reproductive tract when only a few days old and then transferred to the reproductive tract of non-mated ewes (recipients), which give birth to the donor ewes' offspring. It is another method which can be used to disseminate animals of superior genetic merit.

SYNCHRONY OF DONORS AND RECIPIENTS

Both donor and recipient ewes (which may be of different breeds) are oestrus synchronised using sponges, preferably at the peak of the sheep breeding season for best results. At the time of sponge removal in the donor group, the ewes are injected with a follicle stimulating hormone to tighten the synchrony of oestrus and ovulation. Where required, a high dose is used to superovulate ewes, so that more eggs than normal will be shed. Ewes are either mated naturally by superior rams or are inseminated with their semen, for example, using an intrauterine AI technique which will give the highest fertilisation rates.

Meanwhile, recipient ewes will also receive a follicle stimulating hormone (at a lower dose than the donor ewes) to synchronise oestrus accurately. Because of the slightly different hormones used at sponge withdrawal, the onset of oestrus is likely to be 12 to 24 hours later in the recipients than in the donors. Thus, as it is absolutely essential that there is as near perfect synchrony as possible between the two groups, the sponges are removed from the recipients 12 to 24 hours earlier than the donors, depending on the follicle stimulants which have been used. If donors and recipients are out of synchrony, the survival of the embryos will be seriously jeopardised.

Usually around six days after mating or insemination, the donor ewes are operated upon to remove the embryos. Unfortunately, because the cervix of the ewe is difficult to canulate, it is not possible to recover embryos by a non-surgical technique as in cattle. However, the same novel fibre optic technique described above for AI is also suitable for ET, and it allows the eggs to be flushed from the reproductive tract without a major abdominal operation. The new technique is probably less stressful for the ewe and does not result in post-operation adhesions, which may cause considerable pain or discomfort and in some cases eventually prevent the ewe from breeding again. Since embryo transfer may be performed on valuable donor ewes a number of times during the same breeding season, the laparoscopic intrauterine technique is preferable.

THE EMBRYOS

Normally around 70 to 80% of the eggs shed are recovered at flushing. During surgery, or by using the fibre optic laparoscope, the number of ovulation points on the ovary can be counted and compared with the number of eggs recovered. The eggs are examined under the microscope to determine whether they are fertilised and, if so, whether the tiny embryos—only a cluster of cells at this stage—are developing normally and are therefore suitable for transfer to recipient ewes.

The response of donor ewes to superovulation is very variable, but on average around six eggs may be shed, of which four or five should be

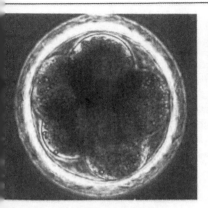

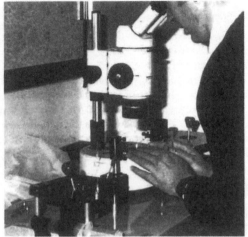

Plate 3.21 (*Above*) A sheep embryo at the eight cell stage. (*Below*) A normal sheep embryo six days after fertilisation at the expanded blastocyst stage and suitable for transfer to the horn of the recipient's uterus. It would be just visible to the naked eye, providing you knew what you were looking for!

Plate 3.22 (*Above*) A micromanipulator. This instrument allows the operator to divide the embryo whilst looking down the microscope. The knife and pipette are held steady and moved by a series of levers for accuracy. (*Below*) Two sets of identical twin Scottish Blackface lambs produced by embryo cleavage and subsequent transfer.

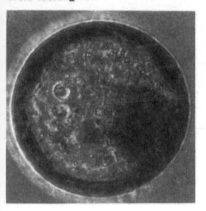

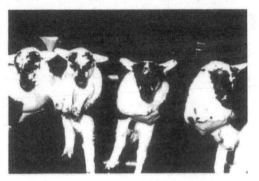

recovered. Of these, between 50 and 90% will be fertilised normally and fit to transfer. Six-day-old embryos will be transferred to the uterus (rather than the oviduct) of the recipient ewe. Usually, two are transferred to each ewe—one to each horn (side) of the uterus—and around 70 to 80% of such double embryo transfers should result in pregnancy and live lambs born (there is obviously a greater chance of pregnancy if more than one embryo is transferred).

Husbandry of ewes

All the factors to be considered in normally mated ewes, such as condition score, feeding in early pregnancy, minimal stress, etc., are equally important in ET donor and recipient ewes. Old 'scrub' animals are quite unsuitable as recipients, just as with ET in cattle. If donor ewes are not to be collected from again during the current season, they can be run with the ram or inseminated at their return oestrus roughly 10 or 11 days after embryo collection (17 days after oestrus) and allowed to lamb down normally. Providing the surgery has not done any permanent damage, the ewes may be collected from again the following season.

REASONS FOR USING ET

Embryo transfer has not been widely practised in sheep in the UK, probably because the economics make little sense in most commercial flocks. There are, however, a number of reasons why it might be considered.

Probably the most common use is by farmers with a small nucleus flock of expensive, exotic ewes who wish to obtain as many offspring from each ewe as possible during the breeding season (or even outside it). ET is the only way of rapidly multiplying up such a flock of breeding females. Ram lambs will also be available for sale, of course.

Embryos may be deep-frozen, and providing they are thoroughly 'washed' (a technique used to remove as much maternal material off the egg shell or zona pellucida as possible), it is fairly unlikely that they will transmit infectious disease. They may therefore be considered more acceptable to importing countries than either semen or animals on the hoof. This method of import–export does not, of course, exclude any diseases of genetic origin. Rare breeds could also be preserved in this way in embryo banks.

ET may be used on valuable old ewes who, for one reason or another (lameness, injury to the pelvis, mastitis, broken mouth) may not be considered fit to undergo another pregnancy, lambing and lactation. Their offspring may be 'carried' by fit, healthy recipient ewes.

WELFARE CONSIDERATIONS OF EMBRYO TRANSFER

In the author's opinion it is difficult to justify the use of a technique which involves a surgical operation—major or minor—sometimes repeated on several occasions during a season and possibly for several seasons in a row, which is not for the benefit of the patient, namely the ewe. These procedures are carried out almost exclusively for financial gain and there is an important welfare issue to be addressed here which will not disappear until a non-surgical approach is developed—and this looks somewhat unlikely at the present time.

Embryo transfer has been and will probably continue to be an important research tool, for example, in the investigation of certain diseases. These procedures are under the control of the Animals (Scientific Procedures) Act 1986, which limits what can and cannot be done to experimental animals and requires justification before such procedures are allowed. No such restrictions apply to ET on the farm, except that under the Veterinary Surgeons Act, such procedures must be carried out by a qualified veterinary surgeon. The technique has been described here so that farmers are informed about what is involved and will be alive to the fact that a number of veterinary surgeons may be unhappy about the morality of subjecting ewes to repeated ET surgery and thus decline to carry it out.

Frequent Lambing Systems

Sheep production in the UK is usually a low input and therefore a low output enterprise. However, if the inputs are increased and sheep systems intensified, then it is quite possible for ewes to rear three lambs per year and continue to do so for a normal breeding life. Increasing the number of lambs reared does not necessarily increase the profitability of the enterprise in direct proportion. Nevertheless, it is possible to achieve gross margins comparable with dairying or cereal growing in well-managed systems.

SUITABLE BREEDS

The number of lambs reared each year can be maximised by increasing the number of lambs born to each ewe at lambing and by increasing the number of lambings per year. Frequent lambing systems attempt to achieve this. In order to do so it is essential to choose a suitable breed of ewe which combines both an extended breeding season and good prolificacy. Amongst British breeds there is none which fits this bill. The only ewe with a significantly extended breeding season is the Dorset Horn but it is certainly not prolific. However, by crossing the Dorset with a prolific breed, such as the Finn, a good compromise is achieved. There are other crosses which can be used, such as the Friesland-Dorset and the Cambridge.

The choice of crossing rams may also be important in terms of producing the right type of lamb for a particular market. It is important that sufficient rams of high fertility are available, especially for the out-of-season matings, in order to achieve high conception rates.

There are a number of factors which limit what can be done to increase the ewe's reproductive performance in frequent breeding systems in the UK. These include the inhibition of breeding during the spring and summer, the time taken for the uterus to recover from pregnancy and the inhibitory effect of lactation and suckling on the return to sexual activity. It is generally accepted that, because of the last two factors, it is unrealistic to expect ewes to breed every six months, since most systems based on this premise have failed. However, there are a number of other options—some of which are too complex and impractical for commercial farm use—which lamb ewes three times in two years, four times in three years or five times in three years.

THREE LAMBINGS IN TWO YEARS

In the UK the only system which has been operated successfully is one lambing ewes three times in two years, developed in Scotland by Dr John Robinson at the Rowett Research Institute and put into commercial practice by Dr Mike Tempest at Harper Adams Agricultural College in Shropshire and a few commercial farms. As ewes are expected to lamb at eight month intervals, there is a tight management schedule. Use is made of sponge synchronisation and induction of lambing to see that all ewes in a group are mated over two days and lamb down together over two days. The eight months are divided into five months of pregnancy, two months of lactation and one month as a preparation for mating.

Table 3.4 **Sequence of events in a frequent lambing flock (three lambings in two years)**

Sub-flock A	Month	Sub-flock B
	December	Mating
Lambing	January	
	February	
Weaning	March	
Mating	April	
	May	Lambing
	June	
	July	Weaning
	August	Mating
Lambing	September	
	October	
Weaning	November	
Mating	December	
	January	Lambing

The flock is divided into two sub-flocks with matings occurring in December, April and August and lambings therefore in May, September and January (see Table 3.4). These timings can be altered slightly to fit in with other enterprises on the farm but are chosen to allow at least two out of the three matings (December and August) to take place within the breeding season of the Finn-Dorset ewe. The dose of PMSG used at

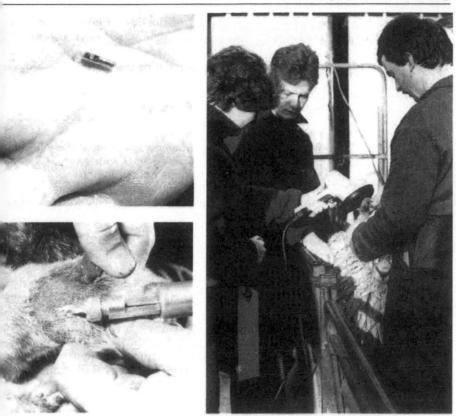

Plate 3.23 (*Top left*) A tiny microchip which can carry up to ten separate pieces of information and is designed to be implanted under the skin. (*Above left*) The chip is implanted under the skin at the base of the ear. (*Right*) As sheep are run through a race, the chip can be read by a wand so as to yield its data for recording purposes. Such a system could be used to record important breeding information.

sponge removal depends upon the season of mating, being highest for the out-of-season April tupping period. Ewes which do not conceive at the service immediately after sponge removal at the April mating do not return to oestrus 17 days later due to the inhibitory effect of day length in the early summer months. Ewes are scanned for pregnancy and empty ewes are allowed to 'slip back' into the next mating group of the complementary sub-flock.

The ewes are injected on day 141 of pregnancy with a corticosteroid drug which induces them to lamb on days 143/144 of pregnancy (see Table 3.5). Lambing takes place indoors and is supervised by skilled shepherds 24 hours a day. Only ewes which have been synchronised and have recorded mating dates can be induced to lamb safely. (Induction of lambing in sheep only rarely has any undesirable side effects, such as retained afterbirth.)

Table 3.5 Breeding programme in a frequent lambing flock (three lambings in two years)

Day	Weekday	Procedure
−14	Friday	Sponges in ewes
−2	Wednesday	Sponges removed, PMSG injected
0	Friday	Rams joined with ewes
3	Monday	Rams removed
+140	Friday	Ewes penned in house
+141	Saturday 6 pm	Ewes injected with corticosteroid
+143	Monday 6 am	
	to	Ewes lamb
	Tuesday 6 pm	

These frequent lambing systems are certainly not for the faint-hearted since they require a very high level of management input with top-class husbandry, stockmanship and attention to detail. They should be attempted only in flocks which already realise above-average results. Feeding lambing management and marketing ability are just three areas of particular importance. Benefits include better cash flow from a more frequent and regular supply of uniform lambs, the more effective use of skilled shepherds over short, intensive lambing periods and higher gross margins.

4

MANAGEMENT DURING PREGNANCY

Early Pregnancy

FERTILISATION

During the act of ejaculation the ram sprays several thousand million sperm onto the cervix or neck of the womb of the ewe. Of these only a few hundred are destined ever to get as far as the oviduct and so stand any chance of fertilising an egg. The first obstacle is the cervix itself, which in the ewe is a tough, muscular structure, with many folds which fit tightly together, leaving only a narrow, tortuous passage through which the tiny sperm must find their way. Assisted by the muscular movements of the uterus they must swim across it and up the oviducts to meet the eggs.

Lifespan of eggs and sperm

The life of an egg is only around half a day, whereas sperm can survive and retain their ability to fertilise for around a day and a half. It is therefore more likely that fertilisation will take place if sperm are either waiting in the oviduct at ovulation or are well on their way there. This would normally take place under natural mating conditions where an adequate number of fit and fertile rams are employed. Ewes are usually in oestrus for about a day before ovulation takes place and may be mated on a number of occasions during this time, before the eggs are shed from the ovaries. The first and possibly fittest sperm take around half a day to complete the exhausting journey and so may be in place before, or shortly after, the egg is shed.

When they are first deposited in the vagina, sperm are still somewhat immature and would be incapable of fertilising an egg. Ram's sperm require about an hour inside the ewe's genital tract to complete their maturity and this takes place during their long journey. Once fully mature the sperm become very vigorous, which is important for fertilisation, but it also tires them out. They very soon lose their power of fertilisation even though they may still be able to swim around. Because there is a large reservoir of sperm in the vagina, a small but steady stream of sperm will reach the oviduct, so

135

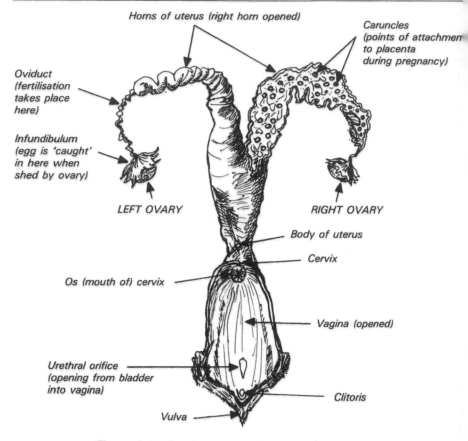

Figure 4.1 Ewe's reproductive tract dissected out.

that a few of them at least will be both mature and vigorous when the eggs arrive on the scene, about half an hour after ovulation.

Fertilisation of the egg

Providing the eggs are 'fresh', only one sperm will be able to penetrate each egg, because a reaction takes place immediately upon penetration which prevents any other sperm from entering the egg. This is important, because if two or more sperm do manage to penetrate, the egg will perish. If fertilisation takes place late in oestrus when the eggs are old and in the process of degenerating, multiple penetration is more likely, since the egg is less able to resist, and normal fertilisation is unlikely.

Fertilisation failure

If animals are stressed around the time of mating, for example by gathering and handling, then the movements of the sperm up the female reproductive tract are inhibited and there is less chance of fertilisation. It is therefore best to interfere as little as possible with ewes during the entire mating period and for several weeks after mating to minimise fertilisation failure and also the loss of embryos. Any procedures which must be done at this time should be carried out with particular care.

It is known from embryo transfer work, where eggs are flushed out of ewes after mating, that fertilisation rates are high—probably in excess of 90% in well-managed flocks. This high success rate is not reflected in ewes lambing to first mating, which averages around 75%. It is estimated that, on average, roughly one-third of all fertilised eggs fail to develop into normal healthy lambs.

In cattle—which normally only shed one egg at each oestrus—it is easier to appreciate these losses since, although the fertilisation rate is high, the calving rate to any particular service in the national dairy herd is less than 60%, highlighting the loss of around a third of pregnancies. However, because most sheep breeds shed more than one egg at oestrus, the 75% non-return rate masks the extent of the losses, which are in fact approximate to those in cattle.

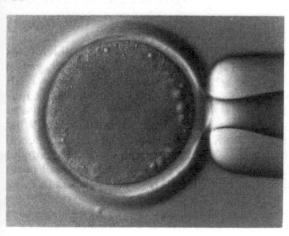

Plate 4.1   A sheep egg (unfertilised) with two pronuclei (at 8 and 9 o'clock) being held by suction with a fine glass pipette (right). For successful single sperm penetration and fertilisation, it is important that eggs are freshly shed and that sperm are not too old.

EMBRYONIC LOSS

Immediately after the egg is fertilised it becomes known as an **embryo** and it takes roughly three days for the embryo to negotiate the oviduct and enter the uterus. During this time and for some weeks longer, the embryo nourishes itself from the fluids secreted by the uterus in which it floats freely. The embryo 'hatches' from its shell when it is about a week old and some losses occur at this time, when it is still very small and only just visible to the naked eye.

Between approximately 15 and 30 days into pregnancy, the embryo becomes attached to the inner lining of the uterus and this is another vulnerable period when losses of embryos occur. Indeed, by the end of the first month of pregnancy, about a quarter of the embryo lambs have perished. After attachment to the uterus they become known as foetuses and by this stage the head, limbs and tiny organs, such as the heart and liver, are clearly visible (see Colour plate 9).

Smaller than expected lambs

If only one embryo is present and it dies, then the pregnancy is terminated and the ewe will eventually return to oestrus. If more than one egg is fertilised but only one perishes, then the pregnancy is maintained and the shepherd is none the wiser! These unseen losses of potential lambs represent very significant reproductive wastage and therefore economic loss to the sheep farmer. Not only are there fewer lambs than there could be, but because the area of the uterus occupied by the dead embryo is not available to the remaining live embryos as they develop, they are smaller than expected when born. So, a single lamb born only the size of a twin, or twins born only the size of triplets, may have originally been twins or triplets respectively which lost a litter mate at an early stage of pregnancy (see Colour plates 10 and 11).

Other consequences of embryonic loss

There are other hidden losses from early embryo death. A ewe which loses her embryo before about day 11 or 12 of pregnancy will return to service around the time she would be expected to do so had she not conceived. That means roughly 17 days after the previous mating and only some four or five days after the embryo died. However, where death of the embryo occurs later than this, the return to oestrus is delayed beyond 17 days. What is more, the older the embryo is when it perishes, the longer is the interval from death of the embryo to the ewe's return to oestrus. For example, death of the embryo at around 3 weeks after a particular mating will mean that the ewe will not come back into oestrus until around 5 weeks after that mating—a gap of two weeks from the death of the embryo. Obviously if a foetus dies, then the return to oestrus will be delayed even longer—perhaps until the following breeding season. (See Chapter 3.)

This delay is because the debris remaining after the death of an embryo has to be eliminated before the uterus is fit to accept a new embryo and therefore oestrus is delayed accordingly. The practical implications are clear, since some ewes will not return to oestrus until the rams have been withdrawn from the flock and will therefore become barreners. Furthermore, those ewes which lose an embryo are often less fertile at the next heat than would be expected.

CAUSES OF EMBRYONIC LOSS

There are many possible reasons why these early embryonic losses occur in ewes. Some are well proven; others may be based only on subjective observations. If the development of the very early embryo is in some way retarded, then it may fail to signal to the ewe that she is pregnant and the ewe may then come into oestrus, so terminating the pregnancy. In a few cases this retardation or abnormal development may be due to some genetic defect. It is better that these are voided at an early stage rather than when the rams have been removed, or much later in pregnancy. Ageing of the egg and penetration by more than one sperm (polyspermy) have already been mentioned as causes.

Feeding

An adequate level of feeding in early pregnancy is crucial to embryo survival. Whilst prolonged periods of starvation are uncommon under UK farming conditions, short periods of semi-starvation may occur from time to time, such as in an early winter snowstorm on the hill. On the other hand, malnutrition due to inadequate energy, protein, vitamin or mineral status is not uncommon. It is crucial that the effects of flushing pre-tupping to maximise ovulation rate are not invalidated by poor feeding in the weeks post-mating. Sudden changes in the quantity, quality or type of food offered should be avoided. The aim should be to keep ewes sufficiently well fed to maintain body weight for at least six weeks after conception. In flocks with a six week tupping period this means for three months after introduction of the rams.

On most true hill farms there is unlikely to be sufficient improved ground to accommodate ewes for longer than the mating period itself and not even that on some farms. Therefore ewes have to rely on the rough grazing of the open hill during the critical early pregnancy period. In some years this can coincide with some pretty atrocious weather conditions and ewes must be supplemented with hay, especially when there is snow cover. On the open hill, ewes are bound to lose weight in winter, but the consequences can be minimised by having them in good condition at mating and by ensuring that there are no periods of starvation during bad weather. Where hill ewes are in poor condition at tupping, then undernutrition during pregnancy is likely to have a profoundly adverse effect upon embryo survival.

Inclement weather, such as prolonged periods of heavy rain, may increase the loss of early embryos through stress, as will gathering the flock and carrying out various husbandry procedures, such as foot treatment or worming—the procedure itself rather than the effect of any particular drug often being to blame. Transportation or moving the flock to unfamiliar surroundings is also stressful.

Dipping

Dipping presents a difficult problem, especially when compulsory dipping periods coincide with either the mating or the early pregnancy period. It can be a particularly stressful procedure and should not be carried out during this high risk period if at all possible. It may even be worth considering an alteration of the mating period so that ewes are at a less vulnerable stage of

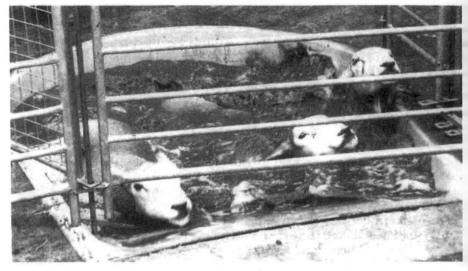

Plate 4.2 Gathering and driving the flock, dipping them and returning them to the grazings can be stressful for the sheep. The procedure should be avoided during mating and early pregnancy to reduce the risk of embryonic mortality.

pregnancy when they have to be dipped. Where dipping in early pregnancy cannot be avoided, the procedure should be performed with the greatest care to minimise losses.

Prolificacy

Naturally prolific breeds, with a few exceptions, have a lower rate of embryonic loss, when expressed as a percentage of eggs shed, than do less prolific breeds. Indeed, their high lambing rate is probably due to a combination of a high ovulation rate and a low rate of embryonic loss. Where multiple pregnancies are concerned, the distribution of embryos in the uterus is an important factor, since crowding of embryos in one area of the womb may predispose to losses. Clearly, the shepherd has no control in this matter.

The generally lower lambing rates in early or out-of-season lambing flocks is due to a combination of lower ovulation rates and higher embryonic losses. This may be exaggerated if ewes have been treated with too high a dose of PMSG following sponging. The excess amount of oestrogen produced by many ovarian follicles may increase the speed at which ova and embryos travel down the oviducts and thereby jeopardise their survival.

Ewe lambs

Ewe lambs can breed satisfactorily providing that, at mating, they are at least two-thirds of the weight of a mature adult ewe of the same breed and

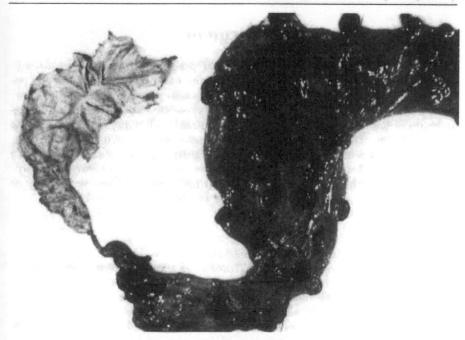

Plate 4.3   Placenta at normal term. The light-coloured portion on the left has been dead for some time, indicating the death of an early foetus. The darker portion (right) is a normal placenta from a live lamb.

are fed preferentially as a separate group, free of competition from ewes. They are generally fertile, but embryonic losses are higher than in ewes. This appears to be due to some defect of the embryo rather than of the ability of the ewe lamb to maintain a pregnancy.

Infection

Some of the infections which cause abortion may also cause the death of embryos in early pregnancy. Toxoplasmosis is such an infection and is dealt with in Chapter 5. Other diseases, especially those which result in loss of condition, such as liver fluke, or a fever, may lead to embryo loss indirectly.

From this discussion it will be clear that a large proportion of the ewes which fail to produce a lamb do so because of no fault of their own. A high proportion of barreners are quite capable of breeding the following season. The decision to retain them in the flock will depend to some extent on the price of barren ewes and upon the willingness of the flockmaster to take a risk by keeping them.

Mid Pregnancy

By the beginning of the second month of pregnancy the embryo already has a beating heart and the other body organs can be clearly identified (see Colour plate 9). Although it is only a few grams in weight, it is very obviously a tiny lamb. It is now called a foetus and has become intimately attached to the inner wall of the uterus by means of a greatly elongated structure called the **blastocyst**. This allows maximum contact with the uterus and will eventually become known as the placenta or afterbirth. At four or five weeks after conception, the forerunner of the placenta is very small, but during the following two months it will grow at an enormous rate, so that by 90 days of pregnancy it will be almost as big as at the birth of the lamb.

THE PLACENTA

The placenta is a truly remarkable organ and has been recognised since ancient times to be of special importance. If the **umbilical cord**—which attaches the newborn lamb to its afterbirth—is examined at lambing, it will be seen to consist of red blood vessels spiralling around a white background of tissue (see Colour plate 12). It is this which is symbolised in the barber's pole to this day since, in medieval times, barbers also acted as surgeons and no doubt became involved in childbirth. The physician's symbol—a staff of life entwined by a serpent—was probably modelled on the umbilical cord.

In the sheep, the foetus has intimate contact with the ewe via the placenta, through a series of structures called **placentomes**, or 'buttons' as they are

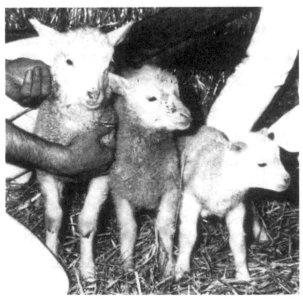

Plate 4.4 Triplet Finn lambs. The discrepancy in size is probably the result of the uneven distribution of embryos in the uterus and the unequal size of their placentae.

more commonly known. This attachment begins just a fortnight after conception and is complete by four to five weeks into pregnancy. There is no direct connection between the blood supply of the ewe and the foetal lamb at these 'buttons', but there is a constant exchange of nutrients and other essential substances from the ewe to the foetus and of waste products from the foetus to the ewe (see Colour plates 13 and 14).

The placenta also produces hormones which are essential for the continuance of pregnancy and hormones which are vital for the development of the ewe's udder and consequently for the amount of milk available to the lambs after lambing. The final size of the placenta largely determines the birth weight of the lambs, and no amount of good feeding of the ewe in late pregnancy will ever fully compensate for poor placental development during the mid-pregnancy period. Each lamb has its own personal placenta and because the total weight of the placentas of twins or triplets will be greater than that of a single lamb, more hormone will be produced. This ensures that ewes with multiple pregnancies will produce more milk than ewes with singles. Placental hormones are also responsible for the bond between the ewe and her lamb immediately after lambing.

Feeding

In order to produce big strong lambs and an adequate supply of milk, it is therefore vital to feed ewes appropriately during mid-pregnancy to ensure maximum growth of the placenta. But what is an appropriate feeding regime? The first thing to appreciate is that extremes of both underfeeding and overfeeding should be avoided. Having ewes in good body condition prior to mating is very important, because during the summer and early autumn body condition can be put on ewes relatively cheaply at pasture, usually without any need for supplementation. The energy reserves laid down as fat at this time are invaluable, both during pregnancy and well into lactation. They can be drawn upon gradually, so that savings can be made on expensive winter feeding stuffs.

A mild degree of underfeeding can be tolerated during mid pregnancy, but only providing ewes were in good condition score (3 to 3.5) at mating and maintained their weight and condition during the first month of pregnancy. This loss of condition should not exceed half a condition score (5 to 10 pounds body weight depending upon the breed and size of ewe) during this two month period.

A problem arises with hill ewes on rough grazings, especially gimmers and twin bearing ewes, since they may lose up to 10 or 15% of body weight. Where possible, these special groups should be given preferential treatment following scanning for pregnancy (see below). This can be done by bringing them down onto better grazings and/or by providing some form of supplementary feed, perhaps as high energy feed blocks for example. A problem arises with gimmers, in that many will not take supplementary feed unless they have been trained to do so—for example, when they come back from the winterings as hoggs.

143

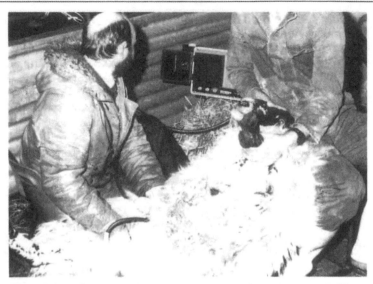

Plate 4.5 Diagnosis of pregnancy by real-time ultrasound. The technique is now normally carried out with the ewe in the standing position.

PREGNANCY DIAGNOSIS BY ULTRASOUND SCANNING

Diagnosis of pregnancy using the real-time ultrasound technique—scanning—takes place during the mid pregnancy period. Real-time ultrasound sends sound waves through the ewe's body tissues and these bounce back to the machine at different rates depending upon the type of tissue (bone, muscle, fluid) they encounter. The machine then converts these returned waves into a picture on a screen from which the scanner operator can determine whether ewes are pregnant and if so, whether they are carrying singles, twins or triplets. This is a highly skilled job and since there is little point in scanning unless the results are accurate, only trained and approved operators should be hired to do the job. Ask your local agricultural adviser for a list of approved contractors.

The accuracy figures quoted as being acceptable are:

- pregnant or not—99%
- empty, single, multiple—98%
- multiples defined as twins, triplets, quads, etc—96 to 97%

Good results partly depend upon the farmer providing the sheep as the operator requests. For example, ewes should be presented at the most appropriate stage of pregnancy and starved overnight. Good handling facilities and adequate help are essential if the job is to be carried out smoothly and with the minimum of stress to the ewes and to the operator.

Scanning 'window'

The number of foetuses present cannot be accurately detected before about seven weeks of pregnancy, and after 14 weeks it becomes more difficult to determine numbers because of the large size of the foetuses. In most flocks (unsynchronised) the rams are likely to be kept in for at least two oestrous cycle lengths or around five weeks. Therefore, for the best results, there is a fairly narrow 'window' when scanning can be carried out. The ewes which return to the ram at the end of the tupping period should be at least seven weeks pregnant before scanning, so the job should not be done earlier than 12 weeks after the rams are first introduced for mating. If the ewes which are served and conceive in the first few days of mating are not to be more than 14 weeks pregnant, this only leaves about a fortnight as the optimum time to scan.

Pregnancy can be detected earlier than seven weeks by identifying placentomes on the placenta. However, the temptation to do so should be strongly resisted because of the risks of causing early embryo or foetal death through gathering and handling ewes at this crucial stage of early pregnancy. The task can be left until later than 14 weeks, but the accuracy

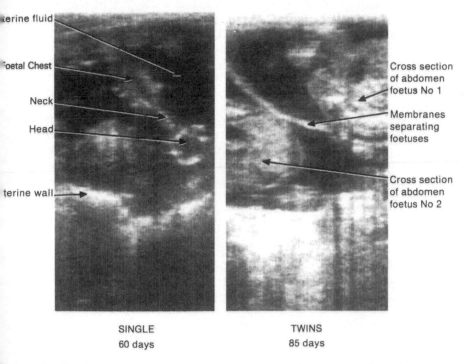

SINGLE
60 days

TWINS
85 days

Plate 4.6   The interpretation of scanning pictures requires a great deal of experience.

145

may suffer. In any case, one of the main benefits of scanning—that of selective rationing according to the number of foetuses present—should be implemented during the final six to eight weeks of the 21 week pregnancy at the latest. Hill ewes carrying twins and hill gimmers will benefit from even earlier preferential treatment, so the nearer to 12 weeks after the rams are introduced that scanning can be done the better. Where the rams are run with the ewes for longer than five weeks, scanning may have to be done somewhat earlier than is advisable for the last ewes to the ram in order to gain maximum benefit for ewes holding to the first and second cycles. In this case, it will be helpful to the scanner operator to have late mated (third cycle) ewes identified where a raddled ram has been used.

Preparation for scanning

The operator will often request that ewes be deprived of roughage overnight before scanning, since a full rumen makes diagnosis more difficult. So, if ewes are brought indoors the night before the job is to be done, they should not be bedded on straw. If they are already indoors, then they should not be given fresh bedding in the day immediately prior to scanning. The operator may also request that belly wool be removed, so that contact can be made between the scanning head and the skin. Ewes may be scanned whilst reclining in a cradle or in the standing position and the speed of operation will depend on the type of scanner used, the skill of the operator, the size of the sheep (when being cradled), the number of people available to handle ewes and the adequacy of the handling facilities. All these factors should be discussed with the contractor beforehand, rather than left to the day of operation, so that things run smoothly for sheep, shepherds and scanners.

Above all, gather and handle ewes with care so as to stress them as little as possible. The results are likely to be less accurate if things are badly organised, and inaccurate results are positively misleading. Take the opportunity to condition score ewes as they come through and shed off any thin ones for special attention. After scanning, each ewe should either be clearly marked as to the number of lambs she is carrying, or shed off at the time into the appropriate group.

BENEFITS OF SCANNING

Scanning costs money, necessitates an extra handling of the ewes and involves changes in management and feeding. These costs have to be recouped in increased productivity and should be carefully considered for individual flocks. Identifying 'empty' ewes means they can be fed at a much-reduced cost if they are to be kept and given a further opportunity to breed the following season. Otherwise, they can be sold immediately— often at a higher price than when cull ewes flood the market—so saving feed costs overwinter. In housed flocks, removing barreners also allows more space for heavily pregnant ewes. In many cases the savings on barren ewes can pay for the cost of scanning before any of the other benefits are accounted for.

By identifying ewes carrying singles, twins or triplets, feeding during the late pregnancy period can be more accurately apportioned. Lowland flocks with a reasonably good lambing percentage may normally feed all ewes as if they were carrying twins. Scanning can identify single bearing ewes so they can be fed less, thereby reducing the risk of oversized lambs and subsequently difficult lambings.

Scanning hill ewes

On the hill, where grazing is in short supply in winter and extra supplementary feed costs can be difficult to justify, the small proportion of ewes carrying twins often become very thin and may be at serious risk of pregnancy toxaemia, especially during snow cover. Lambs are liable to be small and more vulnerable to hypothermia and infectious disease since their dams rarely produce sufficient colostrum and milk for twins. Twin bearing ewes can be kept down on in-bye grazings and fed supplementary concentrates, or in hill enclosures and fed blocks. This has the added advantage that it saves bringing ewes with pairs down off the hill after lambing, which can be a frustrating and time consuming business, especially when the lambs are undersized and weakly. On hill farms, the housing of twin bearing ewes and gimmers prior to lambing makes shepherding easier and will undoubtedly save many lambs.

Prolific flocks

With lambing percentages of around 200%, there will be roughly as many ewes carrying singles as triplets. The latter group can be fed preferentially at relatively little extra cost through the savings made by reducing the rations of the single bearing ewes. There are obvious advantages in identifying twin bearing ewe lambs which need very careful feeding and management.

Alternative methods of pregnancy diagnosis, such as the Doppler technique and the measurement of hormone levels in blood, have been superseded by the real-time ultrasound scanning technique and will not be described here.

Late Pregnancy

The number of lambs which will be born at lambing time is largely determined in the weeks before, during and immediately after mating. Some losses occur during mid and late pregnancy through abortions or conditions such as twin lamb disease, but apart from flocks which have particular problems in this regard, these losses should be small.

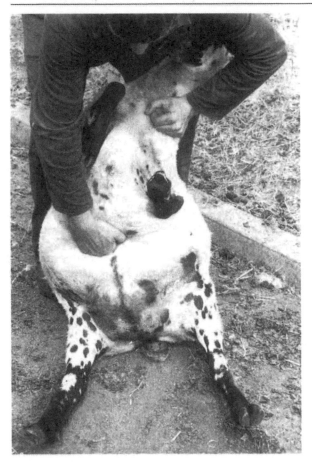

Plate 4.7 In late pregnancy the presence of a foetus(es) can often be detected by gently bouncing the hand into the ewe's lower abdomen (without losing contact with the skin).

FEEDING

As stated earlier, good feeding during the last two months of pregnancy can never totally compensate for a small placenta consequent upon inadequate mid pregnancy feeding. However, it may help to ensure that ewes do not lamb prematurely, that lambs are provided with adequate energy supplies in the form of brown fat, that ewes have a strong mothering instinct and that they produce adequate supplies of both colostrum and milk. No udder development takes place after lambing, so that adequate feeding during the whole of pregnancy is crucial for optimal milk production and therefore lamb growth rates to weaning.

The best quality forage should always be reserved for late pregnancy and the protein level in the concentrate ration adjusted according to the forage analysis. An adequate proportion of the concentrate protein should be in a rumen-undegradable form, such as fishmeal, and the final crude protein evel should be in the region of 15 to 16 per cent. The cereal portion of the ration should not be finely ground since this may lead to digestive upsets (see acidosis). Cereals can be fed lightly rolled but preferably as whole grains. The final ration should be supplemented with an appropriate vitamin, mineral and trace element mixture.

An example of a simple late pregnancy ration would be nine parts of whole barley plus one part of a fishmeal pellet, with a vitamin and mineral supplement added at 2.5% (25 kg per tonne) of the final mix. Oats, maize and wheat can also be used in suitable proportions to supplement barley, and soya, peas, beans, or linseed can be used as part of the protein component. Choice will depend on availability and price, and examples of rations are given in the Meat and Livestock Commission booklet *Feeding the Ewe*.

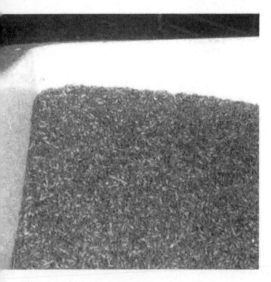

Plate 4.8   Whole barley fed to sheep is less likely than ground barley to lead to digestive upsets such as acidosis.

ENERGY AND PROTEIN REQUIREMENTS

The correct feeding of ewes, particularly during pregnancy and lactation, is so vital to the success of any sheep breeding enterprise that advice from an independent expert is well worth while, preferably in the autumn once the forages have been analysed. The diet should be formulated on the expected or known (scanned) lamb crop and it is important to know the nutrient intake requirements for ewes at the various stages of pregnancy and lactation.

The metabolisable energy (ME) requirements for the rapid growth of the foetal lambs in late pregnancy increase steadily through to lambing. An average sized ewe (70 kg body weight) carrying twins will need only a modest amount (e.g. 350 g/day) of concentrates in the last few weeks of

149

pregnancy if she is receiving ad lib high-quality roughage with an ME value of at least 10.5 megajoules (MJ) per kilogram of dry matter.

However, many roughages are far below this standard, with ME values of 8.5 MJ/kg dry matter, in which case the same ewe would require some 1.2 kg of concentrate daily to meet her requirements for energy and protein. This high level of concentrate feeding is undesirable, since it tends to predispose to acidosis with consequent loss of appetite, which may then lead to pregnancy toxaemia. Providing the cereal portion of the concentrate as whole grains and feeding it twice a day may reduce the risk, but it is probably better to reduce the energy portion whilst maintaining the protein requirements, so as not to jeopardise the viability of lambs and the udder development of the ewes.

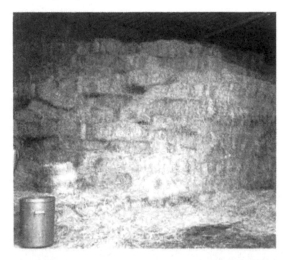

Plate 4.9 The analysis of all forages should be known, and the best ones kept for ewes in late pregnancy when voluntary feed intake declines.

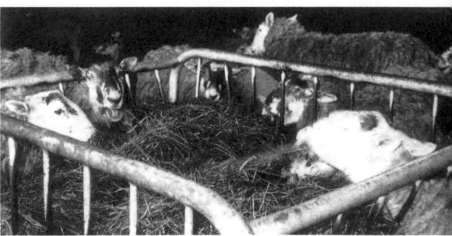

Where concentrates are mixed on the farm, high protein balancers for mixing with carbohydrate-rich constituents give flexibility to diet formulation, since their proportions can be varied to take account of the quality of the forage available and the specific requirements of the flock.

Whilst both energy and protein levels are important, it is unlikely that a diet which contains sufficient energy will be deficient in protein. An exception to this rule might be the prolific lactating ewe suckling fast-growing lambs.) As the foetal lambs grow at an ever-increasing rate in late pregnancy, so too do the ewe's requirements for energy. Also, the conversion of dietary energy into the energy required for the growth of the foetal lambs is a very inefficient process, which further increases the ewe's requirements. In late pregnancy, energy is stored in the lamb mainly as brown fat, which protects it from hypothermia immediately after birth, and this is a further drain on the ewe. It is not surprising, therefore, that in late pregnancy, a ewe carrying twins needs twice the energy, and one carrying triplets three times the energy, of a barren ewe of the same body weight.

It is unlikely that many farmers will supply ewes with their total requirements for energy in late pregnancy, so that they do not lose any body condition. This would be both expensive and unnecessary. Providing ewes are in good condition (around score 3) at 90 days of pregnancy, they can afford to lose up to half a condition score during the last 60 days up to lambing. Any more than this could reduce the amount of body tissue available for ewes to draw on for milk production. At this time there is an even higher energy requirement than in late lactation and voluntary feed intake is unlikely to be able to meet the demands. The energy requirements steadily increase as lambing approaches, hence the use of a step-wise increase in the concentrate portion of the diet and a reduction in the forage intake.

Protein requirements on an energy-adequate diet will usually be met, at least until the last month of pregnancy when some undegradable protein supplementation will be necessary to supply essential amino acids. Soya bean (heat treated) or, better still, fish meal is usually included in the concentrate ration (e.g. 8% fish meal). There is a good measure of interdependence between the components of a ration. Protein cannot be fully utilised by rumen microorganisms unless sufficient energy is provided to fuel the chemical reactions. The rumen fermentation process cannot function adequately without a sufficient supply of roughage. The ratio of roughage (hay or silage) to concentrate will be decided partly on the prevailing costs of each, but care must be taken to make the ration palatable and to see that the amounts required to satisfy the ewe's needs can indeed be consumed.

Feed intake

Voluntary feed intake (VFI) is influenced by a number of factors. Water intake will limit the amount of dry matter which can be consumed.

151

Generally speaking, dry matter intake will be higher when the component of the ration have a high dry matter content (e.g. concentrates) and where drinking water is freely available. Intake will be lower when succulent feeds such as roots are fed, since the water content is 'locked-up' and less available to the digestive process. Voluntary feed intake tends to decline in late pregnancy because the increasing amount of space taken up in the abdomen by the rapidly growing lambs restricts the capacity of the rumen. This situation is more critical in overfat ewes carrying large amounts of abdominal fat. When feed intake is reduced, food tends to spend less time in the rumen than normal and is therefore improperly digested. This may lead to digestive upsets or pregnancy toxaemia. It is obvious, therefore, why there is a need for an energy-dense ration in late pregnancy and why the essential roughage must be of high quality so as not to reduce intake and impair digestion.

Supplementation of hill ewes

Ewes at pasture will always pick away at the sward as long as there is anything there to nibble at, but the contribution of pasture from Christmas onwards is small and is unlikely to supply even a third of the energy requirements of a ewe with twins. Ewes must therefore have free access to hay or silage at this time. Care must be taken in hill flocks where hay is used to supplement poor grazings (e.g. heather hills) that it is of good quality, as poor hay will have the effect of reducing appetite and therefore reducing the intake of natural grazing, which may, in some cases, have a higher nutritional value than poor hay.

Hill ewes can rarely eat sufficient natural forage during pregnancy to maintain body condition and this will prejudice lamb survival. The difficulty arises in how best to supplement them in the most cost-beneficial way. To some extent this depends upon the accessibility of the hill and the availability of in-bye pastures and fields. Hay is often difficult or impossible to make and expensive to buy and, on extensive units with no roads, difficult to distribute. On such farms, feed blocks, although expensive, can be a useful supplementary feed. As well as supplying both energy and protein, they also stimulate rumen fermentation and therefore allow the ewe to make better use of the rough hill grazings. Many blocks contain urea (a non-protein nitrogen source) but this is not a suitable feed for the last few weeks of pregnancy.

There are a number of snags to block feeding apart from cost. They must be sited correctly to allow easy access to all ewes on a hirsel. Even then not all ewes will eat them and it is said that those that do so will tend not to forage so effectively. Ewes vary enormously in the amount of block they consume and this is difficult or impossible to regulate. The high level of salt included is intended to limit intake, but is only partially successful and easy access to fresh clean water is essential. However, blocks have been successful on many hill farms where they have helped to increase the lambing percentage and the survival of lambs by ensuring that ewes have sufficient colostrum and milk available.

Blocks would normally be fed on the hill from New Year onwards. On the more fortunate hills ewes may be fed concentrates, either in the form of cobs spread on the ground, or conventional home mixes or compounded cakes fed in troughs. Hill sheep need to be taught how to eat these feeds and this is best done when they are ewe hoggs. Many progressive hill farms now in-winter their hoggs in sheds, due to the high cost of away-wintering. Under these conditions they become used to feeding, are better grown and generally have a better start in life.

Young ewes

Ewe hoggs or gimmers are still growing when they become pregnant for the first time and therefore have higher requirements than adult ewes on body weight basis. They usually have a lower lambing percentage than adult ewes and those carrying single lambs will require supplementary feeding at a higher level than a single bearing adult ewe, but less than a twin bearing adult. Scanning will be particularly useful in ensuring that twin bearing young adults are fed appropriately so as not to prejudice their lambs or their subsequent reproductive performance. They must not be allowed to lose too much condition in late pregnancy and, as a guide, no more than one-quarter condition score in the last six weeks.

Feeding based on sound principles is all very well and good, but it is essential to monitor the flock throughout to check that they are indeed performing as predicted. Every time that ewes are handled during pregnancy, for whatever reason, they should be condition scored and the feeding adjusted accordingly. Not even the most experienced shepherd can tell by eye how ewes are performing—although it is much easier in housed, winter-reared flocks. Condition scoring at six weeks before lambing and again at three weeks—for example, at the time the clostridial '7 in 1' vaccine pre-lambing booster is given—will provide a good guide as to whether the feeding regime is adequate and allow time for correction if it is not.

It is important to pick out individual ewes which are not thriving as well as they should be and to feed them preferentially. Be aware of the possibility that they may be suffering from some chronic condition, such as liver fluke, in which case treatment will be necessary before better feeding is likely to be effective.

Housing of Sheep and Associated Health Problems

An increasing number of farmers on lowland, upland and hill farms are housing ewes, either over the whole winter period or for a restricted period around lambing. There is nothing new about overwintering sheep indoors, since agricultural historians tell us that probably a smaller proportion of the national flock is housed today than in medieval times. In

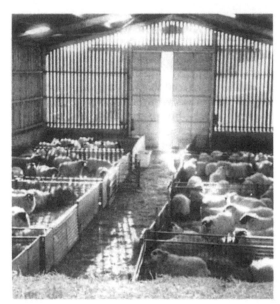

Plate 4.10 A bright, airy sheep shed housing ewes in late pregnancy.

Plate 4.11 (*Below*) It can be difficult to justify purpose built sheep accommodation on economic grounds, but the cost can sometimes be shared with other enterprises. Where suitable housing is provided there are considerable benefits to ewes, lambs and shepherds.

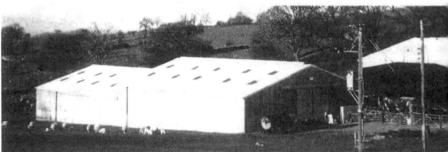

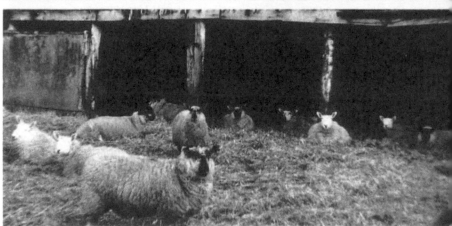

Plate 4.12 Cheap, home constructed sheep accommodation, comprising an open yard with shelter on all four sides. It is essential that drainage is excellent and that there is ample bedding in the open area.

older climates, such as Scandinavia and Iceland, where snow covers the grazing for months at a time, all sheep are housed for a prolonged winter period.

In Britain, winter housing began to decline in popularity some 200 years ago and despite the recent interest, the majority of flocks are still unhoused for any period of the year. This is not necessarily a good thing, since, not surprisingly, the vast majority of both ewe and lamb deaths occur in the short period around lambing time. Close shepherding and protection from the weather would undoubtedly reduce these unacceptable losses very significantly, especially in prolific flocks and in hill situations.

It is the cost of providing shelter for the flock that deters many flockmasters. Certainly the economics of constructing a portal frame, purpose-built house do not make good reading, but there are many alternatives which can provide relatively cheap accommodation for the flock. Existing buildings can often be adapted inexpensively, and new buildings can be constructed to multipurpose specifications—for example, to store grain, fodder, cattle or machinery at other times of the year. Lean-to sheds or cheaper constructions such as plastic tunnels are alternatives, and it is even possible to hire a large marquee in which to lamb the ewes. (One West Country farmer had his daughter's wedding reception in a marquee, then kept it on to lamb the flock and had even begun to construct the lambing pens before the last of the wedding guests had left!) Cheapest of all, perhaps, is a temporary shelter made of bales, hurdles, corrugated sheeting, etc. Some of these constructions are quite astounding examples of the ingenuity of farming people.

There are a number of benefits from housing the flock overwinter or over lambing and these are listed below:

- Housing will allow ewes to be fed more appropriately by grouping them according to body condition, scanning results or lambing date as required. Older ewes generally do better indoors and may be retained for longer in the flock, so reducing replacement costs. There are generally fewer ewe deaths indoors, partly because flock inspection is easier, so that when they are unwell they can be pulled out of the group and treated more appropriately.
- The greatest benefits should be obtained around lambing in terms of the extra number of live lambs born and in a significant reduction in lamb losses through close and constant shepherding and shelter from the vagaries of the weather.
- Shepherding is made easier and more comfortable—few shepherds who have lambed indoors wish to return to outdoor lambing.
- Where ewes are housed early in the New Year through to lambing, there are a number of substantial benefits in pasture management. Poaching by sheep's feet and tractor wheels is avoided and this can mean considerably earlier and heavier yields of better-quality grass in the spring. Growth may begin a month earlier, especially on wet,

155

heavy land, with as much as one-third greater yield in first-cut silage. This in turn means earlier clean grazing on aftermaths for weaned lambs.

- This better quality and quantity of grass allows ewes to attain higher milk yields, which in turn allow lambs to grow faster.
- The grazing available is less heavily contaminated with parasitic worms
- Because there is more grass available, higher stocking rates can be carried on the farm.
- Where desired, lambing can be brought forward because of the earlier grass growth and the protection provided during the less reliable weather early in the year.
- On arable farms running sheep as a break crop and to enhance fertility housing overwinter means that sacrifice pastures will not be required and can therefore be ploughed for winter cereals with their higher yields and margins.

There are of course some disadvantages of housing:

- Ewes kept indoors have lower food maintenance requirements, because they need less energy to keep warm, but since they are not grazing they will eat approximately twice the quantity of roughage as ewes kept outdoors. There are also extra bedding costs involved.
- There may be some fleece damage due to contamination from bedding, from rubbing against troughs at feeding or from disease in the fleece if ventilation is inadequate, thus allowing humidity to rise. All these can reduce the value of the fleece. (See winter shearing below.)
- The costs of providing a building.

SUITABLE BUILDINGS

Before constructing or adapting buildings for housing sheep, it is helpful to consult a specialist in farm buildings and to visit other housed flocks to see and talk over the practicalities. The housing requirements of sheep differ considerably from those of other species. In general terms, for both comfort and good health, sheep require only shelter from wind and rain. The temperature and humidity inside a sheep shed or house should be as nearly the same as outdoors as possible, and draughts should be eliminated at sheep level.

To achieve such conditions, it is important to choose the siting of a new building carefully, or to adapt an existing building accordingly, so that best use is made of natural shelter, whilst at the same time providing protection from prevailing weather. Remember also that constructing a new building amongst existing buildings can radically alter the movement of air and may interfere with conditions in neighbouring buildings.

A good sheep house should be bright, airy, free from stale smells and with not a hint of condensation. In really cold weather, the shepherd should eed a thick sweater and jacket and possibly even a hat and gloves! Ewes which are to be housed over the whole winter period can be shorn as soon s they are housed. To prevent hypothermia if a spell of cold weather occurs oon after shearing, some temporary adjustments such as the hanging of acking or plastic netting may be necessary to reduce wind speed through he house.

To prevent draughts at sheep level in a pole barn, some form of solid onstruction such as blocks, plyboard, stockboard, or even straw bales vill probably be needed around the perimeter of the building to a height f about 1.25 m. The space above to the eaves can be left completely open r infilled with space boarding, perforated metal profile, plastic netting or ther material which will allow a free passage of air whilst cutting down vind speed. The choice will depend upon siting and cost. Many sheep sheds lave one completely open side (away from the prevailing weather) with the thers protected in some way.

Warm air from the sheep and bedding rises and all sheep sheds should lave an open ridge in the roof, preferably a protected one which will prevent ain and snow from entering. Without an open ridge there will be a endency for condensation to form and humidity to rise despite space board-ng around the sides. This will affect the fabric of the building adversely ind may also produce damp bedding. It will also predispose the sheep to espiratory disease in particular. Many farmers are wary of housing sheep ecause of the risks of pneumonia, but providing the stocking rate is not excess-ve and the housing is suitably ventilated, the risk should be no greater

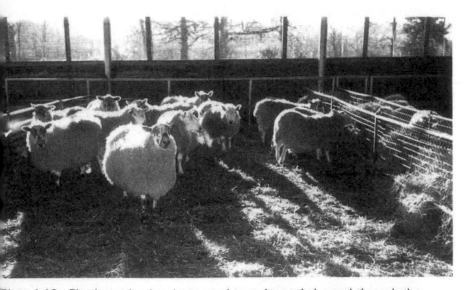

Plate 4.13   Plastic netting has been used to reduce wind speed through the building above.

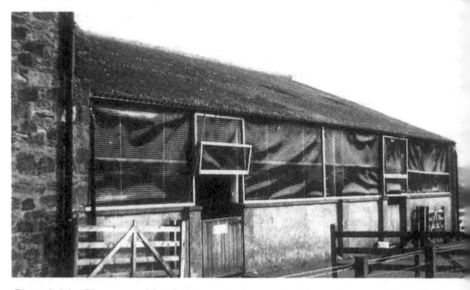

Plate 4.14 The open side of this small sheep shed faces the prevailing wind and has had to be protected by a plastic windbreak.

than for sheep kept outdoors. Sheep indoors with a full fleece cannot lose heat as effectively as they can outdoors and will pant more. Where this is excessive, modifications to the ventilation will have to be made.

A word of warning regarding the storage of hay and straw in the same building as stock. Mouldy material can be hazardous to both livestock and stockmen, since it may contain highly toxic substances (mycotoxins). When bales are moved about, these substances billow into the atmosphere (observe the amount of 'dust' from even clean hay in a shaft of sunlight). When inhaled, these poisons may make animals or humans very unwell and in some circumstances have proved fatal. The author can recall a poorly ventilated calf unit where some very old hay had been stored behind a high wall with a gap at the top between it and the roof. After removal of the bales, many of the calves developed respiratory symptoms and a number died. The stockman who had removed the material—without wearing a protective mask—was also very unwell and required medical attention.

Apart from plenty of fresh air, sheep need a dry bed to walk and lie on, adequate floor space and trough space and fresh clean water constantly available.

FLOORS AND BEDDING

The importance of a dry lie cannot be overstressed. The slightest hint of wetness on entering a pen and paddling about in it is unacceptable (this is often referred to as the 'squelch test'). The type of floor, the amount

158

and type of bedding, the stocking rate in the pens and the humidity in the building will all have an effect. The floor may be of concrete, some form of hard core or simply earth. Providing the area is well drained, hard core and earth are perfectly acceptable, even preferable. They may be damaged at mucking out, but this can be in-filled, and they are much less costly to maintain than a concrete floor is to lay in the first place. Concrete floors must have an adequate slope for free drainage and they do have the advantage of ease of cleaning and disinfection. However, bare concrete floors without bedding are totally unacceptable on a number of grounds, particularly the welfare of the sheep.

Whatever the basic flooring material, adequate bedding must be provided. Straw is much preferable to sawdust or shavings, which may spoil fleeces and are generally less comfortable. There is also evidence from work in dairy herds that sawdust may allow the multiplication of certain microorganisms—for example, *E. coli*—to a greater extent than either shavings or straw. Straw is relatively cheap, except for farms a long way from arable areas, where transport may make it considerably more expensive. Dried bracken, which is sometimes used as bedding on hill farms, is unacceptable because it is poisonous if eaten. Straw is best provided little and often, but the allocation should be generous, especially at lambing time when it can be used to 'bury' and therefore reduce the weight of infection which inevitably builds up. Slaked or hydrated lime spread on an earthen or hard-core floor both dries and acts as a disinfectant. It can be sprinkled amongst the straw when it is not possible to clean out lambing pens between each and every ewe, but it must be covered up with plenty of fresh straw, since animals must not have direct contact with lime.

Slats can be used as a flooring and have some advantages, such as separating the sheep from their dung, so reducing the disease risk. However, they are expensive and are not commonly used for ewes in late pregnancy or over the lambing period, when lambs could break their legs between the slats. They are used more commonly in lamb fattening units.

Floor and trough space allowances

From the point of view of both husbandry and health, it is important to allow ewes sufficient floor area and trough space, taking into account the size of the ewes, whether or not they are shorn and their prolificacy. The latter will affect their body size in late pregnancy and the number of lambs running about in the pens in the few days before turnout to grass. Ewes should therefore be allowed at least 1.2 to 1.5 square metres of floor area, depending upon breed and the other factors mentioned. Around half a metre of trough space will be required for large ewes.

The shape of the pens is important in providing the correct combination of floor area and trough space, long narrow pens with a feed trough down one long side being most satisfactory. It is best to have concentrate troughs only along one side of the pen, since otherwise ewes may dodge from one side to the other. Insufficient trough space causes jostling at feeding and

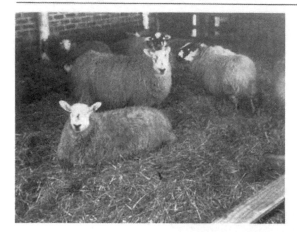

Plate 4.15 Ewes in late pregnancy (*left*) and with lambs (*below*) on deep straw bedding over a well-drained floor providing dry, warm, comfortable conditions. Straw applied frequently and amply helps cover infection.

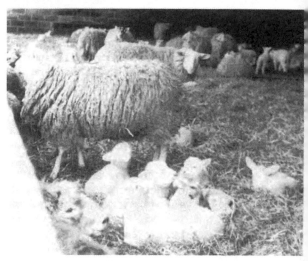

Plate 4.16 (*Below*) The choice of bedding material is often dictated by cost and availability. These weaned lambs in the south-eastern United States are bedded on peanut haulms, which are cheaper and more readily available than straw.

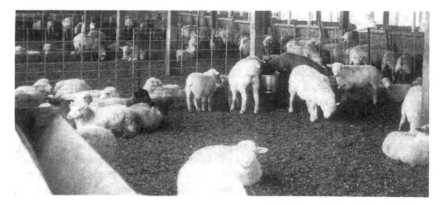

makes the equal distribution of feed amongst ewes more difficult than it is already, with both greedy and shy feeders to contend with. The depth of troughs and their height above ground should be carefully considered bearing in mind the build up of straw.

Keeping too many ewes together in a pen (even with adequate space allowance) also creates problems at feeding time. Ideally, numbers should be restricted to 25 or 30 per pen at most. Walk-through troughs, which also act as pen divisions, make feeding easier for the shepherd and also serve as good observation posts.

It is important to have sheep handling facilities available, either in the building or nearby, and these should include a footbath, preferably of the stand-in type. Hot water and electricity should be laid on with sufficient strategically placed power points for lamb warming boxes and other essential equipment, such as hot water for hand washing and the electric kettle for making coffee at lambing time!

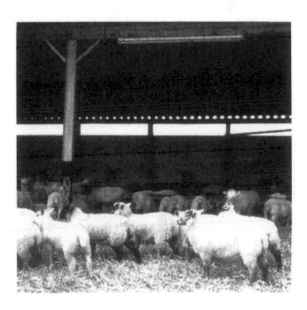

Plate 4.17 Early born lambs finishing in a semi-covered yard. The floor is well drained and deeply bedded, and whilst lambs can get under cover in the wind and rain, adequate ventilation is assured.

Sheep should be dry-fleeced when housed and a cool, dry day is best. House ewes early in the day to allow them to settle down during daylight hours. Subdued lighting at night may be helpful for the first week or so, and at lambing time it is essential.

Water supplies

If intake is not to be restricted, a good clean water supply is vitally important to housed ewes fed a high dry matter diet. Water pipes should be lagged and in frosty weather troughs should be checked and unfrozen if necessary. One flock housing ewes for the first time in old converted build-ings experienced illness and deaths from pregnancy toxaemia brought on because the water supply had frozen up. This had gone unnoticed for long enough to reduce food intake significantly—not to mention water intake! Restriction of water intake and therefore dry matter intake will adversely effect lamb birth weights and survival and reduce milk production in the ewe.

WINTER SHEARING OF EWES

Winter shearing of housed ewes seems a logical thing to think of when watching heavily pregnant, fully fleeced ewes puffing and panting in a shed on a warm spring day. Indeed, as with many techniques, it is not a new idea—it was practised in the Orkney Islands off the north coast of Scotland at the turn of the century and nowhere does the wind blow colder or more persistently than there.

Shearing ewes at housing in January reduces the heat stress on them. Initially, they tend to shiver and huddle together, even when a comb is used which leaves a longer stubble, but most ewes eventually acclimatise. Those which do not will need to be removed to a warmer place or given a 'coat' to wear. The need to keep warm makes sheared ewes eat considerably more than housed, fleeced sheep by some 15 to 20%. The extra costs incurred can be largely offset by the increase in size and strength of the lambs born to shorn ewes, which may be 10 to 15% heavier. This is largely due to the fact that shorn sheep have a more normal length of pregnancy as opposed to unshorn ewes, which, because of heat stress, tend to lamb a couple of days early.

This increased lamb weight is a benefit to most multiple bearing ewes, but with single bearing ewes some rationing may be required to avoid oversized singles which may give difficulty at birth. Another reason for the bigger lambs is that, in shorn ewes, the food tends to remain in the rumen for a slightly shorter time and therefore the protein portion of the diet is less degraded and better utilised. This effect is most noticeable in the smaller breeds of ewe.

Because ewes are physically smaller after losing the fleece they can be stocked at a slightly higher density. It is much easier for the shepherd to assess the condition of shorn ewes and therefore to pick out ewes which are not doing so well for preferential treatment. Ewes which are unwell are more easily identified, as are the signs of impending lambing and the state of the udder, especially when ewes stand eating at the trough.

Shorn ewes tend to be more lively at lambing time and their lambs are quicker getting to the teat, giving them a better chance of survival. Stillbirths and lamb deaths are generally lower in shorn ewes, and when turned out to graze after lambing, shorn ewes usually recover the body condition lost during pregnancy quicker than fleeced sheep, providing the weather is kind. However, if the weather turns nasty after turnout, it may be necessary to

162

rehouse them until conditions improve, and this can prove difficult where there is pressure on accommodation. Certainly, some form of shelter such as plastic netting hung on the fence, or big straw bales should always be provided, not only for the lambs, but also for their shorn mothers.

WOOL SLIP

Wool slip, which has been recognised as a problem for only a short while, is associated with the winter shearing of housed ewes. Normally, the practice is to house ewes, allow them to settle and then shear them. This normally takes place in December or January when the weather may be very cold, even inside a sheep shed full of animals.

Wool slip usually occurs a few weeks after shearing and often affects a large proportion of the flock. The wool falls out in patches, generally over the back, leaving the ewe with unsightly bald patches which grow back only very slowly (see Colour plate 56). The woolclip from affected ewes is significantly reduced and may downgrade its value by some 25%.

Ewes show no signs of illness, but may shiver in cold weather. Winter sheared sheep eat more than unsheared ewes if food is offered ad lib and ewes affected with wool slip eat considerably more again than other sheared sheep. This is obviously in response to cold stress, as in the effort to maintain a normal body temperature more energy is required from food.

The cause of wool slip is unclear. It was originally thought to be due to one of the skin parasites—lice or forage mites for example—but the problem arises in flocks where no external parasites can be identified on sheep. From recent studies it would seem more likely to be a stress-induced condition. Stress is difficult to define, but by measuring the level of certain

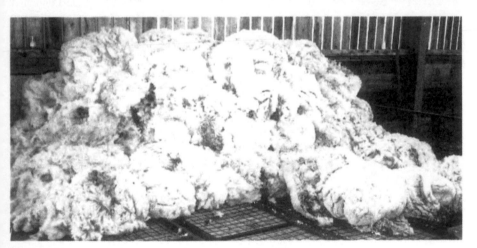

Plate 4.18 Wool slip reduces the value of the clip.

substances, such as cortisols, in the blood, it is possible to get a clue as to how stressed the sheep are. Products similar to the cortisols have been used in Australia to induce sheep to cast the fleece spontaneously, so doing away with the need to shear—so-called 'chemical shearing'. It is thought that stressing ewes by housing and then again by shearing some time later mimics the artificial technique of chemical shearing.

Prevention

In the absence of any other evidence to date, the advice for the prevention of wool slip is as follows:

- Do not winter shear if the flock lambs too early in the year, when the chance of poor weather at turnout is higher. As a general guide, in the north of Britain do not winter shear flocks which lamb before mid-April or in the south before late March.
- Make sure all ewes are in good body condition before housing. Feed a little concentrate (e.g. a quarter pound of mineralised barley) for a week or so beforehand if necessary.
- Try to house ewes during a spell of reasonable, dry weather and clip them immediately they are housed—do not wait for a week or 10 days.
- Do not shear any ewes in poor condition or any which are lame or unwell.
- Do not shear draft hill ewes which have never been housed before, since they are likely to be considerably stressed. These animals may also be unused to eating hard food and this will make them more likely to suffer from cold stress.
- Do not winter shear unless the sheep house is adequately draught-proofed at sheep level.
- Observe ewes carefully in the days following shearing and pull out any which are suffering excessively from the cold. Put them in a warmer place with plenty of bedding and/or provide them with a 'coat' made of sacking until the fleece has grown to a respectable length and/or the weather improves.
- Delay turning out shorn ewes and lambs until the weather is reasonable and choose a naturally sheltered, south-facing field and provide some artificial shelter such as straw bales.
- If the weather turns nasty after turnout, rehouse shorn ewes and their lambs for as long as necessary. If this is not possible, provide coats for the poorest ewes and extra shelter for the rest of the flock.
- Watch out for starving lambs caused by a drop in the ewe's milk yield in bad weather.

Because wool slip presents a welfare problem, serious consideration should be given to abandoning winter shearing if the above methods do not help in prevention.

DISEASE IN HOUSED FLOCKS

The risk of disease in indoor flocks should not deter any good flockmaster from trying the technique. A well-managed, healthy flock at pasture, brought into a good sheephouse after suitable pre-housing preparation, should stay healthy. Indeed, more ewes and lambs should survive after lambing than if the flock had not been housed.

However, if a flock already suffers from a number of disease problems—especially those of an infectious nature—then housing such a flock is likely to magnify the problems. The density of sheep in a house is very high as compared with even the highest stocking rates at pasture. The spread of infectious disease depends to a large degree upon the weight of infection in the environment, whether in the atmosphere (e.g. pneumonia), in bedding (e.g. footrot), in the feed or water supplies (e.g. scours) or by direct contact (e.g. lice). If one animal becomes ill, it is more likely that any infectious agent will spread more rapidly when the sick animal is in close contact with its pen mates. Infection may spread into adjoining pens, or even into adjoining houses, should it be a particularly infectious microorganism.

There are no diseases which are specifically confined to housed sheep. Those listed in the quick reference chart below are the ones most likely to occur or to give rise to particular problems in housed flocks. They are all discussed elsewhere in this book and the reader should consult the index for detailed references. The list is not comprehensive, and from time to time individual farms may experience disease problems not mentioned here.

Sheep which are unwell from whatever cause should be promptly segregated from the rest of the flock and housed in a separate building until they are fully recovered. Examples would be sheep suffering from footrot, eye infections or lice infestations. The stress of housing may precipitate latent infections, so that a close watch on the flock is necessary, particularly in the early days following housing.

QUICK REFERENCE CHART

Disease problems associated with housed sheep

ABORTION

- Immediately identify and isolate offending ewes.
- Search for aborted foetuses and membranes in bedding and remove safely. Beware of the risk of human infection.
- Supply copious amounts of straw bedding to bury any infectious discharges.
- Watch for and act swiftly on any further cases.

- If enzootic (chlamydial) abortion (EAE) disease is present, discuss the implications with your veterinary surgeon before taking the decision to house the flock overwinter. (Vaccination will be necessary and should be given before mating.)

FOOTROT

- Reduce the level of infection in the flock by the usual methods before housing. Any cases which are still active at housing should be segregated and treated. They should not be allowed to rejoin the flock until they are completely free from infection.
- Ewes already on a footrot vaccination scheme should receive a booster dose before housing. Flocks not vaccinating should consider this option early enough to allow time for the primary and secondary doses (four to six weeks apart) to be given in advance of housing.
- Maintain freedom from footrot by regular footbathing throughout the housed period.
- Ensure a dry bed with adequate straw to keep feet dry and clean. Slaked lime spread on the floor will help dry and sterilise the bedding and reduce the risk of spread.

LICE AND OTHER ECTOPARASITES

- Pour-on pyrethroid products are safe and easy to apply and are ideal for use where sheep are to be housed. Treat all ewes before housing. The residual effect may last for the whole of the housed period in many cases.

WOOL SLIP

- See discussion in text earlier in this Chapter.

WORMS (PARASITIC GASTRO-ENTERITIS)

- Ewes should be allowed to settle down after the stress of housing and then treated for worms with a broad spectrum anthelmintic which will cope with inhibited larvae as well as adult worms. Clearing out the worm burden at this time will ensure a better milk supply and reduce pasture contamination for lambs when ewes are turned-out after lambing. (Ewes wormed shortly after housing should not require a repeat dose immediately before turn out with their lambs, as they do not normally pick up infection indoors unless they are turned out onto a paddock by day.)

LIVER FLUKE

- Ewes should be dosed to ensure freedom from fluke infestation on infected farms. This dose can be combined with that for worms (see above).

PNEUMONIA

- Ensure adequate ventilation.
- Avoid overstocking the shed and keeping too many ewes or lambs in a single pen.
- Provide ample trough space.
- If pasteurella pneumonia has proved to be problematical in the past, an extra booster vaccination pre-housing should be employed.
- In outbreaks where poor housing conditions would seem to be the main predisposing cause, the flock may have to be turned outdoors if the faults cannot be rectified.

EYE INFECTIONS AND FACIAL DERMATITIS

- Segregate and treat.
- Increase trough space, as this is where these diseases spread through close head contact.

LISTERIOSIS

- Avoid feeding unfit silage to ewes. Change to hay if there is no alternative.
- Look for early signs of the disease in the rest of the flock and treat promptly on veterinary instructions.

PREGNANCY TOXAEMIA AND HYPOCALCAEMIA

- Ensure that ewes are in good condition at housing and group them in such a way that all in a pen require the same rations.
- Provide an adequate diet with a suitable roughage to concentrate ratio in late pregnancy. Avoid sudden dietary changes.
- The ration should have an acceptable calcium to phosphorous ratio (1:1 to 2:1) and vitamin, mineral and trace element content.
- Provide adequate trough space to ensure all ewes can get their fair share of concentrates. Watch for shy and greedy feeders.
- Water supplies should be clean and wholesome and kept unfrozen during frosty weather.
- Minimise handlings in late pregnancy. If these are necessary, ewes should be handled with care and not deprived of food and water for hours on end.

COPPER POISONING

- Never supplement ewe concentrates with copper or feed products formulated for other species which may contain too much copper.
- Do not provide any mineral mixes or licks which contain copper.

167

- Do not drench, dose, inject or otherwise provide copper to ewes without first checking on their copper status through blood samples sent to the veterinary investigation laboratory.
- Be aware of breed differences in susceptibility to copper poisoning (e.g. Suffolks and Texels are more susceptible and may require specially formulated low copper concentrates when housed overwinter).
- Avoid periods of food or water deprivation.

MASTITIS

- Provide a dry lie and hygienic conditions for ewes kept indoors by the liberal use of clean straw bedding, so that the udder is kept clean and dry.
- Check the udder for mastitis, making sure that hands are thoroughly clean before drawing colostrum from the teats.
- Segregate any ewe with mastitis.
- Where orf is present in the flock, discuss the use of the vaccine with your veterinary surgeon. Orf lesions (see below) on the teats of ewes often predispose to mastitis.
- Do not lamb ewes in pens where a previous occupant has had mastitis or some other infectious disease, without thorough disinfection and the provision of ample straw bedding.
- Do not turn housed ewes and lambs outside in bad weather.

METRITIS

- Provide hygienic conditions for ewes to lamb down in.
- Do not interfere with any lambing ewe unnecessarily.
- Observe scrupulous cleanliness before inserting a hand or implement (such as a lambing aid or rope) inside a ewe.
- Always provide antibiotic cover by injection and/or pessaries after examining any ewe at lambing.
- Ensure ewes are boosted with a combined clostridial vaccine pre-lambing.
- Segregate any ewe which develops metritis in a comfortable hospital area.

ORF

- Do not vaccinate against orf in flocks which are free from this disease.
- Where vaccination is advocated, vaccinate ewes well before lambing (e.g. two months).
- Try to lamb ewes down in a different area from where they were vaccinated.
- If ewes have to lamb down in the area where they were vaccinated, use copious bedding; otherwise lambs may contract the disease from the scabs which fall off the ewes following vaccination.

NEONATAL INFECTIONS OF LAMBS

- Vaccination of ewes pre-lambing with a booster against the clostridial diseases is essential.
- Ensure immediate and adequate colostrum intake for all newborn lambs.
- Stomach tube 'at-risk' lambs with colostrum where necessary.
- Have an adequate supply of colostrum available, stored in small containers.
- Provide hygienic conditions for lambs to be born into.
- Dip navels in tincture of iodine immediately after birth.
- Divide the flock into small groups according to lambing date so that a penful of ewes will lamb down over a relatively short period, thus minimising any build-up of infection.
- Segregate any sick lambs, together with their ewes, in a hospital area.

NB Hypothermia can and does affect indoor lambs.

UROLITHIASIS

- Do not castrate ram lambs if unnecessary.
- Ensure the diet has an appropriate calcium to phosphorus ratio.
- Ensure diets have a low magnesium content.
- Supply good-quality hay to stimulate salivation.
- Add 2 to 3% common salt to the concentrate ration to encourage drinking.
- Ensure that clean, fresh water is freely available (unfrozen) at all times.

5
ABORTION

An abortion is the expulsion by the ewe of one or more foetal lambs before the end of a normal term of pregnancy. Lambs may either be born dead or perish within a few hours. Abortions occur in most flocks from time to time, but should normally be rare and isolated events. If an infectious organism causes abortions in a flock which has not had previous or recent experience of that particular microorganism, then the result can be disastrous, with up to as many as a third or a half of the ewes aborting their lambs. Fortunately these abortion 'storms' are relatively uncommon events and usually occur after the introduction of breeding females purchased from an infected flock. They are probably the most demoralising problem shepherds have to face and one of the most difficult to deal with. Abortion also costs the sheep industry a great deal of money.

The infectious causes of abortion are by far the most important to the sheep farmer, but there are other, non-infectious reasons why ewes may slip their lambs. For example, twin lamb disease (pregnancy toxaemia)—due to problems with feeding in late pregnancy—may cause the death of lambs or the birth of premature lambs which die shortly afterwards. Mishandling of ewes and other events which stress or fatigue them may lead to abortion, although this is often subjective and difficult to substantiate. Certain chemicals and plant poisons may damage the foetal lamb sufficiently to cause its death and abortion. Some drugs used routinely in sheep husbandry, such as certain anthelmintics ('wormers'), may cause problems during pregnancy, especially if ewes are overdosed. Always think twice before medicating ewes at this time and if in doubt consult your veterinary surgeon.

THE RISK OF HUMAN INFECTION

At this juncture it is important to point out that a number of the infectious microorganisms which cause abortion in sheep are also infectious to humans. The two most commonly diagnosed types of abortion are enzootic abortion (EAE) and toxoplasmosis, both of which present a serious risk to pregnant women in particular.

In a number of recent cases, women who have become infected with enzootic abortion have lost their babies and themselves become seriously

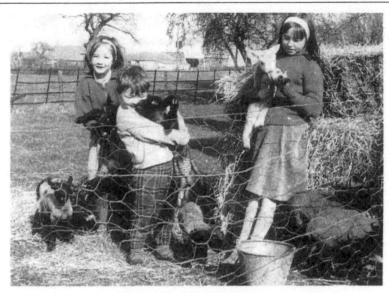

Plate 5.1 Young children should not be allowed to help at lambing time because of the risk of infection through aborting ewes and scouring lambs. Older children should be provided with protective clothing and taught good hygiene practice.

ill, requiring hospital treatment in the intensive care unit. Toxoplasmosis is also a risk, and where it is diagnosed or suspected, a pregnant woman in contact with a flock should inform her doctor and request a blood test for toxoplasmosis as early as possible. If infection with toxoplasma occurs during the woman's pregnancy, then depending upon the stage of gestation, the doctor may ask the woman to consider a termination, since the risk of foetal damage is very considerable. Toxoplasmosis can also be picked up from eating undercooked meat and from an environment contaminated by cat faeces (see below).

Since it is not possible to say which infection is present in a flock without laboratory examination and since a proportion of infected ewes go to full term and produce apparently normal lambs, it is therefore most important that **pregnant women and women of child bearing age who may be pregnant should not be involved with the lambing flock.**

Reducing the risk of human infection

Human infection is not confined to pregnant women, however, and a few guidelines will be helpful on how to minimise the risk of human infection:

- Treat every abortion as if it is infectious and transmissible to humans.
- Wear rubber or plastic gloves when handling aborted ewes or when collecting dead lambs and afterbirths.

172

- Dispose of gloves by burning after using only once.
- Wash hands and arms thoroughly after assisting with **any** lambing.
- **Never give the kiss of life to any lamb,** since weakly lambs are always suspect and a proportion of apparently normal lambs may also be infected.
- As well as pregnant women, **young children should be kept away from lambing ewes and newborn lambs** and should be discouraged from cuddling lambs of any age near their faces. They should also be encouraged to wash their hands after handling any animal.
- Any signs of illness in humans around lambing time—particularly where an infectious abortion known to be transmissible to humans is present in the flock—should be **reported to your doctor without delay. Make him or her aware of any infection amongst the ewes or lambs.**

Whilst there is no reason to become obsessive about the dangers of the lambing shed or paddock, they are real and anyone being asked to work there is entitled to be fully informed of the risks and given every encouragement to take avoiding action.

Apart from enzootic abortion and toxoplasmosis, other infectious abortions of sheep in the UK which are transmissible from sheep to humans (zoonoses) are:

- campylobacteriosis (vibriosis)
- salmonellosis
- listeriosis
- Q-fever (caused by *Coxiella burnetti*)

Notes on these and other infections appear later in this chapter.

WHAT TO DO WHEN ABORTIONS OCCUR

The most important thing for the shepherd to know is what to do if abortions occur in the flock. **The golden rule is always to assume that the cause is infectious and to act immediately:**

- **Isolate aborted ewe(s)** and tag or otherwise mark them permanently for future identification. Keep them separate from the rest of the flock for at least a month.
- **Remove aborted lambs and afterbirths from the lambing area,** but keep them in a clean plastic bag for diagnosis at a laboratory.
- **Wash your hands thoroughly.**
- **Contact your veterinary surgeon** for advice on what to do next.

Constant vigilance is crucial, so that ewes which look as though they may be going to lamb early, those with blood-stained rear ends and freshly aborted sheep can be identified. Most infectious organisms causing abortion infect ewes by mouth. Aborted lambs, placentae and fluids which the ewe expels

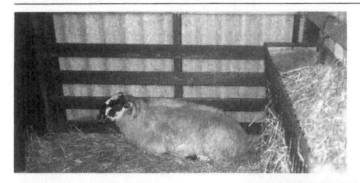

Plate 5.2   Ewes which abort
should be isolated immediately
(*above*) and identified so that they
can be blood sampled (*right*) at a
later date if necessary.

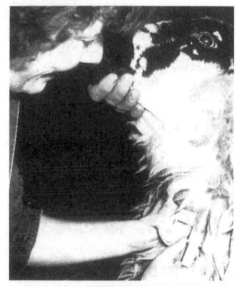

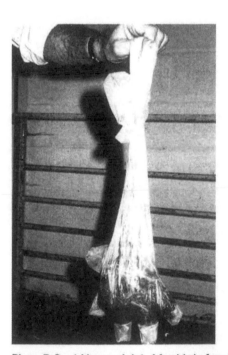

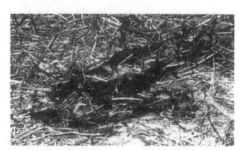

Plate 5.3   (*Above right*) Afterbirth from an abortion. This material plus dead
foetuses should be saved for diagnosis. (*Above left*) Wear an arm-length, strong
plastic sleeve-glove, pick up the infected material, roll the sleeve down your arm
and thus enclose the material without touching it.

for some days or weeks following abortion are often highly infectious. It is most important therefore that the remaining ewes in the flock are isolated from these sources of infection immediately. Whether the ewes which have aborted are removed from the rest of the flock or vice versa will depend upon particular circumstances.

At pasture

Where sheep are at pasture when abortions occur it is often difficult to find the products of any abortions or to relate those abortions to the correct ewes, especially if the flock has a large area to graze over. There is, of course, less risk of other ewes coming across infectious material in these circumstances, but a search should be made nonetheless. At higher stocking rates, such as in small lambing paddocks, the risks are significantly increased and a real effort should be made to find the materials and remove them. Some shepherds wisely dig over the area where dead lambs and afterbirths have been found. If other paddocks are available, the ewes yet to lamb can be moved onto clean ground, but further abortions may still occur, so contaminating the new area.

Indoors

In housed flocks, the risk of other ewes becoming infected increases very considerably. The area of straw bedding where the products of abortion are found should be removed and burned and the offending ewe removed to an isolation area. If there is no alternative area for remaining ewes to lamb in, then the whole area should be very liberally bedded down with fresh straw. Where concreted areas are used, the area should be thoroughly cleaned out and washed down with a MAFF recommended disinfectant before fresh bedding is put down. If abortion takes place in an individual lambing pen, this should not be used for other lambing ewes, or else a special effort should be made to clean it up and bed it down.

DISCOVERING THE CAUSES OF ABORTION

The next thing to do is to obtain a diagnosis, which is based on laboratory examination of the aborted lambs and afterbirths. Blood samples from aborted ewes will also be helpful, even some time after the event, hence the reason for permanently identifying ewes which abort or are abortion suspects. Roughly half the samples submitted to the laboratory do not yield a diagnosis. This may be because of one or more of the following reasons:

- the samples are grossly contaminated with bedding or faeces
- the samples have begun to decompose
- there is insufficient material submitted
- the wrong samples are sent
- the abortions are caused by something other than an infectious agent or by an agent not routinely screened for

175

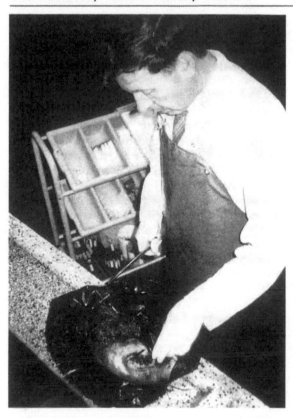

Plate 5.4 A senior veterinary investigation officer examining an aborted foetus and membranes sent in from a farm outbreak. Laboratory examination is essential for an accurate diagnosis. Note that the officer is wearing rubber gloves and a heavy rubber apron over a white laboratory coat to protect against infection.

Apart from samples, your veterinary surgeon will need additional information about the flock and its management to help in arriving at a diagnosis, for example:

- type and size of flock (e.g. hill or lowland—any common grazings)
- management policy (e.g. at pasture or winter housed; 'closed', 'open' or 'flying' flock)
- feeding regime (e.g. source of ingredients for home mixed concentrates and when fed)
- whether female replacements are home bred or purchased (age and source)
- history of abortion in the flock in previous years
- whether enzootic abortion vaccine is used, the frequency of vaccination and the age groups vaccinated
- record of any medicaments which have been used (e.g. monensin feeding for toxoplasmosis or oxytetracycline injections for enzootic abortion)
- predicted start and finish of lambing
- number of abortions to date and in which age group of sheep
- stage of pregnancy when abortions occurred and whether ewes were ill post-abortion

It is quite possible for there to be two or more microorganisms causing abortions in a flock, especially where female breeding replacements are purchased. It is even possible for an individual ewe to become infected by more than one abortion agent at the same time. It is therefore unwise to assume that the results of the first laboratory examination will apply to all abortions which may follow. For example, if the laboratory confirms that toxoplasmosis is present, it does not mean that the next abortion will also be toxoplasmosis—it may be due to enzootic abortion or any of the other possibilities. If the first samples are negative, this does not necessarily mean that there is no infection present in the flock.

Since the future management of the flock will depend on which infection or infections are present, it is essential to continue investigating cases in an outbreak. As a general rule, if more than about one in 50 ewes aborts it is likely to be an infectious agent. At the start of an outbreak it is best to examine material from all aborted ewes to give the laboratory a good chance of identifying the agent or agents and, if abortions continue, your veterinary surgeon may suggest sending samples from one in every four or five. You should **mark every aborting ewe**, so that they can all be blood sampled when the outbreak has subsided or lambing has finished.

WHAT TO DO WITH ABORTED EWES

Generally speaking, ewes which have aborted should be retained in the flock since they will usually be immune to the infection from which they aborted and are therefore unlikely to abort again from that particular infection. However, it does not mean that they will not abort the following year or in a subsequent year from a different infection. There is no such thing as immunity to abortion, only to specific infections.

Aborted ewes must not be used as foster mothers for female lambs which could be retained or sold as breeding replacements, until your veterinary surgeon can assure you that abortion was not due to enzootic abortion. This is because the infection will almost certainly be passed on to the lambs, some of which may then abort when they lamb down as ewe lambs or gimmers.

What the farmer does after a diagnosis has been made will depend on the infection or infections present in the flock. Some of the more important ones will now be described before general and specific control measures are discussed.

Enzootic Abortion of Ewes (EAE)

Enzootic abortion of ewes (EAE) or kebbing is the most commonly diagnosed infectious abortion of sheep in the UK and one of the most problematic. Like most infectious diseases it is more troublesome in lowland, intensively kept and housed flocks, where ewes are concentrated together over the lambing period. The products of abortion are very heavily contaminated with the causal microorganism, so that there is ample opportunity for spread. Ewes become infected by ingesting infected material when they sniff or lick at material deposited by their aborted flock mates, or when they eat concentrates or drink water contaminated by the fluids discharged by ewes. Venereal contact—from ram to ewe or vice versa at mating—is not thought to play any significant role in the spread of EAE although it is theoretically possible.

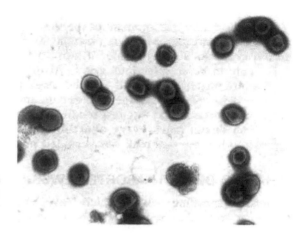

Plate 5.5 *Chlamydia psittaci*—the bacterium responsible for enzootic abortion of ewes (EAE), seen here magnified 20,000 times via the transmission electron microscope.

The microorganism responsible for this infection—*Chlamydia psittaci* (*C. psittaci*)—is a bacterium. It was discovered by workers at the Moredun Research Institute and the Veterinary Investigation Service in Edinburgh in 1950, although the infectious nature of EAE had been known long before this time. The disease is diagnosed in the laboratory by identifying the organism from infected afterbirth. Blood sampling will also give helpful information, but as this is not a foolproof method of diagnosis, it is important to get freshly aborted lambs and uncontaminated samples of afterbirths to the laboratory as soon as practicable.

The vast majority of cases of EAE take place within the last fortnight of pregnancy. Because lambing is spread over several weeks in most flocks, this usually means that a high proportion of abortions will occur either during lambing itself or in the period immediately before, when ewes have been gathered together. Therefore the opportunity for spread of infection is ideal.

In hill flocks the disease is uncommon, mainly because such flocks are usually self-contained or 'closed', breeding their own female replacements and buying in only rams. Also, hill ewes are spread thinly over the grazings, so if infection should be introduced, it is unlikely to be as devastating as it can be in lowland flocks. However, should hill ewes be brought down off the high ground for lambing and put into enclosures or in-bye parks or fields where earlier lambings have occurred, then the risks are obviously increased.

ABORTION 'STORMS'

In unvaccinated flocks which have not previously encountered enzootic abortion, ewes are particularly susceptible to infection because they have no immunity. If breeding females purchased from an EAE-infected flock are allowed to lamb down along with the 'clean' home flock, there may be a few cases of enzootic abortion. The shepherd may well be caught unawares by the first abortions, because they happen 'silently', usually without the ewes showing any signs that they are likely to abort. If shepherds have not experienced an EAE outbreak before, a few premature births or the births of normal term but weakly lambs may not alert them, especially when these are not accompanied by any abortions.

Often there are no EAE abortions amongst the home flock during the first season. Infection is likely to spread from the infected purchased ewes to the home flock around lambing time, despite the vigilance of the shepherd in isolating aborted ewes and their products. These freshly infected ewes will harbour the microorganisms until they become pregnant the following year. The disease will then take-off and cause abortions, premature births and stillbirths in all ages of ewes, apart from first-time lambers which have not been through the lambing quarters previously. As many as a third or more of the ewe flock may abort and this is called an abortion 'storm'.

CHRONIC INFECTION

In subsequent years the pattern of infection in a flock will depend upon what action is taken. If no control measures are implemented, then roughly one in 10 or 20 of the ewe flock will abort each subsequent year. Most of these will be second lambers which became infected in the lambing area during their first lambing season. Most first lambers will not abort because they have usually had no previous exposure to infection. Any newborn ewe lambs surviving out of EAE infected ewes will be infected and will harbour the infection until they become pregnant for the first time as ewe lambs or gimmers, when a proportion of them will abort. The same applies to any ewe lambs fostered onto aborted ewes.

The reason for the year's delay between infection and abortion is that the infection does not normally become established in the pregnant uterus until the last two months of pregnancy. It then takes some five or six weeks for sufficient damage to be done to the placenta to produce abortion. As infection normally occurs during or just prior to lambing, there is usually insufficient time for this process to take place before lambing in most ewes. However, if some of the earliest lambing ewes abort and late lambing ewes become infected, then in flocks with a protracted lambing there may be sufficient time for abortion to occur during the same season.

The infection causes damage particularly to the 'buttons' (placentomes) on the placenta (see Colour plate 16) but does relatively little direct damage to the lambs. At abortion, whilst the afterbirths can be thickened and discoloured, any dead lambs appear fresh. The ewes are apparently unaffected by the infection and only rarely become ill. If they do it is usually due to secondary complications such as retention of the afterbirth. However, ewes do discharge highly infectious fluid from the vulva for up to a month or more after abortion. This can often be seen staining the fleece.

CONTROL AND PREVENTION

This is a problem and generally a compromise. If a flock is free from EAE, then every effort should be made to keep it free. Once a flock becomes infected it will usually remain so and control measures will be required ad infinitum. If breeding stock is sold, enzootic abortion-free accredited status should be worth a premium, and consideration should be given to joining the Scottish Veterinary Investigation Service's Premium Sheep Health Scheme or the ADAS Sheep and Goat Health Scheme. These are monitoring schemes whose aim is to identify sheep flocks free from EAE (and other diseases in the case of the ADAS Scheme). If females must be bought from flocks where the disease status is unknown, it is always wise to buy females which have never bred and are therefore unlikely to have been through a lambing area except when they were born.

When EAE occurs for the first time in a flock, especially when confined to an isolated group of purchased ewes, culling those ewes may be considered, although aborted ewes will not abort again from EAE, nor should they shed the organisms at any subsequent lambing. However, infected ewes which do not abort during the current lambing may do so during their next pregnancy, or may shed infection at an apparently normal lambing.

Limiting the damages with antibiotics

Where infected purchased ewes are lambed amongst the home flock it is inevitable that infection will spread and that many of the home-bred ewes will abort at the following lambing. It is possible to reduce these losses by injecting all ewes with a suitable long-acting antibiotic, such as oxytetracycline, on at least two occasions some two to three weeks apart at around six weeks and three weeks before the first ewes are due to lamb. The dose may need to be repeated for later lambing ewes in a long drawn-out lambing. The drug does not eliminate the bacteria but slows down its multiplication, so limiting the damage. More ewes should go through to lamb 'normally' (although they are still infected) and more live lambs should be born in the flock. This is quite an expensive exercise, but can be cost effective if enough lambs are saved.

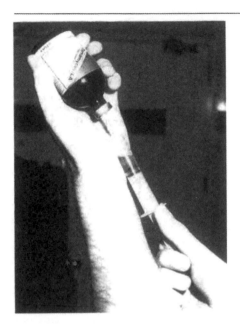

Plate 5.6 Long-acting oxytetracycline may be injected into ewes expected to abort at around six and three weeks before lambing.

This same approach can be used in the face of an outbreak of enzootic abortion, by injecting all the ewes which have yet to lamb in the hope of keeping them going until normal term. It should be appreciated, however, that in either of these circumstances some damage to the placenta will already have occurred and it is therefore inevitable that a proportion of ewes will still abort or produce stillborn, premature or weakly lambs at normal term.

Vaccination

A vaccine is available—Ovine Enzootic Abortion Vaccine (Coopers Pitman-Moore)—based on the original Moredun vaccine of the 1950s. Until about 1980 it gave excellent protection, but in recent years a number of break-downs have occurred. It would appear that part of the problem is that new strains of the chlamydial organism have become more widely established since the vaccine was first introduced. One of these new strains has now been incorporated into a modified vaccine and work is progressing to improve the product further. Nevertheless, vaccination can give a useful degree of protection in most flocks and is a valuable tool in the control of the disease.

Lowland commercial farms which run 'closed' flocks are rare and wherever breeding females are purchased from anything other than an accredited source of enzootic abortion-free sheep, the vaccine should probably be used. Vaccination is unnecessary in hill flocks which have never experienced the infection and which breed all their own female replacements.

181

In the year following an outbreak of EAE, all ages of breeding females should be at least vaccinated a month before tupping. It should be appreciated that vaccinating sheep which have already been infected at the previous lambing will not necessarily prevent all ewes from aborting or from producing stillborn or weakly lambs. If the vaccine is given long after tupping, then there is always a risk that chlamydia already harboured within the sheep will have invaded the tiny placenta of a new pregnancy before the vaccine has had time to protect.

The vaccine should protect ewes for two to three years and possibly for their full breeding life, providing the challenge is not overwhelming. After the first year only the replacement females — both home bred and purchased — need to be vaccinated. Live lambs which are to be bred in the autumn of their first year must be vaccinated before they are tupped. However, although the manufacturer recommends revaccination after three years, it is probably wise to vaccinate annually in flocks where there is a heavy challenge.

Remember that vaccination will not prevent all abortions and that some ewes which lamb normally may still be infected. However, it should reduce the abortions to around 2 to 3% and keep it within these manageable proportions for as long as it is used.

Readers are referred to Technical Notes T144, T187, and T189 published by the Scottish Agricultural Colleges for guidance on the economics of the control, prevention and replacement policy options for EAE.

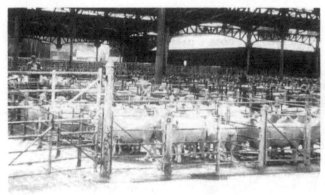

Plate 5.7 Purchasing breeding ewes through a market or from farms of unknown disease status carries a high risk. Vaccination against EAE—for both the home flock and any purchased ewes— is a wise precaution.

Toxoplasma Abortion

Toxoplasmosis is the second most commonly diagnosed abortion of sheep in the UK after enzootic abortion and is just as difficult to control, but for very different reasons. The disease is caused by a protozoan parasite called *Toxoplasma gondii*, which can infect any warm-blooded animal, including humans. Probably around half the sheep population of the UK have been infected with this parasite and thereafter are immune for life. The infection will normally go completely unnoticed in non-pregnant animals, since sheep are rarely ill enough to attract the shepherd's attention.

Infection during pregnancy

However, the problem arises when ewes become infected for the first time during pregnancy and the sequence of events depends upon the stage of gestation when the infection occurs. During the first two months of pregnancy, toxoplasma will kill the embryo or foetus. As the developing lambs are so small at this time, these events will go unnoticed by the shepherd. Ewes will either return to the ram, or if the rams have been removed, they will remain barren. Toxoplasmosis is a widespread infection and is probably a relatively frequent cause of above average barrenness in flocks.

Should ewes become infected during the third and fourth months of pregnancy, then the foetuses may die and become mummified—that is, they shrivel up and become shrouded by the placenta or afterbirth. These may be aborted or they may remain in the uterus until full term. Some ewes may produce dead lambs approximately a week early, whilst others may produce stillborn lambs at full term. Lambs may also be born alive, but small and weak, and, not surprisingly, many of these perish due to starvation, hypothermia or other neonatal problems. Quite often a live lamb will be born alongside a mummified litter-mate.

Ewes infected during the last month of pregnancy will probably lamb normally and the lambs will generally survive but are nevertheless infected. In this case both the ewe and her lambs are thereafter immune to toxoplasma for life.

In an outbreak of toxoplasma abortion, as many as a quarter of the ewes may abort or give birth to stillborn or weakly lambs and there may be further losses due to barrenness. As with any abortion, ewes should be isolated and the dead foetuses and afterbirths handled with care. Toxoplasma infected afterbirths often have small white spots on the 'buttons' but samples must go to the laboratory for confirmation (see Colour plate 17).

CATS AND THE SPREAD OF TOXOPLASMOSIS

It is the domestic or farm cat which is mainly responsible for the spread of this disease amongst sheep. Whilst toxoplasma can infect most animals, it is only in the cat family that the parasite has a unique method of multiplying, during which it produces enormous numbers of highly infectious oocysts (eggs) which are shed in the faeces. Cats become infected themselves by eating toxoplasma-infected rats and mice, although the rodents themselves pose no direct threat to sheep. Young cats are generally not infected until they start hunting. A few days after they catch their first toxoplasma-infected mouse they become off-colour, run a temperature and may suffer from

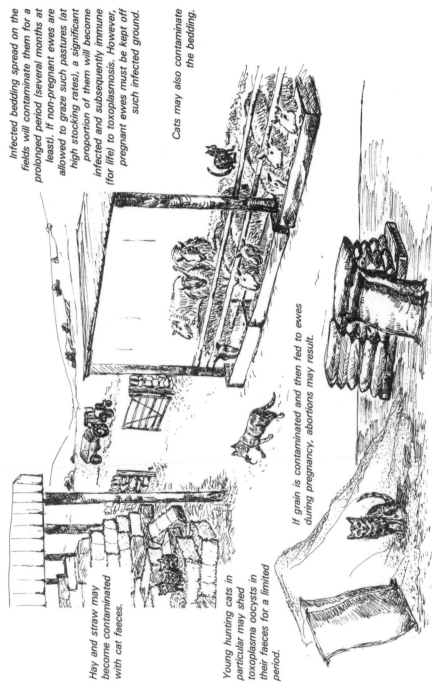

Infected bedding spread on the fields will contaminate them for a prolonged period (several months at least). If non-pregnant ewes are allowed to graze such pastures (at high stocking rates), a significant proportion of them will become infected and subsequently immune (for life) to toxoplasmosis. However, pregnant ewes must be kept off such infected ground.

Cats may also contaminate the bedding.

Hay and straw may become contaminated with cat faeces.

Young hunting cats in particular may shed toxoplasma oocysts in their faeces for a limited period.

If grain is contaminated and then fed to ewes during pregnancy, abortions may result.

Figure 5.1   How cats contribute to the spread of toxoplasmosis in a sheep flock.

mild diarrhoea. For a period of a week to 10 days their faeces are highly infectious—not only to sheep but to any other animal, including man. They may excrete over 200 million oocysts during that time and it only takes a few hundred oocysts to infect a sheep.

Feedstuffs contaminated with cat faeces

Cats, being cats, like to defaecate in comfort and there is nothing they enjoy more than to dig amongst a pile of grain or to settle down amongst the hay or find a nice dry corner in a sheep shed or cattle court. Being creatures of habit they may go back again and again and if there is a litter of young cats they can very soon contaminate an area very heavily. The faeces dry and break up and if deposited in grain they may be incorporated into a home mixed ration to be fed to ewes during late pregnancy. Contaminated hay may be fed at a much earlier stage of pregnancy. Where ewes are housed over-winter, they may also pick up infection from contaminated bedding. Dung contaminated with cat faeces from sheep sheds and cattle courts which is spread onto pastures will disseminate the oocysts far and wide. Oocysts are very tough and can survive for very many months in buildings or on pastures.

Cats, like sheep, become immune to toxoplasmosis after their initial infection and stop shedding oocysts in any appreciable numbers. Adult cats, therefore, do not pose a serious threat to the flock unless they become sick, when they may again excrete large numbers of oocysts.

HUMAN INFECTION

It is estimated that roughly half the UK human population has met toxoplasma by middle age. Fortunately, in most people it is a mild or inapparent infection. However, as with enzootic abortion, **pregnant women are**

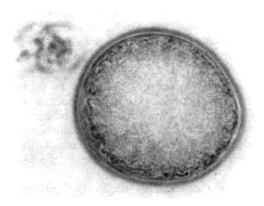

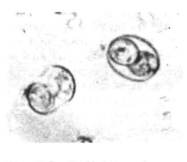

Plate 5.8   (*Left*) A toxoplasma tissue cyst (under high power magnification). These are a source of infection to humans from eating improperly cooked meat. (*Above right*) Toxoplasma oocysts from infected cat faeces. It is this form of the parasite that contaminates feedstuffs.

185

a high risk group and a proportion of them will pass the infection to their unborn baby. This may result in abortion, stillbirth or a number of distressing conditions such as hydrocephalus, epilepsy, eye defects and brain damage. Some of these conditions may not become apparent in the child for years.

The most likely sources of infection for humans are as follows:

- Areas contaminated with cat faeces containing oocysts, such as gardens, children's sandpits or barns.
- The handling of uncooked meat or eating of undercooked meat. Sheep meat and pork are potentially the most dangerous, as they most frequently contain tissue cysts of the toxoplasma parasite.
- The handling of sick animals suffering from a generalised toxoplasma infection.

CONTROL OF TOXOPLASMOSIS

Control of toxoplasma abortion in sheep is problematical. As there is at present no vaccine available in the UK, the sheep farmer must take advantage of the life-long immunity which follows natural infection. In infected flocks, aborted ewes should be retained since they will not abort from toxoplasma again. Between the end of lambing and well before the next tupping, an attempt should be made to infect as many ewes as possible, since infection during non-pregnancy will stimulate immunity and so prevent abortions, stillbirths and the birth of weakly lambs. This is a rather hit and miss affair and will only be partially successful at best.

Since cat faeces is the source of infection, sheep should be exposed to areas thought to be contaminated. Bedding from yards where cats defaecate can be spread on small fields and then ewes grazed over them at a high stocking rate in the hope that they will pick up infectious oocysts in sufficient numbers to protect them. This does, however, contaminate the area for a long time, and care must be taken not to graze pregnant ewes over this ground. Any ewe hoggs, gimmers or bought-in breeding females should likewise be exposed to infection.

On farms where the toxoplasma is already present and also in clean flocks where the disease has never been encountered, it is important to make every effort to protect ewes from infection throughout the whole of pregnancy. This is easier said than done, but it is possible to reduce the risks. Feed stores for concentrate rations should be kept shut to cats. Grain silos must be cat-proof so that they cannot bury their faeces in the corn when the ground outside is frosted.

It is difficult to see how cats can be kept out of most conventional hay barns, but sheep hay could be kept in a cat-proof building on some farms. Keeping cats out of the sheep shed is another matter altogether, but generous straw bedding will help to bury infection. On clean farms, cats should be discouraged from taking up residence or their breeding should be kept under control by castrating toms and spaying queens.

Control of toxoplasmosis by medication

When an outbreak of toxoplasmosis occurs in a flock, there is little that can be done to minimise the losses. However, it is possible to medicate ewes to reduce the losses in subsequent seasons. Work at the Moredun Research Institute in Edinburgh has shown that monensin—a coccidiostat and growth promoter (Romensin, Elanco Products Ltd)—can substantially reduce the number of abortions, stillbirths and weakly lambs when fed to ewes during the second half of pregnancy. Infected ewes treated with monensin may also produce heavier lambs at birth than untreated infected ewes.

Monensin is not licensed for use in sheep, but your veterinary surgeon can prescribe it for this particular therapeutic purpose and will advise you on the dosage and period of use. It is a toxic substance if fed at too high a level, so accurate and thorough mixing of the medication with feed rations is important. It is particularly poisonous to horses, so medicated feed and the raw material should be kept in a safe place.

Monensin is somewhat unpalatable and care should be taken to see that ewes in the last third of pregnancy are not put off their concentrates, as this might predispose them to pregnancy toxaemia. The medication will be less effective if ewes became infected earlier in pregnancy before treatment, so some abortions and other problems may still arise.

Campylobacter Abortion

Campylobacter, or vibriosis as it used to be called, is a bacterial disease caused by *Campylobacter fetus*. It is usually (although not exclusively) introduced into a breeding flock via the purchase of infected carrier animals, which shed the bacterium in their faeces. Ewes are unlikely to abort if they become infected before mating or even during the first three months of pregnancy. However, infection in the last two months of pregnancy will usually result in abortion within two or three weeks of infection.

When the first ewe in a flock aborts, her dead lambs, placentae and discharges will heavily contaminate the area. Despite thorough cleaning up, it is inevitable that other ewes in the same area will become affected. Some will abort if they have more than a couple of weeks to go before lambing, and in a susceptible flock—one which has not experienced the disease previously—up to half the ewes may abort in the worst outbreaks. Great care must be taken by shepherds not to transmit infection from the infected isolation area back into the main lambing flock on their boots, hands or lambing equipment. The disease is also highly infectious to humans, in whom it causes an unpleasant diarrhoea—so beware!

Flocks which have previously been infected and which buy in female breeding replacements that have not met the disease on their farm of origin

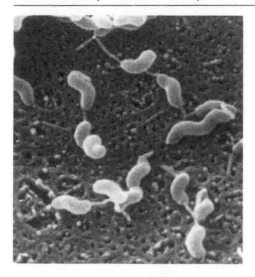

Plate 5.9 Campylobacter bacteria as seen using the scanning electron microscope, magnified 20,000 times.

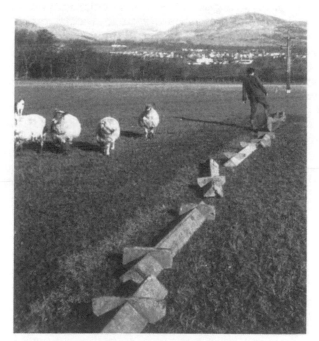

Plate 5.10 Feed troughs should be turned over to discourage birds and other creatures from soiling the area.

188

may experience minor outbreaks every few years amongst the 'newcomers' when they become infected through the faeces of carriers in the home flock. Sometimes campylobacter abortions occur on farms which maintain a closed flock and only buy in rams. However, there is no evidence that this infection can be passed on to the ewes by the ram at mating as there is with the same disease in cattle. It is known that wild animals and birds may become infected and shed the organism in their faeces. Little can be done about this, except to discourage them from feeding from sheep troughs by turning troughs over after the ewes have cleaned up and also by moving the troughs frequently to reduce local contamination of the area.

CONTROL

Once a diagnosis has been made in an outbreak, your veterinary surgeon may consider it worth treating ewes which are yet to lamb but have been in contact with aborting ewes. However, results can be disappointing following antibiotic treatment. This is one situation where the splitting of a flock into two or three separate lambing groups is most helpful in limiting the spread of infection.

There is no vaccine available in the UK to control the disease and since outbreaks do not tend to recur—because most ewes become immune—it is unlikely that one will ever be marketed.

Providing you are completely satisfied that there is no enzootic abortion (EAE) in the flock, ewes diagnosed as having aborted from campylobacter infection can be mixed with ewes which have already lambed, as well as with home-bred and bought-in replacement females. This will spread the infection amongst all non-pregnant breeding females and hopefully stimulate an immunity before the following pregnancy. Mixing must not take place during pregnancy and any bought-in sheep should always lamb in a separate group, since they may be infected with other agents capable of causing abortions, particularly EAE, which could prove disastrous. (Flocks adequately vaccinated against EAE can mix females with less degree of risk.)

Salmonella Abortion

A number of different species of salmonella bacteria may cause abortion in ewes. Outbreaks are relatively uncommon, which is fortunate since they can be most unpleasant. Ewes are often quite ill, either before or after abortion, and deaths are not uncommon. Salmonella is yet another microorganism which will readily infect humans, sometimes with serious results. Cattle, pigs, poultry and other domestic and wild animals can become affected with some of the strains which affect sheep and may occasionally be responsible for outbreaks of abortion in ewes—for example, where infected slurry or dung out of calf pens is spread on sheep ground. Contaminated water courses may also be responsible for spreading infection.

One particular salmonella, which appears to be largely confined to sheep—*Salmonella abortis ovis*—used to be one of the most common, unpleasant and difficult of ewe abortions to deal with, especially in the southwest of England. Fortunately, in recent years it appears to have declined to very low levels for reasons which are unclear.

As with most abortions, the main risk is from the products of abortion being licked or chewed by other ewes. Abortions usually occur in late pregnancy and ewes may develop diarrhoea and a fever. Some lambs are born alive, but are often sick and may die from salmonella blood poisoning, starvation, hypothermia or other diseases such as pneumonia. In an outbreak, antibiotic treatment of ewes which are ill and of all in-contact ewes may be considered, but it may not always be successful.

CONTROL

Following outbreaks of most strains of salmonella, affected ewes do not usually abort again from this cause, although some may become salmonella carriers. Purchased animals may therefore succumb to infection when meeting it for the first time on their new farm. Mixing aborted ewes with ewes which have already lambed and with any replacement females is sometimes practised where EAE is not present or where the flock is vaccinated against EAE.

As with campylobacter infection, feed troughs should be moved frequently and turned over to reduce contamination of the feeding area by wild birds which may carry salmonella infection. If cattle or other species on the farm are known to be infected with salmonella, mixed grazing should be avoided, infected slurry should not be spread on sheep grazings and contamination of water courses should be avoided. (Piped trough water is always safer for grazing stock where this is feasible.) Early, mid and late lambing groups, grazed or housed in separate areas, can be a great help in containing an outbreak, especially when combined with good hygiene practice.

No specific sheep vaccines are available, but your vet may advise the use of pig salmonella vaccines which may give some protection in an emergency situation.

Listeriosis

Listeriosis is a bacterial disease of sheep which may cause abortion, a generalised infection (septicaemia) or inflammation of the brain (encephalitis). Outbreaks of listeriosis have increased in recent years and frequently appear to be associated with the feeding of poorly made or spoiled silage, in which these bacteria can readily multiply. Ewes eating such contaminated silage may abort during the last six or eight weeks of pregnancy. Some ewes may experience difficulty at lambing (dystocia) and become very sick due to an inflammation of the uterus (metritis). Treatment of sick, aborted ewes with antibiotics is not very rewarding and mass treatment of ewes which are as yet to lamb is unjustified, since usually only occasional cases occur rather than outbreaks. Aborted ewes should always be isolated and the products of abortion removed. Prevention depends upon avoiding feeding ewes silage likely to pose a risk.

Listeriosis is yet another zoonosis. Although most human cases arise from sources other than sheep, there is nevertheless a risk from handling the products of abortion, infected animals or contaminated silage, and care with personal hygiene is a wise precaution. Organisms can also be shed in the milk of infected ewes and this presents a public health risk from the consumption of cheeses and yoghurts.

The other forms of listeriosis are discussed in Chapter 6.

Border Disease

Border disease was first recognised in flocks in the English/Welsh Border region—hence its name. It is caused by a virus (border disease virus—BDV) which is usually brought into the flock with persistently infected sheep, such as rams or gimmers purchased at the autumn sales as breeding replacements. Ewes which become infected when they are not pregnant will suffer only a very mild illness which the shepherd is unlikely to detect. The problems arise when infection takes place during pregnancy and the outcome will depend upon the stage of pregnancy at which the infection occurs.

During the first half of pregnancy, infection can result in the death of the embryo or foetal lamb. Some foetal lambs may not die immediately but be aborted at a much later date or presented as stillbirths at full term.

A proportion of lambs survive to full term, some of which are born with a hairy birthcoat and a tremble, because of brain damage caused by the virus. These lambs are known as '**hairy-shakers**' and are a pathetic sight. The majority die because they cannot keep up with their mothers or cannot suck colostrum because of their trembling defect. Other lambs which survive the virus attack may be born looking apparently quite normal. Some will survive but others develop a fatal diarrhoea or waste away within weeks or months of birth. Post-mortem findings closely resemble those of bovine virus diarrhoea or mucosal disease of cattle, as the viruses are very closely related.

All surviving lambs born of ewes infected during the first two or three months of pregnancy will harbour the virus for life. They may therefore infect any other sheep with whom they come into contact. The virus persists in the body because the young foetal lamb does not have a developed immune system and therefore fails to 'recognise' the BD virus as 'foreign' material (see Chapter 1). If any of these persistently infected cases survive to breeding age, then the females may give birth to infected lambs and the rams may transmit the virus in their semen.

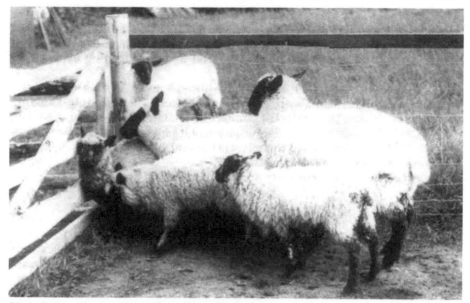

Plate 5.11 Border disease. All these lambs are the same age but those at the front of the picture are stunted because of the infection.

Infection of ewes during the last two months of pregnancy results in most lambs being born normally. Although a few may be weak, the majority survive, do not shed the virus and are immune for life. This is because the older foetal lamb's immune system recognises the virus, produces antibodies against it and thus effectively clears the body of all virus particles before they can cause too much damage.

CONTROL AND PREVENTION

Keeping a closed flock by breeding female replacements at home will obviously help to keep out the disease, but it is still possible to buy in a persistently infected ram. Purchased females should, whenever possible, be kept as a separate flock from mating right through until lambing is over.

In flocks experiencing this infection for the first time, the entire lamb crop must be slaughtered before the start of the next breeding season. Sheep which are suspected of bringing infection into the flock or which are shown to be positive from a blood sample must also be slaughtered, since this is the only way to prevent the disease from spreading. Newly purchased rams should be blood tested and kept isolated until declared free from infection.

In flocks where the disease is already well established, this slaughter-out policy may be unacceptable. In this situation some control may be achieved by identifying persistently infected lambs by blood testing and purposely running them with the non-pregnant breeding flock, including ewe lambs and gimmers, so as to infect as many as possible during this safe period. They should be heavily stocked or housed together for as long as possible, but preferably no later than two months before mating. Ewes which become infected when they are not pregnant will become immune and eliminate the virus from their bodies. They will then present no risk to other susceptible animals.

Ewes must be protected from infection during pregnancy. This means keeping them isolated from any sheep which may be infected with border disease or any cattle which may be infected with bovine virus diarrhoea or mucosal disease. Other species infected with the same family of viruses (pestiviruses), such as goats, deer or pigs, also constitute a risk to sheep.

No vaccine is available at present, although it is hoped that one will eventually be developed. The vaccine could then be used to immunise replacement ewe lambs each year well in advance of tupping. This would provide a greater degree of certainty than the method described above, which cannot guarantee that every in-contact animal will become infected and therefore immune.

Q-fever

Q-fever, or Queensland fever, is occasionally diagnosed as a cause of abortion in sheep. Sheep probably become infected by ingesting or breathing in the organisms (*Coxiella burnetii*) which are contained in minute droplets of fluid (aerosol) which accompany an abortion or an infected lambing. Ewes may also inhale the organisms once they have dried out from infected material and are blown around the lambing area.

Humans may become infected when present at the parturition of any infected mammal. Whilst infection in otherwise healthy humans normally causes only mild flu-like symptoms (which will usually go undiagnosed), in a small proportion of people serious heart complications (valvular endocarditis) and/or pneumonia may develop. The organism is also excreted in the milk of infected animals and is another good reason for not consuming any unpasteurised milk products from whatever species.

Treatment and control are problematical and your veterinary surgeon will advise should Q-fever be diagnosed in your flock.

Tickborne Fever

Tickborne fever can cause abortion when pregnant ewes, previously unacclimatised to tick grazings, become infected after being bitten by ticks. Ewes become ill and run a very high temperature (up to 108°F, 42°C) for as long as a week or 10 days. It is this prolonged fever which causes the

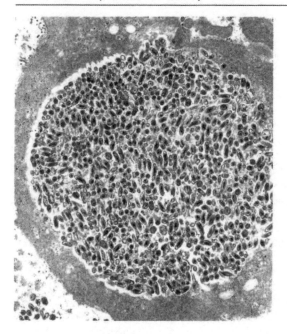

Plate 5.12 *Coxiella burnetii*— the causal agent of Q-fever— packed in their thousands into a cell (magnified 12,000 times) in the placenta of a ewe. An infected ewe may shed as many as a thousand million of these very resistant microorganisms in every gram of infected placenta.

abortion. Unfortunately, aborted ewes may develop a serious infection of the uterus after abortion (septic metritis) and the death rate is high. If, however, ewes have already been exposed to infected ticks before pregnancy, they will not normally abort if bitten again during pregnancy.

Tickborne fever is dealt with in detail in Chapter 9.

ABORTION CHECK LIST

The following is a check list to help prevent abortion from entering the flock, to minimise the damage when it does occur, to protect yourself, your family and staff from infection and to assist planning for the following breeding season. Not all points will apply to all farms. Generally speaking, outdoor lambing flocks with a high stocking density in the lambing area and housed flocks are at greater risk than extensively managed flocks.

GENERAL FARM POLICY
- 'Closed' flocks, breeding their own female replacements, are at much less risk from abortion.
- Rams have to be purchased from time to time in all flocks, but generally present less of a risk than females, since venereal spread of infectious sheep abortion is relatively unimportant. There is some risk from Border disease, so rams should be blood tested.

- Where females have to be purchased, the following precautions should be taken:
  Buy in unbred ewe lambs or gimmers, since ewes which have bred and have therefore been through the lambing quarters present a greater risk.
  Purchase from the safest sources, such as 'closed' hill or upland flocks of known disease status. There is much to be said for buying regularly from the same flock(s) where the owners will value your business.
  Enzootic-abortion-free ewes from accredited flocks will probably command a premium, but this should represent good value for money, other things being equal.
  Avoid buying breeding females from dealers who are known to purchase from numerous flocks of unknown health status.
- After the purchase of breeding replacements:
  Identify purchased animals permanently and isolate them from the home flock for at least a month to allow time for any incubating diseases to develop. It is highly desirable, wherever practical, to maintain this isolation right through until a month after lambing, especially where purchased ewes are not guaranteed free from enzootic abortion.
  Bought-in sheep mated with the home flock and run alongside the home flock during pregnancy must be split off and lambed as a separate flock. It is highly desirable that they are run separately for the last two months of pregnancy, since this is the high risk period for abortions. This will partially protect the home flock from picking up infection brought in with the purchased sheep and vice versa.
  Where enzootic abortion is a risk, as it is in all flocks which purchase unaccredited breeding females, discuss vaccination against EAE with your veterinary surgeon. If you do decide to vaccinate, then do so in the manner and at the time recommended by the vaccine manufacturer.
- Raddle rams at mating so as to identify early and late lambers and run these as separate flocks. Lamb them down in different paddocks or buildings. This will help to break the chain of infection, both with regard to abortion and with the infectious diseases of newborn lambs.

DURING PREGNANCY AND LAMBING

- An unexpectedly high rate of returns to the ram should make you suspicious of the possibility of infection—for example, with toxoplasmosis.
- Be on the look-out for signs of abortion, especially from mid pregnancy onwards. Any ewes with dirty behinds or any debris found in the fields should be thoroughly investigated.
- **Isolate all aborted ewes immediately; collect up dead lambs and placentae hygienically in a plastic bag using plastic gloves and save them for laboratory diagnosis; contact your veterinary surgeon immediately for advice; mark aborted ewes permanently; clean up the area where the abortion took place; wash hands thoroughly after handling aborted material.**

195

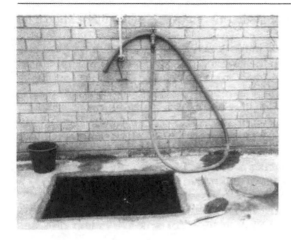

Plate 5.13 Visitors to the farm should be encouraged to wash and disinfect footwear on arrival and departure. Likewise, shepherds and others moving between clean and contaminated areas.

- Shepherds should not move from the isolation area back into the main flock lambing area without a complete change of boots and overalls. If you rely on chemical disinfection of boots, they must be free of any dung or mud before standing in a disinfectant footbath. These rules should apply to **everyone**—including the boss and the vet! Shepherds visiting from other flocks should be excluded from the lambing area unless they wear clean protective clothing and clean Wellington boots provided by you.
- If abortions occur, immediately reduce the stocking rate (outdoors or indoors) if at all possible. Split groups up into early, mid and late lambers to reduce the risk.
- Where an infectious abortion is present in a flock, remember that a number of apparently normal lambings may nevertheless be infected. Therefore take all personal hygienic precautions and avoid spreading infection from ewe to ewe on your hands or on lambing ropes etc., when assisting at lambings.
- **Pregnant women and very young children should avoid the lambing area**. All staff, helpers and visitors should be made aware of the dangers of human infection. (Smokers and nail-biters should take extra care to keep their fingers away from their mouths!)
- A high standard of shepherding is essential, especially when things go wrong, as in an abortion outbreak. Wrong decisions or general careless-ness can be very costly.
- Remember that more than one infection may affect a flock—or even an individual sheep—at the same time. Therefore, continue to submit a regu-lar supply of aborted material to the laboratory. Where enzootic abortion occurs alongside any other infectious abortion, the control measures for enzootic abortion should generally take precedence.
- Depending upon the diagnosis, the mixing of infected sheep (aborters) with clean sheep during the non-pregnant period can sometimes be very

196

helpful in producing a natural immunity. However, **this must never be practised when enzootic abortion is present in the flock** or where there is a possibility of its presence.

- Do not pass on your abortion problems to other sheep farmers by knowingly selling infected breeding stock, either privately or through a market.

6

OTHER DISEASES ENCOUNTERED DURING PREGNANCY

Listeriosis

Listeriosis is caused by a bacterium (*Listeria monocytogenes*) which brings about illness in a number of different ways. The disease has become much more common during the last decade, coincident with the increase in feeding silage to sheep, although it should be noted that sheep can contract the disease other than by eating contaminated silage. It is not new, since it was known as 'Silage disease' in Iceland early in the century and as 'Circling disease' in New Zealand more than 50 years ago.

Listeriosis occasionally leads to abortion in ewes, as mentioned in Chapter 5. It may also cause a diarrhoea and a bacteraemia (when the organisms invade the blood stream), the latter being the most usual form of the disease in lambs. However, the most common manifestation of the disease in the UK is an **encephalitis**, due to the bacteria getting into the brain. Here it forms numerous tiny abscesses and produces nervous symptoms which eventually lead to death in the majority of cases. Ewes are most commonly affected during late pregnancy, often some weeks after the introduction of silage feeding. Consequently, most are diagnosed during February and March, although cases may be seen from December to May and occasionally at other times of the year.

THE SILAGE CONNECTION

Listeria organisms are commonly found in soil contaminated by the faeces of animals, since even normal healthy sheep, cattle and many other species (including man) may harbour the bacteria in the gut without showing any untoward effects. It is probable that disease occurs only when sheep are exposed to a heavy weight of infection, such as in silage which has been contaminated with soil containing the bacteria.

It is difficult to make silage without some soil contamination. Where air is

199

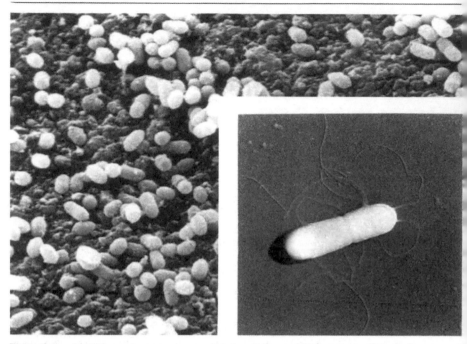

Plate 6.1 *Listeria monocytogenes*—the bacterium which causes listeriosis, seen under the scanning electron microscope, magnified 15,000 times and, in the inset, 60,000 times.

not adequately excluded from a clamp, because of either poor consolidation or imperfect sealing, poor fermentation will allow the pH to rise—that is, the silage will become less acidic or even alkaline. If listeria are present they are able to multiply in these pockets. Even prize-winning silage with a first-class analysis has been implicated in cases of listeriosis, possibly because no clamp is uniform throughout. Big bale silage is a very different product from clamp silage and every bale can be regarded as an individual clamp. The plastic bags are prone to damage by vermin, which leads to spoilage, thereby increasing the risk. However, there is no evidence to suggest that this type of silage is any more hazardous than clamped material. The disease appears to be more common in the north of England and Scotland where, because of the poorer weather conditions, it is generally more difficult to make high-quality silage.

Infected silage usually causes the nervous form of listeriosis (encephalitis) and there is some evidence to suggest that the bacteria travel to the brain via a nerve which supplies the face. The disease is most common in two year olds, older ewes and baby lambs, which may be either losing or cutting teeth. Bacteria may gain access to the tooth socket where there are numerous small branches of the nerve. It probably takes three or four

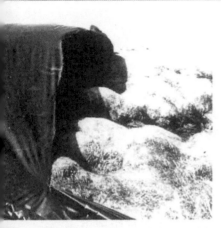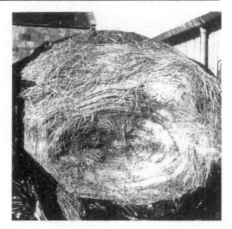

Plate 6.2   Spoiled clamp (*left*) and big bale silage (*right*). Such material should never be fed to sheep.

weeks for the bacteria to reach the brain by this unusual route, so even if suspect silage is withdrawn, further cases may occur for up to a month.

CLINICAL SIGNS

Affected ewes stop feeding and hang back from the rest of the flock. They may stand motionless for long periods with the head drooped or tilted to one side, drooling saliva from the side of the mouth because they cannot swallow. When examined they may have a mouth full of cud tucked between the molar teeth and the cheek. Occasionally ewes may have a drooping eyelid, a cloudy, discharging eye, a sagging lip and a dropped ear, all on the same side. When approached they may appear to be blind and circle to right or left, depending upon which side of the brain is affected. They may fall over and not be able to rise, frequently making paddling movements with their front feet, breathing heavily all the while. Convulsions may occur and ewes eventually lapse into a coma and die. The whole course of the disease lasts for only one or two days.

The disease may easily be confused with a number of others including hypocalcaemia, pregnancy toxaemia, gid, CCN, meningitis and louping ill in tick-infected areas. It is therefore most important to obtain a diagnosis by submitting dead ewes for post-mortem and by sending silage samples for examination.

Lambs can also become affected with listeriosis. This can result from contamination of the navel cord, or it can be picked up by mouth from infected silage in a lambing area or from the products of an abortion due to listeriosis. If the weather is bad or ewes are short of milk, lambs may begin to nibble

201

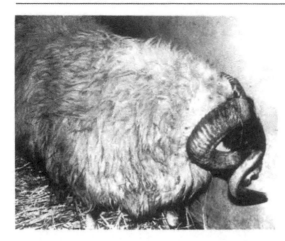

Plate 6.3 Nervous form of listeriosis in a Scottish Blackface ram, seen here head-pressing against the wall. The symptoms are caused by the bacteria multiplying in the brain—encephalitis.

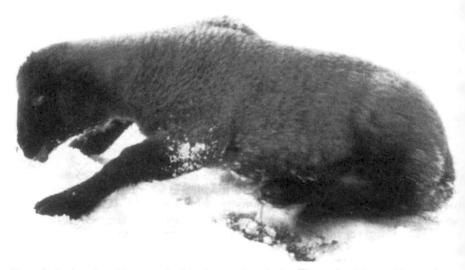

Plate 6.4 Lamb with encephalitis due to listeriosis. The animal is unable to rise. Note how the tongue hangs out of the mouth and how the ears and eyelid are drooped because of loss of nervous control.

silage at a young age and so become infected. Lambs may suffer from both the nervous and the diarrhoeic forms of the disease. Some may be born alive out of ewes with an infection of the uterus.

TREATMENT

Treatment of listeriosis is most disappointing in both adults and lambs. Antibiotics such as tetracycline and penicillin may be successful in a small proportion of animals which are detected very early in the course of the disease, but most die despite careful nursing. Of those that do survive, many are brain damaged and eventually have to be destroyed.

PREVENTION

Prevention of listeriosis is based upon providing sheep with safe food supplies. Soiled feeds such as roots or grazing which are heavily poached during the winter present a risk, but by far the most dangerous is silage. This should not deter flockmasters from feeding this excellent food to sheep, but rather make them aware that there is a risk which can be substantially reduced in a number of ways:

- Control moles and roll grass parks destined for silage.
- Do not cut too close to the ground.
- Cut silage for sheep at the optimum time (full leaf stage) to encourage good fermentation.
- Where applicable, use a suitable silage additive (not formic acid) to lower the pH.
- Take care not to incorporate soil into the silage when filling the clamp. (Pits dug out of a bank side with earth floor and sides are particularly hazardous.)
- Consolidate clamp silage well and seal up tightly after every day's filling and when the pit is full.
- Seal big bales effectively and protect from vermin and bird damage.
- Have the silage analysed before feeding and do not feed it to sheep if the pH is above 4.5 or the insoluble ash (which gives an indication of the degree of soil contamination) is above 1.5%. Beware that silage samples do not necessarily represent the analysis throughout the whole clamp or in other big bales.
- Do not feed mouldy, slimy or otherwise suspect silage to sheep. (Cattle are less susceptible to listeriosis than sheep and can tolerate all but the worst material, but it is much better to discard suspect silage altogether.)
- Where sheep feed at a silage face, tidy up wasted or trampled silage at least daily.
- Big bales are best eaten up in a couple of days; otherwise they dry out and the material lies about and becomes contaminated. Try to arrange for sufficient ewes to eat the bales up quickly.

CASE HISTORY

When cases of listeriosis occur in a flock they are usually all the same form of the disease (e.g. all abortion or all encephalitis) and usually affect only a relatively small percentage of the flock. However, the following history from a farm in the south of Scotland illustrates an extreme case where a very high proportion of the flock were affected and all three forms of the disease occurred together.

A silage pit was excavated out of a bank side and therefore had an earth floor and sides. It was filled with silage harvested in July and inadequately consolidated and sealed. Some 200 Mule and Scottish Halfbred ewes were housed in early January of the following winter when they were in mid pregnancy. For the first couple of weeks indoors, ewes were fed hay. In mid January the silage clamp was opened and the ewes were offered poor-quality, mouldy silage which remained largely uneaten, except for some rather better-quality material offered to two of the pens of sheep. More of the same was put in to the ewes the following day.

On the third day, 20 ewes were unwell and all the uneaten silage was removed from the sheep house and replaced with hay. On the following day the ewes developed a diarrhoea and more ewes became sick. By day five some 40 ewes were ill and 5 dead. By day six there were 80 sick ewes and a further 10 dead. On day seven the whole flock was given antibiotics but by this time a total of 19 ewes were dead. There was some improvement over the next couple of days and most ewes were eating some hay. One ewe aborted at this time and 60 others had a discharge from the vagina. These ewes were separated from the rest of the flock and scanned, which revealed that only one out of the 60 remained in lamb. In the two groups of ewes which had been fed the better silage on those two fateful days, only one aborted and none died.

When lambing time arrived only 80 out of the 174 ewes left alive lambed, the other 94 barren ewes having probably lost their foetal lambs due to listeriosis.

In another group of Mule hoggs housed in a different area of the same shed, six cases of the encephalitic form of the disease occurred about a month after being fed silage from the same pit. These were spotted early, treated with antibiotics and half of them recovered.

The outbreak was blamed on very heavy soil contamination of the silage, which occurred particularly when the clamp was being filled, since the soil apron sloped into the clamp. This was reflected in the very high ash content on analysis, which went up to 172 g/kg dry matter in parts. The pH of the silage varied, but was as high as pH 8.4 in parts, which is alkaline. This would allow any listeria microorganisms present to multiply.

HUMAN INFECTION

Listeriosis is yet another on the list of diseases which are transmissible to humans. Ewes which abort probably present the greatest risk, but contaminated silage is also dangerous, so wash hands carefully. The organism can be excreted in the milk of affected ewes and survive pasteurisation temperatures. It therefore presents a public health risk. Several hundred cases of human infection have been reported in the United States. It can be a serious and potentially fatal disease in humans, particularly in babies, children and older people. Most human infections in the UK occur in townspeople (there are more of them!) and possible sources of infection include improperly cooked meat, human sewage sludge, mud, stream and river water and even hospital sickroom dust.

Acidosis

Acidosis is a dietary condition caused by varying degrees of overeating on starchy foods like cereals and concentrate rations. At its mildest it takes the form of an indigestion with a mild scour, such as may occur if there has been a change in the ingredients of a ration. Providing the problem is corrected these animals usually recover uneventfully. In its severest form, such as when animals break into a feed store, it results in sudden death or in a very severe and distressing illness which ends in death after only a few hours. In between these extremes there are all grades of illness which often have a poor outlook, or may lead to other problems, such as pregnancy toxaemia.

The rumen can be thought of as a large fermentation vat where the bacteria and protozoa responsible for the breakdown of food are in equilibrium. If the diet is changed suddenly, as when concentrates are introduced in late pregnancy, the microorganisms need time to adjust if the delicate balance is not to be drastically altered, so producing a digestive upset. Therefore it is always wise to offer ewes a small amount of concentrate initially and then to build up gradually over a week or 10 days to the correct ration. The sudden introduction of large amounts of starchy food results in the rumen contents becoming more acidic than they should be, which causes an inflammation or rumenitis. This in turn causes diarrhoea, dehydration and sometimes death.

In late pregnancy, because of the rapid increase in the size of the lambs, ewes cannot take in sufficient bulky food to meet their nutritional requirements, hence the reason for feeding concentrated foods. However, rapidly reducing the amount of hay or silage in the diet can in itself cause problems, since a certain amount of roughage is essential for satisfactory rumen function. Simply changing the ingredients of a ration may be sufficient to upset the rumen. An adequate supply of fresh clean water is also essential, but it is surprising how frequently this is forgotten or neglected, either through pipes freezing or water bowls blocking up.

CLINICAL SIGNS

The clinical signs of acidosis are variable, depending very much on the severity. Mild cases will have a dirty rear end but continue to eat. More severe cases stop eating and look miserable, standing or lying with their ears down and grinding their teeth, which is often indicative of abdominal pain. They soon become very weak and exhausted and begin to breathe rapidly which helps them relieve the acidosis to some extent.

The diarrhoea differs between cases depending upon the cause of the acidosis. For example, it may be watery if ewes have been flushed on a barley stubble where a significant amount of grain has been shed. In other cases it may be like thin porridge, but in all cases it has a foul smell. Diarrhoea always leads to a severe loss of body fluids and this dehydration is manifest in a tight, hide-bound skin and sunken eyes. Ewes may stagger about, appearing to be drunk, and may show other nervous symptoms because of brain damage, before finally going down and lapsing into a coma shortly before death.

TREATMENT

Affected animals require careful nursing to get well again. This takes some time since the rumen micro-flora is always seriously upset and cannot be corrected overnight. Bring ewes indoors into comfortable quarters and offer some good-quality, mature hay, plus fresh water. Prop ewes up with bales to prevent bloat. In all cases the suspect diet should be removed and no concentrate of any kind fed.

In all but very mild cases, veterinary advice should be sought promptly, as this is a serious condition and a difficult one to treat successfully. The dehydration must be corrected by the administration of fluids and the excess fermentation checked by the administration of penicillin or the sulpha drugs, either by mouth or by injecting directly into the rumen. The acidity must be reversed by the administration of magnesium hydroxide or sodium bicarbonate by mouth. Other drugs such as steroids and vitamins may also be necessary and in severely engorged animals, the rumen may need to be emptied surgically.

PREVENTION

Preventive measures should include the provision of fresh, clean water with the gradual introduction of a suitable concentrate in late pregnancy. Home rations should be thoroughly mixed to avoid selection by ewes. Grains should be matured before inclusion and should preferably be fed in whole grain form to sheep. Bruised or ground cereals increase the risk of acidosis and are not so well utilised by sheep as the whole grain. (Apparently undigested grains often appear in the faeces, but the rumen flora have usually managed to extract the nutrients despite the appearance of the grains.) Sufficient trough space is essential to prevent bullying and to allow fair shares for all.

This section has dealt particularly with acidosis in the pregnant ewe, but the condition occurs in other classes of stock and especially in feeder and store lambs on cereals or stubbles, particularly where considerable quantities of grain have been shed.

Pregnancy Toxaemia/Twin Lamb Disease

Pregnancy toxaemia or twin lamb disease is a largely preventable condition which affects ewes during the last few weeks of pregnancy. As the name suggests, it principally affects twin or multiple bearing ewes and is encountered most frequently in lowground flocks, although it is also seen in hill flocks, in both twin and single bearing ewes.

The condition occurs as the result of an inadequate supply of dietary energy at a time when the ewe's demands for energy are very high because of the rapid growth of her foetal lambs, which put on four-fifths of their final birth weight during the last two months of pregnancy. There are a number of circumstances which may predispose to pregnancy toxaemia and they differ to some extent between lowland and hill flocks.

LOWLAND EWES

In the more prolific lowland flocks, cases of pregnancy toxaemia may arise from feeding an inadequate amount of concentrate ration during late pregnancy or from feeding an inferior, low-energy feed. This latter situation does not arise only in home mixed rations. The Scottish Agricultural Colleges have recently analysed a number of commercially compounded cakes, manufactured specifically for ewes, which have been totally inadequate in terms of energy, with very low ME values. Farmers should therefore demand a full analysis and if they are not satisfied, have it checked by an independent feed laboratory.

Some farmers feed bulky feeds (such as swedes) to capacity before distributing the concentrate ration. Because of this some ewes may not be able to consume their appropriate ration of concentrate before the rest of the mob have finished it off. Other ewes may be deprived of their fair share of concentrates because of lack of trough space. This is generally more common in housed flocks and less easily rectified by virtue of the design of many sheep houses. As ewes become more heavily pregnant, they take up more room at the trough and this should be taken into account. There is also some stress involved when ewes have to fight or are bullied whilst trying to get into the trough.

If ewes are brought indoors to lamb, there is the inevitable stress of settling down and establishing a pecking order. A change of feed at this time may mean that ewes take some time to adjust and start eating adequately. If these changes occur during the danger period for pregnancy toxaemia, that is, around three or four weeks before lambing is due to begin, then some ewes may succumb.

Overfat ewes appear to have a lower than expected voluntary feed intake during the last third of pregnancy. This may be due in part to large quantities of fat taking up space in the abdomen and restricting rumen fill.

Fat ewes may therefore be more prone to pregnancy toxaemia through partially starving themselves.

Cast hill ewes, such as the Scottish Blackface, brought down onto the better grazings of lowground farms, are quite capable of bearing a high proportion of twins. It is not uncommon for them to refuse concentrate rations, especially if they have never been hand fed on the hill. They may therefore be at considerable risk from twin lamb disease.

HILL EWES

In true hill flocks, probably the most risky situation is where ewes are on a semi-starvation diet, perhaps because they are overstocked and/or are not provided with supplementary feed. Sometimes ewes are retained when they should have been sent off as cast ewes to easier lowland pastures. Old, thin ewes, which may have liver fluke damage, broken mouth or molar disease, may not be able to make best use of what little they can manage to forage under harsh hill conditions.

Hill flocks are often fed as if all the ewes were bearing single lambs. This may be because there is no suitable in-bye ground for gimmers and twin bearing ewes, or because the flock is not scanned and thus the twin bearing ewes cannot be identified. Snowstorms may mean that ewes do not get sufficient forage, and if no supplementary feed is provided, pregnancy toxaemia may occur in both twin and single bearing ewes because of starvation.

The author can recall digging Scottish Blackface ewes out from under snow drifts on the hill over a period of a week or more. Most ewes were still alive, having survived by licking the snow, but many subsequently died from pregnancy toxaemia caused by starvation at a critical time during late pregnancy.

CLINICAL SIGNS

The clinical signs of pregnancy toxaemia are mainly nervous in character. They arise because of a shortage of energy in the diet, leading to low blood sugar (glucose) levels, or hypoglycaemia. This in turn leads to an inadequate supply of energy to all organs of the body, including the brain. If this low sugar state persists, the damage to the brain becomes irreversible. No amount of medical treatment will then correct the situation and the ewe will die. When a case of pregnancy toxaemia occurs, it may be the first warning that there is something radically wrong with the feeding or management of the flock as a whole. Therefore it is important that the shepherd is alert to the earliest clinical signs of the condition. However, it should be noted that isolated cases of pregnancy toxaemia do occur in correctly fed flocks perhaps because of footrot, bullying or other factors which may affect the feed intake of individual ewes.

Affected ewes tend to hang back from the rest of the flock and may tand still or lean against some object for long periods. Others may adopt unusual postures, such as kneeling or sitting on their rear-ends with the hind legs pointing forwards, like a dog. When approached by the shepherd and his dog, they make little or no attempt to escape and may even challenge the dog. When forced to move, ewes may stagger about with their heads pointing up to the sky—often termed 'stargazing' by shepherds. Some convulse after the effort of being caught, so care should be taken (see Figure 6.1).

Ewes often grind their teeth and make licking and chewing movements, although they refuse to eat or drink. There is trembling or twitching of the ears, lips and face muscles. Some ewes appear to be blind, since they do not respond to a hand in front of their eyes and may walk into objects, although the eyes appear normal. Their breath has a sickly sweet smell rather like nail-varnish. This is due to substances called ketones which are formed from the breakdown of body fat into glucose as the ewe attempts to correct her low sugar status (the smell is similar to the lactating dairy cow with ketosis). Breathing may be rapid and the shepherd may suspect pneumonia, especially as some ewes also have a discharge from the nose.

Since ewes stop eating altogether, they rapidly deteriorate and eventually collapse. They lie perfectly still with their heads tucked into the flank or stretched out in front with their chins on the ground. Rumen contents may issue from the nose and mouth, and coma and death soon follow. The whole course of the disease may take up to a week or even longer. (See Colour Plate 18.)

Some ewes may abort their lambs during the course of the illness and since this greatly relieves the demand for energy, the ewe may appear to improve, if only temporarily. Providing no permanent brain or other damage has been done, some aborted ewes may recover with appropriate treatment and good nursing.

DIAGNOSIS

Veterinary advice should be sought immediately the first case is suspected, to confirm the diagnosis and to blood sample a selection of ewes from the flock. Feeding should be improved immediately but gradually, pending the results. A re-sampling some time after the dietary change will show if the corrections have been effective. Despite these changes, further cases may continue to occur for a while, and if nothing is done they almost certainly will occur. As many as one in five ewes has been affected in 'outbreaks'.

Where any cases have arisen, shepherds should gently stir up the flock—preferably without the dogs—so that other cases can be spotted as early as possible. The whole flock should be condition scored and any thin ewes pulled out for preferential feeding, as should any shy feeders, footrot cases or other compromised sheep. Overfat ewes can be given some gentle forced exercise, but their feed should not be reduced abruptly as this may well precipitate the disease.

Pregnancy toxaemia may be easily confused with a number of other conditions which can occur around this time, such as listeriosis, pneumonia and, in particular, lambing sickness or hypocalcaemia.

TREATMENT

Treatment of pregnancy toxaemia is generally very disappointing, the majority of cases dying despite medication. In all cases prompt action is necessary, so shepherds should have a supply of calcium borogluconate solution (preferably containing magnesium and phosphorus) to hand. The treatment of a collapsed ewe with a calcium borogluconate solution will usually revive one with lambing sickness very quickly and will do a ewe with pregnancy toxaemia no harm, since the borogluconate portion will supply a little much-needed energy. Indeed some ewes with twin lamb disease also have low blood calcium levels. Do inform your veterinary surgeon of any treatment you may have given, or better still, consult first over the phone, as such treatment may confuse the diagnosis.

Nursing

Ewes need lots of tender loving care and should be carefully transported back to the steading and put in a warm, dry, well-bedded loose box. Clean fresh water should be supplied daily and placed where the ewe can get at it if she is unable to get up. Pregnant ewes drink a great deal of water and fresh supplies are essential if appetite is to return fully. Ewes that cannot get up must be carefully propped up with bales to prevent them getting onto their sides and dying from bloat.

Energy sources

It is useful to know the approximate lambing date from a raddle mark, since the form of treatment and the outcome may depend in large measure on how far the ewe is off lambing. Your vet may initially treat with glucose injections directly into a vein and leave instructions for you to give either glycerin, propylene glycol, treacle or some other proprietary substance by drench. These products will be converted into glucose by the ewe (glucose itself by mouth is not effective in treating this condition).

Drenching must be done with care, and your vet may add something bitter to the drench so that the ewe can taste it more easily, which will stimulate swallowing. Stomach tubing is an alternative and sometimes safer way with really sick animals, but on no account should any unconscious ewe be drenched or stomach tubed, as she cannot swallow and will probably drown. If the ewe is caught at an early stage in the disease and responds to this treatment, drenching will need to be continued for a period of perhaps a fortnight or even longer, until appetite returns and is sustained. It is claimed that some success has been achieved by stomach tubing valuable ewes with a thin suspension of grass meal in water.

Removing the foetal load

As noted above, ewes which abort may stand a better chance of recovery and to this end some veterinary surgeons may use drugs to abort them artificially. Alternatively, if ewes are reasonably close to their lambing date and not too ill to withstand a surgical operation, caesarean section may be performed to relieve the ewe of her foetal load. Unfortunately lambs are often already dead or may be difficult to revive, but a proportion of ewes recover well after surgery if nursed and fed carefully afterwards.

Ewes which are very ill and in the advanced stage of the disease are unlikely to respond to any medical treatment. This is because the damage to the brain is irreversible and the mechanisms by which the medicines are converted into glucose have usually failed by this stage.

PREVENTION

Avoidance is the only sensible way of approaching twin lamb disease. Prevention begins with having ewes in good body condition score (CS) before mating and maintaining CS as level as possible throughout pregnancy, so that ewes have sufficient reserves to draw upon during late pregnancy. Some moderate undernutrition is acceptable in late pregnancy, however, and providing ewes are around CS 2.5 to 3 at six to eight weeks before the start of lambing, they can afford to lose up to half a condition score by lambing time. However, during late pregnancy there must be an

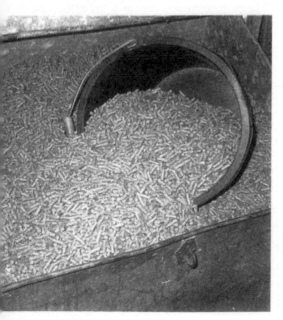

Plate 6.5 Some commercial compound cakes have been found to be of inadequate ME value. Since this could predispose to pregnancy toxaemia, ask for a full analysis before purchase.

increase in body weight of around 10% for single bearing ewes and 15 t
20% for twin bearing ewes. The use of ultrasound scanning is most usefu
in this regard, both in lowground and hill flocks, so that ewes can be fe
according to foetal load.

Forage feeds should be of good quality, particularly in late pregnancy
but beware of silages of proper nutritional analysis which the sheep won'
eat! Concentrate feeds should be formulated to give a balanced ration wit'
at least 16% crude protein. In the last month or so of pregnancy,
proportion of this should be in the form of an undegradable protein, suc
as fish meal. This will not only be more efficiently utilised, but will als
improve digestion and appetite. This in turn should reduce the variation i
feed intake which is often a feature of ewes in late pregnancy and whicl
can predispose to twin lamb disease. Whilst the concentrate feed can b
provided to balance the roughage analysis, careful shepherding is require
to see that the ewes themselves agree with the analysis!

Sufficient trough space is crucially important in late pregnancy an
splitting the concentrate feed into two feeds per day is useful, especially fo
prolific flocks which have a large ration to get through in one feed. Feedin;
large groups of sheep outdoors almost always means that about 20% of th
flock eat too much, 60% eat the correct amount and 20% get insufficient
It is therefore important to separate out thin ewes and shy feeders and fee
them apart from the main flock.

Traditionally ewes have been fed concentrates from around six or eigh
weeks pre-lambing, starting with a small amount of around 0.25 kg (0.5 lb
and increasing to about 1 kg (2.2 lb) by lambing time. Alternate regime
based on a flat-rate system have been introduced recently, in which the sam
total amount of concentrate is fed but in equal amounts daily for a slightl
longer period. It is claimed that this level feeding system is as good or eve
better for ewes in the long term, by reducing the incidence of pregnanc
toxaemia as well as other metabolic diseases such as lambing sickness, gras
staggers and prolapse of the vagina. The birth weight of lambs and mil
yield of ewes also appear to compare favourably. The system is said to b
particularly suitable for small framed, highly productive ewes.

Hill ewes present particular problems. Hill grazings provide a valuabl
source of roughage all year round, but without some form of supplementa
tion, hill ewes may lose up to one-fifth of their body weight during the lat
pregnancy period and this can only mean small lambs, an inadequate mil
supply and therefore high lamb losses, as well as a risk of ewes succumbin;
to pregnancy toxaemia.

This weight loss can be prevented in single bearing ewes left out on th
hill during pregnancy by providing supplementation, such as extra higl
energy/high protein feed blocks. Good blocks are a relatively expensiv
feed but are a most convenient method, especially for inaccessible areas
(Cheap blocks are usually nutritionally inadequate for the purpose—yo
generally get what you pay for.) If blocks are strategically placed about th
hill where ewes can find them easily whilst still continuing to forage, the

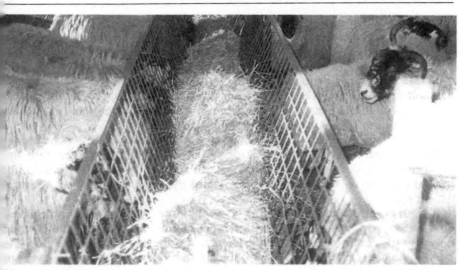

Plate 6.6   Draft hill ewes brought down to lowland farms and housed during pregnancy may refuse to eat if they are not accustomed to concentrates. This will predispose them to pregnancy toxaemia, even if they are carrying only a single lamb. Ample trough space should be allowed and shy feeders separated. High-quality roughage is essential and diseases such as footrot (which may make them reluctant to come to the trough) must be controlled.

will prevent many ewes—older ones in particular—from becoming lean and prone to pregnancy toxaemia.

Twin bearing ewes and gimmers should be brought down onto enclosed areas of rough grazing with shelter and a dry lie and fed roughage (usually hay) and concentrates.

The reader is referred to the discussion of feeding in late pregnancy in Chapter 4.

Hypocalcaemia/Lambing Sickness

Hypocalcaemia is an acute condition of both hill and lowland ewes in late pregnancy and early lactation, and it rapidly leads to collapse and death unless prompt treatment is applied. It is otherwise known as lambing sickness, moss ill, trembles or transport tetany. The symptoms are caused by a fall in the amount of calcium circulating in the blood.

The ewe's requirements for calcium increase dramatically in late pregnancy because of the calcium demands of the rapidly growing foetal lambs. In the last few days of pregnancy, colostrum is being produced and both colostrum and milk are rich in calcium. Even though the lambs are no longer a direct drain on the ewe after lambing, their milk requirements keep up the demand for calcium.

Hypocalcaemia is similar to milk fever in the dairy cow, and like old cows, older ewes are more likely to succumb. This may be partly because, with increasing age and in an emergency, both cows and ewes cannot release calcium rapidly enough from the reserves in their bones. The ability to do this is essential at a time of heavy demand, especially when there is a crisis of some kind, such as a spell of very bad weather.

Calcium is essential in a number of important body processes including the proper functioning of the muscles. When blood calcium levels fall, the poor ewe becomes weaker and weaker until she finally collapses, and if not treated she will die from heart failure, since the heart is a very active lump of muscle.

It would seem that hypocalcaemia is brought on by physical or nutritional stresses to which the ewe cannot respond quickly enough, rather than because of a straightforward deficiency of dietary calcium, since the condition occurs on diets which are considered to contain adequate levels of calcium. Indeed, most diets containing sufficient grass, hay or silage should contain adequate amounts of calcium. But where calcium levels provided in the diet are satisfactory, ewes may succumb because of a sudden demand for calcium through physical (muscular) exertion. Hill ewes driven down off the tops onto lower enclosures or in-bye parks very close to lambing time, or ewes being returned to the hill with their lambs after lambing, may go down with hypocalcaemia within a day or so of being herded.

The risk is increased when ewes are fed diets containing very low levels of calcium. This may occur in lowland ewes on a ration of roots and straight cereal grains, with insufficient good-quality hay or silage, or in hill ewes on a semi-starvation diet of rough forage only, which is often deficient in calcium. Indeed, in the hill situation, ewes may become so depleted that even when the demands of pregnancy and lactation are over, they cannot make up reserves in their skeleton before the next pregnancy and so become more and more depleted the older they get. In some hill flocks, ewes live on a knife-edge and if they are further stressed—such as would occur when they are gathered and penned without food for several hours—then 'outbreaks' may occur a day or so later. In the worst cases, hypocalcaemia may affect up to a third or even a half of the flock.

Diets fortified with extra calcium are sometimes fed. However, these have been shown to make ewes more prone to develop hypocalcaemia. The high levels of calcium appear to exert a negative feedback effect on the hormone which controls the amount of calcium absorbed from the diet through the gut and into the bloodstream. This effectively reduces the amount of calcium absorbed—exactly the opposite of what is required.

Other dietary components may influence the absorption of calcium from the diet. Vitamin D, which is found in sun-dried fodders such as hay and is also manufactured in the skin by the action of sunlight, is essential for efficient calcium absorption and its subsequent deposition in bone. In the

JK, vitamin D levels generally decline to their lowest levels around the late pregnancy—early lactation period in spring lambing flocks. Protein also plays an important role, since if there is sufficient protein of good quality in the diet, ewes can produce normal healthy lambs, even on diets quite low in calcium. If, on the other hand, calcium levels are adequate but protein is deficient, then calcium absorption and deposition in bone will suffer adversely.

Much is made of the importance of the ratio between calcium and phosphorus in the diet of ruminants. However, they appear able to function adequately within quite a range of ratios. Somewhere between 1 : 1 and 2 : 1 of calcium to phosphorus would appear to be most satisfactory, providing the overall levels of each element are within the normally accepted range. In hypocalcaemia, levels of phosphorus in the blood also fall because the two elements are closely associated in bone. If calcium levels are corrected, phosphorus levels will generally follow suit. (Phosphorus deficiency is generally less common in sheep than in cattle.)

The role of magnesium in calcium metabolism is the subject of some controversy. On the one hand, magnesium deficiency is said to make ewes more susceptible to hypocalcaemia, whilst on the other, feeds rich in magnesium fed during late pregnancy—with the purpose of preventing staggers in lactation—are accused of doing precisely the same thing. This anomaly has yet to be resolved, but it is most important to take care that any mineral supplement is formulated to suit the particular requirements of the flock as they alter throughout the year.

CLINICAL SIGNS

The degree of calcium deficiency will, to some extent, determine the rapidity and severity of the clinical symptoms and these do vary between affected ewes. In the earliest stage, ewes may be very excitable and anxious, with startled eyes. This is especially noticeable when they are being caught, and this may make the shepherd suspicious of magnesium staggers. On handling, the ewe will be felt to be trembling, especially over the shoulder muscles, and when released will walk or trot away very unsteadily. As the condition progresses ewes tend to remain stationary and eventually go down due to extreme muscular weakness. They tend to lie on their chests, sometimes with their hind legs stretched out behind them and their heads resting on the ground, saliva often drooling out of the mouth, especially when they become a bit 'blown' (see Figure 6.1). Breathing becomes very shallow, since the weakness also affects the muscles which control respiration, and ewes eventually become comatose and die if not treated promptly. The course of the illness may only be a few hours, but some ewes may resist going down for longer and may take up to a day or even longer to die, depending, presumably, upon the degree of calcium deficiency. Occasionally, ewes may simply be found dead on the morning round.

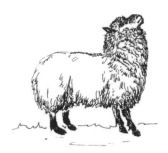

Twin lamb disease
(pregnancy toxaemia)

LATE PREGNANCY   *LAMBING*   *Early — LACTATION — Peak*

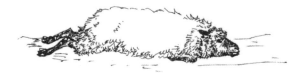

Lambing sickness (hypocalcaemia)

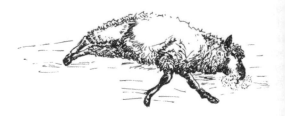

Grass staggers (hypomagnesaemia)

Figure 6.1   Three metabolic diseases of ewes and when they occur.

TREATMENT

Prompt treatment is essential and is usually carried out by the shepherd. As a general rule, when a pregnant or lactating ewe is found in a nervous or collapsed state, it is most likely to be either pregnancy toxaemia or hypocalcaemia if before lambing, or hypocalcaemia or hypomagnesaemia if after. Treat ewes immediately with 100 ml of a 20% solution of calcium borogluconate, with added magnesium and phosphorus, by injection under the skin, dividing the dose over two or three different sites.

Ewes with hypocalcaemia will usually respond rapidly to this treatment and will often pass dung, get up and trot away. They should be held until they are steady and have belched up any gas which may have accumulated if they were 'blown'. If they do not respond, then you should phone your veterinary surgeon for advice before you administer any further treatment. Ewes which recover should be watched carefully over the following week or so, since a proportion may relapse and need further treatment. Lowground ewes can be kept next to the steading, but hill ewes can be temporarily paint-marked for ease of identification. Ewes which cannot get up must be propped up with bales to prevent bloat.

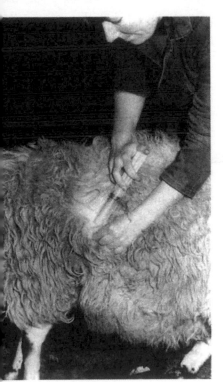

Plate 6.7   Sub-cutaneous injection of 100 ml calcium borogluconate 20% solution, with added magnesium and phosphorus, for the treatment of hypocalcaemia. Where large quantities such as this are necessary, divide the dose and inject at two or three sites to aid absorption. Take full hygienic precautions.

PREVENTION

Prevention of hypocalcaemia depends upon providing ewes with a die containing adequate, although not excessive, amounts of calcium. AFRC recommended levels are between 5 and 10 g per day. As mentioned previously, this should be balanced with phosphorus at a ratio between 1 : and 2 : 1 and should contain sufficient vitamin D and good-quality protein to allow proper absorption of calcium and phosphorus. Ewes should be gradually introduced to the concentrate diet some six to eight weeks before lambing, whether step-wise or flat-rate systems are employed.

Hill ewes should be brought down to enclosures or in-bye pastures as early as practicable. They should be gathered with care and where necessary given adequate rest periods en route. Gatherings for vaccinations or other medications can be combined but only where this is feasible and safe and only in reasonable weather and with a minimum of stress. When snowstorms occur contingency measures should be implemented quickly, so that hill ewes have immediate access to supplementary rations such as blocks.

It is sometimes advocated that lower calcium levels should be fed during late pregnancy and the amount increased towards lambing and during lactation. These matters should be fully discussed with your veterinary surgeon and an independent nutritional adviser before implementation. Ensure that a suitable mineral, trace element and vitamin mix is added to any concentrate feed or provided for hill ewes in feed blocks, liquid feeds or on free access. Where the diet is suitably fortified, do not provide other sources of minerals, such as free access mineral licks or blocks. Long-acting vitamin D injections are sometimes advocated at the beginning of the winter period and can be repeated after a suitable delay where this is thought necessary. Great care should be taken not to overdose with vitamin D.

Hypomagnesaemia/Grass Staggers

Hypomagnesaemia, grass staggers or lactation tetany is an acute disorder of both hill and lowland ewes characterised by sudden death and caused by low levels of magnesium in the blood.

The condition is most common in ewes between lambing and peak lactation, although it occasionally occurs immediately before lambing. In spring lambing flocks this period coincides with the rapid growth of spring grass. Lush swards which have been heavily fertilised and have a low clover content are especially dangerous. Improved marginal land is particularly hazardous to upland and hill sheep. Ewes moved from old established pastures or turned out of a lambing shed with their lambs onto a lush new ley are particularly at risk. If the weather at this time turns cold and wet, as so frequently happens, then outbreaks may occur. As many as a quarter of the ewes may become clinically affected, although the whole flock will be at risk.

Ewes of any age may be affected, but older ewes and those nursing twins
ıd therefore producing more milk are at greater risk, as are cast hill ewes
ı lowground farms. Undernourished ewes, such as unsupplemented hill
ves, are also prone. Other classes of sheep, such as lambs after long-
ıstance transport, may succumb, especially when they are stressed through
ﺇing deprived of food, water and adequate rest.

Grass staggers may occur on swards containing what would be regarded
. adequate levels of magnesium, which makes the point that it is the **avail-
bility** of the element to the animal that is important. Unlike calcium, there
very little magnesium stored in bone. As ewes become older, magnesium
ɛcomes less available in an emergency, the meagre stores being quickly
ɪhausted. Magnesium therefore needs to be assimilated by the ewe on a
ɪily basis.

A number of factors during the period of greatest risk may affect the
ﬠailability of magnesium, and when several factors act together they may
p the balance in favour of the disease. Some of the more important ones
ɾe listed below:

- Young, rapidly growing spring grass is particularly low in magnesium,
  especially when heavily top-dressed with nitrogen fertilisers which
  suppress clover growth and reduce the uptake of both magnesium and
  calcium. (Hypomagnesaemic ewes are also frequently hypocalcaemic).
- Only about one-quarter of the magnesium in the diet is available to the
  ewe, although this depends on the constituents of the diet to some extent.
  Individual ewes vary in their ability to absorb magnesium and this may
  partly decide which ewes become clinically ill and which do not.
- Nitrate fertilisers increase the protein in grass which in turn produces
  excessive amounts of free ammonia in the rumen, lowers rumen pH
  (makes it more acid) and depletes carbohydrate. All these factors
  make both magnesium and calcium even less available to the ewe. The
  imbalance of carbohydrate to nitrogen may also depress appetite, making
  matters even worse.
- Lush spring grass passes through the intestines very quickly, which
  allows less time for magnesium to be absorbed.
- If potash fertilisers or slurry (which is high in potash) are applied
  before grazing in the spring, they will reduce the amount of magnesium
  taken up by the sward and also make it less available to the grazing
  animal.
- Magnesium may be less available on acid soils.
- The level of sodium in fertilised swards is low, which means that the
  ratio of sodium to potassium in the rumen is upset. This interferes with
  the transfer of magnesium from the rumen contents into the blood.

CLINICAL SIGNS

ʾhe clinical signs of hypomagnesaemia usually last for only a very short
ɪme and therefore the shepherd may simply find a dead ewe. Early clinical

signs include a stiff, stilted walk—often with the head held high—nervou twitching of the face muscles and frequent urination. There is an exagger ated alarm to noise or to the sucking of the lambs. Being gathered an caught is particularly stressful and may precipitate convulsions and death so ewes should be approached with care and cunning. As the deficienc progresses, ewes develop a wild-eyed look, and appear to be blind, grin their teeth and eventually go down. They usually lie on their side with th legs stretched out straight, their head thrown back and the neck rigid (se Figure 6.1). Convulsions follow, with rolling of the eyes, chomping of th jaws, frothing at the mouth and wild thrashing movements of the limbs which may dig up the turf, leaving the tell-tale signs often seen beside dead ewe. These convulsions are extremely exhausting and hasten deatl through heart and respiratory failure. Some ewes die within half a hour of showing nervous symptoms, whilst others may last for severa hours.

TREATMENT

The preceding distressing symptoms in ewes during early lactation o fresh spring grass in April or May should always strongly suggest hypo magnesaemia and the need for immediate action. Ewes with grass stagger are often also low in calcium as well as magnesium, and the early symptom may be confused with hypocalcaemia. It is therefore wise to use a combinec treatment of 50 to 100 ml of a 20% solution of calcium borogluconate witl added magnesium and phosphorus given as a sub-cutaneous injection. I hypomagnesaemia is suspected, this treatment should be accompanied b 50 ml of a 25% solution of straight magnesium sulphate, again under the skin. This large volume should be divided and injected at three or fou different sites.

Ewes should be treated where they lie initially and the shepherd shoulc stay with them until they have settled down and stopped convulsing. The should then be propped up on their sternum and supported by bales so as tc prevent bloat. Once ewes look like getting up they should be very carefully transported back to the steading. Their lambs should be fed by hand until the ewe has totally recovered, since attempts to suck may precipitate anothei convulsion. (Veterinarians treating staggers cases may use sedatives tc reduce the risk of convulsions.) Hill ewes present more of a problem, but i possible they should be moved to some temporary shelter or into the neares wood.

Ewes should be made comfortable indoors, especially if the weathei is bad. They should be offered fresh clean water and a little of something tempting to eat, such as greens out of the kitchen garden. Quiet, gentle handling is essential if further convulsive episodes are to be avoided. It is not uncommon for ewes to relapse and require further treatments and these are a poor prospect. If ewes cannot be persuaded to eat, they are much more likely to relapse. To prevent this happening, they should be given a daily

ose of 60 g (2 oz) calcined magnesite by mouth for a week or until they
tart eating. It should then be withdrawn gradually by decreasing the daily
ose.

CONTROL

A sudden death or clinical case of staggers should alert the shepherd to
he possibility of more cases, and a veterinary surgeon should be contacted
or advice and confirmation of the diagnosis. Whilst there is little at
ost-mortem to confirm or reject the diagnosis, a sample of urine from the
ladder of a dead ewe and blood and/or urine from a random selection of
wes may give helpful information on the magnesium status of the flock.
Even before confirmation is obtained, immediate steps should be taken on
he mere suspicion of staggers. The flock should be moved off the danger
rea and onto some permanent pasture or longer term ley which has not
een heavily fertilised. This is usually all that is required in the short term
o prevent further cases, but ewes should not be returned to the offending
asture unless and until appropriate remedial measures are taken. The
implest of these is to restrict the grazing time to a few hours a day and to
un ewes back onto safe ground for the rest of the 24 hours. Hay can be
ffered to ewes as it stimulates rumination and salivation, which prevent
xcessive build-up of ammonia in the rumen and aid magnesium absorption.
However, if there is any picking of new grass growth, ewes are unlikely to
ake much, if any, hay.

PREVENTION

Both short- and long-term measures can be taken to supplement the diet with
magnesium either directly or indirectly. There are a number of ways this
an be attempted and the choice will depend very much on the particular
circumstances of the flock.

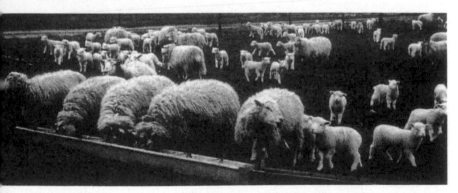

Plate 6.8   Prolific lowland ewes with Texel cross lambs. The ewe's concentrate
ation can be supplemented with magnesium in a number of ways.

Where concentrates are being fed during lactation—as is usually the case in the highest risk group of prolific lowland ewes on intensively managed swards—the rations can be supplemented with magnesium as follows:

● By adding magnesium oxide in the form of calcined magnesite at the rate of 10 g (⅓ oz) per ewe per day to home mixed rations. As magnesium is somewhat unpalatable and it is important not to put ewes off their rations, treacle, molasses or beet pulp can be added to help mask the taste. Do not exceed the dose advised, as excess magnesium can cause scouring which will defeat the purpose.

● By using a manufactured cake with extra magnesium added. Check the analyses and check that all ewes are eating. (A high-energy cake will minimise the need for ewes to break down body fat, which can depress appetite.)

● By feeding concentrates even when they are not usually used, since this is the safest and surest way of providing short-term protection. Magnesium enriched feeds should only be fed immediately before and during the period of risk. For example, introduce the feed gradually during the last week of pregnancy by mixing increasing amounts with the ration and continue to feed for a month to six weeks after lambing, depending upon the estimated risk. It obviously helps if the flock is split into early, mid and late lambing groups.

Where no concentrates are fed, magnesium can be supplied in the following ways:

● As magnesium acetate mixed with molasses and fed from a ball-lick dispenser on free access.

● As magnesium acetate added to the water supply, although this method (which is used for cattle) is not particularly suitable for ewes.

● As magnesium sulphate sprayed onto pasture as a 2% solution every two weeks over the period of risk.

● As calcined magnesite dusted onto pasture at the rate of 10 g (⅓ oz) per ewe per day. This is only practical for small flocks grazing a limited area. (125 kg/hectare will give protection over the risk period during one season—see also below.)

● As a magnesium 'bullet' administered by a balling gun. The 'bullet' lies in the reticulo-rumen (forestomach) and slowly releases magnesium over a period of a month or slightly longer, depending upon rumen conditions. 'Bullets' should be given to all ewes in the flock immediately the problem is diagnosed or just before ewes are due to be turned out onto risky pasture. (As magnesium is not stored for any length of time in the body, there is no point in giving bullets much before the period of risk.)

● As high magnesium minerals in the form of powders, liquids or licks. Some ewes will take more than they should and scour, whilst others will not take enough.

For long-term protection, pastures which are to be managed intensively should be treated in an attempt to increase the magnesium content of the herbage. (The above methods of spraying or dusting merely apply magnesium to the surface of the plants for short-term protection.) Below are some ways of trying to achieve this:

- Clover should be included in new seeds mixtures and encouraged to persist by good grassland management, since it has a much higher magnesium content than grass.
- Potash fertilisers should not be applied immediately before grazing in the spring.
- Slurry should not be spread during the winter on ground destined for grazing by ewes and lambs during early lactation.
- Correct any acid soils by liming with a magnesium limestone which will both supply magnesium and make it more available to the plant.
- Magnesium-rich top-dressings can be applied to ewe grazings.
- Pastures can be dressed with calcined magnesite (at 625 kg/hectare) or with kieserite, both of which are quite costly, but will give long-term protection for several grazing seasons. They are really effective only on sandy or acid soils, however.

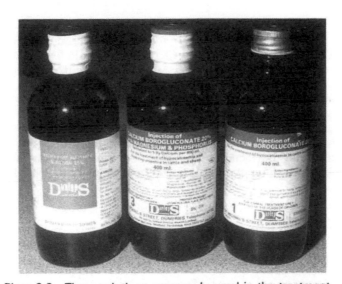

Plate 6.9   Three solutions commonly used in the treatment of metabolic disease in ewes during late pregnancy and early lactation. Left to right: magnesium sulphate 25% (for grass staggers or hypomagnesaemia); calcium borogluconate 20% with magnesium and phosphorus; and calcium borogluconate 20% (for lambing sickness or hypocalcaemia and for twin lamb disease or pregnancy toxaemia). These solutions are sterilised for injection and should be given under the skin.

223

Before applying any of these pasture dressings it is essential to discuss what you are proposing with your independent agricultural adviser so that the most appropriate and cost-effective method for your farm is identified and correct application rates are used. Do not combine any of the methods mentioned above without consulting your veterinary surgeon, since over-dosing or prolonged use may bring its own problems.

Some form of shelter, be it a proper sheep shed, straw bales or simply access to a dry lie in some woodland, should always be available to lambing ewes and lactating ewes and their lambs. Cold, wet weather is physically stressful and may be sufficient to precipitate hypomagnesaemia.

Prolapse of the Vagina

This is a condition which affects ewes during the last month of pregnancy and consists of the vagina being turned inside out and forced out through the lips of the vulva, so exposing the delicate tissues to contamination and damage.

INCIDENCE

Prolapse occurs with widely varying degrees of frequency from flock to flock and from year to year, but it does appear to be most common in prolific lowland flocks and amongst older ewes. Surveys suggest that about half of all flocks never see the condition. In those that do, as few as one in a thousand ewes may prolapse in hill flocks, or as many as one in ten in a few upland and lowland flocks. On average, only one in a hundred ewes prolapses and it is therefore not a condition which has received much research attention, often to the disappointment of shepherds whose flocks are particularly affected. The cause, or causes, of the condition are therefore unknown, although there are almost as many theories as there are sheep farms.

CLINICAL SIGNS

In the mildest of cases, the ewe prolapses a small portion of the vagina only when she lies down, when there is slightly more pressure put on the abdomen. This shows as a pink, fleshy protuberance appearing at the lips of the vulva and can easily be missed. When the ewe stands up the prolapse disappears. Some ewes never progress beyond this stage and lamb normally.

In other ewes, more and more of the vagina prolapses and fails to disappear when the ewe stands up. The delicate tissues become infected due to soiling, then swell up and become subject to further damage and bleeding. The ewe is obviously in discomfort at this stage and tends to strain more

224

and more, further increasing abdominal pressure and making the situation worse.

As more of the vagina protrudes, the pressure may block off the urethra (the tube which leads from the bladder into the vagina), so that the ewe cannot urinate. This eventually leads to rupture of the bladder. Also, the vagina may become so congested and damaged that it may rupture, sometimes allowing coils of intestines to escape with consequent peritonitis (see Colour plate 19). In both these circumstances death occurs fairly rapidly, or else the ewe must be destroyed on humane grounds. Occasionally the lambs may be salvaged. Despite treatment, around one in five affected ewes dies, either directly or indirectly, from prolapse.

CONTRIBUTORY FACTORS

There are a number of factors, which, acting either independently or together, contribute to prolapse of the vagina. It should be appreciated that whilst only the occasional ewe may be affected, this often indicates a general problem in the flock.

Most cases of prolapse occur during the last two weeks of pregnancy and those cases which occur very close to lambing are often associated with a failure of the cervix (or neck of the womb) to open up properly and allow the birth of the lambs. The lambs are frequently presented abnormally and in severe cases may be dead. These ewes often have low blood calcium levels, which tend to decline as pregnancy progresses. Calcium is important for maintaining muscle tone (see hypocalcaemia), and although these ewes may not show any clinical signs of hypocalcaemia, the lack of tone in the muscular walls of the vagina may be a contributory factor to prolapse.

As pregnancy progresses the foetal lambs take up more and more room in the abdominal cavity and if twins and triplets are involved there is very limited room for anything else. Where ewes are given a diet with too high a proportion of roughage to concentrate in late pregnancy, this increases gut-fill and therefore pressure within the abdomen. Ewes in excessively good body condition carry a lot of fat in the abdominal cavity and this may have a similar effect. In both these circumstances, ewes carrying twins or triplets appear to be more prone to prolapse than do single bearing ewes.

This is borne out to some extent in one survey carried out by the Scottish Veterinary Investigation Service in the Borders region of Scotland on almost 1,000 flocks farming a quarter of a million ewes. Prolific hybrid sheep such as the Greyface, when crossed with the Suffolk ram in upland or lowland flocks, had an incidence of vaginal prolapse in the ewe flock approaching 2%. This was higher than in less prolific pure-bred Suffolk flocks under similar management conditions. Scottish halfbred ewes, which are just as prolific as Greyfaces, had a lower prolapse rate of just above 1%, possibly because they are just that bit larger and 'roomier'.

It has been suggested that ewes grazing steep ground may be more at risk, but the previous survey and others have found that there were just as many cases on level ground. Nor was there any difference between housed flocks and those kept at pasture.

TREATMENT

Appropriate treatment will depend upon how severely the ewe is affected and how far she is off lambing. In the mildest cases where only a small amount of vagina is visible when the ewe lies down, it may be sufficient to keep a close eye on the animal (which should be marked for ease of identification) to see that she does not progress to being permanently prolapsed. Because calcium deficiency may be involved, it will be helpful—and will do no harm—to inject 50 ml of a 20% solution of calcium borogluconate under the skin before proceeding with any other form of treatment.

If the prolapse is permanently showing, veterinary attention should be sought. Some shepherds may prefer to, or may have to, deal with uncomplicated cases on their own, but they should be taught how to do so correctly and humanely in the first instance. Wherever possible a second pair of hands will allow the job to be done all the more hygienically and efficiently. The aims of treatment are:

- to clean up the prolapsed vagina with the very minimum of damage
- to replace the vagina to its correct position
- to prevent the ewe from prolapsing again until she lambs

It is important to choose the most appropriate method of retaining the prolapse once it is replaced, and there are a number of methods, some more successful and humane than others. This choice must be made before any attempt to replace the organ. It is preferable to have ewes indoors. Ewes with badly damaged or ruptured prolapses with coils of intestine hanging out should not be moved and should be humanely destroyed where they lie.

Taking the weight of the abdominal contents off the ewe's hind end will stop her from straining temporarily and allow the vagina to be replaced very much more easily. This is done by looping the ends of a short length of soft rope (like a calving rope) just above each hock (not the fetlock) and drawing the ewe's back end up in the air by slinging the rope over the shoulders of the assistant or shepherd, who then supports its weight whilst the job is done.

Cleaning up the prolapse

Any gross dirt should be picked off the surface of the vagina. Copious amounts of lukewarm—**not** hot—water, containing a few drops of a very mild disinfectant, should be used to gently remove any debris (soaps generally have a drying effect on these delicate tissues and are better avoided). Gently dab the tissues dry with a soft towel—do not rub, or bleeding may occur. Then cover the whole of the prolapse with a soothing antiseptic cream or the contents of an intramammary syringe (for treating cows with mastitis), which will both lubricate and help clear up the inevitable infection

226

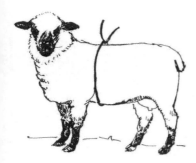

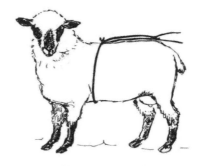

(1) Double a length of cord and loop it around the girth immediately behind the point of the elbow. Tie a knot reasonably tightly over the spine. (Make sure the cord is bedded into the fleece.)

(2) Tie a second knot in the doubled cord over the spine, approximately above the udder.

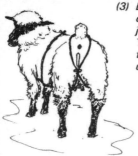

(3) Bring the cord either side of the tail and tie a knot just below the vulva. Take the cords between the back legs and the udder on each side and

(4) up to the knot above the spine. Tie reasonably tightly with a temporary knot. Adjust regularly as required and check for any sores.

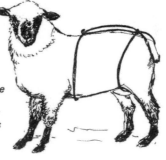

NOTE: The truss should prevent straining but should not make it uncomfortable for the ewe to move about. A prolapse retainer can be anchored to the truss illustrated above.

Fig. 6.2 Applying cord truss to ewe with vaginal prolapse to prevent straining.

which will occur. This is important, because any inflammation will cause the ewe to strain and attempt to prolapse the vagina once more.

Replacing the prolapse

If the prolapse is swollen because of its hanging out of the vulva for some time, then cup both hands around it and with patience apply gentle, steady pressure to reduce its size. This will make it easier to replace and will again reduce the risk of the ewe straining. Then gently push the lubricated vagina back through the lips of the vulva using cupped hands, not finger tips, which might rupture the vagina and lead to peritonitis and death. Feel gently inside the ewe to see that the vagina, once replaced, is back in its proper position. The ewe should then be allowed to stand or be supported and the assistant should grasp wool from either side of the vulva and hold the fleece together in a clenched fist to make sure the prolapse does not pop out again before the next stage of treatment.

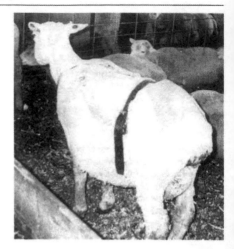

Plate 6.10 A commercial truss made of leather and webbing. In this case no retainer has been used and the truss is preventing the ewe from straining.

Truss

The next job is to apply a truss, which is essential to the success of whatever method of treatment is used. A truss applies gentle but firm pressure on the spine so that the ewe slightly arches her back, which makes it much more difficult for her to push and strain. This is applied with a thin rope or baler twine as shown and described in the series of diagrams in Figure 6.2. It is important to adjust so as to get the tension just right, so that the ewe is reasonably comfortable. (Commercial trusses are available, or they can be made up from pieces of webbing. See Plate 6.10.) This is often all that is necessary to see ewes with mild prolapses through to lambing.

Prolapse retainer

In the more severe cases, the truss can be used in conjunction with a prolapse retainer (see Plates 6.11–6.14), which is made of plastic or a non-corrosive metal. One part of the device fits into the vagina whilst the 'arms' are secured to the truss on either side. Ewes should be watched carefully for signs of lambing so that the retainer and truss can be removed, although some ewes can lamb satisfactorily with a retainer in place. Retainers used without the assistance of a truss are much less successful in all but the least troublesome prolapse cases.

Stitching

The most severe method of treatment is to stitch the lips of the vulva together using nylon or tape. In the author's opinion—although not necessarily that of all veterinary surgeons—this is a less acceptable method when there are others available. It is often used without a truss and if the ewe continues to strain she will be quite capable of tearing out the stitches and prolapsing the vagina once more, often causing severe damage in the process. The stitches, being in a 'dirty' area, frequently become infected

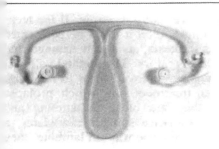

Plate 6.11   A plastic prolapse retainer. This should be attached to a truss as shown in the other plates on this page.

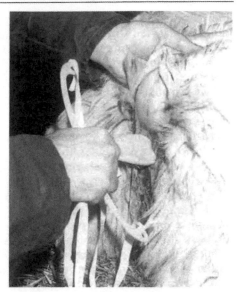

Plate 6.12   Inserting a prolapse retainer. The ewe is supported over bales with her head downhill.

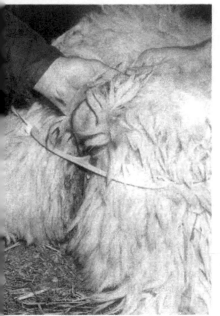

Plate 6.13   The retainer in position in the vagina.

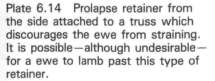

Plate 6.14   Prolapse retainer from the side attached to a truss which discourages the ewe from straining. It is possible—although undesirable— for a ewe to lamb past this type of retainer.

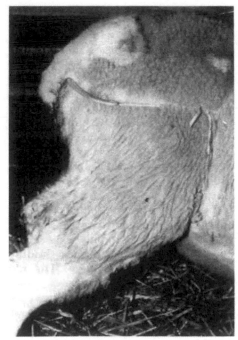

229

and painful and may make the ewe even more likely to strain. If the technique is resorted to because all else has failed, then it **must** be performed
by a veterinary surgeon using spinal anaesthesia, as much damage and
unnecessary pain are inflicted by unskilled operators. The method will not,
therefore, be described here. Stitches must be removed prior to lambing.

Ewes which do not settle down after treatment and which prolapse
again and again are problematical. If they are close to lambing and
your veterinary surgeon thinks they are otherwise suitable candidates, a
caesarean section may be performed. If they are some way off lambing, they
may have to be slaughtered.

Ewes which have sustained damage or infection may suffer from metritis
(an infection of the uterus or womb) after lambing. In a few ewes infection
may spread to the uterus before lambing and this may kill the lambs. In
cases where a rupture of the bladder occurs, or the intestines are prolapsed
through a rupture in the prolapse, the outlook is grim. Most of these cases
die very quickly or have to be destroyed.

There is some evidence that this condition may be inherited, so ewes
which prolapse are better culled and their female progeny sold for killing
rather than being retained or sold for breeding purposes.

PREVENTION

Prevention of vaginal prolapse is not easy. As has already been mentioned,
cases often signify that a flock problem exists, although it may be difficult
to pinpoint exactly where things are going wrong. Feeding ewes carrying
a heavy crop of lambs requires great skill and not a little art. On the
one hand ewes need to be in good condition, though not too fat. They
also require adequate roughage, but not too much. Providing adequate
energy, protein, vitamins and minerals whilst not overfilling the abdomen
is difficult. If the possible reason for a number of prolapses occurring can
be identified, then the feeding—if that is implicated—should be adjusted with
great caution at this late stage of pregnancy. It is so easy to induce
pregnancy toxaemia (see earlier) in the type of flocks where prolapse
most frequently occurs and the outcome of that is likely to be worse than
prolapse.

In future seasons, ewes should not be allowed to become too fat
and should be given gentle forced exercise where this does occur. High-
energy—high-protein concentrate rations of good quality and palatability
should be fed. Including some fish meal in late pregnancy will increase
appetite. Concentrate rations should be fed twice a day, preferably before
ewes fill up with roughage. The roughage itself should itself be of good
quality and should be rationed, especially in the last month of pregnancy.
Despite all efforts, however, the condition will still occur in certain flocks
with unfailing regularity, whilst in others it may appear one season but not
the next.

Hernia or Rupture of the Abdominal Wall

This is a relatively uncommon condition which principally affects older ewes carrying two or more lambs. It occurs during the last few weeks of pregnancy when the weight of the abdominal contents is very substantial. The muscular wall of the abdomen herniates or ruptures, so that the contents of the abdomen—the stomachs, intestines and uterus containing the lambs—come to lie directly under the skin. Affected ewes are sometimes referred to as being 'broken down'.

SYMPTOMS

The result of this lack of muscular support is that an enormous swelling appears, either directly underneath the ewe's belly or to one side. In the former case, the swelling may almost touch, or even trail along, the ground. A swelling to one side makes the ewe lop-sided. In either case the ewe may have difficulty in walking and there is a risk that the abdominal contents will be damaged because of their vulnerability. As the lambs increase in size, the swelling usually increases correspondingly, so that in the final stages of pregnancy ewes may be in considerable distress and some may be unable to rise.

At lambing there is quite likely to be some difficulty, since the lambing process depends on the involuntary muscular contractions of the uterus aided by the voluntary contractions of the abdominal muscles known as 'straining'. Since the abdominal muscles are ruptured, this process will be much less effective and there may be a protracted, difficult or impossible lambing (dystocia). It is, therefore, helpful to know roughly when individual ewes are due to lamb (from the raddle mark) so that they can be observed for signs of impending lambing and given assistance as necessary. Some ewes which become severely distressed can be caesarean sectioned and providing the lambs are not too premature they should survive. Once the weight of the lambs is removed, many of these ewes can manage to suckle lambs successfully.

Possible causes

This is another condition which has not received much research attention because it is relatively uncommon and hence the cause or causes are unknown. It is said that in older ewes the abdominal muscles may be weakened over the years because of bearing the weight of several pregnancies, as well as the extra stretching the muscles receive during the lambing process itself. Previously difficult lambings—such as the malpresentation of a lamb or the presence of dried-up dead lambs, either of which may lead to prolonged straining—are also quoted as the cause on occasion. Prolapse of the vagina before lambing or of the uterus after lambing and an infection

231

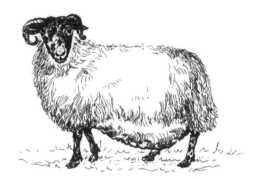

Figure 6.3 Ewe with a ventral abdominal hernia.

of the uterus may all cause prolonged straining, which can weaken the abdominal muscles.

Of course, many ewes suffer these indignities without succumbing to rupture of the abdominal muscles and it is tempting to look for other more convincing reasons—such as an inherited weakness. Calcium is important for normal muscular activity, and deficiency is not uncommon in late pregnancy, especially in undernourished ewes.

There is no corrective treatment for this condition and preventive measures which can be taken are limited to those based on unproven theories. These include avoiding crushing during feeding by providing sufficient trough space and avoiding feeding excessive roughage in late pregnancy to reduce gut fill—all good husbandry in any event. Comprehensive flock records may shed light on whether there is any hereditary basis to the condition in a flock and so give guidance on culling policy. Ewes which herniate will do so again in subsequent pregnancies and should be culled, and it is probably unwise to retain the offspring of herniated ewes for breeding.

Scrapie

Scrapie is a slow-developing disease of sheep and goats which can occur at any time of year. However, spread of infection within a flock occurs principally around lambing time, during the period immediately afterwards and also during the winter housing period preceding lambing.

This fascinating and enigmatic disease has been recognised for more than two centuries in Britain and other European countries. It is suspected of having caused serious losses amongst flocks in England during the 18th century, when sheep were also farmed intensively and many of the breeds we know so well today were being developed. Despite some 60 years of continuing scientific study the disease is still incompletely understood. It

232

s an infectious disease, and although the causative agent has not yet been
identified, much is known about its properties. Usually referred to as the
'scrapie agent', it is a virus-like particle (or virion) which exists in at least
20 different forms or strains. It is a tough organism which can resist many
of the chemical and physical conditions that would kill viruses and is able
to survive for many months on pastures and in buildings.

CLINICAL SIGNS

The clinical signs of the disease are nervous in character and are due
to the multiplication of the scrapie agent in the brain. Different strains of
the agent may cause different symptoms, but the most common syndrome
is an itchy one. The unfortunate sheep are literally tormented to death by
an insatiable urge to scratch, rub and bite whichever parts of their body
they can manage to reach. Their compulsive rubbing against any available
object causes wool loss and skin damage where the rubbing is intense. The
fleece generally becomes dry, bleached and lacklustre. Whilst rubbing or
scraping—hence the name—sheep often have a glazed look in the eye as if
in ecstasy from the temporary relief. They may raise the head, stretch the
neck and perform nibbling and licking movements whilst rubbing. Some
may flag the tail rapidly and urinate and dung without apparent control.
Others sit down like dogs and chew at their limbs (see Plate 6.15).

Animals may be tormented day and night, and although appetite is often
unaffected, they lose condition very rapidly, because constant rubbing
leaves no time for eating. Others may maintain reasonable body condition.

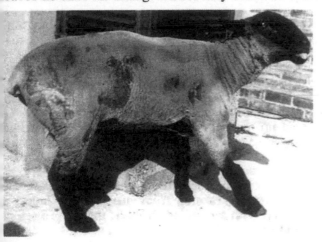
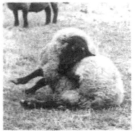

Plate 6.15   Suffolk rams with scrapie. The ram to the left is rubbing and
nibbling (tongue out). Note the severe self-inflicted damage on the rump and
flank. The ram to the right is nibbling at its hind limb—an unusual posture for a
sheep. Both animals are tormented to distraction, and such cases lose body
condition quickly through not eating.

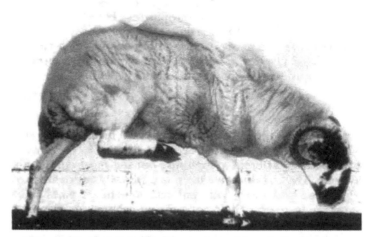

Plate 6.16 Scottish Blackface ewe with scrapie showing abnormal limb movements when it is scratched over the shoulder. This ewe also had an abnormal gait.

These symptoms can persist for weeks or even months if allowed to, but the outcome is always fatal.

Other scrapie agents may produce symptoms of incoordination. Affected animals often graze apart from the flock and may be left behind when the flock is moved on. A strange high-stepping movement may affect the fore legs whilst the hind limbs appear weak so that sheep may sway about (see Plate 6.16). Occasionally steps appear to be missed and animals may fall, especially when they are chased or turned sharply. They may then have difficulty in getting up. Sheep may become unduly alarmed or aggressive at the approach of the shepherd and fine tremors of the head and neck are apparent. Some animals lapse into unconsciousness for short periods.

If ewes go down they may lie all night and have to be helped to their feet in the morning. They can often manage to get about for the rest of the day once they have steadied up. Some sheep may become very slow and sluggish and simply lie about as if in a stupor. Occasionally sheep die very suddenly or after a short illness. Pregnant ewes which lose condition may abort or succumb to pregnancy toxaemia.

In flocks where the disease is established shepherds will recognise the early signs. The picture is often very similar from year to year, unless a new scrapie agent is introduced with purchased sheep or the agent present in the flock mutates or changes.

SUSCEPTIBILITY AND RESISTANCE

Sheep do not necessarily succumb to the disease simply because they become infected with the scrapie agent. Individual sheep react to infection with one or other of the agents in a way which is determined by the animal's genetic make-up. Sheep are said to be either susceptible or resistant to scrapie, although this is probably rather simplistic. The incubation period of the disease—that is, the time between becoming infected and showing clinical symptoms of scrapie—is measured in years. It is thought that resistance to scrapie simply means that some individuals are able to prolong the incubation period, perhaps for so long that the animal dies of other natural causes or is culled before it has time to develop clinical signs of scrapie. On the other hand, susceptible sheep are probably unable to do this and will therefore develop clinical signs much sooner.

However, even in susceptible sheep, the incubation period is usually at least a year and most affected sheep do not show clinical signs until they are from two to five years of age. Cases have been recorded in very old sheep of nine or ten years of age despite the fact that most animals probably become infected with the scrapie agent as lambs or young sheep. This has important practical implications, since it is known that the scrapie agent is present in the products of lambing—that is, the afterbirth and foetal fluids. Whilst an infected ewe may not develop clinical disease for many years, if at all, she may nevertheless infect her own lambs year after year plus any other ewes or lambs which come into contact with the infected material. Meanwhile she may remain undetected as an excreter of the agent.

It can therefore be imagined how contamination can build up insidiously within a flock. Because all ewes have differing abilities to cope with any particular strain of scrapie, the number of ewes and rams in a flock going down with the disease will depend upon the proportion of resistant to susceptible ewes and the strain or strains of scrapie agent present in the flock. Resistance to one strain of scrapie does not mean that ewes will be resistant to other strains. Indeed, it is possible for a particular strain to mutate and then produce clinical illness in ewes previously unaffected.

In most affected flocks the number of deaths from scrapie each year usually averages less than one in 20, but in highly susceptible flocks this may rise to a third or even half the flock. Although there is great variation in susceptibility between individual ewes, there does not appear to be any particular breed susceptibility.

THE PROBLEM OF DIAGNOSIS

Resistance to the scrapie agent is not like resistance to other diseases. With infections such as enzootic or toxoplasma abortion, ewes develop antibodies which circulate in the bloodstream and protect the ewe from further attack by the same organism. By testing blood for the presence of these antibodies it is possible to say whether ewes are, or have at some time, been infected with these microorganisms. The presence of antibodies can be used as a diagnostic test. The scrapie agent, however, does not stimulate any inflammatory response in its host, nor does it stimulate the sheep to produce antibodies. Hence, there is no diagnostic test for scrapie in the living animal. The only way of diagnosing the disease with certainty is to perform a post-mortem on an affected sheep and examine sections of the brain under the microscope for the typical signs of damage. This is a decided disadvantage when it comes to controlling the disease, since because of the lack of a test there is no way that a flock can be declared free from the disease, even in the total absence of any clinical cases. Similarly, there is no way that scrapie can be eradicated from a flock except by slaughtering out the whole flock. Recent research at the Neuropathogenesis Unit in Edinburgh has raised hopes that it may soon be possible, by blood testing, to identify animals which are resistant to scrapie.

Export problems

This inability to declare unequivocal freedom from the disease is a serious impediment to the export of sheep. Many countries wishing to improve the genetic merit of their flocks by importing British breeds are unwilling to do so because of the fear of this insidious disease. Once the disease becomes established in a national flock, such as in Britain, there is no way of eradication. The ADAS Sheep and Goat Health Scheme is unlikely to alter this situation until a good diagnostic test becomes available. Whilst it is possible that many flocks are free from the disease, there is no method of identifying them. Quarantine arrangements are totally impracticable and unacceptable, since sheep would have to be kept in isolation for five years or longer to allow for the detection of cases with a long incubation period. Even if there were no clinical cases during this time, this would not guarantee freedom from infection.

Rams from flocks which are infected with scrapie obviously present a risk to flocks which are free from the disease. Even rams purchased from apparently scrapie-free flocks may have a considerable influence on the number of clinical cases of the disease which occur in flocks which are already infected. This is because a ram may donate genetic material to its offspring which makes them either susceptible or resistant to any particular scrapie agent. For example, if an infected flock is losing an average 3% of the ewe flock annually from scrapie, then the introduction of a new ram which contributes a gene for susceptibility may increase the losses to 20 or 30% without the introduction of any new scrapie agent.

CONTROL OF SCRAPIE

Careful flock recording may allow the identification of families which are either more or less susceptible to clinical scrapie and this information can be used in breeding programmes designed to reduce the incidence of clinical scrapie in a flock. However, this may seriously interfere with or impede progress in improving flock performance, and such breeding programmes are not guaranteed to be successful. Also, fresh blood will be required sooner or later in most flocks and this may lead—albeit unknowingly—to

ιe introduction of new scrapie agents, or to genes conferring susceptibility
ɔ the disease.

Since control of scrapie by breeding programmes is limited, attempts
ιust be made to limit the spread of the scrapie agent within the flock by
ther methods:

- Ewes or rams which develop scrapie should be slaughtered immediately.
  This especially applies to ewes which develop the disease during pregnancy, which should be slaughtered **before** they lamb, since the products
  of lambing contain the scrapie agent and the lambs stand a high chance of
  becoming infected. (It is not known whether lambs are infected at some
  stage during pregnancy or during the process of lambing.)
- Affected or suspicious ewes allowed to lamb must be isolated when
  lambing. Other ewes should not be allowed to lamb in the same area,
  since the scrapie agent is very resistant to physical and chemical disinfection and the area will remain infected for many months. The afterbirth
  and bedding should be destroyed by burning.
- Using a different outside lambing area each year will obviously reduce
  risks. Although it is probably impossible to remove all infection completely from a sheep house, careful cleaning, disinfection and the use of
  generous bedding will help minimise the risk of spreading infection.
- The progeny of ewes which develop symptoms of scrapie—at any time
  during their breeding life in the flock—should not be bred from, but
  sold for slaughter. Unless sheep are individually identified by tattooing
  or tagging and carefully recorded, it will be impossible to identify the
  offspring of previous pregnancies. Remember that ewes may have been
  excreting the scrapie agent for years before showing clinical symptoms
  themselves. All offspring of scrapie infected ewes, including wethers
  and non-pregnant females, may excrete the scrapie agent and infect any
  in-contact sheep grazing or housed alongside them.
- Flocks infected with scrapie should not sell any animals—male or
  female—for breeding purposes. It is well known that a number of
  pedigree breeders with scrapie in their flocks destroy and dispose of
  cases promptly, but continue to sell breeding stock. This is totally
  unacceptable and usually shortsighted, since it will eventually come to
  light and such breeders will lose all credibility.
- Although it is not proven that scrapie can be spread from farm to farm
  on tyres, boots, etc., it remains a possibility, and reasonable avoiding
  action should be taken.
- Where there is a high level of infection, the only answer may be to slaughter
  out the whole flock. The problem remains of how long to leave the farm
  free of sheep before restocking and where to buy in scrapie-free sheep.

There is no vaccine available against scrapie, and because the agent does
ιot stimulate an immune response in the ewe, it is unlikely that there will
·ver be a conventional one.

Research work on scrapie in the UK continues at the Neuropathogenesis

Unit in Edinburgh, which is jointly funded by the Agricultural Research Council (ARC) and the Medical Research Council (MRC). There are similarities between scrapie in sheep and a number of dementias in humans such as Creutzfelt-Jacob disease, and pooling resources may help to throw further light on this important group of 'slow' nervous diseases which pose difficult problems for investigators.

In April 1985, the first cases of a new nervous disease of cattle known as bovine spongiform encephalopathy (BSE), were seen in the UK. This condition closely resembles scrapie in sheep, both clinically and at post-mortem examination of brain material. It is now known to be caused by a transmissible agent. Epidemiological studies have shown that cases probably emanated from a common source and that this was probably commercially produced cattle feed stuffs. The ingredient most likely to have contained the scrapie-like agent is meat and bone meal which contained processed sheep's heads and therefore brains. The infectious agent may have survived processing because of recent changes in the methods of rendering such materials.

There is no evidence that BSE has been transmitted either directly or indirectly from sheep to cattle on farms where the disease has occurred. Research is continuing into this important group of diseases.

Johne's Disease

This is an infectious disease of sheep, cattle and other ruminants such as deer and goats which causes enteritis, progressive loss of body condition and, in the majority of cases, death following a long illness. Not all animals which become infected will develop clinical signs of the disease. Stressful situations, such as may occur during late pregnancy, lambing and lactation, may tip the balance in favour of the infection, and lead to the development of clinical signs. This is especially so where ewes are suffering from some other debilitating disease such as liver fluke, or where they are being inadequately fed.

The disease appears to be less common and less dramatic in sheep than in cattle, where the frothy, foul smelling, watery diarrhoea can hardly be ignored. It is probable that many sheep outbreaks occur as a result of infection from cattle, although sheep do have their own strain of the bacterium. It is possible that the disease may go undetected in some flocks which do not seek veterinary diagnosis, cases simply being put down to other, more common causes of wasting. The disease may apparently 'disappear' from a flock for a year or two, although it is more likely that it remains in a sub-clinical form until conditions alter and losses occur once more.

Carrier animals

Johne's disease is caused by *Mycobacterium johnei*, a bacterium closely related to the one responsible for tuberculosis in man and animals. The bacterium causes an inflammation of part of the gut and is therefore shed in the faeces of infected animals, whether or not they show clinical signs, although the number of microorganisms shed by clinical cases is generally much greater. The bacteria can remain infective in faeces, soil and water for up to a year or more. Apparently normal animals which pass the bacteria in their faeces are called carriers. They play an important role in the perpetuation of disease on a farm and in the spread of Johne's to other farms when they are sold.

This is another disease with a long incubation period, since it may be many months (or even a year or more) between an animal becoming infected and the development of clinical symptoms. Whilst infected animals do not always show obvious symptoms, they may nevertheless suffer some loss of performance due to the low-grade gut infection. These animals cannot be detected because there is no satisfactory diagnostic test available at present.

Methods of infection

Animals become infected by swallowing the bacteria which have contaminated their food or water supply. Where infection has been present on a farm for some time, it is likely that animals will become infected sooner rather than later, probably as lambs or hoggs. For example, lambs born to infected ewes may themselves become infected by swallowing the bacteria when they suck teats contaminated by the ewe's faeces. The ewes do not necessarily need to be showing symptoms of Johne's for this to happen. Ewes which are obviously ill themselves during pregnancy may infect their lambs before they are born. Other sheep may become infected by drinking pond water contaminated by Johne's-infected cattle.

CLINICAL SIGNS

The clinical signs of Johne's disease are largely due to the gut infection which interferes with the digestion and absorption of food and of proteins in particular. This in turn leads to a wasting of muscle, with consequent loss of weight (often despite the fact that most sheep continue to eat), anaemia and eventually death. The illness may last for many weeks or months if animals are not humanely destroyed. Some sheep may appear to recover temporarily, only to relapse and die some time later. Only very occasionally do animals survive after developing clinical signs. Many affected sheep are desperately thin and the fleece often pulls out when they are handled. Watery diarrhoea as in cattle is not very common, but the dung may become soft and lose its pelleted form.

DIAGNOSIS

In flocks where the disease is known to be present, shepherds can usually recognise the early signs. Where it has never been diagnosed previously it

239

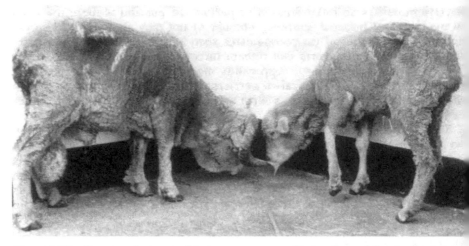

Plate 6.17 These unfortunate Merino rams are suffering from Johne's disease and salmonellosis simultaneously.

may be confused with other wasting diseases, such as liver fluke, worms or trace element deficiencies. However, even if treatment for these other conditions gives some temporary respite, this improvement is short-lived in Johne's cases and animals continue to decline. With many of the other wasting conditions a large proportion of the flock is affected, often across all age groups. With Johne's disease, only the occasional sheep becomes clinically ill and it is usually young breeding ewes of at least one year old.

Dung from suspected cases may contain the bacteria responsible and this is proof of infection. However, as the bacteria are only excreted intermittently in faeces, a negative result does not rule out the disease. Therefore, affected animals should be slaughtered on suspicion and submitted to a full post-mortem.

CONTROL

Johne's disease is incurable and like all diseases with a long incubation period is difficult to control. Its transmission by carriers—that is, apparently normal animals excreting the bacteria in their faeces—further complicates the situation. By the time the disease is first diagnosed, the infection is often well established in the flock and the farm may be well and truly contaminated.

However, as with most infectious diseases, it is sensible to attempt to reduce the weight of infection. The first essential is to slaughter any affected animals or suspicious cases, since they will continually contaminate the pastures and buildings. Unfortunately there is no satisfactory diagnostic test for the detection of carrier animals.

The offspring of affected ewes are very likely to become infected themselves and they will then add to the contamination whether or not they eventually develop clinical symptoms. They should therefore be fattened for slaughter and certainly not retained for breeding.

Sheep sheds, lambing paddocks and other pastures which have been heavily stocked are likely to be heavily contaminated. If feasible, the lambing area should be changed each year. Risky areas can be grazed by adult ewes, since although they will become infected, they are less likely to develop clinical disease than younger ewes. Lowering stocking rates overall will also reduce the risk.

If sheep are part of an arable rotation, ploughing will bury infection, but in the wetter western areas of Britain this is rarely feasible. Where cattle are also farmed it is important to remember that they can infect sheep with Johne's and vice versa. Do not graze sheep over ground grazed by infected cattle or where their dung or slurry has been spread.

It is important to avoid contamination of feedstuffs with faeces. It is particularly important to have a clean fresh supply of water for stock at all times, so that they do not go looking for water in stagnant pools or ditches, which should be fenced off since they present a high risk.

There is a Johne's vaccine for cattle, which can also be used on sheep, but because the responsible bacterium is a close relative of tuberculosis, vaccination creates difficulties with interpretation of the tuberculin test, and special permission from the veterinary authorities is required for its use. Johne's is particularly bad news for flocks with an export trade in breeding animals, since most countries demand proof of freedom from the disease.

Recent research in the UK and USA has strengthened the case for suggesting that the bacterium which causes Johne's disease in ruminants may also be the cause of some cases of Crohn's disease in man.

7

LAMBING TIME

Preparation for Lambing

Whilst it is probably erroneous to suggest that one period of the sheep year is any more important than another, there is no doubt that lambing time should be the climax of the year's work. Unfortunately, in many flocks this is not always the case, often because of inadequate preparation and lack of attention to detail throughout the year.

Birth is the most hazardous period in any animal's life. Since the sheep is a seasonal breeder, a large number of births take place over a relatively short time, putting pressure on both the shepherd and the sheep. It is nevertheless the shepherd's responsibility to minimise losses of both lambs and ewes and to ensure that neither are subjected to any unnecessary stress or hazard. Apart from welfare considerations, it makes sound economic sense to rear as many fit and healthy lambs as possible. It is unfortunate that economic pressures mean that shepherds today often have too many ewes to look after.

TRAINING

All young people who are to be given this responsible job should receive some formal training. Even the most experienced shepherds will benefit from occasional refresher courses, such as those organised by the Agricultural Training Board, to update themselves on the latest techniques of their craft. Any who consider such updating to be unnecessary are almost certainly deluding themselves and probably allowing unnecessary suffering and loss amongst their charges as a consequence. There is, for example, no possible excuse for ignorance of the techniques for preventing and treating hypothermia in lambs, which should be in use on every sheep farm in the land, without exception.

Some deaths amongst lambs and ewes at lambing time are inevitable, even in the best managed flocks, but the huge losses of lambs in the national flock are totally unacceptable because the majority of them are avoidable. Figures of 15% average mortality, or 3 to 4 million lamb deaths per year in the UK are largely meaningless, causing only a momentary raising of the eyebrows. However, if from a 500 ewe lowland flock where 900 lambs are born (180%), the 135 lambs which die (15%) were laid nose to tail, they would stretch for about 50 metres and weigh approximately half a tonne. If they were valued at only £40 each at slaughter, this would represent a potential loss of £5,400 in income.

The hope is that this section of the book will assist in reducing losses of both ewes and lambs to a more acceptable level and also reduce the less obvious losses due to non-fatal and sub-clinical disease.

PRE-LAMBING HUSBANDRY

Among the important tasks which have to be carried out in the late pregnancy period, a pre-lambing visit from your veterinary surgeon who specialises in sheep matters should be most beneficial and cost-effective. It is important to attempt to minimise the number of times that ewes are handled at this time, so a discussion regarding which jobs can safely be done at the same time will be helpful, although some compromises will have to be made. For example, in hill flocks, where gatherings are difficult and stressful for ewes, many shepherds delay booster pasteurella and clostridial vaccinations until the ewes are brought down off the tops to lamb in enclosures or parks. This may be only 10 days or a fortnight before lambing is due to begin and therefore somewhat late for the earliest lambers. Most flocks—both hill and lowland—would benefit from being split into early and late lambing groups, based on ram raddle marks, so that vaccinations could be timed more appropriately. This would ensure that the majority of ewes have sufficiently high levels of antibodies in their colostrum to protect their lambs adequately.

Lowland ewes should be in body condition score of 2.5 to 3 at lambing and hill ewes 2 to 2.5. If any are thin at vaccination time, they should be pulled out and fed preferentially. Any underlying reason for the thinness should be investigated (e.g. teeth, liver fluke).

It is important not to make any abrupt changes in the diet around lambing time, but ewes which are to go onto fresh spring grass with their lambs immediately after lambing will need a magnesium supplement added to their concentrate ration. Magnesium can be unpalatable and should be added in increasing amount to the mixture during the last week or 10 days of pregnancy. (There is no need to supplement pregnancy rations with magnesium otherwise.) Ewes should have been checked for trace element status (copper, cobalt and selenium) earlier in pregnancy and the ration corrected accordingly. The same applies to the major elements (calcium and phosphorous) and to the vitamins (e.g. vitamins D and E).

Crutching the ewes—removing any dirty or excess wool from around the ewe's rear end and from the udder—is important, so that the newborn lambs can find the udder quickly and easily in the crucial first few hours of life.

244

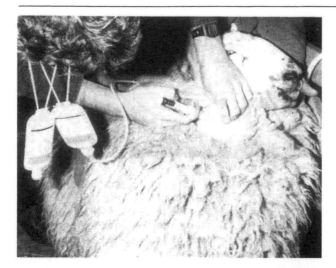

Plate 7.1 (*Above*) The pre-lambing booster vaccinations against the clostridial infections plus pasteurellosis are crucially important if lambs are to be protected via colostrum.

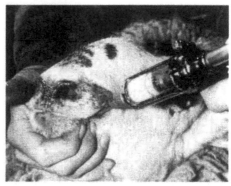

Plate 7.2 (*Right*) Ewes should be dosed with an anthelmintic shortly after housing to eliminate all parasitic worms so that they do not contaminate pastures at turn-out with their lambs.

PREPARATION OF THE LAMBING AREA

Immediately before lambing the flock should be split into early, middle and late lambers and these should, wherever possible, be lambed in separate areas of the house or lambing paddock to reduce the risk of the build-up of infectious disease. In outdoor lambing flocks a different area should be used each year wherever practical, since a number of infectious microorganisms and parasites (e.g. cryptosporidium) may remain infective from one season to another. However, this risk is much less than the risks of the current season, so a favoured sheltered paddock is acceptable if sensible precautions are taken.

Temporary lambing pens built of straw bales have the advantage that they can be burned at the end of the season, thus destroying any infection with them. Individual pens which become infected, by a scouring lamb for example, can also be burned and replaced. It is useful to have pens covered

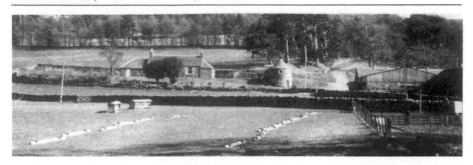

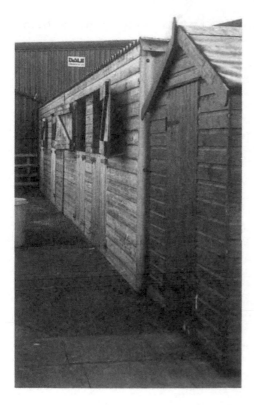

Plate 7.3 For outdoor lambing, a favoured paddock close to the steading is acceptable. It is always best to lamb early, mid and late lambers in separate enclosures where possible.

Plate 7.4 A hospital area for infectious cases should be apart from the main lambing area. Separate boots and overalls should be worn and strict hygiene observed to reduce the spread of infection.

or part covered with corrugated sheeting or something similar, to allow lambs shelter from the rain and wind. It is always wise to have a contingency plan, so that if infection does gain the upper hand, ewes yet to lamb can be moved to a fresh area. If there is no option for flocks lambing indoors but to lamb in the same location each season, every attempt should be made to ensure that the area is scrupulously clean at the start of the lambing.

For outdoor lowland lambings, the area chosen should be in a sheltered position and reasonably close to the farm buildings for handiness and access to water and electricity. Where possible, ewes should be housed at night, since this is so much more convenient for the shepherd and provides protection for both ewes and lambs in bad weather. Only small numbers of ewes should be brought into the lambing area at any one time, since this will make shepherding easier and reduce the risk of mismothering and the build-up of infection.

Young females lambing for the first time should be in a separate area away from the mature ewe flock to protect them from infection and particularly from enzootic abortion of ewes. Keeping them in a separate group also allows them to be fed preferentially, without having to compete with the ewes.

Any purchased ewes should always be lambed apart from the home flock to avoid cross-infection.

Hospital area

Whether the flock is lambing indoors or outdoors, provision should always be made indoors for a hospital area, where infectious cases can be looked after, and also for an intensive care area for lambs with non-infectious conditions such as hypothermia or broken limbs. The latter can be within the lambing area itself, but the hospital area must be distinctly separate. Shepherds should not traipse back and forth between the infectious area and the clean area without washing hands and changing boots and overalls. This may sound overfussy, but sloppy methods on the part of some shepherds are undoubtedly responsible for the spread of infection at lambing time.

Lambing pens

An adequate number of lambing pens should be constructed. As a rough guide 12 pens will be needed per 100 ewes lambing. However, if a flock is synchronised, so that ewes are lambing thick and fast, then 40 pens may be needed per 100 ewes. Teased flocks would come somewhere between these extremes.

Some indoor lambing flocks provide individual pens for every ewe if space is available, and this has a number of advantages. Ewes can be penned before lambing, rather than being moved after the event, and this allows them to settle down, unmolested by the rest of the mob. Providing the pens are lamb-proof, this should mean less mismothering and a better chance of the lambs finding a teat earlier rather than later, especially those born at night when the shepherd may be snatching a little well-earned sleep. Where ewes have been scanned and the number of foetuses is known, single and triplet bearing ewes can be penned opposite each other, so making cross-fostering easier.

For both indoor and outdoor lambing areas, ensure that there is a dry lie for ewes and lambs. Put slaked lime down on indoor earth floors before bedding up with ample straw. Disinfection during lambing is often difficult or impossible and generous bedding is an excellent substitute. In areas where straw is relatively expensive, it is still a very worthwhile investment, as saving even one lamb will pay for a substantial quantity of straw.

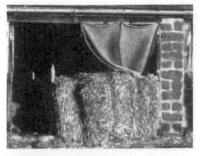

Plate 7.5 Straw bales provide good shelter for lambing pens and can be burned after lambing or after infection in the pens. The plate below shows a large airy building for lambing with ample straw bedding. The building is used for different purposes at other times of the year.

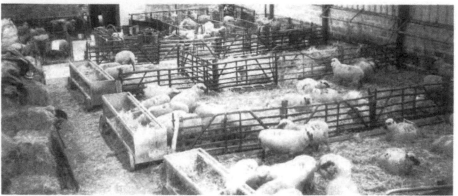

LAMBING PREPARATION ON HILL FARMS

On hill farms, the flock at lambing time is much more at the mercy of the weather, since few farms are able to lamb the whole flock on sheltered in-bye land. For some, the single carrying ewes have to lamb on the open hill and on others the twin bearing ewes also.

It is therefore not surprising that in bad years lamb losses can be nothing short of catastrophic, with death rates of 40 or 50% not unheard of. Shepherding, in the true sense of the word, is often impossible under extensive conditions, being reduced to disaster limitation. It can be very demoralising for a shepherd to set off at dawn to find lambs frozen in the snow, or a ewe which has died in the process of a difficult lambing. On the most extensive farms, the chances of a shepherd ever coming across a ewe in the act of lambing are slim indeed, let alone coming across one requiring assistance in time to do some good.

Many hill farms bring ewes down off the high ground into large enclosures lower down the hill to lamb. In this way the shepherd has some degree of control. Ewes and lambs in difficulty can be brought down to the farm buildings by tractor and box or by an all-terrain vehicle. Some farms invest in a sheep shed for in-wintering hoggs. The hoggs can be turned out in spring to allow gimmers and the older and thinner ewes to lamb indoors.

On farms which have reclaimed ground from the hill in order to increase the stocking rate and the lambing percentage, some form of shelter must be provided for the twins. As these will be born at a lighter weight, they will be even more vulnerable to chilling, and access to a warming box and, therefore, electricity will be essential. Pens for mothering-up and for fostering-on lambs should also be provided, preferably indoors.

Scanning ewes to determine lamb numbers has proved to be of particular benefit on hill farms where there are a significant number of twin bearing ewes, since after scanning they can remain on the lowground in relative safety for lambing time. The shepherd can then use the time more productively than previously, when much of the day was spent bringing ewes with pairs down off the hill—a tedious and time-consuming task.

SUPPLIES OF COLOSTRUM

Once a lamb is safely born into the world, the most important factor for its future survival is an early and adequate feed of colostrum. For one reason or another, some ewes may not have adequate supplies for their lambs. Other lambs may be orphaned, weak or sick and may require supplementary feeds of colostrum. Collection of colostrum from ewes can often be disappointing and it is difficult to judge how much to take from a ewe to leave her with sufficient for her own offspring. Also, supplies must be available right at the start of lambing, and therefore it is essential to collect and store some ewe colostrum from the previous season or to make alternative provisions. The role of colostrum is discussed in detail in Chapter 8.

Goat colostrum and CAE

Goat colostrum is often for sale and is a good substitute for ewe colostrum. However, it it most important to establish that the goat herd is free from caprine arthritis encephalitis (CAE). The virus which causes this disease is closely related to—and cannot be distinguished from—the one responsible for maedi-visna (M-V) in sheep. The virus is shed in goat's milk by which it may be transferred to lambs, which would then react positively to the maedi-visna blood test in later life. This would obviously be highly undesirable in M-V accredited flocks. Also, it is possible for the virus to cause actual clinical illness in lambs, and although this has not been seen in the UK, cases have been reported in New Zealand. A significant proportion of goat herds are known to be infected, but only relatively few are regularly tested, so beware.

Cow colostrum and the anti-ovine factor

Cow colostrum is an acceptable substitute for the ewe product and has the advantage that it can be collected in large quantities for storage in the deep freeze in small quantities of up to 250 ml. A small proportion of cows have an anti-sheep or anti-ovine factor in their colostrum, which leads

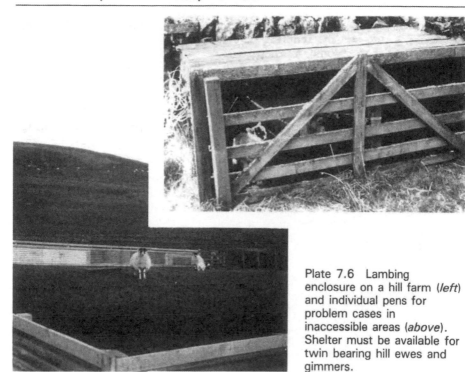

Plate 7.6 Lambing enclosure on a hill farm (*left*) and individual pens for problem cases in inaccessible areas (*above*). Shelter must be available for twin bearing hill ewes and gimmers.

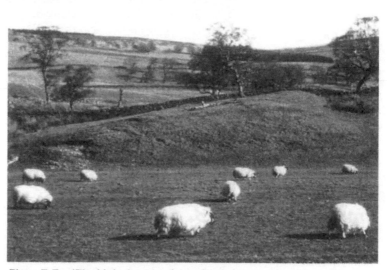

Plate 7.7 'Blackie' gimmers brought down to riverside parks to lamb. Access to areas of open woodland provides vital shelter for ewes lambing on the high, exposed ground.

to the destruction of the red blood cells of any lambs which drink it. This produces a profound anaemia which is usually fatal unless treated early by blood transfusion. Affected lambs initially become very thirsty and some may eat soil. They soon lose their appetite, grow very weak, collapse and die, usually within a day of the onset of illness. The ears and inside of the mouth appear very pale due to the anaemia. If any such cases occur, do not feed any more of that particular cow's colostrum and destroy any that remains, or feed it to calves.

Each pot of stored colostrum must be identified with the cow's name or ear number, as well as the date it was frozen. Where cow colostrum is being relied upon, it is also essential to have supplies from at least two or three cows in case a lamb anaemia problem occurs. Samples of colostrum can be tested in the laboratory to give an estimate of the likelihood of anaemia. This condition is relatively uncommon and the value of cow colostrum to lambs needing it far outweighs the small risk. Pooling colostrum from several cows reduces the risk.

Vaccinating cows against the clostridial diseases of sheep

Cow colostrum is even more valuable to lambs if it contains antibodies against the clostridial diseases of sheep. This can be arranged by vaccinating the cow with 10 ml of a '7 in 1' type clostridial vaccine on three occasions—at three months, one month and a fortnight before calving. Colostrum should be collected from the first two milkings after calving. As colostrum may be needed for premature lambs some time before the onset of the main lambing, suitable cows should be identified and vaccinated for the first time at least four months before lambing. As colostrum freezes satisfactorily, it can of course be collected at any convenient time.

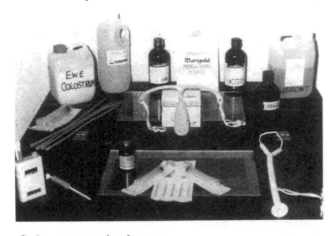

Plate 7.8 A selection of items needed at lambing time arranged on top of a lamb warming box.

Colostrum substitutes

A number of live colostrum replacers or substitutes are now on the market, but it is too early to make any recommendations.

QUICK REFERENCE LIST
Materials required around lambing time

GENERAL

Clostridial and pasteurella vaccines	for pre-lambing booster doses
Fluke and worm medicines	for pre-lambing treatment
High magnesium concentrate or other form of magnesium supplementation	for gradual introduction during the last week of pregnancy and during lactation for the prevention of hypomagnesaemia
Polythene arm-length gloves	for grasping and containing aborted foetuses and afterbirths
Strong plastic bags, ties and labels	for transporting aborted materials to the laboratory for diagnosis
Prolapse retainers (several)	for use on ewes with prolapse of the vagina before lambing
Soft ropes, string, webbing or a commercial truss	for applying a truss in cases of prolapse
Bottles or flexible packs of sterile solutions for injection of:	
calcium borogluconate	for the treatment of hypocalcaemia
calcium borogluconate with added magnesium and phosphorus	for the treatment of hypocalcaemia, pregnancy toxaemia or hypomagnesaemia when the diagnosis is unclear
magnesium sulphate	for the treatment of hypomagnesaemia
glycerine, propylene glycol, treacle or molasses	for administration by mouth for the treatment of pregnancy toxaemia

FOR ASSISTING THE EWE AT LAMBING

Plastic bucket, soap, towel and mild disinfectant	for shepherd's hygiene before and after lambing
Lambing lubricant (or soapflakes)	to avoid damage to the ewe and to assist in the extraction of lambs
Hard margarine blocks	for rubbing into the coat of a 'dry' lamb during a difficult lambing

Lambing aids and soft nylon or rubber lambing ropes (several)	to help in holding a limb or the head in position when assisting a ewe to lamb; an ample supply is required so that a clean sterilised set can be used for each ewe assisted
Milton or equivalent antiseptic and plastic containers with lids	for storage of all sterilised materials such as lambing ropes
Antibiotic injection (e.g. long-acting penicillin) and pessaries	for treatment of **all** ewes assisted at lambing. **NB** All prescription-only medicines (POM) such as antibiotics have to be supplied by a veterinary surgeon who will advise on a suitable product for your circumstances
Syringes and needles	it is important to use the correct size of syringe and needle for a particular purpose
Water heater and heat source (e.g. electric ring)	for cleaning and sterilising equipment by boiling

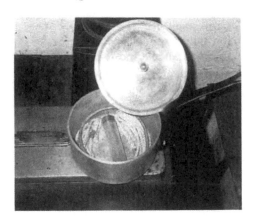

Plate 7.9 Where items have been sterilised by boiling, the water should be drained off and the lid replaced to keep the contents sterile until needed again.

FOR CARE OF THE NEWBORN LAMB

Resuscitator	to suck the sticky mucus from the back of the throat of lambs
Lung inflator	to assist lambs to begin breathing (the 'kiss of life' must **never** be used)

Plate 7.10 A resuscitator (designed for human babies) can be used to suck mucus from the back of a lamb's throat. A shorter, softer rubber tube should be substituted and care taken not to damage the back of the mouth.

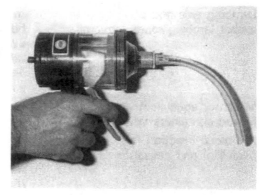

Old towels	an ample supply is required for drying lambs should they be neglected by the ewe (these should be washed immediately after use)
Low temperature thermometer	for the detection of chilled lambs
Lamb warming box (with thermometer of the greenhouse type)	for reviving hypothermic or chilled lambs (*see text*); the thermometer is to check the temperature of the box, especially if it is not thermostatically controlled
Colostrum	an ample supply of frozen ewe, goat or cow colostrum in small amounts for feeding to vulnerable lambs
Stomach tubes and 50 ml syringes	for the administration of colostrum (and occasionally medicines)
Lamb feeding bottles and teats	
Glucose solution	for intraperitoneal injection of lambs
Tincture of iodine (BP) and suitable dispenser	for the treatment of the navel cord and surrounding skin of newborn lambs
Plastic lamb macs or thermal jackets	for the protection of vulnerable lambs out of doors in bad weather
Cardboard grocery boxes	for the construction of an intensive care unit for lambs recovering from hypothermia or illness
Infra-red lamps	as a heat source for the intensive care unit

Electrolyte solutions and glucose powder	for the replacement of body fluids in scouring lambs which have become dehydrated; these solutions may sometimes need to be fortified with glucose
Oral antibiotics	for the treatment by mouth of lambs with an infectious disease; these may be supplied by your veterinary surgeon as tablets, capsules, liquids or pastes. 'Pumps' are a convenient method for baby lambs
Antiseptic or antibiotic sprays, powders or creams	for the treatment of wounds or to prepare the skin for injection
Liquid paraffin (or soapy water)	for administration as an enema to constipated lambs
Beechams pills	for oral treatment of constipation
Eye ointment (antibiotic)	for the treatment of eye infections; only special eye preparations should ever be used in the eye
Michel clips and applicator	for the correction of entropion (turned in eyelids) in lambs
Rubber or plastic handgloves	for handling lambs with orf or other infectious diseases transmissible to humans
Washing soda crystals	for cleaning and disinfecting concrete pens at the rate of 0.5 kg (1 lb) to a bucket of hot water
MAFF-approved disinfectant	for follow-up disinfection after thorough cleaning
Elastrator and rubber rings	for castration and tailing of lambs
Marker spray	for identification of lambs
Fostering crate	
Automatic milk dispenser	for feeding ewe milk replacer to lambs
Ewe milk replacer (EMR)	for feeding to artificially reared lambs
Thermally insulated bag and lamb jackets with heat-releasing gel	for carrying hypothermic or sick lambs down off the hill
'Pour-on' insecticide	for the protection of hill lambs against sheep tick

Shelters for ewes and lambs	strategically placed on the hill, e.g. for fostering-on lambs
Shepherd's hut	for inaccessible areas of the hill, to store equipment and for the shepherd to shelter, rest, eat and drink
Hardback notebook and pencils (which write in the rain)	for recording lambing data

The Lambing Process

Pregnancy lasts for approximately five months in the ewe. The majority of lambings occur between days 146 to 148 inclusive, but even in a pure-bred flock, normal lambings will occur between days 140 and 150. Single lambs are generally carried longer than twins or triplets, which tend to be born somewhat prematurely.

It is the lambs which decide when they will be born, rather than the ewe deciding that it is time to deliver her lambs. The whole lambing process is controlled by a complex series of hormonal changes triggered off by the foetal lambs responding to 'stress'.

INITIATION OF THE BIRTH PROCESS

At the end of pregnancy things are getting very cramped in the uterus, with a large foetus (or foetuses), full-grown placenta (afterbirth) and a large accumulation of fluids which bathe and protect the lamb. The foetal lamb receives its oxygen and nutrients from the ewe's blood supply via the placenta and rids itself of waste materials by the reverse route. In the final stages of pregnancy these processes become critical, since the ewe finds it increasingly difficult to maintain the lambs adequately as their demands increase daily. These 'stresses' stimulate the lamb to produce an increasing quantity of a steroid hormone called **cortisol**, which finds its way into the ewe's bloodstream and is responsible for the initiation of the birth process.

Hormonal changes

All throughout pregnancy it is important that the uterus—which is a large muscular sac—does not contract, since this would jeopardise the life of the lambs. Therefore, the 'buttons' (placentomes) on the placenta secrete the hormone progesterone, which very effectively prevents this happening. Before birth can proceed, the levels of this hormone have to be substantially reduced to allow the uterus to contract and expel the lambs into the world. The cortisol secreted by the lambs causes progesterone to be converted to another hormone called oestrogen, to which it is closely related, but which has very different effects. As progesterone levels fall and oestrogen levels

256

rise, this has the effect of allowing yet another hormone—prostaglandin F2 alpha (PGF2alpha)— to act on the uterus, causing it to contract and thus beginning the lambing process.

Signs of impending lambing

The hormonal changes going on inside the ewe can be detected by the shepherd in a number of ways. As lambing approaches, the udder gradually develops and fills up with colostrum. This can be seen most easily when ewes are feeding at the trough and particularly in housed ewes which are shorn. This feature is extremely variable and whilst udder development is a reliable sign that lambing is relatively imminent, a lack of udder development does not necessarily mean that lambing is a long way off. Some ewes lamb with virtually no udder development, whilst others may have a well-developed udder for a week or more before they lamb. This depends to some extent on the feeding of the flock.

As lambing time approaches, ewes generally take more and more interest in newborn lambs and may attempt to mother and 'steal' them. This behaviour is due to the fact that the fluids spilt at lambing become very attractive to any imminent ewe.

When contractions of the uterus begin, they do so gradually and ewes will tend to isolate themselves from the rest of the mob and may refuse their concentrate rations. As contractions increase in both strength and frequency, they make the ewes uncomfortable, so that they become very restless. They may scratch and scrape around the chosen 'nesting' spot and get up and down frequently, often stretching out their necks and making nibbling and licking movements.

LABOUR

Meanwhile, inside the ewe, another hormone called **relaxin** has been at work, softening up the tough tissues which make up the cervix (the neck of the womb) so that it can be stretched to accommodate the passage of the lamb. The ligaments which hold together the bones which form the pelvis, through which the lamb must pass, also soften up, making this rigid ring of bone more flexible. The strong contractions of the uterus force the fluid-filled sacs surrounding the foetus up against the cervix, which then gradually yields and begins to open up. Within a few hours the cervix becomes fully relaxed and open and the lamb itself is pushed into the birth canal.

Up to this stage the ewe has taken a passive role in the process, having herself no conscious control over the muscles which contract the uterus. However, once the head of the lamb (in a normal forward presentation) engages in the pelvic region of the birth canal, this stimulates the ewe to hasten the process further. This she does by 'straining' or 'pushing'—that is, by contracting the muscles of her abdomen—so significantly increasing the pressure on the lamb. Eventually the shepherd will see the 'waterbag'

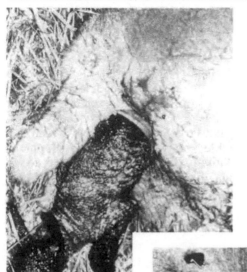

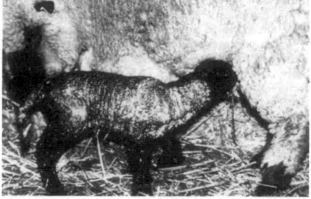

Plate 7.11 A Clun Forest ewe giving birth onto clean straw bedding (*left*), and the lamb taking its first feed of colostrum within five minutes of birth (*below*).

appearing at the now swollen vulva, or, if the waterbag has already burst, perhaps the foot or nose of the lamb poking out. A few more powerful contractions of the abdominal muscles are now necessary to finally expel the lamb, since the uterine contractions become less potent as the lamb passes out of the uterus, through the cervix and into the vagina.

Once the lamb is expelled and the umbilical cord is finally ruptured, the lamb must immediately take on an independent existence. Rupturing of the cord, release from the restricting confines of the uterus, sudden exposure to the considerable drop in temperature of the outside air and hopefully the nuzzling and licking of the ewe, all stimulate the newborn lamb to take its first vital breaths.

'Cleansing'

The birth of the lambs is not the end of the lambing process, however, since the ewe must also expel what remains of the placentae or afterbirths.

This is often referred to as 'cleansing' or 'cleaning'. This may follow very shortly after the lambs are born or even at the same time, but when lambs are born slightly prematurely, as most twins and triplets are, it may be some hours before the afterbirths are voided. Not until this happens is lambing complete. If the lambs get up and suck vigorously, this not only stimulates milk let-down, but also encourages further contractions of the uterus which help to void the afterbirth (both processes are stimulated by the same hormone, oxytocin). The uterine contractions also stem any bleeding from the numerous small blood vessels which are ruptured during the birth process. Eventually the cervix closes up again to prevent infection entering the uterus.

It is most important to appreciate that the lambing process has evolved over many thousands of years and, whilst it occasionally goes wrong, it will proceed normally and without incident for the majority of ewes. Ewes will vary in the time taken to complete lambing. For example, first-time lambers may take considerably longer than older ewes. However, the hormonal changes which control lambing coordinate the process in such a way as to ensure the highest survival rate for the lambs.

ADAPTING TO LIFE OUTSIDE THE WOMB

Consider the changes a lamb must adapt to within a very short period of being thrust into an often hostile world. The foetal lamb's lungs contain fluid, but as soon as it is born it must get rid of these sticky fluids so that it is capable of breathing air. Its blood supply must begin to circulate through its lungs to capture the oxygen. In the uterus it receives all its nutrients from the ewe and is insulated from heat loss by the fluids which surround it, but at birth it must generate its own heat from what energy reserves it has acquired from the ewe during late pregnancy, principally in the form of brown fat.

The lamb must also change from being a foetus of leisure to a vigorous, teat-seeking lamb, able to keep up with its mother in wind, hail, rain or snow. When it sucks colostrum for the first time, its gut must be able to cope with the digestion of a complex food. Its kidneys must also be capable of excreting waste materials and of maintaining the body's fluid balance, and the liver must function in a multitude of ways.

All these organs and systems must be sufficiently mature in order to function satisfactorily and the hormonal influences of the last few days and hours before and during birth are crucially important to the lamb. The corticosteroid hormones which start off the lambing process are also involved in the final stages of maturation of all the lamb's organ systems mentioned above. For example, for the proper functioning of the lungs, a substance called **surfactant** must be secreted into the lung substance to enable them to inflate and thereby allow the lamb to breathe. If surfactant is not present, then the lungs will remain collapsed and the lamb will perish. The same hormones also control the supply of energy (glycogen) to the newborn lamb, by mobilising carbohydrate from brown fat. This process is essential to its survival in the crucial period before it sucks colostrum. Colostrum then takes over as the sole energy source, since the lamb's own reserves rapidly run out.

Any unwarrented interference with the smooth functioning of the birth process will therefore jeopardise the lamb's chances of survival. This particularly includes pulling lambs out of ewes before they are ready to be born. This is an instinct in many shepherds which should be strongly resisted, since it is undoubtedly responsible for the death of some lambs.

THE EWE-LAMB BOND

An important feature of early life for the lamb is the relationship it has with its mother. This ewe-lamb bond needs to be manifest immediately the lamb is born, but in fact is established before and during the birth process. The hormones circulating immediately before birth (particularly oestrogen), together with the stimulus the ewe receives during birth, when the lamb is in the birth canal, stimulate strong maternal instincts in the ewe, so that she protects her lamb and licks it dry. In doing so she identifies the unique smell of her own offspring in the foetal fluids which soak it at birth. If this bond is not established quickly after birth, then the chances of its happening fade rapidly by the hour. In licking the lamb, the ewe not only forms a bond with her offspring, but also stimulates it to breathe, to get up and follow her and to bleat. This in turn reinforces the maternal bond and increases the lamb's chances of getting to the teat to take colostrum early, which is so vital to its survival.

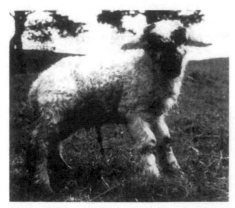 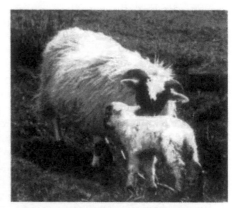

Plate 7.12 Scottish Blackface lamb newly born on a bitterly cold April afternoon at 1,000 feet above sea level. Its survival is totally dependent upon an immediate and close bond with its mother, who must lick it dry and allow it to suck colostrum or it will quickly perish.

260

SUPERVISION OF THE FLOCK AT LAMBING

Whilst the role of the shepherd at lambing time is a crucial one, it should be remembered that the final outcome will have been largely determined by the management of the flock throughout the year. Indeed, a detailed study of a large lambing flock in Scotland, carried out by the workers at the Moredun Research Institute, indicated that more than two-thirds of the lamb losses occurring at or immediately after lambing were attributable to factors determined before birth. For example, the viability of lambs is strongly influenced by their birth weight, which is largely determined by the size of the placenta, which in turn depends upon how the ewe is fed during the first three months of pregnancy. In a well-managed flock, therefore, the shepherd's job at lambing is almost always going to be easier than in a poorly managed flock. However, all the good work put into the flock throughout the year can be undone by poor shepherding at lambing time.

Welfare at lambing

Whilst the profitability of a flock will depend to a large extent upon the number of lambs reared and therefore upon the number of lambs born and kept alive, this should not be the only consideration at lambing. The welfare of the animals—both ewes and lambs—should always come first. There is no place in the lambing paddock for callous or uncaring individuals. Inexperienced staff should be closely supervised by skilled shepherds at all times. Sheep farmers should provide their shepherds with every reasonable facility to make the job easier and should not expect them to cope with too many lambing ewes, as this will inevitably result in stress and suffering for both sheep and shepherd.

It is not possible to put a figure on the number of ewes one person can look after, as this will vary considerably, depending not only upon the capabilities of the individual, but also upon the circumstances of the flock. Long, spread-out lambings should be avoided, since ewes lambing at the end frequently get less than adequate supervision. Shepherds become fatigued, especially when they have to work long hours with relatively little happening in the lambing area, but much to do elsewhere.

It is a salutary experience to record a lambing in detail and in total honesty, recording all lamb and ewe losses and, wherever possible, getting an accurate diagnosis of all deaths and of any disease outbreaks. It will become apparent from such a survey just where and why problems are occurring, how well or badly the flock is being managed and how well the shepherds are coping with the number of ewes allocated to them. Without accurate records of this type it is not possible to make objective judgements, but merely to gain impressions which may be completely erroneous.

In intensive lowground flocks the level of supervision will, to some extent at least, be dictated by the type of organisation at lambing—for example, on whether or not the flock is housed and on the lambing percentage expected.

Increasing the intensity of stocking, either in-house or in the lambing paddock, will increase the risk of mismothering and the spread of infection and this will necessitate a higher level of shepherding. Extra labour will almost always be required, whether it be skilled, semi-skilled, or simply extra hands to fetch and carry. On the hill the level of shepherding will again be determined by whether or not the ewes (or a proportion of them) are brought down off the hill to lamb in enclosures, fields or a sheep shed.

Maximum supervision with minimum interference

The philosophy at lambing should be one of maximum supervision with the minimum of interference. If the ewes have been well looked after, there should be few problems with difficult lambings. If shepherds have to assist a high proportion of ewes—for example, more than about one in 15 or 20—then either they are interfering unnecessarily or there is some other fault in the management or breeding of the flock. Knowing when to interfere is a difficult decision and comes only with training and experience.

It is useful to identify ewes which give problems at lambing and to make a decision on whether to retain such animals and their female progeny for future breeding. Flockmasters in various parts of the world have attempted—often with a degree of success—to breed so-called 'easy care' flocks, which are left completely unattended at lambing time to fend for themselves. This they have done by ruthlessly culling any ewe which has given any trouble of whatever kind at lambing time, whether or not it was the ewe's 'fault'. By so doing it has been possible to reduce the proportion of ewes with lambing problems to a very low level, for example, to around 1 or 2 per cent in some flocks. Whilst there are obviously considerable welfare implications in flocks which are left completely to their own devices, there are, nevertheless, lessons to be learned from such rigorous culling methods.

The lambing shed, paddock or enclosure should be a relatively peaceful place, with the minimum of noise and clamour. A 'softly, softly' approach is desirable, since the less stressed the flock is, the fewer should be the problems. Ewes should preferably be allowed to settle down in the area where they are to lamb and not be shifted from pillar to post. If they are stressed in late pregnancy, ewes may lamb prematurely—so called 'disruption lambings'—and lamb survival may be seriously compromised as a consequence.

Examining and Assisting Ewes at Lambing

There is an important difference between examining a ewe thought to be in trouble and assisting her to lamb. An examination is a necessary preliminary before deciding what to do and may reveal that nothing is apparently amiss, in which case the ewe should be left to get on with lambing in her own good time, but should be observed at frequent intervals of say half an hour. Ewes should not be internally examined repeatedly when lambing is thought to be progressing normally. It is also entirely wrong to pull a lamb away from a ewe before it is ready to be born. A number of shepherds not only do this, but also delve inside and bring away any other lambs which may be present, either to save them the bother of observing the ewe further, or because they feel that by getting it over and done with the lambs will be safe and sound. This is poor shepherding.

A ewe should only be assisted with her lambing if an examination suggests that she is unlikely to lamb successfully on her own, or that by leaving her to do so may jeopardise the life of the lambs. A number of situations call for examination of a lambing ewe, of which the following are some of the most important:

- The ewe is wandering about with a wet or blood-stained rear end, but there is no sign of a lamb. This may mean that the ewe has aborted, given birth to a dead lamb or given birth to a healthy lamb which she has abandoned or which has been 'stolen' by another ewe. Check the approximate lambing date from the ram raddle mark.
- The ewe has been straining her abdominal muscles for an hour or more but there is no sign of a lamb appearing at the vulva.
- The ewe has been straining for some time, with part of the lamb visible at the vulva, but is making no headway.
- Part of a lamb is visible at the vulva, but the ewe has given up straining and is wandering about unconcerned, or lying away on her own.
- The ewe is straining, the waterbag has burst (wet behind) but no progress has been made for some time.
- The lamb is obviously being born in an abnormal position—for example, tail first, or head first but without one or both forelegs.
- A ewe which has prolapsed the vagina and been stitched up or had a retainer and truss fitted is showing signs of being about to lamb.
- A ewe known to be carrying multiple lambs (i.e. scanned) has apparently finished lambing but has not produced the expected number of lambs. (NB: scanning is not foolproof)
- A ewe has been restless and uneasy for an excessively long period, but has not yet begun to strain, or does so only intermittently. Afterbirth may be seen at the vulva but no sign of a lamb.

It is important to keep an extra careful watch on any ewes which have been unwell during pregnancy. They are best penned up in a separate area for ease of observation.

THE EXAMINATION

Wherever possible, it is highly desirable that any ewe to be examined is brought indoors. Whilst some may need no assistance to lamb, others undoubtedly will and it is both easier to practice good hygiene indoors and much more convenient. Also, should things prove awkward, assistance is at

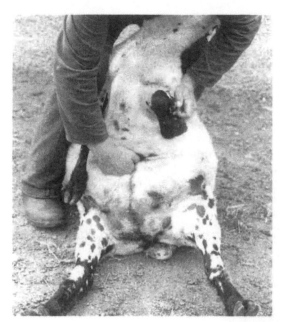

Plate 7.13 Ballotment. By gently pushing the clenched fist into the lower abdomen, it is sometimes possible to determine whether the lamb is alive.

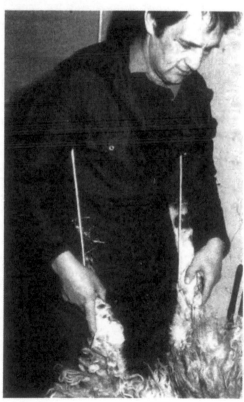

Plate 7.14 Supporting a ewe for vaginal examination single-handed. Ewes must not be held in this position for too long.

hand—for example, to look after lambs which have had a difficult birth. Everything which could be needed to assist a ewe to lamb should be immediately to hand before starting any examination.

Before any internal examination, gently tip the ewe so she is sitting up on her hind end. Examine the udder with clean hands, remembering that absence of development does not necessarily mean the ewe is some way off lambing. Check for any signs of mastitis, but do not draw off any milk at this stage even if you suspect infection, since you will contaminate your hands. In any case never strip any mastitic secretion onto the floor of the lambing area as this will effectively contaminate it for other ewes.

While the ewe is sitting upright, clench a fist and press it gently but firmly against the abdomen just above the udder. By keeping contact with the skin and moving the fist in and out it should be possible to bounce the knuckles gently against the lamb or lambs. If the fist is pushed firmly against a lamb and held there it may also be possible to feel movement, confirming that the lamb is alive and kicking. This technique, called **ballotment**, is also useful for detecting the presence of a twin or triplet after the birth of one lamb, without the need for an internal examination (see Plate 7.13).

Choose a clean, well-strawed area and lay the ewe gently on whichever side will be most comfortable for you to examine her. Except for the most simple examination it is always easier to lift the ewe up on to straw bales to a comfortable working height. Another bale covered with a paper sack can be used as a table for any equipment required. An assistant should hold her down whilst you clean up her rear end with copious amounts of soapy water. Paper towels are useful to mop up excess moisture.

Next, thoroughly wash your hands and arms using clean and preferably warm water. **The importance of cleanliness before carrying out even the most cursory examination cannot be overemphasised.** Even with the greatest care you will inevitably introduce some infection, but careful washing will minimise the risks. Make sure that fingernails are clean and short and if you have hands like shovels, ingrained with dirt, ask someone else to carry out the examination! Use only the mildest antiseptic solutions for washing, at suitably low dilutions, remembering that the delicate tissues lining the vagina are very easily damaged by inappropriate chemicals.

For preliminary examinations and for very simple manipulations the ewe can be restrained on her side as described, but in many cases it is very helpful to have an assistant hold up the ewe's hind end by using soft rope or, better still, a home-made device of narrow webbing, which is slung over the shoulders and attached above the ewe's hocks. The ewe's fore legs are best tied together so that she cannot make a bid to escape. The reason for using this technique is that many manipulations will require the repositioning of the lamb or lambs and to do this they must be returned to the uterus, often against the vigorous straining of the ewe. Therefore, a little help from Sir Isaac Newton (gravity!) is extremely useful. It is much easier to work standing up, easier to keep the area clean and to reach for things. When lubricant is applied, it also runs in the right direction.

However, the weight of the uterus and its contents, plus that of the full rumen, will be pressing on the ewe's diaphragm, which will make it difficult for her to breathe. There is also the risk of regurgitation of rumen contents, which could choke her. She must therefore be made as comfortable as possible and not be upended for too long. Hopefully, most manipulations should be completed in a short time.

LUBRICATION

It is essential to use liberal amounts of a suitable lubricant. Even the smallest lambs are too big to pass through the birth canal without adequate lubrication and for large lambs the journey is impossible without it. The tissues lining the birth canal—the mucous membranes—are very delicate and bruise and tear easily if not handled with the greatest respect. Apart from the discomfort to the ewe, such damage may cause haemorrhage or

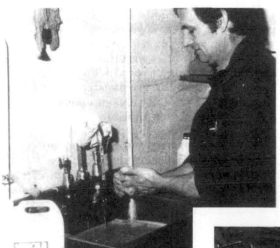

Plate 7.15 Scrupulous cleanliness is essential before lambing a ewe.

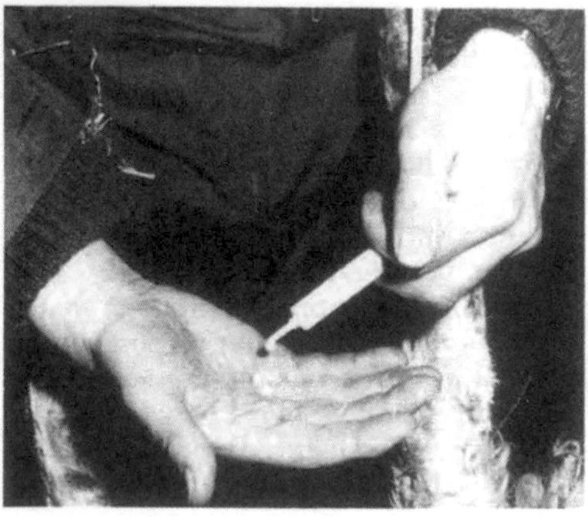

Plate 7.16 Where washing facilities are not available, an antibiotic (cow intramammary preparation) can be smeared onto the hands. The shepherd's hands should be washed at the first opportunity. (Beware of penicillin allergy.)

266

infection, which can lead to her death. The ewe provides her own lubricants, of course, but these fluids may already have been lost if she has been
attempting to lamb for some time. Use only a suitably bland, non-irritant
product, several of which are on the market. Many of the gels are made
more slippery by the addition of clean water. It is sometimes difficult to get
sufficient lubricant past a tightly fitting, dried-out lamb which is stuck in the
pelvis. This is helped by using a short piece of stout rubber tubing with a
smoothed off end, attached to a syringe or to a squeezy bottle with a suitable
nozzle for 'injecting' the lubricant around the stuck lamb. Alternatively, the
hard margarine method often gives excellent results (see below).

Insert one hand very carefully and try to assess the situation. Move
around slowly and gently inside the ewe and keep adding lubricant so that
your hand glides over the tissues. Do not keep pulling your hand in and out
of the ewe and do not change hands without washing again, since the one
you are not using will be heavily contaminated.

It will be obvious immediately if a lamb is already in the birth passage.
It is important to know if the lamb is dead or alive. A live lamb will assist
to some extent with its own birth, whereas a dead lamb is almost always
more difficult for the ewe to deliver. If a lamb has been dead for any length
of time it will inevitably have dried up to a greater or lesser degree and if
any infection is present the lamb may also be swollen. This combination
means that the ewe will inevitably require assistance (see below).

It is not always as easy as it might be imagined to decide if a lamb is
alive. If the lamb moves, then obviously there is no difficulty, but some
may lie perfectly still for long periods, particularly if the ewe has already
been in labour for some time. Slipping a finger into the mouth should elicit
a sucking response. Failing that, pinching the septum between the nostrils
or the skin between the cleats of the hoof should stimulate a withdrawal
response. If you are able to feel the chest wall, it may be possible to feel
the heart beating. If you cannot be sure, always assume that the lamb is
alive.

PRESENTATION OF THE LAMBS

Most lambs are born with both forelegs coming first and partially extended,
with the head pointing forwards and resting on the limbs as shown in
Figure 7.1. This position causes the least problems at lambing and is
considered the normal presentation. Any other position may lead to lambing
difficulties, although not inevitably. Ewes can deliver lambs coming backwards (hind limbs first) or with only one foreleg and a head, for example,
but most other positions are impossible without assistance.

It is crucial to discover not only which way the lamb is presented,
but also whether more than one lamb is present in the birth canal. This is
frequently confusing, especially for inexperienced shepherds, but important,
since extracting two lambs at once is impossible and the attempt is likely
to damage the ewe and both lambs. The secret is to keep the hand in contact

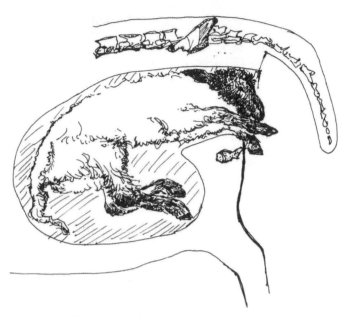

Figure 7.1   Normal presentation of a single lamb. Note how the fore legs are still partially flexed at the elbow.

with the lamb during the examination and to start with a limb—fore or hind— and follow it up, round and down the equal and opposite limb. If necessary loop a lambing rope around the legs identified as belonging to one lamb before starting to sort out any other legs present. In most cases where there are more than two legs present in the birth canal, it will mean that more than one lamb is making a bid for freedom at the same time; however, if only two legs are present they may not necessarily belong to the same lamb. If the 'keeping in contact' method is used, it should be possible to sort out the puzzle.

It is essential to be able to distinguish fore from hind limbs. Where it is only possible to feel the extremities of the limbs, start at the feet and note the direction in which the joints move. In the fore limb, both the fetlock and the knee joints move in the same direction. In the hind limb, the fetlock and hock joints move in opposite directions. Additionally, the shoulder blade can be felt in the fore limb, if this can be reached.

MANIPULATING LAMBS BEFORE DELIVERY

It is important to appreciate that, however small the lamb and roomy the ewe, and however slim, delicate and skilled the shepherd's hands might be, **there is never sufficient room to correct the position of a lamb lying in**

the birth canal. The pelvis is a ring of bone through which the birth canal passes, and although the ligaments between the individual joints of the pelvis become more flexible at lambing, it nevertheless remains a relatively rigid structure. If a hand is introduced into the vagina, even when no lamb is present, it is obvious how little room there is for manoeuvre. Therefore, **lambs must always be returned to the uterus before any corrections are attempted.**

Great care must be taken in returning lambs to the uterus. Whilst it may appear reasonable to assume that if the lamb has come out of the uterus through the cervix, then it should go back, this is not always the case. For example, if a lamb has been stuck in the birth canal for some time, it may have swelled up and the cervix may have begun to close up again, so gripping the lamb tightly. Again, the secret is to lubricate well and to push the lamb back slowly and steadily. Remember that the uterus is a thin, muscular bag at this time and can very easily be punctured by a lamb's foot or a finger, especially if the waterbag has burst and the protective fluids have been lost. Once back in the uterus there will be more room for manoeuvre—but little enough—especially if more than one lamb is present.

If examination reveals that the lambs are in the uterus, it has to be decided if the birth canal is sufficiently dilated and relaxed to allow the passage of the lambs. The vagina itself is a soft, muscular, elastic tube, whereas the cervix is shorter and is composed of much thicker and less pliable tissue, which relaxes and opens up for only a short period to allow the lambs to be born. If the hand is inserted, then depending upon the length of the vagina (which varies considerably from ewe to ewe), the cervix will be located roughly a small hand's length inside the ewe. If the cervix is fully open, then it will be difficult to detect it at all and a reasonably sized, well-lubricated hand will be able to pass straight through into the uterus unhindered. In this relaxed state it is permissible to withdraw lambs which have been repositioned or untangled from each other, if this is thought necessary.

However, if the cervix can be felt as a tight ring of tissue through which it is only just possible to insert a small hand, or indeed only two or three fingers, then the ewe is not ready to lamb. **On no account should any attempt be made to deliver lambs when the birth canal is only partially dilated.** To do so is likely to cause serious damage to the ewe in the form of tearing and haemorrhage and may also injure and compromise the lambs (see below). In these cases it is best to leave the ewe for a half to one hour and then re-examine her. If the cervix is no further open, then it is worth while settling the ewe in a comfortable lying position, inserting a well-lubricated hand and gently working the fingers and knuckles around inside the rim of the cervix in the hope that it might relax and open up. This takes time and patience but is rewarded in a proportion of cases.

It is possible that some affected ewes are hypocalcaemic (calcium deficient), but not so as to produce any clinical symptoms. Therefore it is sometimes helpful to inject 100 ml of calcium borogluconate solution (20%) under the skin. This will do no harm and may assist in some cases. Muscle relaxants (which can only be prescribed by your veterinary surgeon) appear to be largely ineffective in this condition. In most cases the ewe simply needs time and perhaps a little assistance, before the cervix finally yields to allow the delivery of the lambs.

RINGWOMB

This is a relatively rare condition and can be thought of as an extreme form of failure of the cervix to dilate, as described above. True ringwomb cases do not respond to any medical treatment or to gentle manipulation. Affected ewes may have been attempting to lamb for many hours. They are often very restless, getting up and down frequently, and are unable to settle. Occasionally, some afterbirth may be seen trailing from the vulva and on examination, the cervix will be felt as a tight, hard ring through which only one, or possibly two, fingers can be inserted. There are many theories as to the reason for this condition—for example, that it is more common in ewes which have previously prolapsed the vagina—but since none of the theories has been tested, the cause remains unknown.

If an affected ewe does not respond to treatment or manipulation, then any hope of removing the lambs by the normal route should be abandoned and your veterinary surgeon given the case to deal with. Providing the ewe is in reasonable condition and the lambs are alive, then caesarean section is often the best option. Hopefully this will yield live lambs and a ewe capable of looking after them. If, however, the ewe has been trying to lamb for a long time and the placentae have become separated, the lambs may be dead, in which case caesarean section is not usually an option and the ewe may have to be slaughtered. Ewes affected with ringwomb which are successfully caesared should be permanently marked and culled from the flock.

THE USE OF LAMBING ROPES, AIDS AND OTHER DEVICES

These can be most helpful in a number of situations, but care must be taken in their use. It is possible to secure a firmer hold using such items than it is with a well-lubricated hand. However, it is always more difficult to judge when too much traction is being applied than it is with the hand alone. Never pull on ropes without guiding the lamb with the other hand inside the ewe; otherwise grave damage may be done to the uterus and birth canal—for instance, by a foot puncturing the uterus. It is always safer if the same person does the pulling and the guiding—an assistant holding the ewe.

Ropes can be used merely as landmarks to identify the limbs or the head of a lamb—for example, when trying to disentangle twins (different coloured ropes are sometimes useful for this purpose). They can also be extremely useful in holding or guiding part of a lamb during the correction

270

of its position in the uterus. The most common example is when a head keeps flopping back into the uterus as a lamb is drawn forward into the birth canal.

The attachment of ropes must be done correctly so as not to damage the lamb. They are usually provided with a ready made loop in the end so a noose can easily be made. When attaching a rope to a limb, the loop must always go above the fetlock joint and not down around the pastern, since traction at this lower point may damage the joint or pull the hoof off, in which case the lamb will have to be destroyed. When roping the head, the noose should be applied behind the ears and through the mouth, not around the neck, which could obviously strangle the lamb. When pulling on the head, the rope will tend to tilt the head upwards somewhat and also force open the mouth, which can cause some difficulty. Great care must be taken not to dislocate or fracture the fragile jaws of the lamb.

Rubber ropes are kinder to the lamb and have strategically placed 'knots' to prevent the noose from tightening too much. The amount of pull is also modified to some extent by the elasticity of the rubber. They are also easier to clean and sterilise.

Ropes and lambing aids should be washed very thoroughly immediately after use and boiled for 20 minutes before being used again. They are best stored in a mild antiseptic solution, such as Milton, never in a strong disinfectant solution. Keep a plentiful supply so that there are always some sterilised and ready for use. Used ropes left lying around and then used unsterilised on another ewe are an excellent way of spreading infection, not only to the ewe but also to the lambs, even before they are born.

BIRTH TRAUMA

When delivering lambs, with or without the use of lambing ropes, please remember how fragile foetal lambs are and therefore how easily they may be damaged. A very significant proportion of lambs are injured during the birth process, as is demonstrated by detailed post-mortem examination. Even lambs born naturally, without any human intervention whatsoever, may be injured by the crushing pressures bearing down on them during the birth process. Any additional force applied by hand will increase the risk of injury very significantly. Many more lambs die either directly or indirectly through birth trauma than is ever appreciated.

Returning lambs from the birth canal to the uterus and correcting any abnormal posture is most easily done when the ewe is not straining. Upending the ewe is helpful, since her pressing is less effective in this position. When pulling the lamb away, it is best to wait for the ewe to strain unless she has given up. Aim to withdraw the lamb with a smooth, rather than a jerky, action. The ewe may be laid down on her side when actually delivering the lamb, so that her own contractions will assist with the birth.

The delicate tissues of the uterus and birth canal must always be protected from the hooves of the lamb by cupping the feet in the palm of the hand when manipulating them. The lamb's teeth can occasionally cause damage when the head is roped, as this tends to open the mouth. Some lambs, such as Scottish Blackfaces, are born with sizeable horn buds which can cause considerable damage, especially if they are born backwards.

For the purposes of the following discussion it will be assumed that the specific problem facing the ewe and the shepherd has been identified from an initial examination. It is not possible to cover all eventualities, nor is it possible to give anything other than general advice in a book of this type. There is no substitute for on-the-job training, supervised by a knowledge-able and experienced shepherd, backed up by some formal training from the ATB or the local agricultural college. It is also taken for granted that strict hygiene will be observed, that lubricants will be used liberally and that every ewe will be given antibiotic treatment following any interference.

Where a ewe has been examined and the lamb is found to be alive and presented normally, the birth canal is fully relaxed or in the process of opening up and the ewe is correct in every other way, then she should be left to get on with lambing in her own good time. Regular observations—not internal examinations—will show whether she is making progress. Further interference will only be necessary if no headway has been made after an hour or two.

Young ewes

Ewe lambs and gimmers lambing for the first time will generally take longer to deliver than experienced older ewes. They need more frequent observation prior to, during and immediately after lambing, to see that they are looking after their lambs adequately, as the process is a whole new experience for them. The general rule should be to examine young ewes earlier if a problem is suspected, but to allow them more time to lamb if the examination shows that all is well.

Above all, keep calm, for a panicky atmosphere in the lambing area is highly 'infectious' and will upset the ewes at a time when they should be quiet and relaxed. Foolish mistakes are more likely to be made in a panic. There are relatively few situations which constitute an emergency warranting immediate correction. If the lambs are in the uterus or returned to it with their umbilical cords intact, they are unlikely to come to much harm for some time.

Special notes

Do not attempt any corrective manipulations if, from your initial examina-tion, you feel that you will find it difficult to sort the problem out. Do not continue to manipulate inside a ewe for more than five or ten minutes at most. Give first regard to the welfare of both the ewe and the lambs and consider also the value of a ewe with twins at foot. There is no disgrace in being 'beaten' by a difficult lambing, but it is disgraceful to injure or kill animals through a pig-headed attitude that 'no ewe has ever beaten me'.

The sheep specialist in your veterinary practice will be experienced in dealing with every difficult situation. Should a caesarean section be the best option, for example, then one can be performed quickly and simply at the surgery, with a very good chance of a successful outcome, provided that half the parish have not already had a go at lambing the unfortunate ewe.

Generally speaking, the longer the time spent in trying to lamb a ewe, the poorer the chances of success. By success, is meant living, viable, uninjured lambs and a live, undamaged ewe which will not succumb to infection, is capable of milking and looking after her lambs and of breeding again the following year.

Correcting Specific Problems at Lambing and Delivering Lambs

The following are a selection of the more common difficulties which arise at lambing and a guide on how to deal with them. It is assumed that the lambs are alive unless stated otherwise.

OVERSIZED LAMBS

Lambs may become jammed in the birth canal because of their large size in relation to the dimensions of the ewe's birth canal, particularly in the region of the bony pelvis. This may occur especially with a large single lamb in a ewe lamb or gimmer, or with a normal sized lamb in a small ewe. The sticking points come when the head, shoulders or hips of the lamb reach the bony pelvic inlet. These lambs are particularly prone to damage, especially from crushing of the head, which can lead to brain haemorrhage. The easiest cases may only require a gentle pull, whilst in the worst cases there is obviously no way that the lamb can be born per vagina and a caesarean section is the only alternative if the lambs are alive.

Assuming the lamb is presented in the normal forward position and it is judged that it will come with a little help, then very gentle traction should be applied to the fore legs, whilst at the same time rotating the lamb first one way, then the other. Up and down movements may also assist. Great emphasis is often placed on the necessity of pulling lambs out in a downwards direction—that is, towards the udder. However, in practice, using modest leverage and rotation can work wonders, especially where so much **lubricant** is used that the lamb almost floats out! Applying traction to one leg and then the other may also help considerably.

Care must be taken with the feeding of ewe lambs and gimmers to ensure that their lambs—especially singles—do not grow too big and thereby cause lambing difficulties. Late pregnancy feeding can be started earlier than in the ewe flock, but at a lower level. Where ewes are scanned for foetal numbers it is just as important to feed appropriately for singles as for twins or triplets.

273

A problem which occurs with oversized lambs presented backwards (hind limbs first) is that the umbilical cord may become trapped between the lamb's belly and the ewe's bony pelvis and so cut off the lamb's blood supply. The lamb may be stimulated to 'breathe' whilst its head is immersed in foetal fluids as the blood supply is nipped off. This is obviously a life-threatening situation and a difficult one to deal with, since to dawdle is risky and to rush increases the chances of other types of crushing injury. If in doubt, return the lamb to the uterus if possible and seek veterinary advice. Turning a lamb right round in the uterus should **not** be attempted, as there is a considerable risk of damaging the ewe.

FORWARD PRESENTATION WITH ONE OR BOTH LEGS BACK

In a normal presentation the front legs are partially extended so that the feet are forward of the lamb's nose. However, one or both legs may not be as far forward as they should be because the elbows are excessively bent, or they may be left completely behind in the uterus, with only the lamb's head in the birth canal. Where there is excessive bending of the joints, the slender shape of the fully stretched out lamb is lost and the elbow and shoulder regions may stick in the ewe's bony pelvis, so halting progress.

Where the feet are in the birth canal and there is sufficient room, an attempt can be made to draw each leg forward individually, by cupping the hoof in the palm of the hand to protect the birth canal from injury. If this is not possible, slip a lambing rope onto one or both limbs and push the head back just far enough to allow the legs to be drawn forward. Again, protect the ewe from damage by cupping the feet in the hand whilst you are pulling on the ropes. If it is difficult to rope the limbs, then return the lamb to the uterus and draw both feet forward by hand, making sure that the head follows (see the next section).

If the fore legs are left far behind in the uterus (Figure 7.2 and Plate 7.17), so that only the head is in the birth canal, then the head must be returned to the uterus, since there is no room to insert the hand and arm past the head in the passage and at the same time manipulate the legs into position. The legs can then be drawn forward individually into the passage, hopefully followed by the head.

Sometimes the head alone, or the head and one leg, may be poking out of the vulva and the ewe is unable to progress further (see Figure 7.3 and Plate 7.18). It is often possible to lamb a ewe with only one leg forward using gentle traction and rotation, providing the lamb is not too big. If this is not possible, then the lamb should be returned to the uterus and the second leg brought forward in the manner already described.

If the lamb's head has been outside the vulva for some time, it may have become very swollen due to the constriction of the vulva around the neck. Lambs may appear gross, with the eyes bulging and the tongue swollen and sticking out. Although they may appear cold and dead, lambs can nevertheless survive for quite long periods in the 'hung' position. Often the head is

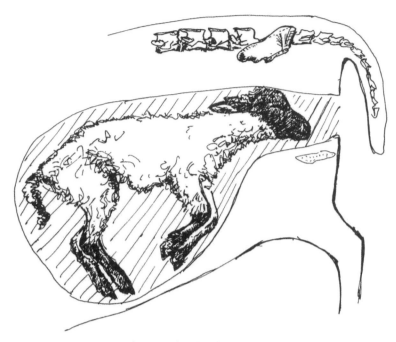

Figure 7.2   Both legs back.

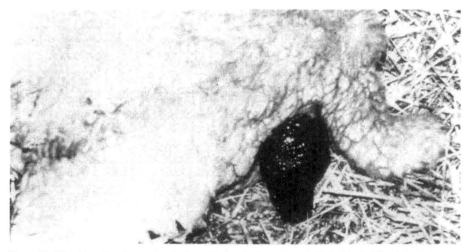

Plate 7.17   Head only presented, with both fore legs left behind. The head must be repelled back into the uterus before any attempt is made to draw the fore legs forward. The situation inside the ewe is diagrammatically represented above in Figure 7.2.

275

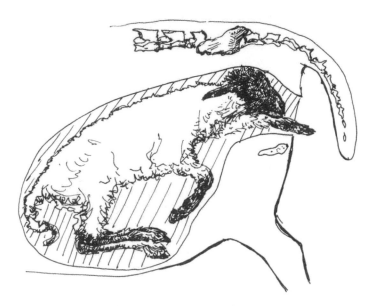

Figure 7.3 A lamb presented with one fore leg back.

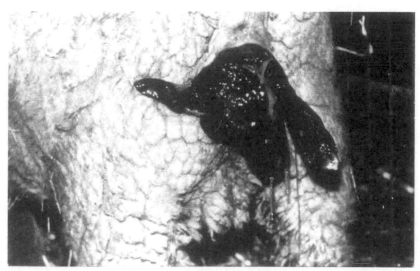

Plate 7.18 Presentation with one fore leg back. With care, this lamb was delivered without drawing the second leg forward. Figure 7.3 above shows the situation inside the ewe.

heavily contaminated with straw and faeces and it must be carefully washed before it is returned to the uterus. The swelling may make it difficult to get the head past the vulva and back into the vagina. Use plenty of lubrication and allow time for the ring of muscles in the vulva to relax, so that tearing does not occur. Try rubbing hard margarine into the hair of the lamb's head and neck, as this is an excellent lubricant which does not get squeezed off during the process. Because the head is so swollen it may be impossible to push it back through the bony pelvic inlet. Patience is needed to simply hold the lamb's head in the vagina of the ewe for some minutes until the swelling subsides somewhat.

Unless the ewe is completely exhausted, she will probably continue to strain and this may help to reduce the swelling more quickly. An assistant should support the ewe in the upended position whilst this is being done, but she can be laid on her side for the delivery. It is best to have the lamb's head roped for easier retrieval. Always bring both fore legs into the vagina before attempting delivery. Once born, the lamb will need careful supervision after its ordeal.

If the lamb is dead, then it is often easier to remove its head before pushing it back into the uterus. However you must obviously be positive that the lamb is dead. As this is a difficult and unpleasant task, it is better to take the ewe down to the veterinary surgery. If you do attempt this yourself, beware that the bones in the stump of the neck can tear the uterus or birth canal unless great care is taken. Therefore, the legs should be brought forward into the vagina and roped individually and the hand used to pinch the loose skin together to cover the stump of the neck. The dead lamb should be withdrawn very gingerly, checking frequently to see that the hooves are causing no damage. Needless to say, copious lubrication is essential.

PRESENTATION WITH THE HEAD BACK

A relatively common and often singularly frustrating lambing problem arises when one or both fore legs are present in the birth canal but there is no sign of the head, which remains in the uterus, twisted around and facing the wrong way (see Figure 7.4). The legs should always be returned to the uterus—having first attached a lambing rope to each—since there is never room enough for the hand to manoeuvre the head through the bony pelvis and into the birth canal.

The head should then be straightened out so that it is pointing in the right direction and resting on the fore legs, as in a normal presentation. Some considerable difficulty may be experienced in doing this and patience is required. **On no account should the jaws of the lamb be used as anchor points to pull the head round,** since they are very easily dislocated and fractured. Lambs with broken jaws cannot suck and will probably perish. Whilst it may sound unlikely, it is much safer to use the hard, bony rim of the eye sockets as anchorage points. Use the thumb and middlefinger—making sure the nails are short—and very gently, but firmly, slip them into

277

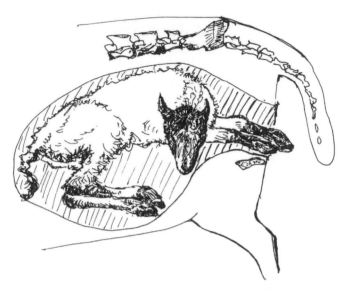

Figure 7.4   Head back. The legs must be returned to the uterus before any attempt is made to bring the head forward. This is often a most difficult and frustrating manipulation and requires patience and great care.

the corner of the eye sockets and draw the head around. This is always more difficult than it sounds.

The temptation is then to draw the roped fore legs back into the birth canal and to hope that the head will follow. However, more often than not, the head flops back into the uterus each time the lamb is drawn forward. (It is almost as if the neck has a permanent kink in it from lying twisted for a long period.) As there is no room for the hand to both draw and guide the head, a rope should be passed behind the ears and looped through the mouth in the first instance. Take up the tension on all three ropes and draw the lamb forward, alternating the pull on each leg. Use the hand inside the ewe to protect her from damage and also to keep the lamb's head coming correctly.

BACKWARDS PRESENTATION

In this position (see Figure 7.5) the lamb is coming hind feet first. In the majority of cases the lamb is the correct way up—that is, its spine is nearest the ewe's spine. (This position is often and quite wrongly called a breech, which is something quite different—see below.) Most ewes can lamb this way perfectly satisfactorily on their own, since it is not an uncommon presentation, especially with twins and triplets.

The important thing about lambs coming backwards is that they are at

278

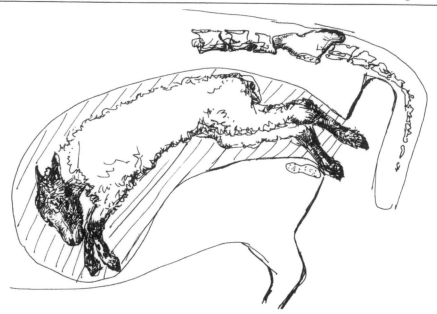

Figure 7.5   Backwards presentation. There is some risk to the lamb with this presentation.

some risk if they get stuck halfway out, due to the umbilical cord being crushed against the bony pelvis (see earlier). Once these lambs have reached the point where the hind limbs are well outside the ewe and the lamb's rear end has 'seen daylight', they should be drawn away if the ewe is not making progress. Pulling on one hind leg at a time has the effect of narrowing the diameter of the lamb's pelvis. Some gentle rotation and up and down leverage of the lamb during withdrawal usually helps. You must supply extra-generous lubrication before attempting to deliver these lambs because of the high risk of suffocation should they become jammed halfway out.

It is a popular misconception that lambs coming backwards must be completely turned around and delivered in the normal forward position. This is both incorrect and unwise, since there is little enough room inside the ewe, especially when another lamb is present, to correct even relatively simple positions, never mind such a difficult and risky one.

BREECH PRESENTATION

This occurs when the lamb is coming rear end first with both fore and hind limbs pointing forwards (see Figure 7.6). Usually the lamb's spine is uppermost when the ewe is standing. The ewe is obviously in labour, but making no progress, and no part of the lamb, except perhaps for the tail, may be showing at the vulva. On internal examination, the lamb's rear end is found to be wedged against the bony pelvis. The aim is to deliver the lamb backwards, so it must first be pushed gently back into the uterus. Then locate a hind limb, grasp the hock and push upwards and forwards very carefully. Slide the hand down to the foot, cup it in the hand and bring the foot up into the birth canal, whilst maintaining an upwards and forwards pressure on the lamb. Repeat with the other hind foot and then deliver the lamb as described above for backwards presentation. Where another lamb is present in the uterus, this is a tricky manoeuvre, so do not hesitate to seek veterinary advice.

Occasionally, only the lamb's hocks may be presented in the birth canal, rather than its hind feet or tail. Ease the lamb gently forwards towards the uterus by pushing on the point of both hocks simultaneously. Then slide a cupped hand under one hoof, whilst at the same time pushing upwards and forwards on the point of the hock, so that the foot can be brought into the birth canal. Repeat with the other foot and then deliver the lamb backwards.

A similar but even more difficult situation arises when the lamb's back is presented at the bony pelvis, so that on examination of a ewe which has been making no headway, only the spine can be felt. Generally speaking these awkward cases should be brought out backwards, since it is usually easier and obviates the need to worry about the head flopping back, as often occurs in a forward presentation.

Upending the ewe greatly assists in correcting the position of all these difficult presentations, even if the ewe is then laid back down on her side for final delivery of the lamb, so that she can assist with her own strainings.

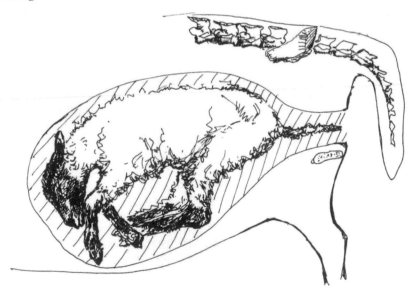

Figure 7.6   Breech presentation.

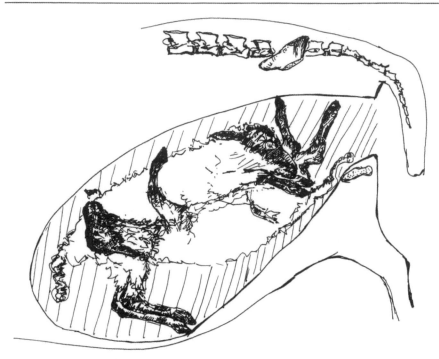

Figure 7.7 Twin lambs, one in a normal presentation, the other coming backwards but upside down. Such entanglements can be difficult to sort out and great care is required to avoid damaging the ewe or the lambs.

MULTIPLES

In the majority of cases of twins and triplets, the lambs come one at a time in a nice orderly fashion, a number of them being born backwards. The relatively smaller size of multiples in most cases means that oversize is generally less of a problem.

However, all sorts of entanglements can occur when more than one lamb tries to enter the birth canal at the same time and the shepherd's task is to decide which bits belong to which lamb and which lamb to deliver first (see Figure 7.7). Sometimes this is relatively simple, but at others it may be particularly difficult, especially against the ewe's straining. Always upend the ewe, since this makes any repositioning of the lambs much easier. Keep the hand in contact with the lamb until you are quite satisfied that you have sorted out which bits belong to which and use lambing ropes to identify heads and limbs. Moderate tension must be kept on ropes or they will tend to slip off, especially if you are using adequate lubrication.

In testing whether you have the lambs sorted out, pull gently on the ropes whilst using the hand inside the ewe to check that all is well and to protect the ewe from damage from the lamb's feet. Tensioning the ropes attached to the lamb to be delivered first allows a second lamb to be pushed back into the uterus, should it be crowding the exit. Obviously, every care must be taken to avoid accidentally pulling two lambs into the birth canal at once, since this is all too easy.

Providing a second or third lamb is presented normally and the ewe has not had a difficult time—which might have exhausted her so that she does not strain—then it need not be delivered by hand. This gives the ewe a chance to lick and mother-up her first lamb and perhaps allow it to suckle before any further lambs are born. The presence of another lamb in the birth canal should re-stimulate the ewe's mothering instincts so that she pays the new lamb proper attention.

In cattle, there is a condition known as freemartinism. This occurs where a bull and a heifer calf, born as twins, share the same blood supply during pregnancy. Male hormones circulate earlier than the female hormones, and thus four out of five of the heifer calves fail to develop a full set of reproductive organs and are therefore sterile. Fortunately—in view of the large proportion of multiple births—this is a rare condition in sheep, since there is usually a separate foetal blood supply for each lamb.

DEFORMED AND DEAD LAMBS

Fortunately, grossly deformed lambs which present a problem at lambing are relatively uncommon. When they do occur it is usually a matter of the lamb being too misshapen to be born through the birth canal. If the lamb is alive, then a caesarean section may be required. If it is dead, then your veterinary surgeon may decide to cut up the lamb inside the ewe (embryotomy) so that it can be removed in pieces. **On no account should this technique be attempted by the shepherd.**

Otherwise normal, although dead, lambs come in a variety of forms. Some are freshly dead and hence still flexible, and many of these can be removed via the birth canal with lubrication and gentle traction. It is almost always more difficult to manipulate a dead lamb, since it lies like a lump and cannot assist in its own birth. If the lamb has been dead for any length of time, then it is quite likely to have become dried up or mummified.

Providing the lamb seems capable of passing through the birth canal, then the secret lies in adequate lubrication. Hard margarine is very useful in many of these cases. Take a walnut-sized lump at a time and rub it well into the dried out coat of the part of the lamb which is in the birth canal. Push the lamb very carefully back inside the uterus and then coat the whole lamb with the margarine. Conventional lambing gel or cream can then be poured into the ewe and the lamb withdrawn, making full use of rotation and leverage to assist in the process. If you feel the slightest 'dragging' on the tissues, stop immediately and provide more lubrication.

Some dead lambs become stiff jointed (ankylosed) and it is usually not possible to deliver these without straightening out the joints (by breaking them) or cutting up the lamb. Your veterinary surgeon should deal with these cases.

Other lambs again may have been dead for some time and become infected. This may be due to a blood-borne infection inside the closed uterus, such as one of the abortion agents, or by infection getting through the open cervix and into the uterus close to lambing. The infection may cause the lamb to swell up and putrefy, and such lambs cannot be delivered by the normal route and must be removed in pieces. Some lambs may come apart when any pull is exerted upon them. It is particularly important that the ewe's uterus—which may be especially fragile due to the presence of infection—is not injured or torn in trying to extract the rotting lamb. Peritonitis would inevitably follow, which would seriously threaten the ewe's life.

Beware of the risk of infection to yourself when dealing with these cases. Use a plastic arm-length glove if this is feasible, but in any case wash extra thoroughly after any such interference. The ewe will, of course, require antibiotic treatment. Remember also that it is not unusual for a live twin to be born alongside a dead one. This may occur with both enzootic abortion of ewes and toxoplasmosis, as well as with other less sinister infections.

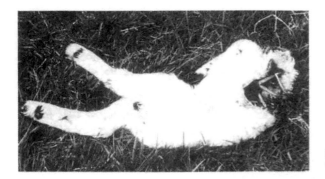

Plate 7.19   A deformed 'headless' lamb.

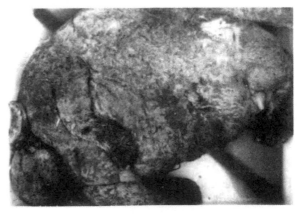

Plate 7.20   A deformed swollen (oedematous) lamb. Such distressing cases can cause serious lambing difficulties and veterinary assistance should always be sought.

283

'TWIST' OR TORSION OF THE UTERUS

Possibly because of the vigorous movements of the lamb as the time of birth approaches, a condition sometimes occurs whereby the uterus and its contents twist around its longitudinal axis through 90 or 180 degrees. The effect of this abnormal movement is to very effectively block the way out for the lambs through the cervix and vagina. The uterus can still contract down on the foetal lambs in an effort to expel them, but there is nowhere for them to go. Hence there is no pressure on the cervix from the waterbag or from the lambs and consequently it does not relax and open. Since no part of the lamb enters the vagina, the ewe is not stimulated to contract her abdominal muscles.

The shepherd therefore sees a restless ewe, which does not settle down or begin to strain. On examination, the birth canal is found to be partially or wholly blocked. The cause may not be immediately obvious, but on careful examination the corkscrew effect in the vagina will be detected. It is important that ewes which have obviously begun the first stages of labour (but are not straining) are examined, since delaying too long may jeopardise the lambs.

Obviously, the twist must be corrected before the birth canal can fully open to allow the lambs to be born. In a number of these cases the cervix does not open properly even after the twist has been corrected, or it may do so only very slowly, since the uterus is often exhausted and has stopped contracting down on the lambs. In these cases a caesarean section is indicated to save the lambs, so it makes sense to take the ewe to your veterinary surgeon in the first place.

If you deal with this problem yourself, on no account should any attempt be made to untwist the uterus by internal manipulation only, as this is not possible and will damage the ewe in the process. The ewe herself must be rolled around the twist. This is done by laying the ewe on her back and having an assistant rock her gently from side to side whilst you keep your lightly clenched fist in the vagina to detect when the twist is corrected. If it is then possible to insert the hand through the cervix, then do so to see if the lambs are alive. If so, allow the ewe time to fully relax and open up the birth canal. This may take several hours and will involve the ewe straining, so she should be observed frequently. The majority of ewes will lamb satisfactorily if given time.

If it appears that no progress is being made, then re-examine the ewe internally. If the birth canal is still only partially open, or if the afterbirth has begun to separate, then refer the case to your veterinary practice, so as not to threaten the lamb's survival any further.

Aftercare for Ewes Assisted at Lambing

If a ewe has required assistance at lambing, this interference will have put her at risk in a number of ways. Firstly the normal lambing process has been interrupted, so it is important to know if any more lambs are yet to be born. Do this simply by feeling inside once more with a clean hand. If any remaining lambs are alive and presented normally, then leave the ewe to complete the job on her own, but keep her under close observation. If there is anything untoward, such as a second lamb coming backwards or a dead lamb, then deliver any lambs which remain.

HAEMORRHAGE

Lambing is normally a surprisingly bloodless affair, so if abnormally large quantities of fresh or clotted blood are present in the birth canal or on the bedding of the pen, it is probable that the ewe has been damaged. Call out your veterinary surgeon immediately—do **not**, on any account, transport a haemorrhaging ewe to the surgery. Do not repeatedly insert the hand into the vagina or pack it with cotton wool, since this will disturb any clotting which may be taking place. Simply pen the ewe up with her lambs and leave her undisturbed until help arrives. Damage to the uterus or birth canal is serious and if these tissues have been ruptured or badly bruised then the outlook is poor.

INFECTION

However hygienic you have been, any ewe which has been examined internally will have had potentially dangerous microorganisms introduced into the reproductive tract. There is therefore a risk that the ewe will succumb to infection, especially at a time when her immune defences are low, as they are around lambing time and during lactation. If dirty hands are inserted, then the risk is increased. If the lambing has been a difficult one and tissues have been bruised or torn, the risk of infection is even greater.

Therefore, it is always safest to assume that infection will occur and to give the ewe's own body defences a helping hand by treating her with antibiotics. This can be done immediately after assistance by inserting large antibiotic tablets (pessaries) into the uterus, where they slowly dissolve. However, these are often voided by the ewe along with the afterbirth. It is therefore better to inject antibiotics under the skin or into a muscle. Your veterinary surgeon will be able to supply you with a suitably long-acting preparation to cover most eventualities. If long-acting antibiotics are not used, then daily or twice daily injections will be required for at least three or four days.

PARALYSIS

Occasionally, when a ewe has had a prolonged or difficult lambing, she may not be able to rise. This may be due to sheer exhaustion, in which case rest and 100 ml of 20% calcium borogluconate for injection will do wonders. However, in some cases the ewe may have suffered damage to a large nerve—the obturator nerve—which passes through the pelvis. The nerve may be crushed or bruised during the birth of a large lamb or by the shepherd's large hand during the manipulation of a malpresented lamb. This nerve supplies the muscles which prevent the hind legs from splaying apart. Paralysed ewes may therefore be unable to rise, or if they can do so, they may stagger and fall about. Paralysed animals are usually keen to eat and obviously not sick, which helps to differentiate them from those with other conditions such as milk fever or mastitis. However, care must be taken not to confuse them with fractures or spinal injuries.

The ewe should be made comfortable and provided with food and water within easy reach. A small pen is preferable so that she cannot go too far and get into difficulty. The hind legs can be tied together loosely with some soft rope in a figure of eight, so as to allow the ewe to rise if she can, but to prevent the legs from splaying. If the ewe tends to lie on her side she must be supported by bales to prevent her becoming bloated. Most animals recover within a week, and if they do not the diagnosis should be reviewed.

Meanwhile, the lambs will not be able to suck and lambs must be given colostrum and then milk by stomach tube (not by bottle). They should be kept close to the ewe, but protected so that she cannot fall on them.

Metritis

This is an inflammation of the uterus due to infection with microorganisms. The condition can occur following an assisted lambing where strict hygiene has not been observed, or where the ewe has not been covered with antibiotics after internal interference. Metritis may also occur following a prolapse of the uterus (see later) or where the afterbirth has been retained, particularly when the ewe has been kept in filthy conditions over lambing. It may also occur following abortion with particular microorganisms (such as salmonella), or where the lambs have died and putrefied in the uterus.

One particularly dangerous and usually fatal form of this disease is **gangrenous metritis** or gas gangrene, which is caused by one of a number of clostridial bacteria. Ewes which are housed or kept in heavily stocked lambing paddocks are at greatest risk. The hind end of the ewe may become very swollen and dark red in colour. There is usually a blood-stained discharge with an unpleasant smell from the vulva. Ewes may breathe rapidly and develop a diarrhoea shortly before they collapse and die; others may simply be found dead. Once this disease has appeared in an unvaccinated flock, more and more cases will appear as lambing progresses. Ewes which have had human assistance at lambing are especially at risk, but the disease also occurs in ewes which have not yet lambed.

CLINICAL SIGNS

Metritis, apart from the clostridial form mentioned above, is usually a chronic condition which grumbles away, possibly for weeks, with small amounts of thick pus discharging from the vulva from time to time. These ewes would probably attract little attention from the shepherd, since they may show no signs of illness. However, some ewes become acutely ill shortly after lambing or aborting, and they stop eating and become very dejected. There is often a putrid smell about them, due to an unpleasant discharge which contaminates the surrounding area. The infection produces a fever and the rectal temperature may reach 106 or 107°F (41°C). Milk production declines rapidly and the lambs therefore become hungry and neglected. Some ewes may become lame due to a laminitis associated with the infection. If the uterus has been ruptured during lambing, then a peritonitis will follow.

TREATMENT

Metritis is a life-threatening condition which must be treated promptly by your veterinary surgeon using injectable antibiotics and other supportive treatments. Do not be tempted to remove any afterbirth hanging from the vulva and do not put your hand inside these ewes or insert pessaries, since the inflamed tissues are very easily damaged and this would make matters worse.

Bring the ewe indoors with her lambs and make her as comfortable as possible in a dry, warm pen. Feed the lambs by stomach tube or bottle, but leave them with her, or close by, so she can see them. Tempt her with small quantities of tasty food, offered fresh and at frequent intervals. Be sure to provide clean, fresh water where she can reach it if she is down. Keep the pen well bedded and check her udder (hygienically) for any sign of mastitis. These ewes need careful nursing and treatment for a prolonged period.

Unfortunately, some ewes will die despite the most tender loving care and supportive treatment. Others will recover in time, but their milk yield will never fully recover and their lambs will not grow as well as they should.

PREVENTION

The condition is a costly one to the sheep farmer and measures should be taken to reduce the risks of it occurring. To this end, always lamb ewes down in clean, dry, comfortable conditions. Do not interfere unnecessarily at lambing (see earlier). If you have to help, then do so with the strictest hygiene and with the greatest care. Always cover ewes with antibiotics afterwards. If abortions occur in the flock due to an infection likely to cause a post-abortion metritis, your veterinary surgeon will advise you on a suitable antibiotic to use on all aborting ewes. Any ewe which gives birth to dead or rotting lambs should be given a course of antibiotics as a routine. Ewes which have a prolonged or difficult lambing should be observed closely in the days following for any sign of trouble. Ewes which retain their afterbirth should be given antibiotic treatment (see below). Clostridial vaccination should be routine in all flocks and this will help protect them against gangrenous metritis.

Retained Afterbirth

The lambing process is not technically over until the placenta or afterbirth has been voided. In most ewes this occurs within minutes or a few hours of the lambs being born. The placenta is attached to the inside of the uterus at the placentomes or 'buttons' and it is a very intimate connection, involving the intertwining of blood vessels. The tissues separate as a result of the contractions of the muscular wall of the uterus during the lambing process. This squeezes blood out of the blood vessels, so weakening the attachment and allowing the placenta to peel away. This normally starts at the tips of the two horns (or arms) of the uterus and the afterbirth is turned inside out as the separation proceeds.

The separation begins during the second stage of labour, that is, when the uterus is contracting and the lambs are being expelled (this is one reason why it is important that lambing is not held up for too long, since the lambs will die if total separation occurs before they are delivered). Although the ewe normally stops abdominal straining after all the lambs are born, the uterus nevertheless continues to contract for many hours afterwards in order to rid itself of the placenta and other debris. The ewe may resume abdominal straining for short periods, stimulated by the presence of a large portion of the placenta in the birth canal.

The separation process can be halted or delayed for a number of reasons which may lead to the retention of the placenta. The factors listed below are some of those thought to be primarily responsible:

- infection of the uterus from, for example, abortion agents
- the presence of dead and putrefying lambs in the uterus
- premature births, including a proportion of multiples which tend to be born somewhat early; with twins and triplets the lambing process is also prolonged and the muscular wall of the uterus becomes fatigued, so that it may fail to contract effectively
- prolonged lambings which exhaust the ewe—for example, where there has been some abnormal presentation of the lambs, such as a head back
- ringwomb cases, or other causes of inadequate relaxation of the birth canal
- assistance by the shepherd during the lambing process, due to physical factors—such as removing lambs before they are ready to be born or damaging the uterus during the process of manipulating the lambs—and the introduction of infection on the hands or lambing ropes

- low blood calcium levels (hypocalcaemia or milk fever), vitamin E and/or selenium deficiency, debility of the ewe through poor feeding or disease, all of which reduce or halt the contractions of the uterus

The retained afterbirth will eventually decompose and is usually voided within a week or ten days. Many ewes show no untoward signs during this time so that the shepherd may be unaware that the placenta has been retained, especially if there is none showing at the vulva. Other ewes may be a little off colour and a few may be downright ill from an infected afterbirth causing a metritis (see above).

TREATMENT

Any ewe which does not get rid of the placenta should be treated with long-acting antibiotics by injection until she does so. **On no account should the afterbirth be forcibly removed**, as this will cause damage to the 'buttons' and possibly reduce the number available for future pregnancies, which would adversely influence the size of the lambs. In the short term it may also lead to haemorrhage. There is nothing wrong in applying a very gentle pull on any placenta which has been hanging out of the vulva for several days to see if it is ready to come away. If it does not flop out with the greatest of ease, then leave it well alone. It will do no harm provided the ewe is treated with antibiotics.

If a significant proportion of ewes in a flock retain the afterbirth, then refer to the above list to see if one or more of the factors mentioned may be involved. There is little that can be done in the case of twins and triplets or the birth of dead lambs, but many of the possible causes are avoidable.

Always promptly remove any placentae or dead lambs from the lambing area. It is not good practice to allow ewes to eat the placenta, as it is highly indigestible. Use ample bedding to cover up any discharge if the pens are not mucked out after each ewe.

Prolapse of the Uterus

This occurs when the whole of the womb is turned inside out and pushed out through the birth canal by the abdominal strainings of the ewe. Immediately after lambing (which is when most prolapses occur) the uterus is a large organ, so it hangs down to the udder as a dark red mass. The cotyledons or 'buttons' are clearly visible on the outside surface, since it is now inside out. It is therefore very vulnerable to damage from being stood on, squashed, torn or otherwise injured. It also becomes heavily contaminated with faeces, mud or straw. The weather is rarely warm at lambing time and the greatest immediate risk to the ewe is usually from shock, because of the rapid loss of heat from the exposed organ.

TREATMENT

It is highly desirable that your veterinary surgeon should deal with this emergency. Meanwhile, the shepherd's immediate concern should be to protect the uterus from further heat loss, injury and infection. This is best done by wrapping the organ in a clean piece of old bed sheeting. If the ewe must be left on her own for a while, then slip the sheet between the ewe's legs and under her belly and tie the ends over her spine. Take the other end and bring it up between her hind legs, enveloping the uterus, and tie the other two corners of the sheet to the knot over the spine. It is preferable if an assistant can restrain the ewe from moving about.

Replacing the prolapse

If you feel confident about replacing the prolapse yourself and have had professional instruction, then the following guidelines may be helpful. Before beginning, inject 100 ml of a 20% solution of calcium borogluconate (with or without added magnesium and phosphorus) under the skin of the ewe (50 ml on each side), since a proportion of affected ewes have low blood calcium levels.

The ewe may be straining, and if not, she certainly will when the prolapse is being returned. Therefore, it is essential that an assistant should up-end the ewe as described in the lambing section—this is always a two-person job. (Your veterinary surgeon will also be able to administer an anaesthetic around the spinal nerves—an epidural—to prevent the ewe straining for an hour or two; this technique will be unavailable to the shepherd.)

If some or all of the afterbirth is still attached to the uterus, then see if it will come away easily—if not, then leave it well alone. Wash as much gross dirt off the prolapse as possible without causing bleeding or further damage. This is best done using large quantities of lukewarm (**not hot!**) water, without any disinfectants or antiseptics in it, as they might cause further damage to the delicate tissues. Pour the water over the prolapse until it is as clean as is reasonable. Do not attempt to remove any engrained dirt, as this may cause haemorrhage. Gently dab the organ dry with a soft towel or paper towels which don't stick. Do not wipe it dry, as this will also cause bleeding.

Squeeze the contents of two or three intramammary antibiotic tubes over the surface of the uterus and gently distribute it evenly. This acts both to lubricate the organ and also to counteract the inevitable infection which will occur when the uterus is returned inside the ewe.

Using both hands to cup the uterus, gently squeeze it to try to reduce its size, at the same time pushing it back inside the ewe. This is not as daunting a task as it is in the cow, but at times it may seem that it will never go back in. Be patient and take great care not to break off any 'buttons' and not to push any fingers through the uterus, which could be fatal. Work with the ewe, pushing when she stops straining and holding when she does.

When the uterus finally disappears inside the ewe, you are only halfway there. The organ must be turned completely outside in, including the full length of both its horns or arms. Again this will have to be done patiently in between the ewe's strainings. If this is not achieved satisfactorily, the chances are that the ewe will attempt to prolapse the uterus once more and she will probably succeed, whatever you do!

The ewe should be allowed to stand up at this stage and a truss should be applied to try to stop any straining. A prolapse retainer tied to the truss may also help. Stitching the lips of the vulva is not recommended and is in any case a veterinary job. If the ewe decides to prolapse again, stitches will not stop her. She will simply strain and burst the stitches out and be left with a painful, irritating wound which will stimulate her to strain even more.

The secret is to get the uterus positioned correctly and to control infection with long-acting antibiotics given by injection, so that any irritation is reduced to a minimum as quickly as possible. The longer the ewe goes without attempting to prolapse again, the less likely she is to do so. Ewes which do prolapse a second or third time have a poor outlook. Keep the ewe close to home and under frequent observation.

If the prolapsed uterus has been ruptured or torn, it is quite possible for coils of intestine to escape through the prolapse. These cases are always fatal and the ewes should be humanely destroyed on the farm. (See Colour plate 19.)

Prolapses may occur if damage has been done in assisting a ewe to lamb, if infection has been introduced or, in some cases, if the afterbirth has been retained. Acute metritis or vaginitis may cause constant straining and eventually prolapse. Hypocalcaemic cases appear to be more prone to the condition and older ewes are probably more likely to prolapse than younger sheep. Culprits should be marked for culling before the next breeding season.

Mastitis

Mastitis is an inflammation of the udder or mammary gland caused by infectious microorganisms which get into the udder via the orifice at the end of the teat. The disease is frequently disastrous in sheep, because at worst the ewe will die or have to be destroyed and at best she will survive but with a useless half or whole udder. Most have to be culled as being unsuitable for breeding, since they are unable to rear their lambs satisfactorily.

Most cases of mastitis occur immediately after lambing and during the first month of lactation, according to a recent survey carried out by the Royal Veterinary College in London in collaboration with the Veterinary Investigation Service in England and Wales. It would also appear that relatively few mastitis cases occur in the period immediately following weaning. Most of the apparently 'new' cases observed at the pre-mating culling examination probably occurred in the early lactation period. Cases are missed at this time, probably because in many instances the ewes are not obviously ill. It is estimated that, on average, around one in 20 ewes succumbs to mastitis, although in some flocks the figure may be two or three times higher than this.

Mastitis in the ewe—as in the dairy cow—costs the farmer dear. There are costs incurred from ewe deaths, for replacements for ewes culled, from lamb deaths due to starvation, from drugs for treatment and from the restricted growth rate of lambs sucking ewes with sub-clinical mastitis.

CLINICAL SIGNS

In milking flocks, where the udders of ewes are examined twice daily as in the dairy cow herd, cases of mastitis should be spotted quite promptly, and if treatment is implemented immediately then some halves may be saved. However, in most other flocks, cases are often well established before the shepherd is aware of the problem. In fact, the first sign may be lambs looking hungry, or a ewe apparently lame behind, as she attempts to keep her leg away from a swollen and painful gland. In acute cases the affected half of the udder and surrounding area is red, hard and hot (see Colour plate 20). The ewe will probably resent having her udder handled and any examination must be done with care and gentleness. At this acute stage, many ewes will die or become so sick that it is only humane to have them destroyed. In very acute cases, the ewe may simply be found dead.

Following this acute stage, the udder changes colour to purple, then black and becomes cold, clammy and sticky to the touch. The gland frequently becomes gangrenous and large portions of it may fall off (slough), exposing the severely damaged tissues underneath, which will take many weeks to heal over. Ewes which survive this unpleasant process are obviously unsuitable for future breeding, since the affected parts of the udder are either lost or rendered useless for milk production.

In the acute stage, when the udder is red and hot, the ewe will usually run a high temperature, but in ewes which are dying, the body temperature will fall drastically in the late stages. There is usually very little secretion in the udder—it cannot be called milk—and as the condition is very painful, no attempt should be made to strip-out the gland. (See Colour plate 21.)

In less severe cases the udder may be swollen but the extreme symptoms just described are absent. The contents of the gland are very variable. In some cases blood and pus may be present and in others a thick or watery secretion. Some may contain something vaguely resembling milk with clots in it. The udders become hard and often contain abscesses which can be detected as hard lumps at a weaning or pre-mating examination. Some of them burst to the surface and pus may leak all over the skin of the udder. This will attract flies in summer and the author has seen such wounds seething with maggots. In some cases the whole of the affected gland may appear to be one huge abscess and pus leaks out of the teats, which may appear twice their normal size. Because the two halves of the udder are

292

completely separate entities, one may remain apparently normal whilst the other may be totally destroyed.

TREATMENT

Treatment of severe mastitis is very unrewarding in the majority of cases and should be aimed at saving the ewe's life, since it is rarely possible to save the udder. If at pasture, the ewe and her lambs should be brought indoors and made as comfortable as possible in a dry pen with deep straw bedding. It is often best to take the lambs away from the ewe, even if only one half of the udder is affected, since it is painful for her to have lambs attempting to suck and there is often insufficient milk in the good half to rear them. The lambs will therefore need to be artificially reared unless they can be fostered-on. Beware, however, that the lambs are not infected with orf, which may have been responsible for their mother's sorry state, in which case they should not be fostered-on to other ewes.

Prompt treatment with injectable antibiotics immediately the condition is detected will be necessary to save the ewe's life. Treatment with intra-mammary preparations is usually unsuccessful in severe cases. Where there is an accumulation of pus or other toxic secretion in the udder, then your veterinary surgeon may consider surgery to remove the teat or part of the udder (this should on no account be attempted by the shepherd). Antibiotics must be given by injection and a high level of the drug sustained by twice daily injections for several days. Since it seems that the vast majority of cases of mastitis occur during the first month of lactation, shepherds should be especially on the look out for suspicious signs at this time. Undoubtedly, many more cases could be saved if they were detected early and given prompt and vigorous treatment.

PREVENTION

In order to prevent mastitis with any degree of success, it is necessary to understand how and why it occurs, but at present this remains largely a matter of speculation. As in the dairy cow, the udder is likely to be more vulnerable to infection around the time of birth for a number of reasons. It is usually well stocked with milk and there may be some leakage, allowing bacteria easier access to the gland via the teat orifice. Lambs may cause damage to the teats with their sharp teeth, and such wounds become contaminated with bacteria which then act as a reservoir of infection. Orf, spread to the teats from the mouths of infected lambs, may be particularly severe and mastitis is a very common sequel. Vaccination of ewes against orf two months before lambing should be considered where such problems have occurred in previous seasons. (See Colour plate 59.)

Shepherds themselves may spread infection, particularly when they tip ewes up immediately after lambing to see if there is adequate colostrum

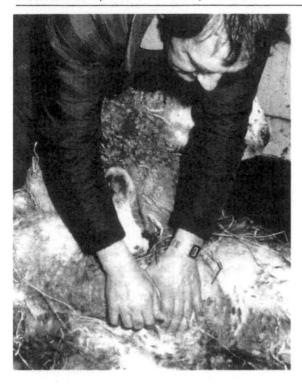

Plate 7.21 Clean hands are essential when examining a ewe to see whether she has milk for her lambs— otherwise the shepherd may spread mastitis from ewe to ewe.

and milk for the lambs. The hands should be washed before examining each ewe, especially if ewes with mastitis have been examined previously. If the hands cannot be washed, then it is best to leave the udder examination until later.

It is important to reduce the risk of contamination of the udder by faeces. In housed conditions, ewes should not be overcrowded and should be provided with very generous amounts of clean, dry straw bedding, especially in the lambing pens. A layer of slaked lime on the floor of the pen, under the bedding, will help to both dry and disinfect the area. If a lambing pen has been occupied previously by a ewe with mastitis, it should be mucked out and disinfected, limed and well bedded before being used again. The microorganisms causing the majority of mastitis cases—staphylococci, streptococci, coliforms and pasteurellae—are common wherever sheep are found. Obviously, if an area is highly contaminated, as when there has been leakage from a mastitis-infected udder, the risk of infection of other ewes is much greater.

Mastitis in ewes is commonly caused by *Pasteurella haemolitica*, a bacterium which also causes pneumonia in sheep. It is commonly found in the tonsils of perfectly healthy lambs and it is thought that the organisms may be transferred to the ewe's udder when she suckles her lambs. In some circumstances this may lead to mastitis and it appears to be more common in ewes suckling twins or triplets. In milking flocks where lambs are weaned early, pasteurella mastitis is less prevalent. However, mastitis due to *Staphylococcus aureus* is common in ewe milking flocks—just as it is in the dairy herd—being a microorganism which can survive almost anywhere, including on the skin of the udder, on the milker's hands, on milking equipment and in milk itself.

Ewes which have lambed indoors and been turned out to pasture in very poor weather—particularly when it is cold and wet—appear to be at greater risk, especially if they have been excessively crutched. The ewe's defences against disease are lowered around lambing and during much of the lactation period. Therefore, every effort should be made to reduce the risk of infection through good hygiene and husbandry and by reducing stress on the ewes as much as possible.

Vaccination against mastitis is not practised in the UK, although there is some interest in this technique in Europe and elsewhere. *E. coli* and *Pasteurella haemolytica* vaccines for protection against diseases other than mastitis are available in the UK, but there is no evidence that ewes so vaccinated are also protected against mastitis caused by these bacteria.

SUB-CLINICAL MASTITIS

Sub-clinical mastitis refers to a form of the disease in which there are no outward clinical signs. The ewe is perfectly well and the milk appears to be normal in every respect. However, there is a low grade infection of the udder which causes sufficient damage to lower milk yield. The effect of this is to reduce lamb growth rates very significantly. For example, there could be as much as 4 or 5 kg difference in 8 week weights between lambs from uninfected ewes and those with sub-clinical mastitis. As many as a third or more of the ewes could be affected in some flocks. As in the dairy herd, it is thus possible that this form of the disease could be responsible for even greater production loss than the obvious clinical forms of mastitis.

Dry ewe therapy (DET) administered at weaning may help to eliminate these infections, but this has yet to be proved. This technique is discussed in the section dealing with the health of ewes from weaning until mating in Chapter 2.

PUBLIC HEALTH ASPECTS

It is most important that mastitis control and dairy hygiene are rigorously practised where products are sold unpasteurised. *Staphylococcus aureus*, for example, which is a common contaminant of ewe's milk, may cause serious food poisoning, and there is a long list of organisms which pose an even greater risk to human health.

In the UK there is a small, although vociferous, lobby which insists that ewe and goat milk and milk products should remain unpasteurised, so that the consumer may 'benefit' from their true, natural taste. The facts are that, far from being a 'health food', these products often pose a considerable health risk. To continue to allow the sale of unpasteurised milk flies in the face of sound public health hygiene. The virtual elimination of tuberculosis and brucellosis from the national dairy herd, together with the pasteurisation of cow's milk, has averted untold misery and death amongst the human population. The level of hygiene in many ewe and goat units selling milk and milk products to the general public falls far below acceptable standards, and the sooner legislation is introduced to prohibit the sale of unpasteurised sheep and goat milk and milk products, the better.

8

THE CARE AND WELFARE OF NEWBORN LAMBS

Vulnerable lambs

The majority of lamb deaths which occur at birth or in the first few days of life stem largely from the management of the ewe flock during the preceding six to eight months. Nevertheless, many of the lambs which are born disadvantaged can be kept alive and reared satisfactorily through good shepherding and attention to detail at lambing time.

The principal aim of the shepherd should be to observe as many lambings as possible, to identify lambs which are in difficulty and to offer prompt and effective assistance. Particular attention should be paid to various special categories of ewe. Young ewes lambing for the first time may be poor mothers, mainly as a consequence of being inexperienced. Occasionally they may even drop their lamb and disappear into the distance. Others may fuss around the lamb, but fail to lick it dry or allow it to suck. Old, sick or thin ewes may have insufficient colostrum and milk for their lambs. Ewes which have had a difficult or prolonged lambing may be damaged or exhausted and so be unable to mother their lambs adequately during the crucial first few hours of life.

In any flock some lambs will be more vulnerable than others. Small lambs—whether they be triplets from a well-fed ewe or singles out of a sick

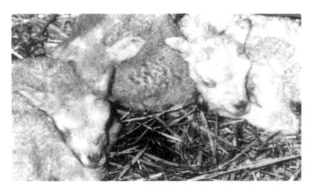

Plate 8.1 Finn triplets dozing after a good feed of colostrum. Despite their small size they stand a very reasonable chance of survival since they have a responsive mother, energy and antibodies from colostrum, a dry lie and shelter. Also, Finns are particularly vigorous and good at sucking.

297

or inadequately fed ewe—are generally more prone to chilling and are also less likely to get a satisfactory feed of colostrum than larger lambs. Triplets are at particular risk since there is the added factor of competition. Some deformed lambs, such as those with cleft palate or under- or overshot jaw, may be unable to suck satisfactorily. Other conditions, such as swayback or border disease, may prevent lambs from getting up and following the ewe so that they starve to death.

BIRTH TRAUMA

Prolonged and difficult lambings, with or without human intervention, are responsible, either directly or indirectly, for a significant proportion of lamb deaths. The pressures exerted upon the lamb from the contraction of the muscles of the uterus and from the ewe straining are very considerable. These pressures force the lamb through the ewe's bony pelvis, the tightest point of its journey to freedom. If the lamb is large and/or the pelvis is narrow, this disproportion further increases the pressure on the foetal lamb. The greater the pressure and the more prolonged the birth process, the greater the risk of damage to the lamb. As for human interference, a simple pull can increase the pressures enormously, and any further manipulation can cause additional damage to the lamb.

Brain damage

The greatest risk to the lamb during the birth process is from brain damage, due to haemorrhage caused by the pressures applied to the soft bones of the foetal skull. In the most severe cases the lamb will die during the birth

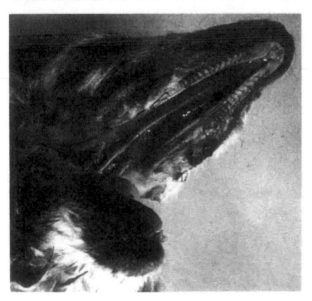

Plate 8.2 Cleft palate. This lamb would not have been able to suck had it survived.

process and so become a stillbirth statistic. If the haemorrhage is less severe, then the lamb will be born considerably compromised. Such brain-damaged lambs are generally much slower in getting to their feet—if they can rise at all—and have difficulty in keeping up with the ewe. If they manage to get to the udder, they will often have difficulty in sucking and they may have a poor appetite. Many of these lambs therefore starve or die of hypothermia, since they are much more vulnerable to low temperatures than normal lambs. Prompt attention will save a proportion of the less severely affected cases, but many will die sooner or later because of the effects of irreversible brain damage.

Hypoxia

Prolonged and stressful lambing may cause pinching of the umbilical cord. Where this is severe and particularly in lambs coming backwards, it may cause the death of the lamb during birth or immediately afterwards because of the restricted blood, and therefore oxygen, supply to the brain. Where the oxygen starvation or hypoxia is less severe, the lambs may be born alive, but the brain damage produces problems similar to those of brain haemorrhage described above. In hypoxia, however, careful nursing—including drying the lamb thoroughly, feeding it with colostrum by stomach tube and keeping up its body temperature in a warming box—will often result in a fully recovered lamb.

Some unfortunate lambs suffer from both brain haemorrhage and oxygen deprivation and their chances are very slim indeed. Oxygen shortage may also be a consequence of a small placenta due to inappropriate feeding of the ewe in the first half of pregnancy.

Liver rupture

The liver may be ruptured during the lambing process, since it is a particularly friable organ, protected only by the thin abdominal wall, and is therefore easily crushed. These cases will normally only be diagnosed at post-mortem, death being due to haemorrhage.

Fractures and dislocations

Other injuries occur during the birth process particularly—although not exclusively—following human intervention. Fractured ribs are common, making breathing difficult, restricting movement and thus putting lambs at further risk. Occasionally the sharp broken ends of the ribs actually puncture the lungs; this causes haemorrhage and is usually fatal. Most rib fracture cases should be humanely destroyed.

The lower jaw is frequently dislocated or fractured during an assisted lambing, especially when the head of the lamb is back. It is a serious injury since it is very unlikely that the lamb will ever be able to suck effectively. Some of these cases go unnoticed and perish through starvation. If it is known that the jaw has been damaged or is deformed, the lamb should be humanely destroyed. Your veterinary surgeon may attempt to repair jaw

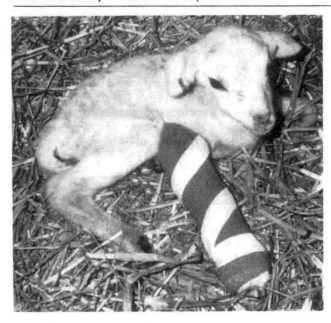

Plate 8.3 Newborn lamb with splinted fracture caused through being trampled by its mother.

fractures in particularly valuable animals, where this is feasible. Such lambs need to be stomach-tubed for a prolonged period and need a lot of attention. They must not be allowed to fend for themselves until they are completely healed.

Dislocations of the limb joints and even limb fractures can occur during assisted lambings, although these usually happen after birth. These are painful injuries and if suspected the lambs should not be subjected to further injury or discomfort by prolonged manipulation to find the break! There is no place for amateur orthopaedics and **all** cases should be taken to the veterinary surgery for repair.

There are far too many fractured limbs amongst lambs of all ages, due in large measure to rough and careless handling, often by people who ought to know better. Literally throwing or dropping lambs over fences onto concrete floors or into trailers is a frequent form of abuse. The pain and discomfort suffered by lambs in the name of saving the shepherd a few minutes (which are probably lost many times over in arranging and carrying out fracture repairs) are totally unacceptable and represent a considerable welfare problem in some flocks.

PREMATURE LAMBS

These are lambs which are born early and therefore in an immature state. Generally speaking, the earlier they are born, the less their chances of survival, especially if they are not found by the shepherd more or less immediately after birth. They are very small and particularly vulnerable to cold, predators and disease. Often they do not respond to the ewe's mothering attentions and are frequently abandoned.

Some premature births are due to infection, probably caused by one of the many microorganisms responsible for abortion in sheep, and this should always be borne in mind. Where this is a possibility—which means in most open flocks which purchase female breeding replacements—the ewe and her lamb should be promptly isolated in the hospital area and any placental remains removed. If the lamb dies, a laboratory post-mortem is advisable to check for abortion.

Prematurity may also be brought on by non-infectious causes. A small placenta may not be able to sustain a pregnancy to full term and a ewe which is stressed during late pregnancy—for example, by being gathered and handled roughly—may lamb prematurely.

Whatever the cause, an untimely birth means that the smooth change-over in hormone status described earlier, which ensures adequate udder development and a relaxed birth canal for the passage of the lamb, may not necessarily take place. The birth process does not normally present too many problems—the lamb's being small helps in this regard—but the lack of colostrum and milk production merely confounds the difficulties for the unfortunate lamb.

Where ewes are marked by weekly ram raddle marks, it may be possible to judge roughly how premature the lamb is, but in most cases this is academic. Because of the rapid growth rate of lambs in the last weeks of pregnancy, even lambs which are only a week early are noticeably small and sleek looking due to the undeveloped fleece. Features such as the unerupted teeth, the excessively soft cleats, the domed forehead and the narrow face are all the more exaggerated the earlier the lambs are born. Also, the lack of udder development and colostrum production in the ewe is a helpful indicator.

Surfactant

Premature lambs have premature organs, including the lungs, and this presents the most immediate problem for many of them. During the last few days of a normal pregnancy a substance called surfactant is produced in the foetal lamb's lungs. The surfaces of the foetal lungs are firmly 'glued' together by surface tension forces and could never expand in the absence of surfactant, which overcomes this surface tension effect.

If a premature lamb is born before any surfactant has been produced then it will perish, since despite artificial respiration the lungs will not expand and function. The muscles of the chest wall may be contracting and expanding the rib cage in an attempt to expand the lungs and the little heart may be beating furiously, but all to no avail. The lack of breathing means no oxygen supply and the lamb quickly dies.

In lambs born not quite so early, there may be sufficient surfactant to expand the lungs partially. These lambs can survive with help, but are very vulnerable because their oxygen supply is limited. This means that they are very slow and sluggish and because of this they do not generate any body heat by moving about and so are very prone to chilling. Even if they can follow the ewe they are poor suckers, since sucking the teat means that breathing has to be temporarily suspended and they must spend every second breathing just to keep going. Blood circulation problems also occur in premature lambs, further jeopardising their survival.

Lambs born with an adequate supply of surfactant can fully expand the lungs but they are still left with the problems of small size, low brown fat energy reserves and a poor sucking instinct. Their most immediate problem, therefore, is that of hypothermia. This common problem is not confined to premature lambs and the techniques for dealing with it are discussed fully later in this Chapter.

Treatment

Premature lambs should be kept indoors alongside their ewes and fed colostrum and milk by stomach tube until they are strong enough to suck the ewe—if indeed she produces any milk. If not, then they should be artificially reared rather than fostered, especially if there is any suspicion of infection. If a lamb dies, the ewe should not be used as a foster mother unless she is known to be free from infectious abortion and particularly enzootic abortion of ewes (EAE).

Unfortunately, despite careful nursing, a high proportion of these lambs die sooner or later, as they are particularly prone to infection. An adequate feed of colostrum—50 ml per kg body weight, at least three times during the first day—is essential if they are to stand any chance of survival. Obviously, husbandry tasks such as castration and tailing must be delayed until the lambs are stronger and the weather is reasonable.

The majority of lamb deaths in a flock arise from the same ewes each year. The ability of a ewe to give birth without difficulty and subsequently to rear her lambs successfully is, in large measure, inherited. It therefore makes sense to operate a fairly rigorous culling policy amongst young ewes lambing for the first time and to avoid retaining female replacements out of ewes which have a difficult lambing.

Colostrum and Lamb Survival

The most important thing a lamb must do in its whole life is to take a large feed of colostrum as soon after birth as possible. Colostrum will provide the lamb with energy to protect it from cold and with protection against certain specific diseases which the ewe has encountered on the farm or against which she has been vaccinated. Colostrum is also a very effective laxative.

When human babies are born they already have ready-made protective antibodies against specific diseases which have been transferred to them in the womb via their mother's blood supply. However, in lambs, calves, kids and foals this is not the case, since antibodies cannot transfer across the placenta, except in certain abnormal circumstances. Newborn lambs are therefore born completely vulnerable to disease. Since they become infected with a host of microorganisms immediately they are born—some of which will be capable of producing disease—it is crucial that they consume colostrum at the earliest opportunity and at frequent intervals thereafter. It is obviously important that they get food quickly too, since they are often born into a cold and hostile environment which will quickly kill them if they cannot keep warm by digesting colostrum and liberating the energy contained in it to produce heat.

Healthy, well-fed ewes and especially those which have been given booster vaccinations in the weeks before lambing will transfer large quantities of special proteins called immunoglobulins—better known as antibodies—into their colostrum. (Whilst this process somewhat depletes the ewe's own resistance against infection, adults are much better able to cope with invasion from microorganisms than newborn lambs.) The levels of antibody in colostrum at lambing will be about six times greater than the levels circulating in the ewe's own bloodstream, volume for volume.

The lamb is able to transfer these antibodies from its gut to its bloodstream for only a very limited time of around 12 to 15 hours after birth. It is important that antibodies reach the blood so that they can be transported to all parts of the body where infection might gain entry—for example, to the lungs for protection against pneumonia. However, the antibodies swallowed after this time are not wasted since some of them will be specifically designed to cope with gut infections such as lamb dysentery.

COMPOSITION AND YIELD OF COLOSTRUM

Colostrum is a thick, yellow secretion which has a high feed value. It contains rich sources of energy in the form of fats and lactose, plus proteins (other than antibody protein) and vitamins. It is produced only in the last few days of pregnancy and for perhaps the first 18 hours after lambing. The udder secretion then gradually changes to milk, which has a less concentrated feed value and contains ever-decreasing levels of antibodies as the days pass.

The amount of colostrum and milk produced depends largely upon the level of feeding the ewe has received throughout the whole of pregnancy. Good feeding in the second and third months of gestation will ensure good growth of the placenta and therefore adequate levels of placental hormones. These hormones, together with proper feeding during the last two months of pregnancy, will ensure good udder development and therefore adequate colostrum and milk production. The number of lambs conceived and carried also affects the total weight of the placenta and the amount of colostrum and milk produced.

Ewes which are inadequately fed may produce little or no colostrum

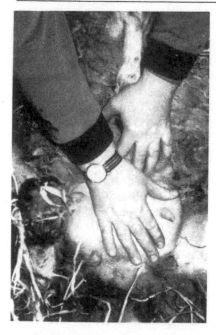

Plate 8.4 Ewe with a large udder and good supply of colostrum. The yield of colostrum and milk is dependent upon the size of the placenta and therefore upon feeding throughout pregnancy as well as during lactation.

by lambing time. Even if feeding is boosted immediately after lambing, it will take a long time before colostrum is secreted and the amounts are likely to be only half what they would be on good feeding throughout pregnancy. This is of little use to the lambs, which need colostrum immediately they are born. Consequently they will have to be supplemented with colostrum from another ewe (or from a cow) by stomach tube until the ewe's supplies come on line, if indeed they ever do so. It is useless attempting to induce milk let-down with hormones if there is nothing present in the udder to let-down.

The amount of colostrum ewes produce is very variable, even on an adequate level of feeding, and obviously there are significant breed differences. Ewes carrying only a single lamb but which have been well fed should produce sufficient colostrum and milk to feed twins. Therefore, in well-fed prolific flocks where there is a proportion of triplets, single bearing ewes can be used for fostering. Unless a really milky breed is particularly well fed, few ewes will be capable of rearing triplets satisfactorily and it takes very skilled management to achieve this. Inadequately fed ewes carrying twins and triplets are handicapped because the drain on the ewe's nutritional resources due to rapid foetal growth in late pregnancy is very heavy. This means that not only are the lambs born small and weak, but also they have less brown fat energy reserves and less colostrum and milk are available to them.

Ewes carrying twins which have not been fed adequately during pregnancy will not produce sufficient milk, and both lambs will need colostrum

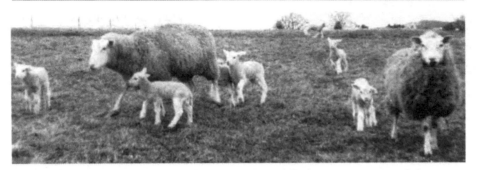

Plate 8.5   Colebred ewes with triplets. It takes skilled management and the right breed to rear triplets successfully on the ewe.

supplementation by stomach tube during the first day. These ewes should be able to respond to better feeding after lambing, but this will be limited by the amount of udder development, which is determined before lambing. No amount of good grazing during lactation will make up for a deficiency in feeding during pregnancy, but it will help to make the best use of what milk secretory tissue is present. If there is obviously insufficient milk, then one of the twins should be fostered. The problem in poorly fed flocks is that most other ewes will also have inadequate supplies of milk.

THE LAMB'S REQUIREMENTS FOR COLOSTRUM

The lamb's requirements for colostrum are frequently underestimated by farmers and shepherds. If a lamb gets sufficient colostrum to meet its nutritional needs, it will be getting enough to meet its needs for antibodies,

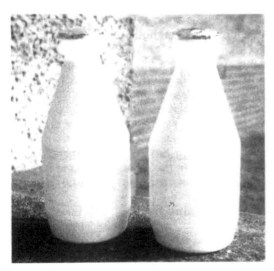

Plate 8.6   An average-sized lamb will require approximately 1 litre (2 pints) of colostrum during the first 18 hours of life. This will fully supply its energy needs and furnish it with antibodies to ward off infection.

305

providing the ewe has been adequately vaccinated. So the important thing is to meet the lamb's nutritional needs fully and this will depend upon its birth weight and upon the weather conditions prevailing at the time it is born. Obviously the colder, wetter and windier it is, the more colostrum will be needed to ensure that the lamb can maintain its body temperature and so avoid becoming hypothermic.

An average-sized single lamb of around 5 kg (9 lb) in weight, running outside in poor weather, will need 1 litre (2 pt) of colostrum from the ewe (or by stomach tube) distributed evenly over the first 18 hours of life. If the same lamb is housed, ¾ litre (1½ pt) will probably suffice, providing the bedding is dry and generous and it is not desperately cold outside. A large lamb will obviously need substantially more. As a general guide, out-door lambs require roughly 210 ml of colostrum for every kilogram of body weight (3½ fl oz/lb). (Note that these amounts must be multiplied by the weight of the lamb in kilograms. For example, the 5 kg lamb at pasture needs 5 × 210 ml = 1,050 ml, i.e. just over a litre.)

These amounts may seem high, but they are well within the amounts that vigorous, healthy lambs will suck from ewes with an adequate milk supply. Obviously, lambs which are compromised in any way or which face strong competition from litter mates may not get enough. Some breeds of lamb are better at getting colostrum than others. Finns, despite being small, frail-looking lambs, are particularly vigorous and even triplets take in large amounts of colostrum and milk for their body weight. Cheviot lambs are particularly efficient in this respect, whilst many other breeds are relatively less vigorous and consume correspondingly less colostrum per unit of body weight.

EWE-LAMB BOND

Lambs needs a good bellyful of colostrum as soon after birth as possible, followed by repeated and regular supplies throughout the day and night. How much the lambs actually get depends not only upon how much is available from the ewe and upon how vigorous a sucker the lamb is, but also on the strength of the ewe-lamb bond. The ewe which licks her lamb dry quickly, gets it to its feet, guides it to shelter and allows it to suckle frequently stands a much greater chance of rearing her lamb successfully. With multiples, it is obviously crucial that the ewe bonds equally strongly with all of her lambs, and the shepherd can assist here. Ewes fed inadequately throughout pregnancy, apart from having less milk, are also poorer mothers, being generally less attentive to their lambs. This is largely a hormonal effect due, once again, to the inadequate placental growth during pregnancy.

It is relatively easy to tell if a lamb is starving, since it will lie about or stand and bleat and will get left behind. If the lamb is picked up the belly will be flat and empty instead of plump and full. The lamb's temperature will fall rapidly and it will become more and more sluggish until it lapses into a coma and dies of hypothermia. A high standard of shepherding is required to identify lambs which are getting just enough milk to survive, but not sufficient to thrive and grow to their full potential.

COLLECTING COLOSTRUM FROM EWES

Storage of supplementary frozen colostrum is an absolute essential for every flock, and its provision has been discussed earlier, in Chapter 7. At this point it is worth considering how to collect ewe's colostrum if no frozen supplies of ewe, goat or cow's colostrum are available. The first thing is to decide from which ewes to collect colostrum. Do not use colostrum from a ewe that has aborted late (when some colostrum may be present) or has lost her lamb but is possibly infected with one of the abortion agents. Do not collect colostrum from a ewe with twins or triplets, as there is rarely enough, if any, to spare. Well-fed ewes with single lambs which are not required for fostering are the best source of colostrum.

Up to about six times more colostrum can be milked from a ewe if she is first injected with oxytocin—a hormone she herself produces when the lamb sucks—to encourage milk let-down. Contact your veterinary surgeon

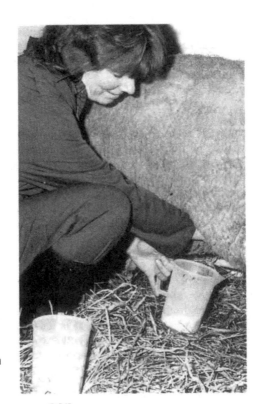

Plate 8.7   Milking colostrum from a Suffolk ewe, which was injected with oxytocin a few minutes before milking began. Note how the ewe is standing quietly. More than a pint has been collected at this stage.

before lambing and request advice on its use, as it is a prescription-only medicine.

Handle the ewe very gently and quietly and do not up-end her, in order to stress her as little as possible. Have an assistant restrain her up against some railings or, if single-handed, use an old fan belt to secure her head and offer her concentrates or something tasty to eat. Inject 10 iu (international units) of oxytocin into the muscle for a small ewe, 15 iu for a large breed. It will take two or three minutes for the drug to work, so in the meanwhile carefully wash your hands and the ewe's udder with lukewarm water containing a mild antiseptic (as would be suitable for washing dairy cows' udders) and dry it with a paper towel. Apply a little hand cream or vaseline to the teats and gently begin to milk into a large milk jug. As the drug works, the colostrum will flow freely, and a pint or even more may be collected at a single session with a milky ewe handled quietly. Wipe the udder again after milking with a clean damp paper towel to remove any lubricant, which may put the lamb off sucking. Do not apply teat dip solution for the same reason. This method, using oxytocin, is very effective and does no harm to the ewe. Indeed, the more colostrum that is removed from the gland, the more milk will be produced.

Ewes can be milked up to three times in 24 hours, but it is essential that the ewe's own lamb gets its requirement of colostrum. Therefore, see that the lamb is full immediately before milking the ewe. The ewe need not be fully milked out, of course, or only one half of the udder could be milked at one milking and the opposite side at the next. Needless to say, good hygiene is essential so as not to introduce infection which might lead to mastitis.

Storing colostrum

Colostrum can be used fresh or kept chilled in a refrigerator for up to two days. It must be deep-frozen in small containers the size of yoghurt pots if it is to be kept for longer and will be perfectly satisfactory for up to a year. Do not thaw out and refreeze colostrum, as this will destroy the antibodies. Microwave treatment is not satisfactory because of the risk of overheating, which would destroy the antibodies. Thawing is best done by placing the container of colostrum into a larger vessel containing hot water.

Using cow colostrum

Cow colostrum can be used fresh or frozen, and although it will not provide the same specific protection against disease that ewe colostrum will, especially if the cow was not vaccinated against the clostridial diseases, it is still a very valuable food. You will need to feed about 30% more than you would of ewe's colostrum, as it is less concentrated in solids. This may mean more frequent feeding, since you should not feed more than about 50 ml per kilogram of the lamb's body weight at any one time. There is no need to feed colostrum for more than the first day of life.

Remember that it is particularly important to ensure that lambs which are to be reared artificially receive colostrum by stomach tube for the first day of life. Likewise, lambs which are to be fostered should be given colostrum if necessary—for example, if the foster ewe has been lambed so long that the colostrum has become well diluted with milk.

Young ewes

Another group of lambs needing special attention are those out of ewe lambs or gimmers, since young ewes tend to transfer fewer antibodies to their lambs via colostrum than older ewes. Their lambs are therefore likely to be somewhat more prone to disease. This may be partly because young ewes are not such good mothers and partly because there is relatively less udder development. Ewes generally become more efficient at transferring antibodies to their lambs the older they get, up to about six years of age, after which they become less efficient.

SEASON OF LAMBING

The time that lambing takes place affects the amount of antibodies absorbed by lambs. Generally, the later in the spring that lambing occurs, the less disease protection is transferred. This may be because lambs born in colder weather earlier in the year take in more colostrum in order to keep warm. However, lamb survival tends to increase the later lambing takes place. This is partly because, in the kinder weather later in the spring, fewer lambs die of hypothermia—the most common cause of death in newborn lambs in the UK. Remember that disease is responsible for a relatively small proportion of lamb deaths in well-managed flocks where lambs receive ample colostrum early in life.

In multiple litters of mixed sexes, the ewe lambs will generally get less colostrum per kilogram of body weight than ram lambs, which means they may be more vulnerable to both chilling and disease should the ewe's supply of colostrum be less than adequate.

It is possible to breed for better lamb survival by selecting flock replacements from ewes which consistently rear all their lambs successfully and at rapid growth rates. Crossing with a breed which is known to transfer colostral disease resistance more effectively will also bring about improvement.

Whilst colostrum is of paramount importance in keeping lambs alive, it is obviously important to pay heed to the other important husbandry factors which influence lamb survival. Adequate shelter is essential to assist lambs that may not get an adequate feed of colostrum to maintain their body temperature.

MINIMISING THE DISEASE CHALLENGE

Every effort should be made to keep the lambing area as disease-free as practical, as no amount of colostral antibody can protect against an overwhelming weight of infection. The protection afforded by colostral antibody is finite—that is, antibodies are used up as they 'mop up' invading micro-organisms which get into the gut, the lungs or the blood stream. If they all become used up, the lamb must depend upon its own immune system to ward off infection. It must manufacture its own antibodies in response to the antigens of the invading microorganisms. This takes a long time and is a much less efficient process in young lambs than in adults. Consequently the invading organisms will have had time to multiply virtually unhindered and will overwhelm the lamb before it has time to muster its defences. Hence the vital importance of ready-made antibodies in colostrum.

Always take veterinary advice before administering vaccines to young lambs. Using them inappropriately may in fact reduce the lamb's resistance to disease rather than increase it. This is due to the interaction between the ready-made antibodies donated by the ewe in colostrum and the antigens in the vaccine and is explained in more detail in the section dealing with clostridial vaccination in Chapter 9.

Hypothermia or Chilling of Lambs

Of the millions of lambs which perish each year in the UK, almost half die through becoming severely chilled or hypothermic. Some years ago, workers at the Moredun Research Institute in Edinburgh investigated this distressing condition. They discovered the causes, identified lambs which were particularly at risk, developed simple and effective treatment techniques which were tried and tested on commercial farms and suggested corrective husbandry for the prevention of hypothermia.

This information has been made widely available and there can be few shepherds or flockmasters who have not been exposed to it. Indeed,

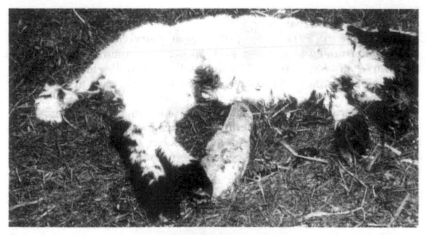

Plate 8.8 This lamb died of hypothermia or chilling—the single most common cause of death in UK sheep flocks.

many have taken up these methods and significantly reduced the suffering of lambs and substantially increased the profitability of their flocks in the process. However, there are still hundreds of thousands of lambs which die unnecessarily and in great distress and this is totally unacceptable. Any flock owner who does not supply some form of approved warming box and any shepherd who does not carry and use a thermometer regularly, or who is not thoroughly familiar with the techniques for detecting and treating hypothermic lambs, could, quite reasonably, be accused of negligence. The days of shoving lambs in the kitchen oven or of barbecuing them under an infra-red lamp are long past!

BODY TEMPERATURE

A hypothermic lamb is one whose body temperature has fallen significantly below normal. Normal for a newborn lamb is around 39 to 40°C (102 to 104°F), and it is important that this temperature be maintained within a degree or so. Should the lamb become chilled by only a couple of degrees—down to 37°C or below—this will be sufficient to prevent it from sucking colostrum, which is its only supply of energy after the first few hours of life. From then on its temperature will continue to fall, often at an alarming rate in bad weather, until, at around 20°C (68°F), it will perish. Under the most harsh weather conditions a newborn lamb could be dead from exposure in less than half an hour, whilst a hypothermic lamb indoors, or out at pasture in reasonable weather, may take several hours to die.

HEAT LOSS

Consider just how vulnerable a newborn lamb is when it is first dropped by its mother, even on a reasonable day. It is both very small and soaking

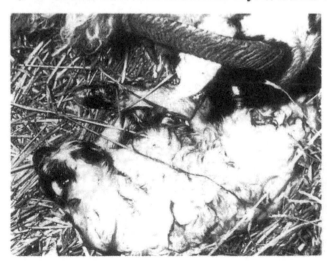

Plate 8.9   A newborn lamb, soaked in birth fluids, being licked dry by its mother—a vital protection against heat loss.

wet from the birth fluids. Its small size means that, relative to its body weight, it has a very large surface area from which to lose heat. The outside temperature in the UK is always well below body temperature at lambing time, even indoors, so cooling will occur quickly unless the lamb can generate enough heat of its own. If the ewe does not lick the lamb dry, the cooling process will be greatly accelerated, since extra heat will be drawn out of the lamb to evaporate the birth fluids. (Just leave a cup of boiling hot tea standing outside to see how quickly it cools, even on a hot summer's day.) If the weather is snowy or frosty, then the lamb will lose heat that much faster, since apart from evaporation, heat will also be lost to the ground and the air through conduction. Wet and windy conditions are particularly hazardous because of the chill factor. A dry lamb, although less vulnerable, is still at risk because the birth coat, especially in some breeds, provides very poor insulation against cold.

BROWN FAT

How do any lambs survive such formidable odds? Most lambs out of ewes which have been well fed during pregnancy will have accumulated depots of energy-rich brown fat, which lie between the muscle layers of the trunk and around the kidneys. When the lamb is born, the drop in temperature it experiences stimulates an enormous increase in blood flow to the brown fat. The blood transports the heat and energy generated by the breakdown of the fat all around the body, and this has to fuel the lamb so that it can get up, follow the ewe and suck colostrum, all of which are very energy-consuming for a small newborn lamb. Colostrum then has to be digested—a process which itself requires fueling—before it can yield its energy. Since the brown fat reserves will run out within less than six hours in harsh weather conditions, it is obvious why it is so important that the lamb gets a stomachful of colostrum as early as possible after it is born.

BLOOD SUGAR

The newborn lamb is therefore totally dependent upon its mother licking it dry quickly and thoroughly, guiding it to shelter and supplying it with adequate colostrum at the first opportunity. The blood sugar or glucose level of most lambs during the first few hours of life is generally high, showing that they are 'burning' brown fat to provide energy. However, if the ewe does not mother the lamb effectively and particularly if the lamb does not get colostrum to replace the fast-depleting energy reserves, the blood sugar levels will fall rapidly and the lamb will die of exposure to the weather, since it will be losing heat much faster than it can generate it.

In bad weather, most lambs which do not get sufficient colostrum quickly will perish before they are five or six hours old. Surprisingly few lambs die between six and twelve hours of age, and death from exposure alone is uncommon in well fed lambs older than six hours. However, lambs which survive for twelve hours are not yet out of the wood, because they are then entirely dependent upon an adequate and frequent supply of colostrum and milk as their sole source of energy, as their brown fat supplies are likely to be exhausted. Unlike younger hypothermic lambs, whose blood sugar levels are satisfactory, older hypothermic lambs have low blood sugar levels, indicating that starvation is the cause of their losing body heat. The reason why some hypothermic lambs last for so long is that they become less and less active. All their bodily functions slow down, so that they expend a minimum of energy, using what little there is in a vain attempt to maintain body temperature. However, because hypothermic lambs cannot suck, they are doomed unless the shepherd finds them in time and treats them promptly and appropriately.

Low sugar fits

It is crucial to appreciate the importance of the low blood sugar levels in older hypothermic lambs. If they are warmed up before they are supplied with energy, this will merely hasten their death, since the warming will speed up all their bodily functions with the result that their blood sugar levels will fall at an even faster rate. The brain is particularly susceptible to a shortage of sugar and the result is that the lamb suffers from a hypoglycaemic or low sugar fit. The symptoms of this will be all too familiar to shepherds and their families who have ever warmed up lambs—a stretched-out neck with the head thrown back and the legs thrashing or paddling about in an uncoordinated way, with death following very rapidly.

Even in flocks which take all reasonable measures to reduce the incidence of hypothermia, a proportion of lambs will always succumb. In hostile weather conditions every lamb born outdoors is in jeopardy. It is therefore essential that all shepherds become skilled at detecting lambs with hypothermia.

USING THE THERMOMETER

There are relatively few occasions when taking a sheep's temperature is of much help to a non-professional. However, lambing is a most important exception, when every shepherd must carry a thermometer, whether outdoors or indoors, and must use it frequently. Every lamb in any way suspect should have its temperature taken immediately. It is much better to err on the side of overcaution rather than to be neglectful and leave a lamb until the next inspection of the flock, when it may well be dead or much more difficult to salvage.

Because the use of a thermometer is so important, it makes sense to purchase a robust model which has a rapid action and is easy to read. There are various models on the market. The Moredun lamb thermometer (Medata Ltd) works on a traffic-light sequence which is helpful for the busy shepherd. The probe is inserted into the lamb's rectum and switched on. After less than half a minute a red, amber or green light will flash.

313

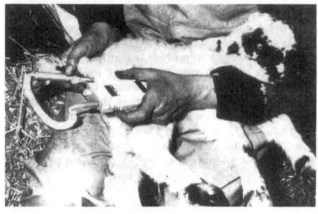

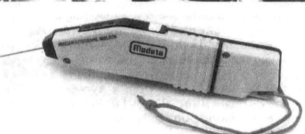

Plate 8.10 Taking the temperature of a lamb with a thermometer which gives a rapid reading on a display that can be seen in the dark. The plate below shows the Moredun hypothermic indicator.

The green light indicates that the temperature is above 39°C, therefore normal or above normal (a fever). An amber light indicates a temperature of between 37 and 39°C, indicating that it is slightly hypothermic and must be attended to. If the red light flashes, the temperature is below 37°C, the lamb is dangerously hypothermic and it requires prompt treatment.

Whichever type of thermometer is used, care should be taken to get an accurate reading and not to damage the lamb. Insert the business end of the thermometer into the rectum, using a little lubrication if necessary. Gently incline the thermometer to one side so that it is resting against the wall of the rectum, rather than in the middle of any faeces present. Allow sufficient time for the thermometer to register a steady temperature. Always wipe clean after each lamb with a tissue soaked in antiseptic. Place in a suitable receptacle to avoid damage in the pocket. If a simple mercury clinical thermometer is used, the mercury will remain at the last registered temperature, so it must be shaken down immediately after use; otherwise a sick lamb could be missed if its temperature is taken after one with a normal temperature.

DETECTING LAMBS IN DIFFICULTY

The approach to shepherding the flock at lambing time has a profound effect upon the efficiency of detecting lambs with a problem, of whatever kind.

The shepherd who rushes around the flock with the dogs, disrupting family groups right, left and centre, has no chance of ever detecting lambs in the really early stages of difficulty, when help is likely to be most effective. Many severely hypothermic lambs are perfectly capable of standing and following the ewe and may go unnoticed in the general confusion. Ideally the shepherd should wander amongst the ewes and lambs, disrupting them as little as possible, so that suspect lambs can be identified much more easily. It is often necessary to arouse lambs if they are resting to see that they are able to get up and follow the ewe adequately and to generally observe their behaviour. Fit, healthy lambs which are disturbed will always rush to the ewe and attempt to suck whenever danger threatens them. The ewe may well walk away ignoring their demands, but if the lambs do not show such an interest in the ewe then they should be treated with suspicion, caught and examined.

The case with which a lamb is caught and its attitude when handled is an important indicator of problems. Handle them with care and respect. Sheep are not very demonstrative beasts, but this should never be taken as an indication that they are not feeling discomfort or pain. Whilst anthropomorphism should not be taken to extremes, it is as well to ask yourself how you would feel about being heaved and pummelled about if you were unwell or had a fractured leg. Always give the animal the benefit of the doubt.

Taking the temperature of an unwell lamb is essential but does not, on its own, provide a diagnosis of what is wrong. If the temperature is above normal (e.g. 41 °C or 42 °C), then the lamb has a fever and is probably suffering from an infection. Alternatively it may have been overheated under an infra-red lamp, in which case it will die of hyperthermia—above normal temperature—very much more rapidly than it would from hypothermia. Even a normal temperature can be misleading since it may be on the way down from a fever and may continue to decline, hence the necessity to check frequently to see whether the temperature of suspect or sick lambs is rising or falling.

Low body temperature may be the result of exposure to bad weather or to starvation as described above, but it is important to realise that the lamb may have some underlying problem which has made it more susceptible to hypothermia. It is always necessary to examine a suspect lamb thoroughly, since treating the hypothermia may revive the lamb only temporarily if an underlying problem remains. Similarly, treating an illness, but ignoring the fact that the lamb is also hypothermic, is equally neglectful, since hypothermia is frequently the final or contributory cause of death in many diseases.

EXAMINING LAMBS

After identifying any lambs with very obvious problems, such as a fracture, take the temperature and then examine the lamb carefully from head to toe. Take note of its general attitude—for example, whether it struggles and bleats or just lies quietly. Examine the eyes, nose and mouth for any sign of discharge, damage or other abnormality. Note whether the ears are pricked up and if the lamb had a sprightly appearance. Check all four limbs for breakages and for any swelling or pain around the joints. When holding the lamb around the chest, note any discomfort or difficulty in breathing which might indicate broken ribs, a respiratory infection or—if it is a newborn lamb—that it is possibly premature and is not yet breathing properly.

Handle the abdomen very carefully because the little organs, such as the liver and kidneys, are very fragile and easily damaged. Also, any inflammation of the gut may be extremely painful. The navel is a danger area for lambs (see later), so note if it is still wet and possibly bleeding, or swollen and painful. Sometimes a loop of gut may herniate through the body wall at the navel, in which case your veterinary surgeon will have to deal with the problem surgically and promptly, as this is a life-threatening condition.

Note particularly whether the outline of the abdomen is nicely rounded and plump when the lamb is held up by the forelegs, indicating that it has a good stomachful of colostrum or milk. It is possible to get confused between this desirable state and a gas-filled stomach, such as might be encountered in a case of watery mouth. They do have a distinctly different feel and the lamb's demeanour will obviously be very different.

Meconium

The rear end of the lamb can reveal a lot. The very first faeces passed are called meconium, which has a thick, sticky, light brown appearance. It is sometimes difficult to void and some lambs may strain, especially if it gets clogged up in the wool, dries and effectively bungs-up the lamb. The dung should be gently removed so as not to damage the skin, or soaked off if it has dried and already caused inflammation of the skin. Great relief should follow such treatment, as constipation, although uncommon, can make lambs very depressed and uncomfortable and if not treated may stop them suckling the ewe. The anal region of constipated lambs will probably be dry and clean and the lamb may require an enema to soften up the faeces and get rid of them. This is a simple job and consists of gently squirting between 10 and 20 ml of warm (not hot) soapy water into the rectum by means of a short length of soft rubber (stomach) tubing attached to a disposable syringe. Normally, faeces will be voided within a few minutes, but the process can be repeated after 20 minutes if nothing has happened.

Imperforate anus

Very occasionally a lamb will be born without an anus, which is a decided disadvantage! It is quite amazing how old some lambs are before this is noticed—usually because the abdomen swells up. Do not on any account attempt to deal with this yourself, but take it into the veterinary surgery.

Some are simply dealt with, but in others quite a long section of the lower bowel may also be missing and these lambs have to be humanely destroyed.

Incorrect castration and tailing

Check that the lamb has been correctly castrated by the rubber ring method. If the ring has been wrongly applied it may have trapped the tube which carries the urine from the bladder to the exterior via the penis. Occasionally a loop of gut may herniate into the scrotum (scrotal hernia) and if this is not noticed when the rubber ring is applied it will cause acute pain and the death of the lamb. In both these situations the lambs will obviously be in pain and the ring must be cut off by placing a key or some such object under the ring and cutting down onto it. Any painful condition, including castration and tailing itself, will delay or prevent the lamb getting colostrum or milk and greatly increase the risk of hypothermia.

Do not assume that the first thing you find wrong is the only problem, since it is quite easy to miss something in a cursory examination during a busy lambing. The ewe should also be examined to see that she does not have mastitis and has adequate milk for the lambs she is rearing. Never leave a suspect lamb to fend for itself. If you cannot find anything wrong, bring the ewe and lambs back to the steading where they can be closely observed. Lambs which have a problem never get better on their own, but usually deteriorate rapidly if they are not given prompt and proper attention.

The most important diseases and disorders of lambs are dealt with in detail in the following chapters.

TREATMENT OF HYPOTHERMIC LAMBS

Lambs suffering from hypothermia should always be brought inside for treatment. If it is intended that the lamb remain with its mother, the ewe and any other lambs should also be brought indoors. It is preferable to remove all the lambs from the ewe and feed them by stomach tube whilst the hypothermic lamb is being treated. This enables all the lambs to return to the ewe together, so reducing the risk of rejection of the chilled lamb.

Treatment is based on sound research and there are a few simple, although important, rules. Because lambing time is usually extremely busy it may be tempting at times to cut corners, but this should be resisted. It is also easy to forget things when under pressure. Therefore, it is helpful to have the rules posted up on the wall above the warming box for rapid reference. This is also most helpful for students or any others who are brought in to help at lambing and may not be familiar with the regime.

Treatment depends principally upon the temperature of the lamb and its blood sugar level, which is largely dependent upon its age. (It is assumed that any underlying problem which may have contributed to the hypothermia, either directly or indirectly, will also be treated appropriately.) Experience has shown that lambs under five or six hours of age will have reasonably high blood sugar levels and will not need to be given glucose

317

before they are warmed. If the age of the lamb is not known, always assume it is older than six hours and deal with it accordingly—see below.

Lambs with a body temperature of 39°C (102°F) or above must not be warmed; otherwise they will die from hyperthermia very quickly. If they are obviously unwell, it will be necessary to look for another reason for their condition, such as an infection.

Moderate hypothermia

Lambs with a temperature between 37 and 39°C (99 to 102°F) are suffering from moderate hypothermia. They do not normally require warming providing they are thoroughly dried, given a feed of colostrum by stomach tube, returned to the ewe in a place of shelter (preferably indoors initially) and observed closely until there is no doubt that they are fully recovered, properly mothered up and getting sufficient milk. Lambs should be dried with old towels since nothing else will get them anything like dry enough. If they are left wet, they will chill further due to evaporation. Never put a wet lamb under an infra-red lamp, which may cause serious scalding should the birth fluids or rainwater in the fleece actually boil on the skin.

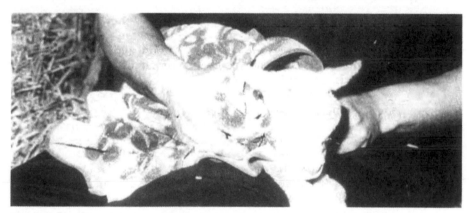

Plate 8.11   Towel drying a lamb to prevent heat loss by evaporation.

Severe hypothermia

Lambs whose temperature is below 37°C (99°F) are in grave danger because they will not suck the ewe and their temperature will always fall further unless they are warmed up. However, the treatment given will depend upon the age of the lamb and upon how seriously chilled it has become. Lambs less than five hours old should be towel dried and placed in a warming box until they reach a body temperature of 37°C (99°F). They should be stomach tubed with colostrum at 50 ml per kilogram of bodyweight (e.g. 200 ml for a 4 kg lamb). If the lamb recovers fully, it can be returned to the ewe providing she has sufficient milk and the lamb is able to suck her successfully and is not rejected. Otherwise, the lamb must be

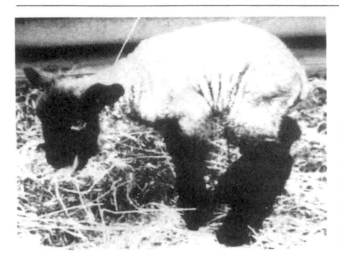

Plate 8.12   A hypothermic lamb of around 12 hours of age whose condition is due to starvation. Such lambs must be given energy before they are warmed up; otherwise they will die in a hypoglycaemic fit.

kept in an aftercare unit (see below) for a while longer and fed colostrum initially and then milk at the above rate at least three times daily until fit.

Lambs over five hours of age are likely to have low blood sugar levels and must on no account be warmed before they have been given a supply of energy. This can be in the form of either colostrum by stomach tube or sterile glucose solution by injection. This is to prevent the onset of a hypoglycaemic fit which would kill the lamb.

Conscious and unconscious lambs

The choice between giving colostrum by stomach tube or glucose by injection before warming depends on whether the lamb is fully conscious and able to swallow satisfactorily. This is indicated by its being able to hold its head up, which will depend on just how cold and short of energy the lamb has become. A 15-hour-old lamb with a temperature of around 35°C (95°F) may still be able to hold up its head, be aware of its surroundings and be able to swallow reasonably well. However, a lamb of the same age whose temperature has fallen to 32°C (90°F) will almost certainly be unable to hold up its head. It will probably be semi-conscious or unconscious and unable to swallow a stomach tube. Below this temperature most older lambs will die, whereas lambs less than five hours of age, who still have some brown fat energy reserves remaining, might be able to hang on to life at even lower temperatures. The Moredun workers have successfully revived lambs with temperatures below 20°C (68°F).

FEEDING BY STOMACH TUBE

Stomach tubing is the simplest, safest and quickest way to feed any conscious lamb which can hold up its head and can sit up on its own without support. Have a jug beside you containing the correct amount of

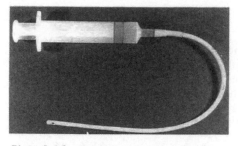
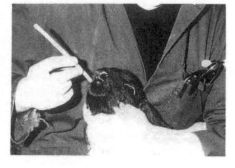

Plate 8.13 Rubber stomach tube for lambs with syringe attached.

Plate 8.14 (*Above right*) Inserting a stomach tube down the oesophagus of a lamb.

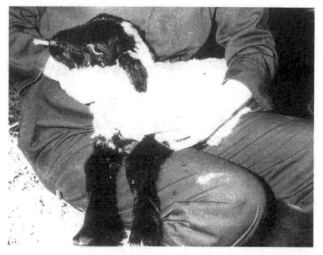

Plate 8.15 The end of the tube is now in the stomach. Note how the lamb is held and how relaxed it is. If the tube is put down the windpipe in error, the lamb will cough and struggle violently.

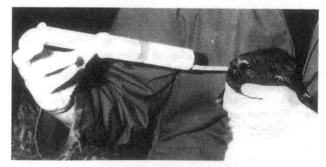

Plate 8.16 Delivering colostrum by stomach tube. The syringe can safely be emptied to a slow count of twenty. This technique must only be used in the conscious lamb which can 'swallow' the tube.

320

colostrum (or milk) for the size of lamb and warmed to blood heat (37°C). Fill a clean 50 or 60 ml disposable syringe ready for use. Sit comfortably on some bales and lay the lamb across your lap, supporting its head with your hand and stretching its neck slightly. Slip a sterilised lamb stomach tube into the side of the lamb's mouth and slowly feed it down its throat, allowing it time to swallow the tube as it disappears. The lamb should show no signs of discomfort as the tube slips down the oesophagus and into the stomach. If it coughs, splutters, rolls its eyes, struggles and calls out as you are introducing the tube, then withdraw it immediately as this means you have managed to put it down the windpipe by mistake. Obviously, to syringe colostrum into the lungs would drown the lamb. It is really quite difficult to get the tube down the wrong way, but don't be put off if it happens first time. Reposition the lamb if necessary, lubricate the tube by dipping it in colostrum and try again. Lamb stomach tubes are made to a length so that two or three inches will be left sticking out of the lamb's mouth when the tube is fully inserted. The lamb will probably chew on the tube but should lie quietly when the tube is in place.

Attach a full syringe to the tube and empty it to a slow count of 20. Exchange the syringe for a full one and repeat until the correct amount has been delivered. Remove the syringe and tube at the end of the feed and set the lamb down. It may cough a little if a drop of milk has got into the windpipe on withdrawal of the tube, but this will do no harm.

Do remember that the lamb must be fully conscious. If not, then it is much more likely that the tube will be introduced into the windpipe, since the unconscious lamb cannot swallow and cannot react by coughing and struggling if the tube goes down the wrong way. Also, unconscious and seriously hypothermic lambs are unable to digest food adequately, since all their bodily functions have slowed down through lack of energy to fuel the chemical reactions. They lie flat out and some of the feed may be regurgitated up the oesophagus and down into the lungs. Note here, too, that weakly newborn lambs should never be fed by feeding bottle and teat, since their sucking reflex will be very poor and their coughing reflex will also be dulled, thus preventing the expulsion of any milk that may dribble down into the lungs.

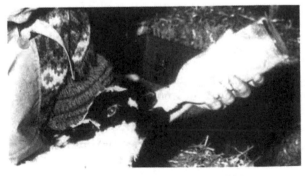

Plate 8.17   Bottle feeding is inappropriate for hypothermic lambs since they are more likely to choke than when stomach-tubed. Bottle fed lambs which have to be fostered are less likely to suck from the ewe's teat than stomach-tubed lambs.

Hygiene

A good supply of stomach tubes and disposable syringes will be needed so that they can be sterilised, either with dairy detergents or by boiling, and then left ready for use in a suitable antiseptic solution such as Milton. It will be necessary to stomach tube any infected lambs from time to time and it is essential not to spread infection on the stomach tube to other susceptible lambs. Treat the lambing area like a maternity ward in terms of hygiene, since lambs are born even more vulnerable to infection than human babies, who at least have a supply of protective antibodies before they are born.

Warning: Colostrum must be collected from ewes, goats or cows in a hygienic manner to minimise contamination; otherwise bacteria will multiply in it, especially if it is left at room temperature. It should be kept in a fridge for use within one or two days or immediately frozen. Grossly contaminated colostrum may actually kill lambs rather than protect them from infection.

Electrolyte solutions

Hypothermic lambs suffering from watery mouth or any of the infectious diarrhoeas should not be fed with colostrum or milk as they cannot digest it. They do need fluid replacement treatment, however, and can safely be given electrolyte solutions by stomach tube if they are conscious and can sit up. There are a number of such products on the market designed for treating diarrhoeic farm animals, and you should consult your veterinary surgeon about how to increase the glucose content for lambs to around 10% of the made-up product. If this is not done, lambs which have to be fed such fluids for two or three days when they are scouring will not get sufficient glucose and become hypoglycaemic as a result. (These products are designed primarily for calves, hence the discrepancy.) Electrolyte solutions can be used as a vehicle for oral antibiotics where these are prescribed.

Frequency of feeding

Lambs require at least three feeds per day at the recommended rate of 50 ml of colostrum per kilogram of body weight. The smaller the lamb, the more frequent should be the feeds to avoid overloading. Also, generally speaking, animals make better nutritional use of food if it is given little and often. For example, a small 3 kg lamb requires a minimum of 3×150 ml, three times per day = 450 ml per day. This would be better spaced out at five feeds of 90 ml each if time allowed. Spread out the feeding times so that there is no long spell when the lamb will not be fed. For example, on a three feeds per day regime, feed at eight hour intervals such as 6 am, 2 pm and 10 pm and on four feeds per day at 6 am, noon, 6 pm and midnight.

INTRAPERITONEAL INJECTION OF GLUCOSE

Lambs more than five hours old which become so weak and cold that they cannot even support the weight of their own heads, or are semi-conscious or unconscious, must be supplied with energy before they are warmed up. This can be given in the form of a sterile glucose solution injected directly into their body cavity. This is the potential 'space' in which organs like the liver, kidneys, gut and bladder are all suspended, and it is lined with a very sensitive membrane called the peritoneum. Care must be taken not to damage the organs within the body cavity, nor to introduce infection which might lead to peritonitis (inflammation of the peritoneum), and with reasonable precautions this can be avoided. Intraperitoneal injections, as they are called, must never be given to lambs with any gut infection such as diarrhoea. Glucose solutions must never be given into muscle or under the skin.

It is essential that your veterinary surgeon instructs everyone who might need to use the technique, as this will reduce the risk of doing any damage to lambs. It is important to use the correct equipment, particularly the right length (2.5 cm) and gauge (19) of needle. A relatively large dose of glucose is required—10 ml of a 20% solution for each kilogram of body weight. A large syringe (50 ml) is therefore essential, as it is undesirable to have to change syringes whilst delivering the full dose. Typical doses would be 50 ml for an averaged sized single lamb of 5 kg, 40 ml for a medium 4 kg twin lamb and 30 ml for a small 3 kg triplet. (It is always important not to under- or overdose lambs with drugs of any kind, and a small accurate spring balance for weighing lambs is useful.)

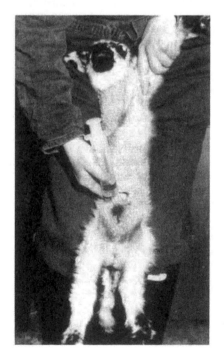

Plate 8.18   Intraperitoneal injection in a lamb. A glucose solution has been injected into the body cavity to supply energy to a lamb over five hours of age which is chilled and cannot hold up its head. Note thé angle of the syringe and the tincture of iodine at the injection site.

Making up the glucose solution for injection

Glucose for injection is usually supplied as a 40% solution which has to be diluted with an equal volume of water to produce a 20% solution. It is important to use boiled water, which is sterile, and—very conveniently—equal volumes of cold 40% glucose solution and freshly boiled water mixed together in the syringe produce a 20% solution of glucose approximately at blood heat, which is exactly what is required. Insert a needle through the rubber cap of the 40% glucose bottle. Attach a syringe and draw out half of the final amount of solution required (e.g. 20 ml of 40% glucose for a 4 kg lamb requiring 40 ml of 20% solution). Detach the syringe from the needle and draw up an equal quantity of the freshly boiled water. Make sure the solutions are thoroughly mixed by rocking the syringe backwards and forwards. Attach a new needle to the syringe, with the needle guard in place until immediately before use. The solution is now ready for injection, so wrap the syringe in a towel to hold it at blood heat. Needless to say, hands should be clean and the actual needle should not be touched.

Hill shepherds can carry boiled water in a small thermos flask to mix the solution on the hill for collapsed hypothermic lambs they find miles from home. This will fortify them until they can be brought back for immediate warming. Thermal lamb jackets which generate heat are also useful for hill lambs during transit.

Method

Lean up against some bales with everything to hand and hold the lamb by the forelegs, letting it hang down to rest against your legs. The site for injection is approximately 1 cm to the side of and 2.5 cm below the navel. Sterilise the site with tincture of iodine or an antibiotic aerosol. Remove the needle cover and point the needle downwards (with syringe attached) towards the lamb's tail head, that is, at approximately 45° to the skin. New needles are very sharp, so slide the needle through the skin for its full 2.5 cm length. If the lamb struggles, wait until it settles down before injecting and count slowly to 10 or 15 whilst emptying the syringe into the abdominal cavity. You should feel absolutely no resistance. If you do, stop, withdraw the needle immediately and reassess whether you are injecting at the correct site and angle and with the proper size of needle. You will find that many lambs urinate during the procedure, but this is normally nothing to worry about.

The used needle should be discarded safely with its guard on and the syringe rinsed out and sterilised by boiling. Never use a needle more than once—disposable needles are cheap. As a precaution against peritonitis, it is sensible to inject the lamb with a long-acting antibiotic, which can be given under the skin of the neck or over the ribs, but **not** into the abdominal cavity along with the glucose.

Once the older hypothermic lamb has had its blood sugar levels raised by either of the two methods described above then, and only then, can it be safely warmed up in a proper warming box to restore its body temperature to normal.

WARMING UP LAMBS

The warming of hypothermic lambs must be done with skill; otherwise lambs may suffer or even die through carelessness or ignorance. The aim is to raise the lamb's body temperature gradually back to around 37 or 38°C. This may take only half an hour if the temperature has dropped only a few degrees, but it will take several hours to bring an unconscious, cold, clammy lamb with a temperature of only 20°C from death's door.

The safest and most effective way to do this is to use hot air between 37 and 40°C in a thermostatically controlled warming device such as that devised at the Moredun Research Institute (Moredun-Medata Lamb Warming Box, Medata Ltd). The lamb is placed on a metal grid half way up the depth of the box and warm air, supplied from below, surrounds the lamb on all sides. The lamb's temperature should be taken every 20 minutes or so, and when it reaches 37 or 38°C the lamb should be removed from the box and given a feed by stomach tube. Once the lamb is up and about again it will be able to raise its own temperature the extra one or two degrees to bring it up to normal (39°C, 102°F).

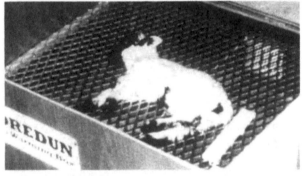

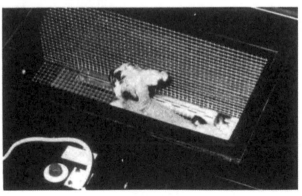

Plate 8.19   A severely hypothermic lamb (*above*) and a fully recovered lamb (*below*) in Moredun warming boxes which are thermostatically controlled. Warm air is blown from underneath the metal grid.

325

Any lamb which gives the slightest cause for concern should immediately have its temperature taken and *be thoroughly towel dried, if wet.*

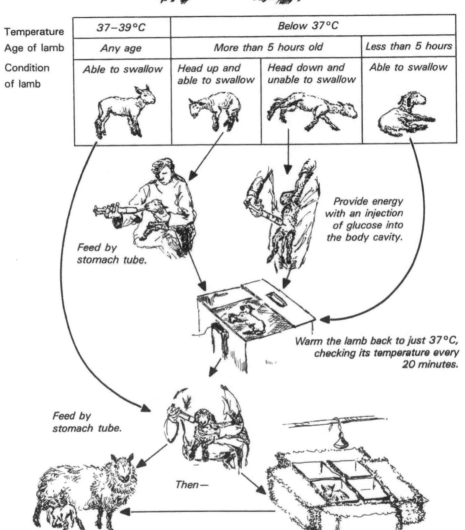

Temperature	37–39°C	Below 37°C		
Age of lamb	Any age	More than 5 hours old		Less than 5 hours
Condition of lamb	Able to swallow	Head up and able to swallow	Head down and unable to swallow	Able to swallow

Feed by stomach tube.

Provide energy with an injection of glucose into the body cavity.

Warm the lamb back to just 37°C, checking its temperature every 20 minutes.

Feed by stomach tube.

Then—

if the lamb revives and is able to suck its dam effectively, keep them close to home for frequent observation.

if the lamb is still weak, keep it in an aftercare unit and feed it regularly by stomach tube until it is strong enough to rejoin its mother.

Figure 8.1 Detecting and dealing with hypothermic lambs.

326

Keep the warming box clean by removing the wire grid and scrubbing it with a disinfectant solution. The whole box should stand on old paper sacks, which should be replaced frequently as they will become soiled with urine and faeces.

It is obviously possible to construct home-made warming boxes or bale warmers, and local farm colleges and the ATB will be able to provide construction details. Do take particular precautions against the fire hazard, especially with bale warmers. Always make sure that any box is large enough and provided with adequate ventilation flaps to avoid overheating lambs.

AFTERCARE FOR REVIVED LAMBS

Most lambs recover from their ordeal well and are fit and strong enough to rejoin their ewe, in which case the family unit should be kept close by in a sheltered position so that the lambs can be observed closely. It is a sad fact that many lambs are revived and then forgotten in the hurly-burly of lambing, only to succumb again. They may not be so lucky the second time. It is important, therefore, that the underlying cause for the hypothermia is identified and corrected if possible. For example, if the lamb was starving because the ewe has mastitis, then it is pointless returning the lamb to its mother. Instead, it should be fostered or reared artificially. On the other hand, if the chilling was due to appalling weather conditions, then temporary shelter to allow the recovered lamb time to mother-up may be all that is necessary. Obviously, such lambs should not be put straight out again into the wind and rain.

Lambs which have recovered from the initial hypothermia but which require further intensive care because of disease or injury should not be returned to the ewe, but kept in a suitable aftercare unit. (The ewe and any siblings of the sick lamb should be allowed to go, since it is unlikely that the ewe will accept a lamb which has been away from her for several days.)

Aftercare unit

An aftercare unit should be provided for lambs thought not to be infectious and another constructed in the infected hospital area. These should consist of a collection of individual cardboard grocery boxes lined with newspaper for insulation. A fresh box can be provided for each lamb and used boxes burned. The whole area can be surrounded by bales of hay or straw to keep out draughts. A series of infra-red lamps should be placed above the boxes so that there is a distance of at least 1.2 m (4 ft) between the bottom of the lamp and the back of a standing lamb. It is very important to observe this precaution because far too many lambs (and calves and piglets) are 'bar-becued' alive. Lambs that cannot turn themselves over must be turned by the shepherd; otherwise one side will get cooked.

Always feed weak lambs by stomach tube rather than by feeding bottle and teat, since they are unlikely to be able to cope with this form of feeding and may choke or drown. Feed lambs at least three times daily on ewe milk replacer, since they should not have colostrum for more than a couple of days at most.

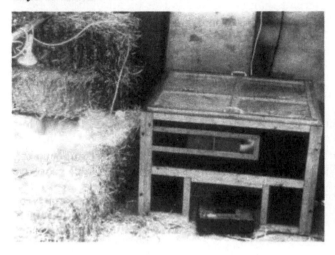

Plate 8.20 A home constructed warming box (with a domestic electric heater as a heat source) alongside an aftercare unit made out of straw bales and cardboard boxes. Fire is a hazard in such an area.

Overheating lambs

Hyperthermia will kill lambs very quickly indeed and should be avoided at all costs. If a lamb in a warming box begins to puff and pant, remove it immediately and take its temperature. If it is above 40°C, it is hyperthermic. Stand the lamb in a few inches of lukewarm water and pour it over the lamb, stopping to take its temperature frequently until it has fallen to around 40°C. Towel dry the lamb thoroughly, place it in a cardboard box in a warm place but away from any direct heat source and check its temperature until you get a series of steady normal readings of 39 to 40°C. Be careful not to overcool it. Hyperthermia is most likely to arise in warming boxes which are not thermostatically controlled or are too small, or in any warming box if the lamb is forgotten about. Noisy timer clocks set at 20 minute intervals are a helpful reminder to check lambs.

Whilst infra-red lamps have a place in the aftercare unit, they are totally unsuitable for warming up hypothermic lambs initially since they cannot be adequately controlled. They heat only one side of the lamb and there is a high risk that the lamb will be burned or scalded if it is still wet. The kitchen warming oven (**not** main oven) should only be used in an emergency, and the lamb must not be burned through direct contact with metal. Its temperature must be taken every five minutes or so, since most ovens will be far too hot and lambs must not be warmed too rapidly. As it is obviously all too easy to overheat lambs, someone should stay with them every minute they are in an oven. The same rules apply whatever warming method is used, namely that lambs must have an adequate energy supply and be thoroughly dry before they are warmed.

Shelter for lambs

Provision must be made for shelter of ewes and lambs in the form of housing, by the erection of barriers against the weather or by allowing the flock access to woodland. Even the simple provision of straw bales or plastic netting hung over a fence out in the lambing fields can be a real life-saver. If vulnerable lambs can get out of the wind and rain, then chilling will be less rapid and they will have more time to reach the teat and get a feed of colostrum before they become too cold to suck or simply to get about.

If ewes and lambs are housed over the lambing period, they should on no account be turned outside until they are mothered-up and it is certain that they have had adequate colostrum and are continuing to get plenty of milk. With litters this applies to all the lambs. If a triplet is not doing too well indoors, it will probably perish outdoors. Obviously lambs must never be turned outside if the weather is inclement.

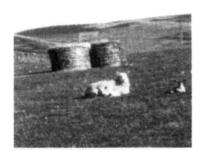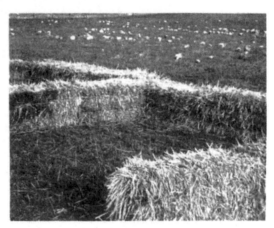

Plate 8.21 Large or small straw bales provide shelter for lambs should the weather turn nasty.

MOTHERING INSTINCT

Newly lambed ewes must be observed closely to see that they are willing and able to mother their lambs. It is not sufficient that they do so with their first-born, but they must treat each new arrival in the same way. When there is a reasonable gap between births, the ewe will have ample opportunity to lick the lamb dry, guide it to shelter if necessary and allow it to suckle. The sucking will stimulate further let-down of colostrum for following lambs. The presence of a new lamb in the vagina will re-stimulate the mothering instincts of the ewe. If births follow in quick succession, inexperienced ewes may pay all their attention to one lamb at the expense of the other, or may be confused and inadequately mother both lambs.

329

Sick, thin or young, inexperienced ewes are less likely to mother their lambs adequately. These groups are also less likely to transfer as much protective antibody to their lambs, which will leave them more susceptible to disease as well as to hypothermia. Similarly, ewes which have had a difficult lambing may be injured, infected or exhausted, or indeed all three, and are at a very distinct disadvantage so far as looking after their lambs is concerned.

PUTTING BACK THE LAMBING DATE

The time of year when lambing takes place has a significant effect upon the survival rate of lambs for a number of reasons. The death rate drops the later lambing occurs, with highest lamb survival and rearing rates in April lambing flocks. Where deaths from hypothermia are unacceptably high, it may be worthwhile to consider lambing later, when the extra lambs reared should compensate to an extent for the lower prices received for lambs sold later in the year.

Fostering and Artificial Rearing of Lambs

Even in the best managed flocks there are likely to be a small proportion of lambs which will need to be fostered or reared artificially. In poorly managed flocks the proportion is likely to rise—for example, because ewes have insufficient milk through inadequate feeding. It is important that the shepherd can recognise early on which lambs are going to need assistance from one of these techniques and that he or she is skilled in applying them. Unfortunately, the success rate generally is not good, especially with artificial rearing. This is often because shepherds are busy and cannot devote sufficient time to the task. The very highest level of stockmanship and attention to detail is essential if lambs are to be artificially reared successfully.

LAMB BANKS

Locally organised 'lamb banks' identify farms willing to purchase orphan and other lambs for artificial rearing and farms which have such lambs for sale because they cannot cope with them. This can work reasonably well if organised properly. However, purchasers should beware of the risks of introducing disease—such as abortion agents or the infectious diarrhoeas—into their flocks in this way. On no account should lambs be offered for sale at the farm gate to the general public since this is totally irresponsible on a number of counts. Very few non-farming people are likely to have the facilities, let alone the knowledge or skills, to rear lambs successfully. This means that a high proportion of such lambs will perish and this presents a welfare problem. There is also a risk that lambs may be carrying any one of a number of infections transmissible to humans, such as orf, cryptosporidium or even enzootic abortion. This is particularly important, since children are likely to have been the ones to pressurise parents into taking such foolish action as buying pet lambs and will be at particular risk through handling and cuddling these appealing creatures. A number of city veterinary surgeons have horror stories of clients who have brought sick or failing lambs into their surgeries, having purchased them during their Easter country holiday, with not the faintest clue how to feed or look after them.

LAMBS AT MARKETS

As there is not a national lamb bank in operation at present to cover all areas of the country, a large number of orphan lambs are still sold through markets. This is unfortunate because the present arrangements are not always in the best interests of lambs. Markets should provide hygienic, comfortable, well-bedded, draught-free, under-cover accommodation. Lambs should have as short a stay in the market as possible. All should have had a full day's colostrum feeding prior to sale and be in good health. No sick lambs should ever be sent to market and any which are found to be ill whilst they are there should be removed to a proper, well-bedded sick bay immediately and seen by a veterinary surgeon.

Lambs should never be overcrowded and should be sold in the pens, not through an auction ring. The auctioneers should make every effort to sell lambs as soon as possible after they arrive at the market. Once sold, lambs should be taken home as soon as possible. The longer they are left in contact with sheep from other farms, the greater is the risk of their picking up infection—especially diarrhoeas—to which they may not have any specific protection via their mother's colostrum.

Lambs should only be marketed once and should be suitably marked to ensure that they are not resold.

Fostering

Generally speaking, fostering is a very much better proposition than artificial rearing. If the ewe has sufficient milk and can be persuaded to take a 'foreign' lamb and mother it well, then the lamb's chances of survival are generally higher than if it has to be artificially reared. Good ewes will always be able to give their lambs much more attention than the most diligent shepherd.

If the lamb's real mother has sufficient colostrum to give all her lambs a first feed, then they should all be allowed to take as much as possible, since the colostrum of the lamb's own mother is usually the most beneficial. Alternatively, colostrum from another ewe, or cow's colostrum, can be used, and the pros and cons of this are discussed earlier in this chapter.

331

SUITABLE FOSTER MOTHERS

There are a number of ways that lambs can be fostered-on and shepherds have their own preferences. However, to be successful, the ewe chosen for fostering must be suitable. She must have adequate milk to take on an extra lamb. If she has a single lamb of her own and has only been fed for a singleton, she may not have sufficient udder development to be capable of producing sufficient milk for twins, however well she is fed during lactation. On the other hand, a ewe which was fed for twins and has lost one lamb may yield sufficient to take on an orphan. Generally, it is better to choose middle-aged ewes, since both younger and older ewes may be less good mothers and may also produce less milk. Obviously ewes must be fit and healthy with no udder disease and with two functional teats. The temptation to use ewes which have aborted late in pregnancy as foster mothers to female lambs should be resisted, however much milk they may have, because of the risk of enzootic abortion (see Chapter 5).

The orphan or multiple to be fostered should be fit and healthy. Sick lambs pose a risk to their new litter mates and also are unlikely to be either strong enough or eager enough to persist in following the ewe to seek out the udder. If there is a choice, it is probably better to leave a weaker lamb with its mother (providing she has sufficient milk) and to foster a stronger one.

EARLY 'RUBBING ON'

The most successful fostering technique entails catching a potential foster mother in the act of lambing. Restrain the ewe gently and check her udder before proceeding. Withhold her lamb or lambs from her in the meanwhile. The foster lamb should be dry, so if it is newborn itself, it should be thoroughly towel dried to remove its own birth fluids. Any ewe's birth fluids become compulsively attractive to a ewe in the last few days before lambing—one reason why they try to steal lambs—but at lambing, the ewe's own fluids are particularly attractive to her. The foster lamb should be rubbed in these fluids, particularly the head and tail region which the ewe tends to nose first of all.

The foster lamb and the ewe's own lamb should be placed in front of her, and then the ewe can be allowed to get up. She should be kept in a restricted area until the shepherd is confident that the ewe has accepted all the lambs. Frequent observation in the early stages is essential, since starvation hypothermia is a distinct risk in rejected lambs, or where ewes turn out not to have sufficient milk. It may be necessary to feed the lamb or lambs by stomach tube to supplement their requirements in the early stages, but if it is apparent that the ewe is not going to accept the foster lamb, then it is much wiser to abandon the attempt sooner rather than later, to reduce the risk to the lamb.

If the foster mother has been lambed for some hours, but it is possible to identify her afterbirth (as in a lambing pen), it is sometimes worth considering late fostering, even though it it usually less successful. The ewe's own lamb should be removed and placed in a large, clean, strong cardboard box along with the foster lamb. Both lambs should be smeared with the afterbirth. The box can be placed in the corner of the ewe's pen so she can see, smell and hear them. Let the lambs back in beside the ewe after about an hour, when they should be hungry and keen to suck, and observe them closely.

Skinning

In cases where the ewe's own lamb has died at birth or immediately afterwards, the dead lamb can be skinned and the skin carefully fitted over a towel-dried foster lamb. Keep the ewe and lamb penned closely. Remove the skin after a day and observe. If the ewe rejects the lamb replace the skin for another day and stomach tube the lamb with colostrum meanwhile. If after this time the ewe will not take the lamb, then abandon the idea. **This method should never be used when the ewe's own lamb has died of diarrhoea or any other infection.**

Fostering crates

Lamb adopters can be purchased or home made. They generally have a poorer success rate than the rubbing on method, but are worth a try where rubbing on is not applicable. These contraptions should allow the lamb to suck without being crushed or beaten up by the ewe, since the ewe's head is restrained—food and water being provided in front of her. The method requires close supervision and is less successful the longer the ewe has been lambed.

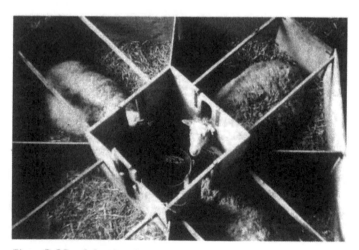

Plate 8.22   A lamb adopter.

333

General guidelines

Whichever method of fostering is employed there are some general guidelines which are helpful. Lambs should be a little hungry when first introduced to the ewe so that they are keen to suck. They must always be fed by stomach tube whilst awaiting a foster mother and never on the bottle, which tends to make them less likely to suck from the ewe's teat.

Ewes can be particularly savage and may inflict severe injuries on fragile newborn lambs, sometimes leading to their death either directly or indirectly. Broken ribs and punctured lungs are common injuries. On no account leave a defenceless lamb to fend for itself, but get it out and give up the attempt if it is likely to be unsuccessful. On the other hand, do not harass the ewe with dogs or by using physical violence. Such aggravation is likely to hinder milk let-down and will rarely persuade a reluctant ewe to accept a lamb.

Try to match lambs up for size where possible, even if it means fostering the ewe's own lamb and replacing it with two equally matched 'foreign' lambs. Always mark foster families clearly so they can be spotted from a distance in case of mismothering or abandonment.

Artificial Rearing

When all else fails—that is, when a lamb cannot be reared by either its own mother or by a foster mother—then it will have to be artificially reared. In milking flocks where lambs are weaned soon after birth, artificial rearing is the only alternative.

This husbandry system requires the very highest level of stockmanship and dedication if lambs are to be reared successfully. Unfortunately, these skills are rare and there tends to be a high death rate amongst lambs artificially reared—mainly because of digestive upsets and infectious disease. No apology is made for mentioning yet again the vital importance of colostrum to the survival of lambs reared artificially, since they are especially vulnerable to infection. This is because lambs are raised together in close proximity at a stage in their lives when they are most vulnerable to infection.

If lambs come from a variety of sources, this greatly increases the risk of introducing new infections to highly susceptible animals. It should also be borne in mind that this presents a risk to the flock as a whole. For example, if a flock is free from orf, the introduction of a single orf-infected lamb from another flock will change the situation overnight. It is therefore essential to allow lambs to suckle their mothers during the first day of life or otherwise supply them with colostrum by stomach tube where this is impossible or impractical.

A thorough knowledge of the feeding regimes for artificially rearing lambs is required and specifications for these can be obtained via the agricultural advisers of the Colleges in Scotland or from ADAS in England and Wales. Debate continues over the relative value of feeding ad lib cold milk replacers versus warm milk replacers, the age to wean and the methods of doing so. These discussions are outside the scope of this book. There are, however, some specific points in regard to the health and welfare of lambs which will be addressed here.

It is important that a suitable person is given the responsibility of rearing lambs. Apart from good stockmanship, much patience and dedication are necessary. Women frequently make a better job of it because they are often more sympathetic. Also, it is considerably easier to give an adequate degree of attention to orphan lambs if the person in charge does not have the responsibility for lambing the main flock, since rearing lambs is very time consuming. There is also the risk of transferring infection to and from the flock to consider.

QUARANTINE

Only healthy lambs which have had adequate colostrum should join a group of lambs. Lambs from other farms or separate flocks on the same farm should be quarantined for several days to allow time for the appearance of any latent infection. Sick lambs should be kept and reared apart and should never be allowed to join healthy lambs. Groups of lambs should be restricted to eight or ten until weaning, because this reduces competition at feeding and limits the spread of infection should it occur.

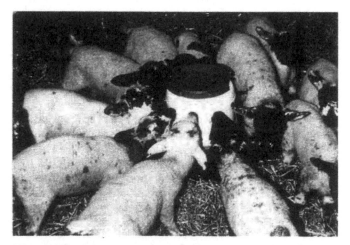

Plate 8.23   A healthy group of evenly matched artifically reared lambs. It is best to keep group sizes small and to ensure that a sufficient number of feeders are supplied so that lambs do not gorge themselves when they are filled up. Feeders should be thoroughly cleaned daily.

335

Match lambs for size and age, as it is always a bad idea to mix different age groups.

Initially, baby lambs should be kept in a small, well-ventilated, although draught-proof area of a building. Supplementary heating should be available if required. Good-quality, mould-free straw bedding should be used on a well-drained floor to provide comfort and warmth. Fresh straw should be added frequently to bury dung and reduce the weight of any infection.

Divisions between groups of lambs should be solid—e.g. metal sheeting or straw bales—and the stockperson should take hygienic precautions so as not to spread infection from one pen to another. If a problem such as diarrhoea occurs in one pen, that group should be attended to last and extra precautions taken. Any sick lambs should always be removed from the group immediately and given special attention in a hospital area. Always assume that other healthy members of the group are likely to become infected, even though the sick lamb has been removed, and take preventive action where appropriate.

HYGIENE

Hygiene is of paramount importance and is often sub-standard. Pens should be mucked out frequently and freshly bedded and should be given a thorough disinfection between batches of lambs. Straw bales used as pen divisions should be burned after each batch.

Milk dispensers should be cleaned daily, using a mild dairy detergent such as hypochlorite, and should be rinsed well before use. Teats must be washed free of milk and then sterilised, by either boiling or suitable chemical sterilisation. An ample supply should be available and those not being used should be stored in a solution such as Milton. The teats on automatic dispensers provide an ideal way of spreading infection by mouth, especially for highly infectious agents such as the virus causing orf, so extra care should be taken. The feeders themselves are best moved daily so that no one area of the pen becomes wet and soggy through a build-up of urine, faeces and spilt milk.

Fresh, uncontaminated water should be available at all times, even though lambs may ignore it for some time whilst solely on milk substitute. Water troughs or bowls must be at a suitable height and should be cleaned out twice daily. Concentrate feeds are likely to be available to lambs from about one week old. Only sufficient feed should be put out so that the lambs can finish up in one day. Any left over should be removed and replaced with fresh. Feed which is left in for some days becomes stale and caked through lambs salivating in it and rapidly becomes contaminated, mouldy and unpalatable.

EWE MILK REPLACERS

As far as ewe milk replacers (EMR) and concentrate feeds are concerned, always go for quality, as cheaper products are generally inferior. Only feeds specially formulated for lambs should be used. Feeds prepared for another species, such as calves, may pose a real danger to lambs, principally because of the inappropriate mineral or trace element content. The commercial concentrate mixtures are generally more suitable and palatable for young lambs than home-mixed rations.

Digestive disorders are probably the commonest problem arising in artificial rearing units and a frequent cause is the inappropriate way that EMR is used. It is of paramount importance that EMR is accurately mixed and fed strictly according to the manufacturer's instructions, which should be followed to the letter, as responsible manufacturers will have gone to considerable trouble and expense to ascertain the correct concentration to give the best results. The most common problems arise through guessing at the amount of powdered milk, so that large errors are made. Weak concentrations of EMR mean that lambs fail to grow or even lose weight. Such undernourished animals are also more prone to infections. If EMR is made too concentrated, lambs do not receive sufficient fluid and become dehydrated. Also, the concentrated feed often causes digestive upsets which lead to diarrhoea. This in turn may exacerbate the dehydration through further fluid loss. Relief stockmen who help out from time to time must be informed as to the strength of EMR being used, since even one day's improper feeding may prove disastrous.

Lambs must be trained to drink, which is a time-consuming but crucial procedure requiring infinite patience, especially in the case of 'slow' lambs. They must be observed frequently to see that they are feeding properly. Difficult lambs can be colour marked for ease of recognition. They must be handled to see if their bellies are full and weighed to see that they are putting on weight. Problem lambs must be withdrawn from the group and tended separately. They must not be left to fend for themselves, as they will slowly (or rapidly) starve. Obviously, sufficient teats must be provided, depending upon the system used.

WEANING

Weaning must not take place until the shepherd is confident that lambs have been eating compound feed for a fortnight or so and that they are taking in at least 250 gm per day—more for large lambs. Because lambs are group fed, this can only be estimated. This, of course, is where good stockmanship and observation come in, since it is important to identify lambs which are not feeding properly. They may not do so because they are unwell, because eating is painful (as in severe cases of orf), because they are not drinking sufficiently well or for a number of other reasons.

If lambs are not drinking water properly, they will receive considerably more of a setback when weaned than they will simply because of the sudden withdrawal of milk. Any suspect lambs should be dealt with individually.

Lambs should always be weighed prior to weaning. As a guide, triplets should weigh not less than 10 kg (22 lb) and a big single 15 kg (33 lb). It is unlikely that many lambs will be less than a month old before they reach these weights.

Weaning is a stressful time and lambs should be closely observed during the following days. Some lambs will remain indoors on concentrates until slaughter, whilst others will eventually be turned out to clean, leafy grazing for finishing. In the latter case it is essential not to turn them out until they are adequately grown and at least two months old. Even then, the weather must be good and the forecast reasonable. Adequate shelter must be provided at pasture. Do not hesitate to bring lambs back indoors if the weather turns nasty.

From weaning, lambs should be offered top-quality hay to stimulate rumen activity well in advance of expected turn-out, so as to minimise digestive upsets. Concentrates should be gradually withdrawn as the lamb's intake of grass increases. If the weather turns nasty or grass growth is impaired, concentrates should be continued for as long as necessary to minimise any setback. Lambs will probably weigh around 18 kg at this stage. Lambs at pasture should grow well providing the grazing is worm-free or they are routinely wormed if no clean grazing is available. Grazing should be kept leafy by adequate grazing pressure or topping, together with strategic fertiliser applications according to the season. Lambs reared artificially should not be grazed alongside other lambs of a different age.

HEALTH

With the exception of urolithiasis (see Chapter 11), the health problems of artificially reared lambs are much the same as those which affect all classes of lambs, such as the infectious diarrhoeas, coccidiosis, pasteurella pneumonia and orf. Because lambs are reared in groups, infections tend to spread rapidly to affect most if not all members of the group. Orf is a particular menace in this regard. Furthermore, once it appears in a group it will almost inevitably spread to all other groups as well, despite careful precautions.

Lambs should be closely and frequently observed for signs of illness. Suspect lambs should always be dealt with promptly, since in almost all cases they will have worsened by the next visit. Separate them promptly from their pen mates and house in extra comfort in a hospital area. If many lambs become ill more or less simultaneously, leave them where they are and consider the whole pen as infected. Take care to minimise the risk of spread to other pens by scrupulous hygiene and by dealing with infected animals last. Separate boots and overalls should be used for infected areas.

Castration of Lambs

Castration can be carried out by a number of methods, all with the aim of either completely removing the testicles or of causing them to become non-functional. The testicles produce both sperm and male sex hormones. By destroying testicle function, male lambs can be rendered sterile and therefore incapable of getting females pregnant, so enabling the two sexes to be run together safely after the age of puberty. This is required in some systems—for instance, where lambs are to be stored over the winter period.

Castration is a painful procedure by whatever method is chosen and should not be carried out where it is unnecessary to do so—for example, where lambs are expected to be sold fat before they are around four months of age. Before this age there should be no unfavourable tainting of the meat from male hormones and entire lambs of this age are still eligible for grading. Entire lambs have slightly better weight gains and food conversion than castrates (wethers), have a leaner carcass, do not suffer any setbacks due to the pain and discomfort of castration or run the risk of complications following the procedure. All these benefits make a good case for not mutilating lambs unnecessarily.

CASTRATION AND THE LAW

There are certain requirements in law which farmers and shepherds must be aware of. No person under the age of 17 may castrate lambs of any age by any method. After the age of three months, lambs must be castrated by a veterinary surgeon using appropriate anaesthesia. Although not a requirement in law, all persons who have to carry out this operation should receive formal training from a veterinary surgeon—for example, through the aegis of the Agricultural Training Board. Unfortunately, far too many lambs are improperly castrated, through either ignorance or carelessness, which is totally unacceptable, particularly in view of the additional unnecessary pain, discomfort and even death that may ensue.

GENERAL PRECAUTIONS

Whichever method is used, there are some general rules which should be observed. Lambs should never be castrated if they are not 100% fit and healthy. If you are in any doubt, delay as long as necessary.

Do not castrate any lamb which has any abnormality of the scrotum or testicles. An important example is a scrotal hernia, where a loop of gut has worked its way through the same gap in the abdominal wall that the testicles descended through en route to the scrotum from their foetal position close to the kidneys. This can be felt as a soft, movable swelling within the scrotum, which may appear larger and lop-sided. Any method of castration could prove fatal in these cases, since the loop of gut would be 'strangulated' by the rubber ring, crushed by the Burdizzo or would cascade out onto the ground if the lamb was cut by the surgical or open method. Your veterinary surgeon should always deal with these abnormal cases. It is helpful to prepare to castrate male lambs before tailing them, so that if castration has to be postponed or abandoned, the tail can be left on, so simply identifying the uncastrated lambs, which can otherwise be forgotten.

Castrating should never be carried out in bad weather, nor should lambs born indoors be rubber ringed just before they are due to be turned outside, since this may compound any mismothering problems. In short, with newborn lambs in particular, it can be a death sentence to castrate if they are compromised in any way, or to carry out the procedure at an inopportune time. The convenience of doing lambs at a particular time should be forgone and the lamb always given the benefit of the doubt. If compromised lambs are identified it is simple enough to castrate at a later date.

All methods of castration carry a risk of infection, since even though the rubber ring and the Burdizzo methods should not break the skin when initially applied, they both deprive tissues of their blood supply. This can predispose lambs to infection caused by those microorganisms which thrive in conditions where there is no supply of oxygen—the clostridial infections being the most important of these in sheep. Tetanus is probably the most common problem in the case of rubber ring castrations. Lambs must be protected and for newborn lambs this means via colostrum from vaccinated ewes. Where ewes are unvaccinated or where lambs have not had colostrum, then they must be protected with clostridial antiserum containing a tetanus component (see Chapter 9). Unprotected older lambs which are to be castrated by Burdizzo or the open method should either be vaccinated well in advance (so that the second vaccination occurs at least two weeks before castration) or given antiserum about two days before castration.

HYGIENE

Cleanliness is obviously important when cutting lambs; it is also important when using the ring or Burdizzo methods. As many as two-thirds of lambs may develop a septic area under the rubber ring and it is preferable that contamination of the neck of the scrotum is kept to a minimum. Lambs should always be set down into clean surroundings following castration, particularly after cutting.

Castration by cutting is always a two-person job because the operator must keep clean and not handle lambs. Likewise the Burdizzo method can only be done responsibly by two people. It is preferable that elastration with rubber rings is done likewise, but it is appreciated that one of the advantages of the method is that it can be done singlehanded in the lambing shed or paddock during the first week of life, when the lambs are near at hand and in a relatively restricted area for catching. With practice and care it is possible to do a good job singlehanded. There are no prizes for doing the job in record time, only penalties and additional pain for the lambs.

ELASTRATION—THE RUBBER RING METHOD

Elastration is the most commonly used method in the UK and is restricted by law to use in lambs during the first week of life only. Tight, thick rubber bands are placed around the neck of the scrotum using an instrument called an elastrator. This deprives the whole scrotum and the testicles inside it of their blood supply. Consequently, the tissues die and fall off within a few weeks.

Lambs should be at least 24 hours old before the rubber rings are applied, as this method causes pain and discomfort for some hours, which discourages lambs from sucking over the most critical period of their lives. This may predispose them to hypothermia and also to disease, in particular to watery mouth.

Method

If you are working singlehanded, hold the lamb with its back to your thighs, and if you are seated or kneeling, make sure the lamb cannot get a purchase with its hind feet. To minimise struggling, restrain the lamb gently but firmly with the forearm, as this leaves both hands free. First, examine the scrotum with care, checking that there are no abnormalities and that both testicles

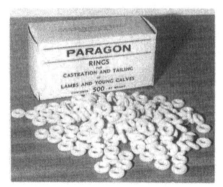

Plate 8.24   Castration and tailing rubber rings.

Plate 8.25   (*Right*) Before releasing the ring, check that the testicles are still in the scrotum and that the ring is not too high up and likely to trap the urethra.

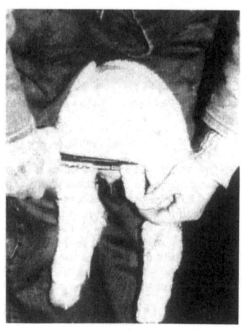

are in the scrotum or can be brought down easily.

Assuming all is normal, place a ring on the elastrator. Open the elastrator, so stretching the ring, and slip it over the scrotum, with the four points of the instrument pointing towards the lamb's belly. Draw the scrotum gently downwards and check that both testicles are present below the position the ring will occupy on the neck of the scrotum. If the scrotum is handled roughly the testicles will be withdrawn up towards the belly out of harm's way, quite understandably! Once you are sure the testicles are in position, release the handles of the elastrator slowly until the ring is in the correct position. Before removing the instrument and completely releasing the ring, finally check that both testicles are in position, as they have a sneaky way of doing a disappearing act at the very last minute. It is important not to leave a testicle behind and vital not to trap one or both beneath the ring which causes great pain.

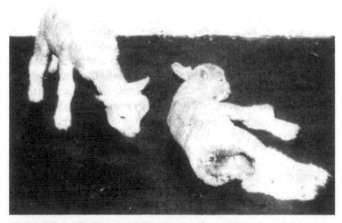

Plate 8.26 Tailing and castration by rubber ring is legal only within the first week of life and is a painful procedure. One of these twin ram lambs has been ringed and is in discomfort on the ground.

Male lambs have rudimentary teats and these must not be trapped behind the ring, because this causes discomfort. If the ring is placed too high up the neck of the scrotum, close to the body wall, there is a danger that the urethra (the tube carrying urine from the bladder to the penis) will become trapped in the ring. This can have disastrous results if it is not spotted, since the bladder may rupture as it fills with urine and this will kill the lamb.

If it is obvious that something is wrong after the ring is released, get it off without delay. Do not drag it off with the points of the instrument, but cut it with a knife using the elastrator or a key slid under the ring to cut down on. (Always use fresh unperished rings since having an unknown number of uncastrated lambs in the flock can be somewhat tedious.) If, at a later date, it is discovered that a testicle was left behind and it is found lying under the skin tight up against the body wall, then a veterinary surgeon should remove it surgically.

Lambs should not be released into dirty conditions—such as muddy, dung-laden sheep handling pens—because they often lie down and stretch out following ringing. Soil and faeces contain tetanus organisms and will contaminate the skin and increase the risk of infection. Set them down in a clean, well-bedded pen indoors, or onto a clean area of grazing outdoors.

Because rubber rings are applied to lambs under a week of age, make particularly sure that lambs get properly mothered-up again. If in doubt, act promptly, so as to avoid cases of starvation hypothermia.

EMASCULATION BY THE BURDIZZO METHOD

The Burdizzo emasculator is a precisely engineered surgical instrument, developed by an Italian veterinary surgeon for the castration of cattle. Small size models that can be operated with one hand should be used to emasculate rams, since the cattle-sized models are quite unsuitable. The Burdizzo consists of a pair of heavy, blunt, metal jaws, which come together very precisely but do not actually touch. The jaws are attached to two handles through a series of pivoted levers. The force applied to the handles to close the jaws is thereby multiplied very considerably and the levers also allow the jaws to be closed very slowly and smoothly. It is essential that the Burdizzo is well maintained and handled with care; otherwise it may become distorted or damaged, which may lead to improper castration and injury to the animal. It should be washed and dried after use, smeared with a light oil and stored away in a clean, dry place with the jaws left partly open.

Before use, the Burdizzo should be tested to see that it is functioning properly. The common way of doing this is to place a stem of unflattened straw between a sheet of folded paper and close the jaws of the instrument. The straw should be severed whilst the paper remains intact because the jaws do not actually meet. This is a fairly crude test but if the instrument fails it should not be used, but returned to the manufacturer for repairs. Burdizzos were never designed to chop off lamb's tails, and such an expensive instrument should never be used to do this, since it is unsuitable and may be damaged in the process.

The principle of the Burdizzo is that when the jaws are closed over the skin of the neck of the scrotum, the blood vessels which run in the spermatic cord will be crushed, so depriving the testicles of their blood supply. This will cause them to shrivel up and die. Whilst the skin of the scrotum is severely bruised in this process, the method is designed to leave a sufficient blood supply intact to ensure that the scrotum itself remains alive. Because the skin should not be broken, only crushed (by a well-maintained and undamaged instrument), infection should not occur. However, if the machine is not well maintained and if it is left uncleaned with the jaws closed between use (which may mean a whole year), then the skin of the

343

scrotum may be broken. In this case infection is inevitable, since the jaws will squeeze infection into the wound, often with serious consequences.

The author can recall being asked to treat a group of calves, kept in filthy conditions, which had been emasculated using a buckled and corroded Burdizzo which was stored on the leaking window ledge of the calfhouse. Every animal in the group was very sick with a fever and all were in considerable pain because of a hugely swollen and septic scrotum. Some were so bad that they had to be destroyed. Whilst the rest recovered with treatment, they received a very severe setback from which they never fully recovered.

Method

The handler should sit comfortably on a bale and restrain the lamb by holding a front and a hind leg in each hand so that the operator has easy access to the scrotum and will not be kicked. The skin of the scrotum should be clean, since if it is caked with hard faeces this might cause the skin to break and introduce infection. Before proceeding, check that two testicles are present and that there is no sign of a scrotal hernia. Open the jaws of the small, singlehanded size Burdizzo and place lowermost the jaw which has lugs or 'cordstoppers' at each end—that is, have the lugs pointing upwards towards the operator. (Burdizzos are made without lugs, but these are unsuitable for lambs, since it is too easy for the spermatic cord to slip from between the jaws when they are closed.)

It is imperative that each side be emasculated separately. Draw one testicle down into the scrotum with one hand and feel for the cord which runs from the top of the testicle up towards the body wall. Manoeuvre the cord to the outer edge of the neck of the scrotum. Position the Burdizzo jaws above and below the neck of the scrotum whilst maintaining your hold on the spermatic cord. The blades should be at right angles to the cord. Only the smallest amount of skin should be bruised consistent with crushing the cord effectively. Therefore slide the blades of the Burdizzo along so that only a small length of blade will be pinching the skin when the jaws are shut. (One cordstopper should be out of sight underneath the neck of the scrotum.) The jaws should now be partially closed so they are just touching, but not pinching, the skin. Position the spermatic cord so that it is caught in the angle of the cordstopper and cannot slip to the other side of the scrotal neck when the jaws are shut. Hold the cord in this position using the finger and thumb immediately below the Burdizzo. Now clamp the jaws firmly shut and count slowly up to ten before releasing them. The spermatic cord should be crushed in this procedure, although not necessarily severed. Resist the temptation to maul the already damaged tissues any further in an attempt to locate the severed ends. Merely confirm that the cord was caught between the jaws of the instrument.

It is preferable that the cord is crushed twice on each side. Therefore the first crush should be high enough on the neck of the scrotum to allow sufficient room for a second crush to be applied below the first (to reduce

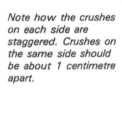

Note how the crushes on each side are staggered. Crushes on the same side should be about 1 centimetre apart.

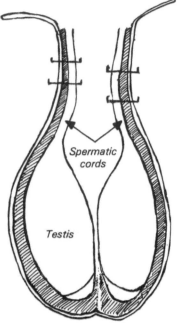

To avoid damage to the penis or urethra, the Burdizzo should be applied well below the body wall—

and well above the testes.

Spermatic cords

Testis

It is vital that a minimum of tissue is crushed. On no account should the instrument be applied across the full width of the neck of the scrotum.

Figure 8.2   Crush positions on the neck of the scrotum following castration by the Burdizzo.

pain to a minimum) but well above where the cord attaches to the testicle. The first crush should not be so high up the neck of the scrotum as to risk pinching the urethra. It is also important to stagger the double crushes on each side so that they do not overlap, thus leaving an area of unbruised skin down the centre. Consider this when sliding the Burdizzo across to make a double crush on the opposite side. **On no account must the Burdizzo be placed across the whole width of the scrotal neck in one crush.** This will deprive the whole scrotum of its blood supply (in a much more severe way than the rubber ring) and cause great pain. Infection of the wound will lead to a very sick lamb.

Even when the technique is performed correctly, the damage to tissues and to the blood supply causes considerable swelling of the scrotum, and animals are obviously in discomfort, the swelling taking two or three weeks to subside in some cases. The method requires a high level of skill and care, and much unnecessary damage and pain can be inflicted by unskilled or uncaring hands. Also, poor technique can mean that lambs may not be castrated correctly. Animals should always be checked some weeks afterwards to confirm that the task has been carried out properly, as judged by the shrivelled up scrotum.

All in all this is an unsatisfactory method of castration for lambs, since too many things can go wrong. This may lead to both management difficulties in the flock and welfare problems for the lambs. For these reasons it is not recommended where an alternative can be used.

SURGICAL OR OPEN CASTRATION

Lambs may be left until they are older before castration, either through choice or because they could not, for one reason or another, be rubber-ringed during the first week of life. In these circumstances the surgical, so-called open method of castration, is preferable to the Burdizzo. In this technique the scrotum is cut and the testicles completely removed. Because an open wound is created, strict hygienic precautions must be taken, and it is imperative that lambs are protected against clostridial diseases beforehand. Open castration should preferably not be performed in fly weather because of the risk of blowfly strike.

Method

The most satisfactory method is to remove the whole of the bottom of the scrotum and to remove both testes without cutting them in any way; otherwise they may be difficult to extract without causing pain and increasing the risk of infection. It is important to cut the bottom off the scrotum so that the wound will drain adequately, which reduces the risk of abscess formation.

Chose a dry day and a clean area to do the job, so that lambs can be set down onto clean straw indoors, or run out onto a clean field with their mothers. It is essential to have an assistant to hold lambs in the method described for Burdizzo emasculation. Hot water should be available near at hand and you should wash and dry your hands after dealing with each lamb and should avoid handling the lambs during the operations. The cut in the scrotum should be made with a scalpel (surgeon's knife), which has detachable blades. These should be changed frequently so that the scalpel is razor-sharp at all times, as this will cause the least pain. Use a large-size blade (e.g. No. 24) and keep a spare scalpel in case one is dropped on the ground. Leave the scalpel in a shallow plastic tray containing an iodophore antiseptic solution between each lamb. On no account must a shepherd's pocket knife be used for this task, since it cannot be sterilised between lambs and is never sharp enough.

If the skin of the scrotum is clean, swab it with cotton wool soaked in alcohol. If it is dirty, it must be washed and dried (this is important) before being swabbed. Excessively dirty lambs, such as those which have been scouring, should be left to one side and done last, to avoid gross contamination of the area and operator (some of these will need clipping up before being washed). Check every lamb before proceeding for any abnormality such as scrotal hernia, since to castrate such a lamb would entail the intestines spilling out onto the ground and would almost certainly mean a dead lamb. Ensure also that both testicles are present in the scrotum.

Use the finger and thumb to pinch the very bottom of the scrotum (not the testicles) and draw it downwards so there is gentle tension on the purse. The testicles will be left behind, well out of the way of the cut. Draw the scalpel confidently across the scrotum in a single stroke, roughly one or two centimetres above the fingers. It is important to cut sufficient away, as this will allow the testicles to be removed easily and give good drainage for the wound. The testicles should now appear at the wound. One hand should hold the neck of the scrotum up towards the body wall, whilst the other hand grasps one testicle at a time. Draw each testicle downwards out of the wound with a firm, steady pull until the cord breaks. On no account should the cord be cut, as this will cause haemorrhage which may bleed the lamb to death. When both testicles have been removed, hold the skin of the scrotum so as to open the wound and puff in a suitable wound dressing powder. A fly repellant product should be used if there are flies about. This will reduce the risk of infection and help stop any minor bleeding. Do make sure that any product used is suitable for application to an open wound.

From the welfare point of view, open castration has some advantages over the other methods mentioned. Providing a sharp blade is used, the initial cut is swift and relatively painless. Drawing the testicles out can be done swiftly by an experienced operator. Providing the job has been done hygienically, the risk of infection is slight and a clean wound will heal quickly. Therefore, the period of afterpain is likely to be substantially shorter than when using either the rubber ring or the Burdizzo.

Haemorrhage

The procedure is a remarkably bloodless one, but should a lamb drip blood to any extent, then keep it aside in a clean area where the amount of bleeding can be assessed, for example by putting newspaper or paper sacks on the floor. If the blood does not gradually stop dripping but persists in running out, then phone your veterinary surgery and either request a visit or arrange to take the lamb in, depending on the severity of the bleeding. A small bulldog paper clip can be used to close the wound temporarily and this may allow blood to clot in the scrotum. In any case the lamb should be kept close by the steading with its ewe for observation. Haemorrhage causes the lamb to become very weak and unwilling to get up. Its gums, the inside of its mouth and the membranes of the eyes will be very pale. The lamb's heart can often be felt beating furiously against the chest wall when the blood loss is severe. Fortunately, however, bleeding is rarely a problem in properly castrated lambs.

Walk round the lambs immediately after the job is completed and repeatedly for the rest of the day—especially last thing at night. Bring any problem lambs inside and attend to them promptly. Ensure all lambs are correctly mothered-up. If the hygiene has not been adequate or lambs have been kept in dirty conditions, some may become infected in the wound.

These may walk stiffly or spend a lot of time lying down, whilst others may be frankly ill. Always check their temperatures as well as examining the wounds. Where infection is present the scrotum will probably be very swollen and painful and may contain large amounts of pus with a disgusting smell. Avoid handling the scrotum, bring the lamb indoors and telephone your veterinary surgeon for advice.

TAILING OR DOCKING LAMBS

Lambs are tailed or docked—that is, they have a portion of their tail removed—to protect them against blowfly strike. When lambs are 'wormy' or on lush grazing, their dung is often very loose and the tail becomes coated. This creates attractive conditions for flies wishing to lay their eggs. All lambs which will be on the farm over the fly season are usually tailed, except for ewe lambs on hill farms which are to be kept as breeding replacements, where the tail is left to protect the udder against bad weather conditions.

Excessive docking can lead to problems, since a very short tail provides no protection to the anus or vulva from flies or adverse weather conditions. Some years ago at an agricultural show almost a third of the animals in a group of short docked ewes waiting to be used for a dipping demonstration were suffering from inflammation of the vulva and vagina and a number appeared to have been fly struck around the vulva. A reasonable length of tail at least allows the sheep to 'flag' and keep flies at bay. Much short docking used to be done to conform to the fashion of the particular breed— much as happens in the dog world and just as ridiculous. The law now states

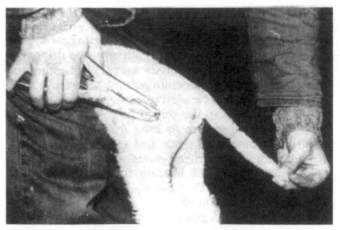

Plate 8.27   Tailing by rubber ring. The law requires that sufficient tail be left to cover the anus in rams and the vulva in females and that, as with castration, the task is performed before the end of the first week of life.

that sufficient tail must be left on males to fully protect the anus and in females to fully cover the vulva.

Tails can be removed by the rubber ring or the scalpel blade, the most common being the rubber ring. (The Burdizzo should **not** be used since it causes unnecessary damage to the bone in the tail, which may lead to painful infected tail stumps and will also damage the Burdizzo.) The tail can be cut off at a joint between vertebrae with one swift stroke of the scalpel by an experienced hand. The tail vein may spurt blood for a short while, but this soon stops in the majority of cases. Large lambs have occasionally bled to death, so they must be observed closely during the first day. To arrest serious bleeding, tie a bandage around the stump of the tail for a few minutes until the bleeding stops, reapplying if necessary. As with open castration, good hygiene must be observed and the task should not be carried out during the fly season if possible.

Castration and tailing are routine tasks carried out on most farms, and because of this the welfare aspects are hardly ever considered. However, no mutilation should ever be carried out unnecessarily, so consider carefully whether it is absolutely necessary to castrate all your lambs. It is your duty to ensure that anyone entrusted to castrate lambs has been properly trained and is closely supervised until fully competent. (Males should consider how they would feel about being castrated by an untrained or uncaring 'surgeon' by any method—with or without the use of anaesthetic!) The law which applies to castration also applies to tailing.

Research is currently being carried out in Scotland to assess the level of pain inflicted on lambs of different ages by the methods described here, with a view to developing more humane techniques to improve the welfare of lambs.

9

DISEASES OF NEWBORN LAMBS

The newborn lamb comes into contact with microorganisms as soon as it pokes its head into the hostile environment of the outside world. During the birth process—maybe even before it has taken its first breath—the lamb will have become contaminated with a host of different organisms, many of which are harmless or even beneficial, whilst others will be potentially dangerous, disease-producing agents. The hindquarters of the ewe, the pasture, the soil or the bedding of a lambing pen, all harbour protozoans, bacteria and viruses which pose a threat to the vulnerable newborn lamb.

These microorganisms have to get into the lamb in order to cause disease. This they may do by a number of routes, the most important to the newborn lamb being via the nostrils, the mouth and the navel. Gaining entry into the lamb does not mean that disease will inevitably follow. However, if the newborn lamb has not sucked the ewe and obtained an adequate amount of good-quality colostrum very early in its life, it will remain vulnerable to infection. The antibodies contained in colostrum and early milk are vital in terms of whether or not the lamb will survive the first weeks and months of life.

There are other factors involved in this battle, however, such as the weight of infection—that is, the number of organisms which infect the lamb. If the lambing area is so grossly contaminated that massive numbers of microorganisms invade, then even if lambs have had a good feed of colostrum, with high levels of antibody, they will still be at some risk due to the sheer numbers of infectious particles.

Lambs which have not received adequate amounts of colostrum may succumb to infection even in very clean surroundings and in the face of a low level of infection. Imagine only a small number of E. coli bacteria entering the digestive tract and each dividing every 20 minutes. Within only a few hours, under ideal conditions for the bacteria, the situation in the lamb's gut can become equivalent to an overwhelming infection. If, however, there is sufficient specific antibody from colostrum to combat the particular E. coli, then they will be inactivated and destroyed and infection will be prevented.

INFECTIOUS DIARRHOEAS IN LAMBS

The infectious agents which cause diarrhoea in lambs gain entry through the mouth by contamination from the faeces of previously infected animals. A lamb sucking a ewe whose udder is contaminated with faeces from a diarrhoeic lamb which previously inhabited the pen, or a lamb simply nosing around in the bedding, may ingest large numbers of infectious organisms and so be at risk of becoming infected itself.

There are many different microorganisms which can cause diarrhoea in lambs. These include bacteria, such as *E. coli*, *Salmonella dublin* or *Clostridium perfringens* type B (responsible for lamb dysentery); protozoans such as cryptosporidium; and viruses such as rotavirus. These may cause damage to different areas of the gut or disease of a different character and may therefore produce slightly different clinical symptoms in affected lambs. However, to all intents and purposes—from the shepherd's point of view—they are scouring lambs and it is not possible to distinguish one infection from the other without careful veterinary detective work supported by laboratory tests.

It is possible to reduce the incidence of scour in a flock by taking general precautions, even in the face of an outbreak. But in order to take more specific and effective measures to prevent further cases or to prevent outbreaks in subsequent years, it is important to obtain a diagnosis. This means identifying the specific infectious agent or other cause. It is quite possible, of course, to have more than one agent causing diarrhoea in a flock, or even in an individual lamb, at the same time. No national surveys have been carried out to identify the relative importance of the various agents causing scours in lambs, but the Quick Reference Chart at the end of this section gives information on those thought to be most important in the UK.

Lamb Dysentery

Lamb dysentery is one of the clostridial diseases of sheep which are characterised by causing rapid death, usually before the shepherd notices that the animal is sick. Despite the fact that excellent and inexpensive vaccines have been available for many years, this type of diarrhoea is diagnosed all too frequently at veterinary investigation laboratories.

The serious losses from lamb dysentery, particularly in the south of Scotland, were one of the stimuli which prompted a number of Scottish farmers, with help from various farming organisations, to found the Animal Diseases Research Association at the Moredun Institute in Edinburgh in the 1920s. Here the cause of lamb dysentery was eventually discovered and the first antitoxin to combat the disease produced.

The infectious agent responsible for lamb dysentery is a bacterium,

Clostridium perfringens (type B), which is found in soil, faeces and the gut of some animals. In soil, the bacteria can survive for very long periods in a resistant form called spores. In areas of the farm where sheep congregate and especially in lambing paddocks, the soil may be heavily contaminated. All newborn lambs are unprotected against diseases such as lamb dysentery. If their mothers have been vaccinated and the lambs suck colostrum in sufficient quantity soon after birth, they will receive passive protection in the form of antibodies which will protect them well beyond the period of risk, which is up to about three weeks of age.

Once inside the gut of the susceptible newborn lamb the bacteria multiply rapidly. They produce a powerful toxin which destroys the delicate lining of the small intestine. Consequently, areas of the gut lining die and become detached, leaving raw surfaces which bleed at the edges (see Colour plate 24). Blood may appear in the faeces, often in a partly digested form which gives the scour a brownish colour. (The word 'dysentery' means blood loss from the gut with or without accompanying diarrhoea.) Many lambs will die without showing any symptoms, and shepherds on their early morning inspection of the flock may find one or more lambs lying dead. Often it is strong lambs from milky ewes which are affected, since the bacteria multiply best in the presence of a good supply of carbohydrate in the intestine.

CLINICAL SIGNS

Lambs which survive long enough to show signs tend to hang back, stop sucking and spend long periods lying down in obvious discomfort. Handling such lambs is distressing for them and when they attempt to dung it is obviously difficult and painful. The faeces may appear normal at first but soon become fluid, brownish in colour and they sometimes contain some fresh blood. Lambs become fouled around the anus and there is an unpleasant smell of decomposing blood and scour. Lambs which are forced to move do so reluctantly and cannot keep up with the flock. They often stand still with their backs arched, bleating plaintively. As in the terminal stages of many diseases the lambs may feel very cold. Eventually they collapse, lapse into a coma and die within a few hours. Post-mortem examination will reveal a severely inflamed gut with ulceration and a particularly foul smell, but laboratory tests are essential to confirm the diagnosis.

TREATMENT

In the early stages of an outbreak of lamb dysentery the cause of deaths will not be known. Unfortunately, whatever treatment is attempted it is unlikely to effect a cure due to the drastic and rapidly fatal nature of the disease. Indeed, once the diagnosis is known then the most kindly course of action may be to have very sick lambs humanely destroyed so as not to subject them to further unnecessary suffering.

Where treatment is attempted it is most important to make the lamb comfortable. Always check its temperature and if it is abnormally low then follow the rules for treatment of hypothermia in Chapter 8. Lambs which have scoured are likely to be dehydrated and will require special electrolyte solutions to replace fluid and salts which are lost, but on no account should these lambs be given intraperitoneal glucose injections. Without fluid replacement and warming where necessary, lambs stand little chance of recovery from lamb dysentery (or any other form of diarrhoea) whatever antibiotics or other medicines are given.

Penicillin or the tetracycline antibiotics are effective against the bacterium responsible, but by the time symptoms are seen the bacteria have already produced large quantities of toxin, against which antibiotics are ineffective. Where lamb dysentery is suspected, early cases should be given antibiotics by mouth and by injection. Antiserum against lamb dysentery is available, often in combination with other clostridial antisera (e.g. lamb dysentery, pulpy kidney and struck). However, these products are designed for the prevention of disease and because the toxin has often caused damage by the time treatment is started, antiserum is usually ineffective.

Medicines containing kaolin or chalk are often used in cases of diarrhoea. They sooth the inflamed gut, absorb toxins and if morphine is included (e.g. kaolin and morphine) slow the movement of the gut.

CONTROL AND PREVENTION

Whilst treatment of this very unpleasant condition is most disappointing, some measure of control is possible when the disease occurs in a flock, and almost complete protection is possible by vaccinating ewes and by ensuring that lambs receive sufficient colostrum immediately after birth.

In the face of an outbreak of lamb dysentery it will usually be the case that the ewe flock is unvaccinated or incorrectly vaccinated (e.g. the pre-lambing booster for ewes may have been forgotten or given too early or too late). Therefore, lambs already born but as yet uninfected and lambs due to be born are all at risk.. The risk will increase as lambing progresses if measures are not taken, due to the contamination of the lambing area by affected lambs.

Antiserum

In these circumstances all unaffected lambs should immediately be injected with lamb dysentery antiserum or preferably with a combined lamb dysentery, pulpy kidney, tetanus and struck antiserum. All newborn lambs should be similarly treated as soon after birth as possible. This will give only short-term protection for two or three weeks, but will cover the danger period for lamb dysentery.

Vaccination of newborn lambs

Lambs from unvaccinated ewes will also need to be protected from the other clostridial diseases, particularly from tetanus and pulpy kidney. They should therefore also be vaccinated, preferably with a combined clostridial vaccine (i.e. '7 in 1' type). Two doses of vaccine are required, the first to be given at the same time as the antiserum, but on the other side of the body. A second vaccination will be needed four to six weeks later and it will be some days after this before lambs will be fully protected.

Lamb dysentery may occasionally occur in flocks where ewes have been properly vaccinated, including a pre-lambing booster. If a lamb does not receive colostrum from its mother or receives an insufficient amount early in life, then it will be susceptible. Newborn lambs from properly vaccinated ewes should not be vaccinated too early in life, since the antigens in the vaccine will combine with the antibodies derived from colostrum. These antibodies will then be unable to destroy the bacteria causing lamb dysentery or the other clostridial diseases when they invade the lamb. Also, the antibodies from colostrum will prevent a proper 'take' of the vaccine.

When lamb dysentery occurs in a flock, apart from the specific control measures described above, there are other general hygiene and husbandry measures which can be taken to contain the outbreak. These are detailed at the end of this diarrhoea section. However, vaccination of the ewe flock is the most effective way of preventing losses due to lamb dysentery and it is also the cheapest. Combined vaccines which cover all the clostridial diseases affecting sheep should be used. Antibodies from the colostrum of vaccinated ewes will protect lambs for up to three months or more. Lamb dysentery does not usually affect lambs over about three weeks of age.

Colibacillosis

Colibacillosis is the name given to the diarrhoea caused by the bacterium *Escherichia coli*. (It should not be confused with the condition known as watery mouth, which is a distinctly separate disease.) The bacterium—*E. coli* for short—is extremely common, being found in the gut of all farm animals, from which it is shed in astronomical numbers in faeces, so contaminating

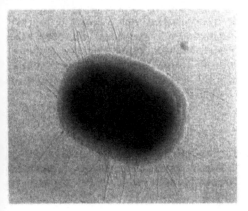

Plate 9.1 This is *E. coli* magnified 60,000 times by the electron microscope. Note the hair-like structures on the surface (pili) which enable the bacterium to hang onto the gut lining.

food and water supplies, bedding, the ewe's udder and hence the lamb.

There are very many different types of *E. coli*, but only relatively few are capable of causing disease. These pathogenic strains possess hair-like structures on their surface known as pili (see Plate 9.1), which allow the bacteria to anchor themselves to the wall of the intestine. There they produce a toxin which causes a diarrhoea. These coliforms are fairly hardy and may survive for months in moist conditions like an indoor lambing area. They will eventually be killed by drying out and/or by sunlight outdoors. During a lambing season, there is a build-up of infection in the lambing area so that a greater and greater proportion of lambs from the later lambing ewes succumb to the infection because of overwhelming contamination. The disease is therefore most common in intensively managed lowground or housed flocks and is rare in hill flocks, except where ewes are brought down to lamb on in-by ground close to the steading.

CLINICAL SIGNS

Some toxins produced by these coliform bacteria reverse the normal chemical reaction which controls the movement of fluids and electrolytes through the lining of the gut. This results in fluids pouring into the gut, rather than from the gut into the body tissues. These events produce the clinical symptoms of a profuse greyish-yellow diarrhoea which leads to extreme weakness and lassitude. The skin is tight and dry due to dehydration and lambs may also become hypothermic. They collapse and die in a very short time in the absence of treatment and often despite it.

Other strains of *E. coli* may damage the gut sufficiently to allow them to enter the bloodstream where they multiply rapidly, producing a bacteraemia which allows them access to all parts of the body. Bacteria may invade the brain and cause meningitis, with accompanying nervous symptoms. Some lambs become incoordinated, whilst others collapse with the head bent back and the legs making paddling movements. Such lambs soon lapse into a coma and die. Occasionally lambs survive a bacteraemia, but may develop joint-ill due to *E. coli* settling out and multiplying in the joints.

Once an outbreak of *E. coli* scour has occurred on a farm it is very likely to do so again in future years, especially if the same lambing area is used year in and year out. The number of lambs which become infected and die may reach appalling proportions in some outbreaks. It is essential to send the carcasses of freshly dead lambs to the veterinary investigation laboratory to establish a diagnosis.

TREATMENT

Treatment of individual lambs will depend upon how quickly cases are detected. Hypothermic and dehydrated lambs should be dealt with appropriately (see Chapter 8) and it should be stressed that this supportive treatment is much more important than any antibiotic treatment.

In the face of an outbreak the most important task is to prevent further cases occurring. All unaffected, in-contact lambs should be treated immediately with an appropriate antibiotic, as should newborn lambs at birth. Shepherds should ensure that all lambs have a good suck of colostrum from the ewe immediately they are born. Twins and triplets should be stomach tubed with ewe or cow colostrum if there is any doubt that they have sucked.

If no cases of scour have arisen, try to resist the temptation to use antibiotics on all newborn lambs. Unnecessary use increases the risk of resistant strains of bacteria arising which may then be difficult or impossible to treat at a future date.

Vaccines

Vaccines for ewes are available which contain a selection of the most common *E. coli* causing scour in lambs and these may sometimes be helpful providing the *E. coli* which are going to cause the scour next season (which may be different from the present season) are included in the vaccine. It is, of course, vital that the lambs get adequate colostrum from the vaccinated ewes. The vaccination regime is similar to that for the clostridial vaccines, but the two should preferably not be given together.

General measures for preventing diarrhoea in lambs are given later in this section.

Salmonellosis

There are many different types of salmonella capable of producing disease in farm animals. Whilst some types may cause specific diseases predominantly in one species—for example, abortion in ewes due to *Salmonella abortus ovis*—all are capable of causing infection in many species, including man. As an example, *Salmonella typhimurium* may cause a severe

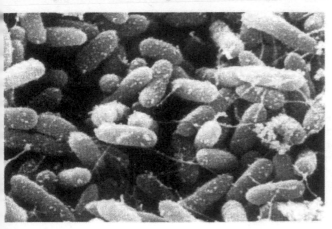

Plate 9.2
Salmonella
typhimurium—seen
under the electron
microscope,
magnified 15,000
times. This bacterium
is capable of causing
serious disease in
animals and humans.

357

gastroenteritis or life-threatening bacteraemia in cattle, sheep and humans. Salmonellosis is therefore classed as a **zoonosis**—that is, a disease transmissible between animals and man. For this reason **it is important to stress the importance of personal hygiene.** Hands should be thoroughly washed after dealing with scouring lambs. When an outbreak of scour occurs, it is likely to be some time before the infectious agent is identified and it should always be borne in mind that salmonellosis, or some other zoonosis, may be the cause.

Fortunately, salmonella infections are less common in sheep than they are in cattle. *Salmonella dublin* and *Salmonella typhimurium* are the most frequent types identified from salmonella diarrhoeas in lambs and ewes.

Sources of infection for sheep are:

- other infected sheep, such as purchased ewes with lambs at foot
- other farm species, particularly calves bought-in from markets
- recovered animals, which may continue to shed the bacteria in their faeces from time to time without showing any clinical symptoms themselves—so-called carrier animals

This last group is particularly dangerous, since carriers cannot easily be identified. Even a negative laboratory test on faeces is meaningless because of the intermittent excretion of the salmonella in dung. Because of the possibility of cross-infection between different farm animal species, it is wise to keep sheep away from cattle known to have been infected and particularly important to avoid lambing ewes down in areas where calves have been reared.

Salmonella can survive for long periods in soil and can contaminate water courses via natural drainage. They also survive indoors in bedding and lambs pick up infection in much the same way as they do *E. coli*—from the contaminated udders of their mothers, bedding, foodstuffs and water supplies.

As with other infectious agents, the higher the stocking rate, the greater the risk. Scouring lambs soon heavily contaminate the lambing area and adult ewes may also become infected, as well as other lambs. Ewes in late pregnancy and those recently lambed are particularly susceptible to salmonellosis and both these groups may be in contact with infected lambs in the lambing area.

In ewes, salmonellosis may produce a bacteraemia and very sick animals, a significant proportion of which will die. So, unlike many of the other infectious scours—where clinical disease is mainly confined to lambs—with salmonellosis the infection is often a flock, or even a farm problem, with cases in more than one species.

CLINICAL SIGNS

The first sign of salmonellosis in a flock may be sudden deaths amongst lambs and/or sick and dying ewes. Lambs which do develop symptoms stop sucking and may develop profuse and sometimes blood-splashed diarrhoea with a foul smell. In sudden lamb deaths the hindquarters may show a pale yellow staining. Some lambs develop a bacteraemia causing any of a number of symptoms depending upon which organs become involved.

If measures are not taken to control the outbreak, the number of lambs born which become infected can reach alarming proportions and a substantial percentage of infected lambs will die despite treatment. Those that do recover may take weeks to do so and never fully compensate for the damage done.

TREATMENT

Treatment of salmonella infection consists of the general measures designed to counteract dehydration and hypothermia. In addition, antibiotics or other drugs given by mouth may help, and lambs with a high temperature should be given antibiotics by injection also. Veterinary advice will be essential in arriving at a diagnosis, in the choice of drugs and in deciding upon a course of action to control the outbreak.

Treatment of both lambs and ewes can be very disappointing, the disease often taking its course in a flock despite vigorous medication of ewes and lambs. Once the strain of salmonella has been identified by laboratory testing, vaccination of all ewes at risk may be attempted but only if an appropriate vaccine containing the identified strain of salmonella is available. This may check the outbreak, but is not without risk, since animals already incubating the disease may react adversely to the vaccine.

PREVENTION

In deciding on appropriate measures to prevent this serious disease occurring at future lambings, or indeed in other classes of stock on the farm, it is essential to try to identify how the infection arose in the first place and also what classes of stock and areas of the farm may harbour the bacterium. This is more easily said than done and will necessitate some sophisticated detective work, involving the local veterinary investigation service along with your own veterinary surgeon. Advice will, of necessity, be specific to the particular farm involved, but the basic rules for prevention of scours still apply.

Fortunately, salmonellosis tends not to recur year after year in sheep flocks unless the disease is reintroduced to the farm from, for example, purchased market calves. Sheep need not be in direct contact to become infected. They need only graze pasture or be housed in an area contaminated with dung from infected calves.

Vaccination of flocks which have never been affected is not justified and even where flocks have experienced the disease, vaccination of ewes is of doubtful benefit, especially as the disease tends, in the main, not to be a persistent problem in sheep flocks. This, and other preventive measures, should be fully discussed with your veterinary surgeon following a thorough investigation of the immediate disease outbreak.

Virus Diarrhoea

Only in recent years has it been established that certain viruses are implicated in both lamb and calf scour outbreaks. Surveys of scour problems in calf units have shown that one particular virus—rotavirus—is the cause of a large proportion of outbreaks. It is known that rotavirus causes scouring in lambs, and although the extent of infection in UK flocks with this virus is unknown, it is likely to be significant.

Lambs are affected during their first week of life, the virus causing extensive damage to the lamb's small intestine, so that it cannot cope with its mother's milk. Food speeds through the gut to produce a profuse diarrhoea which may last for several days, severely dehydrating the lamb. Laboratory tests are necessary to confirm a diagnosis.

Unfortunately, there is no specific treatment available for rotavirus or any other viral scour. Treatment must therefore be based on alleviating symptoms, such as the dehydration and hypothermia. No vaccines are available at present against the viruses responsible for lamb scours and so prevention must rely on the general measures given at the end of this section.

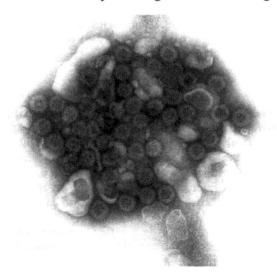

Plate 9.3 A group of rotavirus particles magnified 120,000 times under the electron microscope, from a sample of diarrhoeic faeces. Note the wheel-like appearance which gives the virus its name.

Cryptosporidiosis

Cryptosporidium is a protozoan parasite from the same group of organisms that includes the coccidia, which produce scouring in older lambs. Like the viruses, these organisms have only recently been implicated in lamb and calf diarrhoeas. They also produce disease in humans, especially in immunocompromised patients (e.g. with AIDS), those on steroid drugs and those undergoing cancer therapy. Care should therefore be taken with personal hygiene.

The infection in lambs does not usually become apparent until lambs are at least three or four days old. They become dull, stop suckling and develop diarrhoea. Lambs are often stiff and reluctant to move and some will die within a day or two. Others continue to scour for up to a week, becoming severely dehydrated. Those that survive take several weeks to recover due to the extensive and serious gut damage caused by this organism (see Plates 9.4 and 9.5). Again, laboratory tests are required to reach a diagnosis.

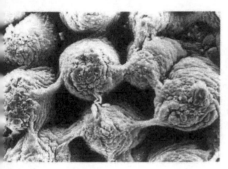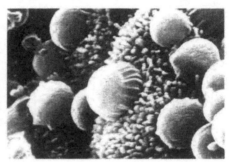

Plate 9.4 (*Above left*) Villi of the gut damaged by cryptosporidia (800 magnifications under the electron microscope). The villi are stunted and joined together by scar tissue formed during the healing process. (Compare with the normal gut in Plate 12.4.)

Plate 9.5 (*Above right*) Fruiting bodies of cryptosporidia on the gut surface (scanning electron microscope, 26,000 magnifications).

The infective stages, or oocysts, are passed in enormous numbers in the faeces of affected lambs and soon heavily contaminate the area, presenting an increasing danger to lambs as lambing proceeds. Also, the very short three to four day life cycle contributes to the very rapid build-up of infection. It is not known precisely how long the oocysts can survive in buildings or at pasture, but they are very tough and it is likely to be long enough to present a problem in the same area at the next year's lambing. Also, the organism is resistant to most disinfectants and it is therefore difficult to make infected areas safe again.

There is no specific treatment for this disease, and the drugs used against coccidiosis are not effective against cryptosporidium. Affected lambs have to be nursed back to health by treating the symptoms of the disease, such as the dehydration and hypothermia. Similarly there is no specific preventive measure such as a vaccine for use in subsequent seasons.

QUICK REFERENCE CHART

Common infectious diarrhoeas in newborn lambs

DISEASE	LAMB DYSENTERY	COLIBACILLOSIS	SALMONELLOSIS	VIRUS DIARRHOEA	CRYPTOSPORIDIOSIS
Infectious agent (type)	*Clostridium perfringens* (bacterium)	*Escherichia coli* (ETEC-K99) (bacterium)	*Salm. dublin* or *Salm. typhimurium* (bacterium)	Rotavirus, coronavirus, etc. (virus)	Cryptosporidium (protozoan)
Age of lamb affected	Up to three weeks	One to three days	Any time, but especially the first week of life	First week of life	Three days to two weeks
Clinical signs	Stomach pain – stops suckling – bloodstained diarrhoea – collapse – death. Also sudden death	Profuse diarrhoea – weakness – dehydration	Dull – stops suckling – severe diarrhoea – dehydration. Also septicaemia – death	Profuse diarrhoea – dehydration	Dull – stops suckling – diarrhoea – dehydration – reluctant to move
Treatment	None satisfactory – symptomatic only (lambs usually die)	Antibiotics or sulphonamides by mouth – if septicaemic, by injection also	Antibiotics or sulphonamides by mouth – if septicaemic, by injection also	No specific treatments are available. Lambs should be treated symptomatically (fluid replacement for diarrhoea, etc.) and nursed	No specific treatments are available. Lambs should be treated symptomatically (fluid replacement for diarrhoea, etc.) and nursed
Control in the face of an outbreak	Antitoxin and vaccine to all newborn lambs	See general measures in the main text	Possibly vaccination or medication of ewes yet to lamb	No specific measures are available. See 'Husbandry measures for reducing infectious disease in newborn lambs', p. 377	No specific measures are available. See 'Husbandry measures for reducing infectious disease in newborn lambs', p. 377
Prevention for future years (specific)	Combined clostridial vaccination of ewes with pre-lambing booster dose	*E. coli* vaccination of ewes may help	Specific treatment (e.g. vaccination) rarely necessary		

NOTES: Some agents such as salmonella and cryptosporidium are transmissible to man, so strict hygienic precautions are necessary. Lambs may become afflicted with more than one infection at the same time, with even more serious consequences.

Coccidiosis and nematodirus infections occur in slightly older lambs.

Lambs with pulpy kidney do not usually live long enough to develop diarrhoea.

362

ESTABLISHING THE CAUSE OF DIARRHOEA IN A FLOCK

It is almost inevitable that cases of diarrhoea will occur during the lambing period. The difficulty from the shepherd's point of view is that the symptoms in all cases of scour, nutritional or infectious, present a similar picture. Therefore, all scouring lambs should be treated as if they were infectious and isolated (with their dams) as soon as possible. Isolation means that the sick lamb should get more attention. If the scour is infectious, as most will be, then the lamb will not be contaminating the main lambing area with copious amounts of highly infectious faeces.

It is most important to obtain a diagnosis, that is, to identify the micro-organism responsible in the case of an infectious scour. This is necessary because it will help in deciding upon the treatment of both affected lambs and lambs in contact. It will also help in deciding upon appropriate preventive measures for the lambs yet to be born in the current lambing season, and for subsequent lambing seasons. For example, in the case of a diagnosis of lamb dysentery, little can be done for lambs already ill, but all newborn lambs can be protected in the short term with lamb dysentery antiserum and in the long term by vaccination. In future years ewes can be vaccinated pre-lambing to protect lambs via their colostrum. However, in the case of a diagnosis of rotavirus or cryptosporidium, there are no specific treatments or preventive measures available to date and so reliance must be placed on a high standard of husbandry and hygiene.

In order to obtain a diagnosis it is essential to let your veterinary surgeon have fresh material. This may mean a freshly dead lamb or, ideally, the

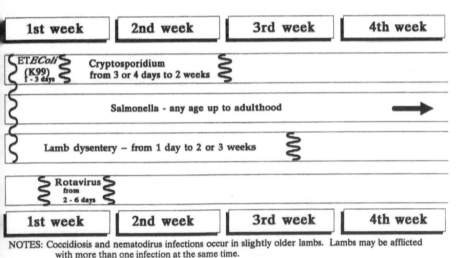

NOTES: Coccidiosis and nematodirus infections occur in slightly older lambs. Lambs may be afflicted with more than one infection at the same time.

Figure 9.1   The important diarrhoeas of newborn lambs and when they occur.

363

sacrifice of any very sick lambs for immediate post-mortem at the veterinary investigation laboratory. Samples of faeces—about an eggcupful in a clean jar—and/or swabs from the rectum of a number of lambs which are scouring will also help with the diagnosis of an outbreak.

It is always worth remembering that there may be more than one cause of infectious scour in a lambing flock at one and the same time. For example, rotavirus and cryptosporidium or rotavirus and *E. coli* may infect lambs simultaneously, usually with quite disastrous results. It is therefore sensible to submit as many freshly dead lambs as possible when outbreaks occur. A farm visit by your veterinary surgeon early in the course of an outbreak will be advantageous, to see how the lambing is organised, to advise on the collection of suitable samples and on the control of the present outbreak, and to suggest preventive measures for future years.

Watery Mouth

This is a very distressing and rapidly fatal disease which affects lambs only within the first two or three days of life. Recent research at the Moredun Institute suggests that the symptoms are caused by a toxin produced by the rapid multiplication of *E. coli* bacteria in the gut. Many of the *E. coli* strains isolated from cases of watery mouth had not previously been recognised as capable of producing disease.

Colostrum protects

The most important observation has been that lambs which receive an adequate supply of colostrum within the first few hours of life do not succumb to watery mouth. Therefore, the standard of management—especially in regard to ewe feeding and shepherding skills—is likely to play an important role in the occurrence of this disease in a flock.

Outbreaks of watery mouth appear to have been on the increase in recent years. From being a condition recognised only in flocks in the Scottish Borders, it is now diagnosed in most parts of the UK. It occurs most commonly in intensively managed lowland and upland flocks and is rare in true hill flocks. However, where hill ewes are brought down off the tops into enclosures or fields for lambing, the disease does occur. In the worst outbreaks every second or third lamb may be affected, the majority of cases dying despite treatment.

The *E. coli* bacteria capable of causing watery mouth are found literally everywhere in the newborn lamb's environment. Most are harmless residents of the gut of all animals and man—harmless, that is, except to the newborn lamb that has not sucked sufficient colostrum immediately after birth, to which they are apparently lethal. Even when lambing is conducted under the most strictly hygienic conditions and in an area where lambings have never taken place before, all lambs born will inevitably become contaminated with *E. coli*, since every thimbleful of faeces contains astronomical numbers of the bacteria.

Vulnerable lambs

All lambs that do not get sufficient colostrum very soon after birth are at risk. Young, inexperienced ewes may neglect their lambs or fuss around them but not let them suck. Ewes which have been inadequately fed through-out pregnancy may have little or no colostrum, or may produce small, weakly lambs which are slow to the teat. Such ewes often have a poor mothering instinct, which may further delay lambs getting a drink. Twins and triplets out of such ewes have to compete with each other and are therefore at greater risk. Sick ewes and older ewes may also produce inadequate supplies of colostrum.

Lambs which have a prolonged or difficult birth or which are injured during the process are likely to be slower to the teat or may be unable to suck properly when they do so. Lambs which are castrated and tailed within the first few hours of life may be in such discomfort that they lie about and fail to reach the teat until it is too late to protect them against watery mouth.

CLINICAL SIGNS

Affected lambs may show the first symptoms before they are even 24 hours old. They stop sucking and become very depressed, with drooping ears and hung heads. In some cases the abdomen becomes very swollen and tense, which is due to the formation of gas in the stomach from the fermentation of any colostrum which may have been ingested. The swelling presses on the diaphragm, which makes breathing difficult and may prevent the lamb from swallowing its saliva, which drools from the mouth in long strings and gives the disease its name. The gas in the stomach may make a rattling sound when the lamb is picked up and has led to the alternative name of rattlebelly.

Many affected lambs produce normal faeces, others scour, whilst the remainder may not have got rid of their first motions or meconium. It has been suggested that this failure to void the meconium is the cause of watery mouth, but this is not the case. The gut movements of normal lambs slow down during the first day of life. This is exaggerated in cases of watery mouth and may be the reason why the meconium is not voided in some cases.

Lambs may become dehydrated and hypothermic and eventually collapse into a coma and die within only a few hours of the onset of the first symptoms.

TREATMENT

Once lambs are showing abdominal discomfort or are drooling saliva, they are likely to die despite the best treatment and nursing. Early cases will

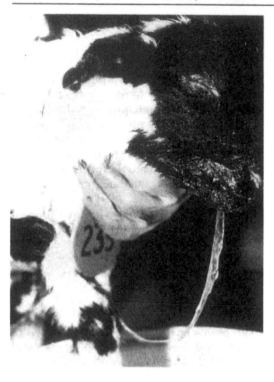

Plate 9.6 A lamb with 'watery mouth'. Note the thick drools of saliva which give this distressing disease its name. This lamb was humanely destroyed.

require antibiotic treatment, both by injection under the skin and by mouth. Since lambs soon stop sucking and may become dehydrated, they should be given fluid replacement in the form of electrolyte solution (not milk) by stomach tube. This solution should be fortified with glucose (10 g per 100 ml solution) to supply extra energy and an appropriate soluble antibiotic can also be incorporated. Such solutions (50 ml per kg bodyweight) should be given at least three or four times a day at well-spaced intervals. Hypothermic lambs will need to be put in a warming box following the guidelines given in the section on hypothermia in Chapter 8.

Constipated lambs or those which have not passed the meconium can be given a Beechams pill by mouth, liquid paraffin (4 or 5 ml) by stomach tube and/or a soapy water enema. The last consists of 10 to 20 ml of lukewarm water containing a few drops of liquid soap or Fairy Liquid, squirted through a sawn-off stomach tube into the lamb's rectum over 5 to 10 seconds. This should give relief within a quarter of an hour, but if not, it can be repeated.

Lambs suffering from watery mouth may be in considerable pain and discomfort, especially if the abdomen is swollen. They should therefore be handled with the greatest care and respect. Very sick lambs should be humanely destroyed, as they are unlikely to recover.

CONTROL AND PREVENTION

When an outbreak of watery mouth occurs in a flock, something has to be done immediately to prevent further cases occurring. If ewes are lambing down with inadequate supplies of colostrum, then all vulnerable lambs must be supplemented immediately they are born.

If supplies of ewe's or cow's colostrum are not available, the shepherd must resort to the use of antibiotics. All lambs should be dosed by mouth as soon as possible after birth with a suitable prescribed formulation. The easiest to administer are in paste form in a syringe, or suspensions in an oral doser. Tablets or capsules are equally effective but are less easy to administer. It is not necessary to inject antibiotics when the aim is to prevent the condition, and injections should always be avoided wherever possible. Indeed, mass medication with antibiotics carries the risk of producing strains of bacteria which may be resistant to one or a range of antibiotics and should be avoided except where there is no alternative. (Probiotics are widely advertised as an alternative, but to date there is no scientific evidence that these products provide any protection against watery mouth or, indeed, against any other disease.)

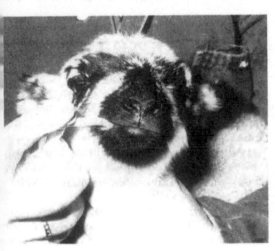

Plate 9.7   Dosing a lamb with an antibiotic liquid from a pump type applicator. Squirt the dose into the side of the mouth slowly and allow the lamb time to swallow.

Preventive measures are those which aim to ensure:

- that ewes give birth to strong, well-grown lambs
- that ewes secrete adequate supplies of good-quality colostrum
- that ewes mother their lambs attentively
- that all lambs get to the teat very quickly after birth and suck adequate amounts of colostrum

Appropriate feeding throughout pregnancy is essential, along with good organisation and skilled shepherding for as near 24 hours a day as possible during lambing in intensively managed flocks. With the tightening of margins in sheep enterprises, the tendency is to give shepherds responsibility for more and more ewes. This is unfortunate and could have serious welfare implications, particularly at lambing time. It is possibly one of the reasons why watery mouth appears to be reported more frequently.

In flocks where this disease has occurred at previous lambings, the level of shepherding should be upgraded, either by taking on extra skilled shepherds or by employing semi-skilled labour to relieve the shepherds of the more routine work, so allowing them to concentrate on the really important task of keeping lambs alive and well.

A vaccine is available, containing a number of *E. coli* frequently isolated from outbreaks of diarrhoea in lambs (see colibacillosis above), which some shepherds use as a preventative against watery mouth. However, it is likely that this disease can be caused by a large number of *E. coli* strains which are not normally associated with diarrhoea and are therefore unlikely to be included in the vaccine. It is doubtful whether this vaccine provides any more additional protection against watery mouth than colostrum from unvaccinated ewes does. The essential thing is to see that lambs get colostrum and, if the vaccine appears to work, it is probably because shepherds are ensuring that this happens.

NAVEL INFECTIONS IN YOUNG LAMBS

The freshly severed umbilical cord of the newborn lamb is wet and sticky with blood. As the lamb drops into the bedding of a lambing pen or onto the pasture, the cord is immediately coated with dirt, which contains microorganisms harmful to the lamb. Since blood is an ideal medium for the multiplication of many bacteria, infection of the navel is a common occurrence, especially when the naval cord is not treated with an antiseptic astringent (see below). At first the cord may look quite normal, but as infection proceeds the cord thickens and a painful abscess may develop close to the body. This condition is called navel-ill.

Bacteria may track along the navel cord, which acts like a wick (see Plate 9.8), and via the blood vessels inside the cord the bacteria may reach any part of the body, such as the liver, kidneys, lungs, spinal cord, brain, or the joints of the limbs. The symptoms which develop in the lamb will depend upon the organ affected. Limb joints frequently become infected and an inflammation of the joints—arthritis—develops, which produces a painful lameness known as joint-ill. If an abscess forms in the spinal column, the pressure on the spinal cord may produce paralysis.

Treating the navel cord

Any of these conditions is serious and may result in death, since treatment is often unsuccessful or only partially successful. Lambs which do recover invariably fail to thrive. Prevention is therefore the only practical way of

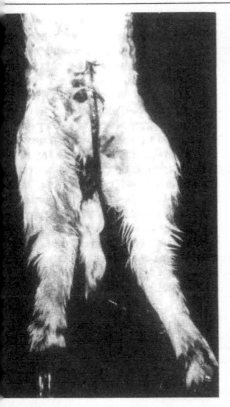

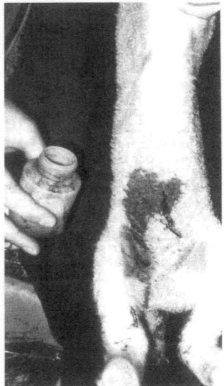

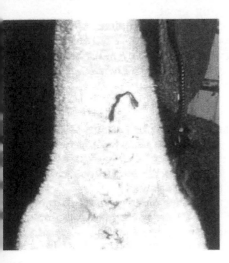

Plate 9.8   (*Above left*) The wet navel cord of a newborn lamb which acts as a wick, allowing infection to enter the body.

Plate 9.9   (*Above right*) Applying tincture of iodine to the navel to disinfect and dry it out.

Plates 9.10   (*Left*) Dry, shrivelled navel cord. There is little chance of infectious microorganisms tracking along this cord.

369

dealing with navel infections. The most important measure is navel dressing (see Plate 9.9). This should be the shepherd's first job, immediately the lamb is born, or at the very first opportunity. The aims are to dry and shrivel-up the cord and to disinfect it. By far the best solution for this task is tincture of iodine BP, which fulfils both of these aims. There are a number of products available which contain iodine, but only the tincture, which is a solution of iodine in alcohol, is suitable for navel-dressing.

The solution should be held in a suitable container, such as a dairy cow teat-dip cup. Although this method of application is more cumbersome than using an aerosol-type preparation or a garden sprayer, it is far more efficient, since it is important to thoroughly soak the cord and surrounding skin. This is rarely achieved with the sprays or aerosols. Moreover, these rarely have the drying (astringent) effect which is of paramount importance. By drying the cord, bacteria are deprived of the conditions they require for multiplication and are less likely to track along the cord into the body.

It is important that lambs are born into a dry, well-drained pen, amply bedded with clean straw. This will reduce the level of contamination from soil and faeces and also speed the drying of the cord. If, after some hours, the shepherd should notice that the navel is still wet, the iodine dressing should be repeated.

Shortening the cord

If the cord is very long or even trailing on the ground then it should be shortened. When the lamb is born naturally, the cord gently tears apart as the lamb struggles to get up or as the ewe moves round to lick the lamb. The gentle tearing action produces a ragged end which self-seals and prevents bleeding. Therefore, when shortening a navel cord, never cut straight through using a sharp knife. It is safer to very gently stretch the cord between the fingers until it breaks, taking great care not to pull the cord away from the body-wall which could produce a rupture. Alternatively, clean tape dipped in tincture of iodine can be used to tie off the cord about one inch from the body and the remainder removed by using a side to side action with a clean scalpel. Dress the navel cord with tincture of iodine immediately after it has been shortened.

Colostral protection

Lambs which suckle early and get a good supply of colostrum will be much better able to withstand the challenge from bacteria which invade via the navel. However, even colostral antibodies will not be able to protect a lamb which is subjected to an overwhelming challenge from filthy conditions in the lambing area, especially if the navel is untreated.

Under such circumstances, infections via the navel can reach epidemic proportions as lambing progresses. Once cases begin to occur, affected lambs further contaminate the lambing area, so presenting a greater and greater challenge to newborn lambs. For example, abscesses of the navel or in the joints may burst and contaminate the bedding. Once an outbreak occurs, the general measures necessary to reduce further cases occurring should be implemented immediately. Moving ewes as yet to lamb to a fresh lambing area is a most important first step in breaking the chain of infection.

The various bacteria which cause navel infection are present on all farms, in the soil, in faeces or on the skin of normal animals. It is not possible to eradicate them but it is possible to reduce the risk of infection both by good hygiene at lambing and by employing some specific measures which are discussed under separate headings below.

Fusobacterium Necrophorum Infection

One organism commonly associated with liver abscesses following infection via the navel is also one of the two organisms responsible for causing footrot in sheep, namely *Fusobacterium necrophorum*. The risk of infection with this organism can thus be substantially reduced by ensuring that all ewes are clear of footrot infection well before lambing. Ewes affected with footrot should not be allowed into the general lambing area, since the conditions under foot will inevitably lead to a rapid spread of the disease amongst other ewes and their lambs. *F. necrophorum* can survive for long periods away from infected feet, in soil or bedding, hence the importance of providing ample fresh straw and of treating lambs' navels promptly.

The bacteria destroy areas of the liver where they settle out and multiply. These can be seen at post-mortem as whitish areas, contrasting with the rich brown of normal liver (see Colour plate 26). A typical case would be a lamb of a week or 10 days of age, off colour, not sucking, tucked up and reluctant to move. Examination of the lamb might reveal a thickened navel cord and in some cases a swollen abdomen. Lambs usually find it painful to be handled and should be treated very gently. Most die within a few days or weeks despite treatment. Those that do survive fail to thrive or may eventually succumb to other fatal infections.

Erysipelas Arthritis

Erysipelothrix rhusiopathiae is the same organism which causes erysipelas in pigs, but the disease in lambs is not confined to farms where pigs are kept and can even be a problem on upland or hill farms where pigs have never ventured. The bacteria live in the soil and may contaminate the navels of newborn lambs, or the wounds made when castrating and tailing lambs of any age.

CLINICAL SIGNS

The bacteria grow and multiply in the navel cord or wound and then enter the bloodstream, from which they are carried to all parts of the body. They

371

tend to settle out and multiply in the limb joints particularly, where they produce a painful arthritis. Unlike some other forms of joint-ill, little or no swelling of the joints is seen, but manipulation of the joints is very painful and should therefore be avoided. A lamb may develop arthritis in several joints in any or all of its limbs. Sucking lambs may get left behind by their mothers, and some die from starvation or pneumonia. Those which survive become progressively more lame and the limbs may become deformed as the arthritis progresses.

TREATMENT AND CONTROL

By the time the shepherd realises that a number of lambs have this form of joint-ill it is likely that many more will be in the early stages of the disease. It is important to obtain a diagnosis so that appropriate action can be taken. Very early cases may respond to a full course of treatment with penicillin or some other suitable antibiotic. However, when lambs are badly crippled, treatment of any kind is usually hopeless and the worst cases should be humanely destroyed. (Joint infections are generally difficult to cure, due largely to the relatively poor blood supply carrying the drugs to the joints.)

Apparently unaffected lambs and all newborn lambs can be given erysipelas antiserum in the face of an outbreak. This should protect them for a few weeks and thus may reduce the number of new cases arising. Lambs already infected before treatment will not be protected by antiserum.

Moving ewes which are as yet to lamb to a clean lambing area and following the other guidelines for control of infections in the face of an outbreak will help reduce the number of new cases and help to prevent infection in subsequent years. Most important of these measures is the dressing of the navel. With older lambs which are to be castrated and tailed by the scalpel, scrupulous hygiene is essential. These jobs should be done on a dry day and, to avoid contamination of the wounds, the area where the task is to be carried out should be well bedded up with straw, especially where lambs are to be set-down after castration or tailing.

In flocks where a diagnosis of erysipelas has been made it is quite likely that it will recur in future lambing seasons. Therefore, you should consult your veterinary surgeon regarding vaccination of the ewe flock. Ewes will require primary and secondary doses initially, with a gap of two to six weeks between, and then a booster dose three weeks before lambing on an annual basis. This regime can be organised to coincide with the clostridial vaccination scheme. Lambs which suckle vaccinated ewes should be protected until they are around two months of age at which time they can be vaccinated themselves should this be considered necessary—for example, in flocks where late castration by the scalpel is practised.

Erysipelothrix rhisiopathiae may also cause lameness and death in sheep dipped in contaminated baths. This is discussed in detail in Chapter 13 under the heading of post dipping lameness.

Tetanus

Despite the widespread use of clostridial vaccine, tetanus still occurs on too many farms. This distressing and fatal disease may be due to inadequate clostridial vaccination programmes, or to lambs not getting enough colostrum for one reason or another.

The widespread use of rubber rings for the castration and tailing of lambs produces conditions which are ideal for the multiplication of the bacterium which causes tetanus—*Clostridium tetani*. This technique works by depriving the testicles and the tail of their blood supply so that they eventually drop off. The oxygen-starved tissues under the rubber ring are an ideal site for the tetanus bacterium, which can only multiply under such conditions. When the bacteria themselves die, they release an extremely potent toxin, which affects the nervous system, causing the classical symptoms of tetanus and eventually the death of the animal. Other wounds, especially deep, penetrating ones and badly damaged tissues, such as may occur in the ewe's vagina following a difficult lambing, may also allow the growth of tetanus organisms in inadequately vaccinated or unvaccinated animals.

Tetanus organisms form very tough, resistant spores which are found in dung and soil. Although some farms may never have experienced the disease, it is prudent to assume that all farms are likely to be contaminated. Obviously, areas where sheep or other species congregate and dung are usually more heavily contaminated than extensive grazings. Hill lambs may become affected, however, although poor soils at high altitudes are generally less heavily contaminated.

Tetanus bacteria may also be taken in by mouth on contaminated feed or soiled herbage. Although conditions in the gut are not suitable for its rapid multiplication, some toxin is produced in the rumen of adult animals. This low level of toxin is insufficient to produce disease, but it is thought to stimulate some immunity. It may be that unvaccinated adult sheep are less susceptible to tetanus than lambs because they have had time to build up a protective level of immunity.

Infection with tetanus following assisted lambings is another reason why strict hygienic precautions should be taken and why ewes should always be protected with a long-acting antibiotic despite being vaccinated. Penicillin is effective against the tetanus bacterium and this, or another suitable antibiotic, should always be used if sheep are wounded, for example at shearing.

CLINICAL SIGNS

Following infection of a wound, one or two weeks generally pass before any symptoms develop. At first, lambs walk somewhat stiffly and a few lambs may never progress beyond this stage and recover. However, most become progressively more stiff to the point of rigidity. The tail sticks out, the ears are erect, the face has an anxious appearance and the third eyelid closes partway across the eye. Lambs find it difficult to eat, since the muscles of the jaw are also in spasm (lockjaw). Lambs may also become bloated.

In the final stages of the disease the head is thrown back, the nostrils are flared and the limbs become so stiff that the lamb falls over in a permanently rigid posture (see Plate 9.11). Any sudden noise, movement or handling may provoke convulsions. Animals usually die because the muscles responsible for breathing go into spasm and they suffocate.

Death usually occurs within a few days of the appearance of first symptoms, but on occasion the disease may last for weeks. It is a most unpleasant condition and lambs showing the severe signs described above should be humanely destroyed, since the majority will die despite treatment.

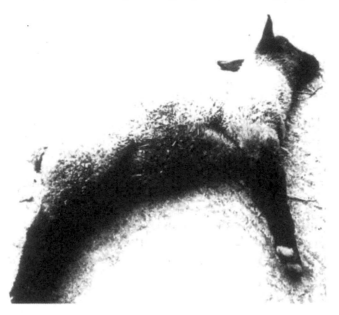

Plate 9.11 A lamb with tetanus. Note the rigidity of the limbs and how the neck is extended and ears pricked.

TREATMENT

A small proportion of very early cases may respond to veterinary treatment. Tranquillisers are sometimes used to reduce the frequency of convulsions and penicillin will kill the bacteria and so stop the production of further toxin. Tetanus antiserum, whilst a most useful product for preventing tetanus, is disappointing in the treatment of established cases. The wound, if apparent, will require local treatment and other symptoms such as hypothermia, or dehydration through not sucking, will have to be corrected. Animals which cannot suckle or eat will need to be force-fed by stomach tube with the greatest possible care because of the difficulty in swallowing and the risk of choking.

Treatment may have to be continued for many weeks. Disappointingly, some lambs will still die, either from tetanus or from some secondary condition, such as pneumonia, despite the best treatment and tender loving care.

PREVENTION

On some farms and under certain conditions of management, many lambs may become affected and in these circumstances it is important to identify the reason for the outbreak. It may be that the flock is unvaccinated against the clostridial diseases, or that the condition of ewes, or the management at lambing, is poor, so that lambs are not getting sufficient colostrum. It may be that hygiene at surgical castration or tailing is inadequate or that the technique for rubber ringing lambs is being carried out incorrectly (see Chapter 8). It is important that this operation is done hygienically. Even though no wound is made at the time the rings are applied, cracks in the skin do appear after they have been on for several days. If rings are applied to lambs when they are older than a week (which is illegal), then the fleshier tissues mean that there is a greater risk of tetanus. Once lambs have been ringed they should not be set down into filthy conditions in the lambing shed. If they are at pasture, they should not be ringed on cold, wet, muddy days.

Where cases of tetanus occur in a flock associated with this technique, consideration should be given to abandoning it and using another, more suitable method. Indeed, if lambs are being fattened quickly, it may be unnecessary to castrate or tail them at all.

Vaccination and the use of antiserum

The best prevention for tetanus is by clostridial vaccination of the ewe flock, with the pre-lambing booster dose being most important, so that lambs obtain a high level of protective antibodies via colostrum. Where cases have occurred in a flock it is possible to give short-term protection for two or three weeks by injecting at-risk lambs (or adults) with antiserum—for example, as soon as lambs are ringed. This may have to be repeated to extend the period of cover as necessary. Antiserum is expensive and inconvenient, but may sometimes be worthwhile, especially with particularly valuable animals.

Tetanus does not affect all species equally. Sheep are moderately susceptible, whilst horses and humans are very susceptible. It is most important that everyone—and particularly those who work on the land—is vaccinated against tetanus and has regular boosters as recommended by the doctor. Also, any serious wound, especially a deep penetrating one, should be attended to by a doctor immediately. There is no particular risk from handling and nursing animals affected with tetanus.

Any animals which die, from whatever cause, should be buried, burned

375

or otherwise responsibly disposed of immediately. Tetanus cases left to rot in the fields will mean that the bacteria in the carcass will form resistant spores, which will be washed into the soil and so become a danger for very many years to come. Mammals and birds which eat the rotting carcass may also distribute the bacteria far and wide in their faeces.

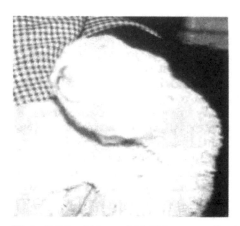
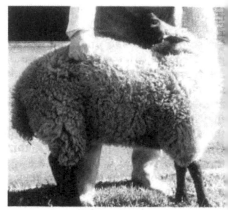

Plate 9.12 (*Above left*) This young lamb has encephalitis—an inflammation of the brain due to a bacterial infection which probably gained entry via the navel cord or some wound.

Plates 9.13 and 9.14 (*Above right and below*) This older lamb has a brain abscess (diagnosed at post-mortem) and is unable to stand unsupported. Note how the head is thrown back to rest on the withers. The infection that caused the abscess may have gained entry to the body just as described in Plate 9.12.

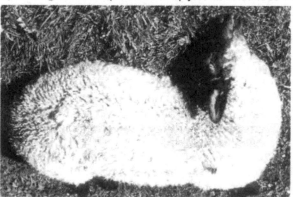

HUSBANDRY MEASURES AIMED AT REDUCING INFECTIOUS DISEASE IN NEWBORN LAMBS

It will have been noted from the previous pages that it is possible to control or prevent some infectious diseases of young lambs by measures specifically aimed at a particular infectious agent. For example, clostridial vaccination of ewes will protect sucking lambs against lamb dysentery and tetanus. However, it is not possible to protect in this specific way against all infections: there is no vaccine or medicine which is effective against diarrhoea due to cryptosporidium, for instance. The following are reminders of both specific and general measures aimed particularly at controlling the level of infectious disease in newborn lambs. See also 'A husbandry and health programme for a spring lambing flock' in Appendix 1.

PRE-LAMBING PREPARATION

● Split the flock into early and late lambing groups and prepare separate lambing quarters for each. (In large flocks, three or more groups may be appropriate.) This has the effect of breaking the chain of infection should it occur. If possible, choose a fresh lambing area each year.
● Crutch ewes so that lambs can find the udder easily.
● Provide some form of shelter for outdoor lambing flocks. In lowland conditions this may be elaborate or simply a construction made from straw bales. On the hill, ewes may be confined in large enclosures in more sheltered areas.
● Where ewes are closely confined, either indoors or outdoors, provide an adequate number of individual lambing pens. This will depend on the size of the flock and the duration of the lambing period, but one pen per six or eight ewes should suffice. (More will be needed in synchronised flocks.)
● It is essential to provide a hospital isolation area with intensive care facilities for sick ewes and lambs away from the main lambing area.
● Ewes which are to be housed or closely confined outdoors should be treated for footrot immediately before confinement. This will help prevent the rapid spread of the disease amongst ewes and will reduce the risk of navel infections in lambs caused by one of the bacteria which produces footrot.
● Group and individual pens should be well drained and liberally bedded with straw as this simple measure will greatly reduce the level of contamination. Individual pens should be mucked out between every two or three lambing ewes at least. Temporary lambing pens made of straw bales should be burned at the end of lambing or earlier if they become heavily contaminated.
● Prepare all lambing equipment and collect appropriate drugs from your veterinary surgeon at least two weeks before the first lambs are due.

- A colostrum bank, of ewe or cow origin, is essential and shepherds should be trained in the use of the stomach tube and other life saving techniques

AT LAMBING

- It is important to have an adequate standard and level of shepherding. In teased or sponged flocks with a compact lambing, it will be necessary to give 24 hour cover.
- Before assisting a ewe at lambing, the shepherd's hands must be thoroughly clean and all equipment adequately sterilised.
- Keep interference at lambing to a minimum. Be very gentle and use copious amounts of a suitable lubricant.
- After assisting a ewe at lambing, always use antibiotics preferably by injection.
- As a general rule when lambing ewes, if at first you don't succeed—give up, and seek professional veterinary help early. Ewes injured or infected at lambing are less likely to look after their lambs properly and less likely to milk well. Lambs injured or compromised after a long, difficult lambing are more likely to succumb to hypothermia and/or infection.
- Check udders of all ewes immediately after they lamb or as soon as possible, to see that there is ample colostrum. Be gentle and hygienic (clean hands) when doing this; otherwise mastitis may follow.
- **Make sure all lambs get a sufficient supply of colostrum within the first few hours of life.** This is the single most important shepherding job of all. Any vulnerable lambs should be given colostrum by stomach tube at the earliest opportunity.
- Apply tincture of iodine BP to navels of lambs as soon as possible after birth. This will disinfect, dry and shrivel up the cord and help prevent infection via the navel. (Many commonly used aerosol type products are unsatisfactory for this job.)
- If lambs have to be injected for any reason, do so with great care and use the subcutaneous method (under the skin) if possible, rather than intramuscular (into the muscle). Disposable needles and syringes are preferable. The shepherd's hands must be washed and the injection site must be clean and dry.
- Avoid castrating and tailing lambs with rubber rings during the first day of life if possible. Castration is particularly uncomfortable and may discourage lambs from sucking vital colostrum and so predispose them to infection. **Never** apply rubber rings to injured or sick lambs or apply them in bad weather.

WHEN INFECTION OCCURS IN A FLOCK

- Isolate all sick ewes and lambs in a distinctly separate hospital area. Very sick animals should be humanely destroyed and not allowed to suffer unnecessarily.

- Shepherds should not move from an infected area to a clean area without adequate disinfection and a change of boots and overalls. Hands should be thoroughly washed.
- Carcasses of dead ewes or lambs should be buried or responsibly disposed of immediately (it is a legal requirement). If left lying around, they are a reservoir of infection.
- On no account should the skins of lambs which have died from an infectious disease be used as 'coats' in an attempt to foster-on orphan lambs.
- If ewes whose lambs have died from any infectious scour are to be used as foster mothers, it is essential that the orphan lambs are protected with colostrum (by stomach tube) from a vaccinated ewe or cow.
- Ewes which have aborted should not be used as foster mothers for ewe lambs intended as breeding replacements.
- In the face of an outbreak of infectious disease such as diarrhoea, move the ewes which have yet to lamb to a fresh area. If lambing indoors, move outdoors if weather conditions permit, as this will help to break the chain of infection.
- Consult a veterinary surgeon early in an outbreak of disease to establish a diagnosis so that appropriate control and prevention methods can be implemented.
- Hypothermia and dehydration are common life-threatening conditions associated with many infectious diseases of newborn lambs and especially in outbreaks of diarrhoea. Always check the temperature of suspect lambs and follow the guidelines in Chapter 8.
- Hospital pens should be thoroughly cleaned and disinfected between cases and liberally bedded with straw.

Remember that many infectious diseases, especially some abortions in ewes and scours in lambs, are transmissible to humans. Wash hands thoroughly and **never apply the kiss of life to any lamb under any circumstances.**

Entropion

Entropion is an inherited condition seen in young lambs, in which the lower eyelid of one or both eyes turns inwards. This causes the eyelashes to brush against the eyeball, causing damage to the cornea, the thin transparent layer covering the surface of the eye. This constant irritation produces a keratitis (an inflammation of the cornea) which may result in blindness if left untreated.

Normally, the tautness of the skin just below the eye prevents the eyelids and lashes from rolling inwards onto the eyeball. In entropion cases, there is a variable degree of 'looseness' of this facial skin. In mildly affected lambs the eyelids may turn in and then out of the eye, giving short periods of relief. In the worst cases the eyelids are constantly inturned, the damage is severe and the pain unrelenting.

CLINICAL SIGNS

Affected lambs have watery eyes, with tears running down the face. A
the condition progresses lambs may partially close their eyes and the wa'
they hold their heads indicates that the eye is painful and vision impaired
If shepherds have not encountered the condition before, they may not notic
the inturned eyelids and therefore assume that the reddened and weepin;
eyes are the result of an infection (which is partly true), treat them with a
eye ointment and wonder why they continue to get worse. In cases whicl
go unnoticed or are incorrectly treated, the cornea becomes progressivel
more 'cloudy' and in the worst cases corneal ulcers—red, raw areas—ma
develop. Blindness in one or both eyes is not uncommon.

The author recently came across a case of inexcusable ignorance o
neglect in a lamb of about two months of age that bumped into him whils
walking across an upland farm. It was totally blind in both eyes due to

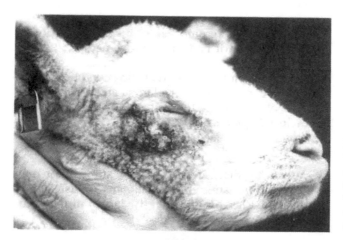

Plate 9.15   A lamb
with its eye almost
closed and with tears
causing encrusting of
the wool below the
eye due to a painful
eye infection.

Plate 9.16   Applying
eye ointment. Hold
down the bottom lid
and squeeze a small
amount (e.g. 1 cm)
inside the lid, taking
care not to touch the
surface of the eyeball
with the tube. Hold
the eyelids shut for a
few seconds to allow
the ointment to melt
and spread over the
surface of the eye.

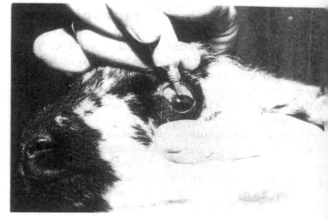

evere ulceration of the corneas. The lamb had obviously been able to find
s mother to suck, but must have suffered very considerable pain quite
nnecessarily, since the condition is simply treated.

TREATMENT

Treatment is aimed at turning the eyelids and lashes out of the eye and
keeping them out. In the very mildest cases this may mean simply 'rolling'
them outwards, by using the thumb to drag down the skin just below the
eye. Some eye ointment should be applied twice daily for several days,
if only to ensure that the eye is looked at frequently. If the eyelid turns
inwards again, then one of the treatments described below must be used.

In more severe cases, minor plastic surgery is required to take up some
of the slack in the facial skin just below the eye. Your veterinary surgeon
will either snip out a piece of skin and stitch up the wound, or else apply
a surgical (Michel) clip to draw the skin together. Ewes with their affected
lambs should be kept close to the farmstead and eye ointment applied twice
daily until the clip is removed after about a week. In severe cases the
corneal damage will take much longer to heal, but further eye ointment
applications are unlikely to be necessary. Some lambs may be left with
imperfect, although adequate, vision.

Occasionally, 'outbreaks' of entropion occur in a flock. Although this is
not an infectious disease, a new ram may be responsible for the condition
in a proportion of his offspring. Apart from the distress entropion causes to
lambs, a high proportion of cases means unwelcome extra work for a busy
shepherd at lambing time. If this should occur, your veterinary surgeon
may supply you with Michel clips and an applicator and demonstrate how
to correct the defect. It is important to take neither too little nor too big a
'bite' of loose skin.

When cases occur in a flock there are likely to be more. Lambs should
be checked at birth, since prompt treatment will prevent unnecessary
suffering. Affected lambs, whether male or female, must be marked and
should not be retained for breeding. If it is possible to identify a particular
ram as the sire of affected lambs, he should be culled.

Daft Lamb Disease

This is a distressing, although fairly uncommon, nervous condition affecting lambs of certain breeds—notably the Border Leicester, Scottish Blackface, Scottish Halfbred, Greyface and Welsh Mountain in the UK. In Canada,
Australia and New Zealand, lambs of the Corriedale breed may be affected.
The cause of the disease is unknown, but there would appear to be some
genetically inherited susceptibility.

Lambs may be born afflicted or develop symptoms within the first few
days of life. Because cases can be confused with other nervous disorders

381

affecting newborn lambs, such as swayback, it is important to distinguish daft lamb disease through post-mortem examination of the brain (which will be improperly developed) so that appropriate control methods can be put into effect in the flock.

CLINICAL SIGNS

In the worst affected lambs the head is bent backwards to such a degree that the poll may be touching the withers. In less severe cases the head points upwards in a stargazing posture. The head also tends to bob from side to side continuously and this makes it very difficult for lambs to walk, or even to maintain their balance when standing still. They therefore often stand with their feet spread well apart or they may kneel down to prevent themselves from falling. The most severe cases may never be able to get to their feet in the first place and even if they are helped up they topple over.

Obviously such a severe disability means that many affected lambs have difficulty in following their mothers. Even though they may be keen, they often cannot find the udder or are unable to suck if they do so. Therefore most of these cases quickly perish through hypothermia and starvation unless the shepherd finds them first and feeds them by stomach tube. It is probably kinder to submit severely affected lambs for post-mortem in order to obtain a diagnosis and to avoid unnecessary suffering, since many of these lambs damage themselves—and their eyes in particular—from banging their heads on the ground or on other solid objects. If the less severe cases are assisted initially, they may learn to suck from the ewe. However they never do well and can always be picked out by their poor condition and unsteady walk, especially when they are stressed, as at gatherings.

Daft lamb disease is untreatable and the cause unknown; thus no specific advice on prevention can be given. Where the condition suddenly appears in a closed flock it is likely to be due to the introduction of a particular ram. If it is possible to identify the culprit he should be culled, as should any ewes which give birth to daft lambs. Rams should not be purchased from flocks where the disease is known to occur. Mildly affected daft lambs, or suspects, should be fattened for slaughter and not kept for breeding.

DISEASES ASSOCIATED WITH THE SHEEP TICK

The sheep tick (*Ixodes ricinus*) is the only tick of economic significance in the UK. The biology and control of this important parasite is discussed in detail in Chapter 13 and should be read in conjunction with this section. Here, we will discuss the three important diseases of sheep which are associated with the bite of the sheep tick: louping ill, tickborne fever and tick pyaemia.

Ticks feed on sheep's blood for only about a week in each of the three

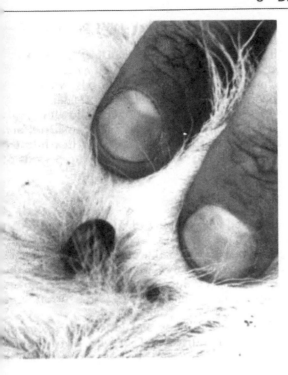

Plate 9.17   A partially engorged tick (*Ixodes ricinus*) continues to suck blood from its host sheep. Tickborne fever, tick pyaemia and louping ill are all transmitted by the tick in the UK.

years of their life cycle. Most ticks feed in the spring and so the diseases they transmit may affect young lambs, hence their inclusion here. In some western areas of Britain there are also some ticks which feed in the autumn.

Sheep can become infected with these diseases only if they graze over tick-infested ground and this means principally the upland and hill areas of Britain where the ground cover is suitable. Not all ticks are infected with the virus which causes louping ill and so this disease does not occur in all tick-infested areas. On the other hand, it is thought that all, or at least the vast majority of, ticks carry the organism responsible for tickborne fever and so all sheep bitten by ticks will become infected. The bacterium responsible for tick pyaemia (*Staphylococcus aureus*) is very widespread and probably contaminates the skin of all animals.

Louping Ill

Louping ill is a virus disease transmitted by the bite of the sheep tick, *Ixodes ricinus*. It affects most domestic animals including sheep, cattle, pigs, horses and dogs, but it is in sheep that it causes most problems for farmers. Whilst it is infectious, louping ill cannot spread directly from sheep to sheep. For sheep to become infected they must be bitten by a sheep tick which is itself infected with the virus.

It should always be born in mind, however, that the disease can occur temporarily in areas assumed to be tick-free—or tick-infested but free from louping ill—due to the movement of sheep at periods when ticks are still feeding on them. When satisfied, the ticks drop off and if there is appropriate ground cover they may survive until the following year, when the adult ticks can feed on highly susceptible, unacclimatised and unvaccinated sheep, often with serious results. Sheep from tick-infested areas should never, therefore, be moved to 'clean' areas during periods of tick activity.

Susceptible animals

Sheep of any age can become infected with louping ill. However, those that have been previously infected and have survived become immune for life, and sheep which have been effectively vaccinated are also solidly immune. Lambs that suckle colostrum from immune ewes are also protected for the first two or three months of life. The most vulnerable sheep are those moved from a disease-free area to a louping ill area and also sheep in a 'clean' area into which tick-carrying sheep are moved (see above).

Rams purchased from non-tick-infested areas and moved to a louping ill farm are very likely to succumb to the disease. They may die or be left partially paralysed and so preventive measures must be taken if the breeding programme is not to be seriously disrupted.

The pattern of disease in flocks grazing over louping ill country will depend on a number of factors, and the management of such flocks to minimise losses is complex. The tick has a three year life cycle as larvae, nymph and adult (see Chapter 13). Infection with louping ill cannot pass from the adult female tick to her eggs and so infection dies with the adult tick. Larval ticks may become infected at their first feed if they bite an infected sheep, but they will not be able to infect a sheep until the following year, when they feed as nymphs, or a year later as adults.

Reservoirs of the virus

Whilst other species of warm-blooded animals—both wild and domestic—may be bitten by ticks, they are, with a few exceptions, less susceptible to louping ill than sheep, and the quantity of virus in their blood is thought to be too low to infect ticks when they bite. They are, therefore, unlikely to play an important role in the continuation of infection on a farm. Red grouse were at one time regarded as being important in the persistence of louping ill on infected farms. However, recent research has shown that the infection is very severe in grouse and that most infected birds die from it. They are, therefore, not thought to provide a reservoir of the virus.

From this and other evidence, it would seem that the sheep is essential for the maintenance of the infection on a farm. In the absence of sheep, other species of mammal may be important in maintaining the tick population by providing nourishment in the form of a blood meal. If sheep are totally removed from an area for more than two years, louping ill will probably disappear, although ticks may remain abundant. However, ticks too will tend to die out if alternative large mammalian hosts are not available to provide a blood meal for their adult stage.

Sheep can infect ticks only when they have high levels of virus in their blood, that is, when the virus is multiplying in the blood stream (viraemia). This occurs only for a day or two following initial infection. If a sheep survives the infection, it becomes solidly immune for life and the virus totally disappears from the body. Such animals cannot therefore infect ticks.

Lambs which are protected by antibodies from the colostrum of immune ewes are likely to be immune from infection for sufficiently long to protect them over the period of spring tick activity, although they may be susceptible at an autumn tick rise. Certainly by the following spring their colostrum derived immunity will have waned and they will be completely susceptible to infection. It is this age group of sheep (hoggs) that provides the main source of louping ill virus for ticks. If a louping ill-infected tick bites a susceptible hogg it will infect the sheep, the virus will multiply in the sheep's blood and all ticks subsequently feeding on that sheep during the period of viraemia will become infected and so perpetuate the infection on the farm.

Replacement hoggs account for approximately 20 per cent of the flock. Since the viraemia in sheep lasts for just a short time, only a very small proportion of ticks will be exposed to infection. It is, therefore, not surprising that less than one in a thousand ticks carries the louping ill virus. However, this is sufficient to perpetuate the disease in a flock, since many thousands of ticks may feed off a ewe during her lifetime on the hill.

Most of the areas where ticks occur are rough grazings where flocks are generally self contained and female replacements are rarely, if ever, purchased. Only rams are bought in as required and therefore there is only a small risk of introducing louping ill under these conditions.

CLINICAL SIGNS

Clinical signs of disease are only likely to occur at times of tick activity, that is principally in the spring but also in the autumn on some farms. Following a bite by an infected tick the virus is injected directly into the bloodstream of the sheep, where it then multiplies. Sheep experience a fever within a few days of the tick bite but this usually goes unnoticed, even in young lambs.

The virus then invades the central nervous system, where it multiplies, and in animals which are unable to fight off the infection it causes severe nervous symptoms (meningo-encephalomyelitis) and frequently death. Animals become dull and reluctant to move and may rest their noses on the ground. Trembling is a common symptom and some sheep walk with a strange high stepping movement. They may stagger sideways or circle and fall and may be unable to rise.

Occasionally some sheep develop an unusual hopping movement due to a progressive paralysis which is referred to as 'louping' (Scots for leaping), from which the disease gets its name. Convulsions follow, with animals lying on their side, paddling and slobbering at the mouth. Sheep eventually lapse into a coma and die. The whole course of the disease takes only a few days from the onset of symptoms, or even just a few hours in the most acute cases.

Sucking lambs which become affected may wander off from their dams and die of starvation. Some sheep become partially paralysed and survive for a few weeks before succumbing. Those in which the damage to the nervous system is limited may survive and develop a lifelong immunity.

All ticks are infected with the tickborne fever organism, and in sheep which become infected with this disease and with louping ill at the same time, the symptoms of louping ill are very much more severe and this inevitably leads to a rapid death.

Diagnosis of louping ill on farms where the disease is known to be present is not too difficult, but may come as a surprise if the disease has not been encountered for some years. It can also be more difficult on farms previously assumed to be free of the disease. Post-mortem examination will be helpful in confirming the diagnosis. It will then be a matter of discussing with your veterinary surgeon the reason for the outbreak and devising a suitable control strategy.

Treatment of louping ill is disappointing. The milder cases may be saved if brought indoors and nursed. Severe cases should be humanely destroyed, as predators will attack them when they are in the final stages of the disease. Because of the risk of human infection through consumption of actively infected animals, these cases should go to the knacker, not to the slaughter house.

CONTROL AND PREVENTION

Control is based on attempting to achieve a high level of immunity in all classes of sheep, since eradication of the disease by eradicating the tick is usually impractical. If ewes have a good immunity and lambs suckle sufficient colostrum, they will be protected over the danger period of tick rise in the spring of their birth. Replacement ewe hoggs, some of which will have been away-wintered, will, in the majority of circumstances, be highly susceptible at the tick rise which occurs around the time of their first birthday. They should, therefore, be vaccinated at least a month to six weeks before they are likely to be bitten. This should be carried out early in the year. Only where losses can be anticipated in the autumn should vaccination be employed in the late summer. Lambs should not be vaccinated at too young an age, since the protective antibody they acquire from colostrum may interfere with the 'take' of the vaccine.

Vaccination

The Moredun-type (inactivated) louping ill vaccine (Coopers Pitman-Moore) should protect sheep for a period of two to three years following a single injection. In flocks where the disease is known to occur, replacement ewe hoggs should be vaccinated and this will protect them and their lambs (via colostrum) up to and including their second or third lambing. The decision then has to be taken on whether to re-vaccinate these two and three crop ewes before their next lambing and advice should be taken from your veterinary surgeon. Bought-in rams should always be vaccinated when moving to a louping ill farm and should not graze tick-infected pastures until at least one month following vaccination. Follow the vaccine instructions carefully.

If sheep carrying louping ill-infected ticks are moved to previously louping ill-free grazings and mixed with unacclimatised sheep, in the following season there are likely to be losses in the unprotected sheep. Losses will not be substantial in the first year, but there will probably be an insidious increase in the proportion of ticks carrying the virus over the next year or two. This may be followed by an explosive outbreak affecting all age categories of sheep, a situation that should be avoided. If there is no alternative, then all sheep—those already on the farm and purchased animals—should be vaccinated prior to the next tick rise.

All sheep purchased from non-tick or non-louping ill farms should be vaccinated a month before the tick rise if they are moving on to an infected farm. In the case of sheep which have never experienced the tick this is particularly important, because the combination of tickborne fever plus louping ill is likely to produce catastrophic losses.

Theoretically, by vaccinating all animals for two or three successive years the infection should be eliminated from the flock, since the infection dies with the adult tick. However, this would only apply providing there is no other source of infection for the tick population, and unfortunately this is not usually the case.

Attempts have been made to eradicate the tick or to substantially reduce its numbers on heavily tick-infested farms, since apart from louping ill, substantial losses also occur in lambs from tick pyaemia and occasionally in ewes from abortion due to tickborne fever. However, even if this is achieved—for example, on a section of improved ground—great care must be taken to see that the flock is managed in such a way as to avoid contact between ticks and unvaccinated, susceptible sheep. The management of flocks on louping ill-infected grazings is a minefield for the inexperienced and full of surprises even for the experienced!

THE RISK OF HUMAN INFECTION As mentioned earlier, the infection can occur in species other than the sheep and this includes cattle, horses, goats, dogs and humans. The louping ill vaccine is also licensed for use in cattle and goats. It is noteworthy that the virus is found in high levels in the milk of goats at the time the virus is multiplying in the blood. Kids sucking infected milk become very ill and it is therefore highly likely that humans drinking infected goat's milk would become infected with this most dangerous and frequently fatal disease. Where goat's milk is to be drunk on louping ill infected farms, goats should always be vaccinated on an annual basis.

It has been demonstrated that the virus is similarly concentrated in the milk of ewes, which explains why some cases occur in lambs of a few days of age. Ewe's milk is usually made into cheese or other products and these processes are likely to reduce the risk of infection. However, there is still some risk to humans milking infected ewes or churning their milk because of the aerosol effect created which allows the virus to be inhaled. Milking ewes should therefore be vaccinated annually on louping ill farms. Pasteurisation of milk will not destroy the virus.

Human beings can also become infected from the bite of infected ticks, although this is probably rare in the UK. Veterinary surgeons and slaughterers are at some risk from blood or other tissues when handling infected carcasses from animals at the height of the fever. Laboratory workers and others employed in the manufacture of the vaccine have occasionally become ill, and this has halted vaccine production a number of times.

DOG INFECTION Sheepdogs may become infected by the bite of the tick and although the louping ill vaccine is not licensed for dogs, your veterinary surgeon may advise it in some circumstances, such as for very valuable dogs. The vaccine is likely to produce quite a large sterile abscess at the site of the injection. Two injections will be required for dogs, three to four weeks apart, to give adequate protection. (Sheep require only a single vaccination.)

Tickborne Fever

Tickborne fever (TBF) is an infectious disease which affects almost all sheep which graze tick-infected pastures. It is caused by a microorganism called *Cytoecetes phagocytophilia*, a rickettsia which is transmitted via the bite of the sheep tick.

As they are born in the spring and usually during a period of peak tick activity, lambs on tick-infested ground are usually bitten soon after birth. They inevitably become infected with the agent of tickborne fever since there are no protective antibodies in colostrum against this disease, even though ewes may themselves be immune. Affected lambs often go unnoticed because the symptoms of infection are often vague, despite animals running a high fever which persists for about a week.

TBF in lambs

It is usually assumed that illness and deaths in lambs due directly to this organism are uncommon. However, it is conceivable that young lambs with a high fever, feeling unwell and lagging behind their mothers in the frequently severe weather conditions met with on the hill during lambing time, may well fall foul of starvation hypothermia, pneumonia or predators and perish. Nevertheless, most lambs undoubtedly survive the initial infection.

The infectious agent remains in the white blood cells for periods of up to two years or more, however. This is called the carrier state, and carrier animals cannot become re-infected with the particular TBF agent present on that farm. They are immune whilst the parasite is present in their blood (there are a number of different TBF agents in the sheep population). Such animals also act as a source of infection for any ticks which bite them, so it can be seen why the vast majority of ticks and sheep become affected. If the carrier state wanes, due to lack of natural challenge by ticks, then it is possible for animals to become re-infected, but the symptoms and consequences are usually very mild and are likely to go unnoticed.

TBF in ewes

The fever which occurs after initial infection may lead to abortion in pregnant ewes from a non-tick area which are moved to a tick-infested farm. This is likely to be a rare event on most hill farms, but such movements should be avoided. Ewes will not abort if they are infected before becoming pregnant, since it is the fever which causes the abortion rather than direct damage by the rickettsial organism itself. Some ewes that abort become very sick and a substantial proportion die (see Chapter 5).

TBF in rams

It has been reported that a period of infertility may occur in rams, lasting for up to two or three months, due to the fever caused by tick-borne fever. Certainly it is feasible that a rise in body temperature, especially for a prolonged period, may interfere with sperm production and perhaps also libido. Rams from tick-free grazings moved in late summer or autumn to tick-infected ground in western areas where there is an autumn rise of tick activity are very likely to be compromised. They may even die if louping ill is also present in the tick population.

CONTROLLED INFECTION

The most important feature of infection with tickborne fever is the effect the rickettsia have on the immune system of the sheep. The organisms invade certain of the white blood cells which play an important role in combating infection. By doing so they compromise the sheep's natural defence mechanisms and so make the animal more likely to fall victim to other infections, particularly tick pyaemia, louping ill and pneumonia. So, tickborne fever can be indirectly the cause of very considerable loss of life and production, especially in hill and upland areas.

No vaccine is available against tickborne fever. Control of this disease depends on making sure that sheep are infected (via the bite of the tick) at a time when the fever and the effects on the blood are least likely to put the sheep at risk. Hill sheep are generally hefted, that is, they are born, reared and bred on the same area of the hill. If the hill is tick-infested, then they will be bitten and challenged with tickborne fever at every period of tick activity and so will come to no harm from TBF, since constant re-infection will protect them. As stated earlier, care should be exercised in introducing unacclimatised sheep to tick grazings and in particular rams or pregnant ewes.

Where hill and upland ground has been improved the sward is often altered dramatically so that it may no longer support ticks because of lack of suitable cover. These grazings are often used to lamb-down a proportion of the flock, usually gimmers. In consequence, this may protect their lambs from tickborne fever during the first few weeks of life, which is also the greatest risk period for tick pyaemia. Lambs—particularly those which are to be retained for breeding—should then be returned to the tick-infested hill with their mothers so that both can be challenged with TBF before the end of the tick rise. Ewe lambs which remain on improved tick-free areas or are away-wintered may become quite ill when they are eventually returned to the tick-infested hill, since they are totally susceptible. This age group of sheep is usually more seriously affected by tickborne fever than are young lambs.

Other methods of protecting young lambs from tickborne fever are discussed under the heading of tick pyaemia, since it is the role of the former in predisposing lambs to the latter which is of such great importance.

TREATMENT

It is possible to treat affected animals with antibiotics such as the tetracyclines, although only infrequently do animals become ill enough to warrant treatment. Tetracyclines can also be used to prevent the infection over short risk periods by using the long-acting preparations. It should be pointed out, however, that treatment will render the sheep virtually free of the rickettsia so that it will then become susceptible to subsequent challenge.

Tick Pyaemia

Tick pyaemia or 'cripples' is a serious condition of young lambs on tick grazings, and it is said to kill or disable in excess of a quarter of a million lambs each year in the UK. It is certainly one of the most important causes of loss of lambs, and therefore of profitability, on hill and upland farms. From the lamb's point of view, it can be a most painful and debilitating condition due to the formation of abscesses in almost any part of the body and poses a considerable welfare problem for the farmer. The bacterium which causes tick pyaemia, *Staphylococcus aureus*, is found on all farms and is frequently the cause of abscesses and skin infections in many species.

Early workers at the Moredun Research Institute in Edinburgh observed that cases of tick pyaemia coincided with the spring period of tick activity on affected farms. They carried out work to show that lambs affected with tickborne fever, whose body defences against infection were therefore severely compromised, were much more easily infected with tick pyaemia.

It is thought that lambs bitten by ticks soon after birth become infected with tickborne fever and develop a high temperature. The damage caused to the protective white cells in their blood is detectable only in lambs of two weeks of age or older. The staphylococci responsible for tick pyaemia, meanwhile, may have entered the body via any of the normal routes in newborn lambs, such as the navel cord, through wounds caused by castration or tailing with the rubber ring, or through any cut or abrasion to the skin or lining of the nose or mouth. It is also possible for the bacteria to gain entry via the bite of the tick itself, since, although staphylococci do not survive for long inside ticks, they are commonly found on the skin of lambs and may simply be pushed through the skin on the mouthparts of the tick.

Whichever way the staphylococci gain entry makes little difference since they may be carried to any part of the body via the bloodstream (pyaemia means pus in the blood). Because the white cells in the blood, which would normally attack and devour them, are in very short supply, the bacteria multiply virtually unhindered and produce abscesses wherever they settle.

CLINICAL SIGNS

The symptoms of tick pyaemia are very variable, depending upon where the abscesses are situated. One of the most common sites, and certainly the most obvious to the shepherd, is in the joints of the limbs, which fill up with

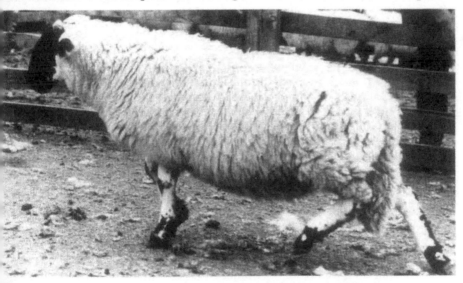

Plate 9.18   This lamb has an abscess in the spinal canal similar to the one shown in Colour plate 28. Note how the right hind limb is dragging. As this is a hill lamb, tick pyaemia must be a possible cause.

pus and become very swollen. This causes severe lameness ('cripples'), which is usually permanent, despite treatment. Affected lambs tend to lag behind their mothers and may lose condition rapidly.

Abscesses may also occur in the liver (see Colour plate 27), kidneys, lungs, spinal cord, brain or indeed any other site. Abscesses in organs such as the liver may produce vague symptoms, giving lambs an unthrifty, tucked up appearance. If abscesses develop in the spinal column, lambs may have difficulty in walking or become completely paralysed. Brain abscesses may also produce paralysis, blindness or any one of a number of nervous symptoms depending on the site of the abscess. The majority of cases occur in three to five week old lambs, and few cases develop before lambs are a fortnight old or beyond three or four mouths of age.

TREATMENT

Hill farmers generally ascribe the majority of losses amongst lambs between birth and weaning either directly or indirectly to tick-associated diseases and tick pyaemia in particular. Because of the difficult terrain and the extensive shepherding, cases of tick pyaemia are often well established by the time they are detected. This often means that treatment is unrewarding. However, if early cases are treated with a suitable antibiotic preparation and lambs and their ewes are brought down from the high ground so that lambs can be given appropriate care, a number will be saved. Despite recovery many lambs fail to thrive because of the irreparable damage done. Severely affected lambs should be humanely destroyed.

CONTROL

Because tick pyaemia occurs as a consequence of tickborne fever infection, the control of these two conditions must be considered together. Tick control is obviously of importance and although the complete eradication of ticks is impractical on all but a small proportion of farms, a reduction in their numbers may still be of considerable help. This is normally achieved by a number of measures as described in Chapter 13. No single technique, or combination of techniques, gives full protection against this disease, but a degree of control is achievable, albeit with a considerable amount of effort and some expense.

Deliberate infection

There are no vaccines available against either tick pyaemia or tickborne fever. It is possible to infect sheep with tickborne fever by injecting them with a small amount of blood from a carrier animal, preferably from the same farm. This has been investigated on a number of occasions, but the results overall have been disappointing. The idea is to inject lambs deliberately with infected ewe's blood well before they are sent to tick-infested hill ground, after having been born on improved, in-bye ground considered tick-free. The theory is that lambs will develop a fever but should recover from the worst effects of tickborne fever and become immune before being bitten by ticks on the hill. This presupposes, however, that the only way lambs can become infected with the staphylococci which cause tick pyaemia is via tick bites, but this seems unlikely (see above). The disappointing results of some trials using this technique may be due, in part, to this fact. There is also the added risk that certain other diseases may be transmitted via blood from other animals. The method cannot, therefore, be generally recommended, although individual farmers and their veterinary surgeons may have found it satisfactory on occasion.

Dips, pour-ons and antibiotics

There may be some long-term benefit from using pour-on insecticides on lambs or by dipping ewes before lambing, since, over a number of years, such methods should help reduce the tick population overall. There is some evidence on farms where pre-lambing dipping has been abandoned that the incidence of tick pyaemia is higher than on similar farms which still practise spring dipping or apply pour-ons.

The dipping of newborn lambs is not a popular technique amongst hill farmers for a number of reasons. Gathering ewes and newborn lambs is difficult and time-consuming and can present problems of mismothering. There is also very little fleece on newborn lambs to hold dip and therefore the residual effect lasts for only a short time. Nevertheless, dipping or, better still, double dipping of lambs at three week intervals should reduce the number of cases of tick pyaemia in flocks where this disease has caused a major problem in previous years. Lambs may be lowered into a small drum of dip and if they are done in small groups and given time to mother-up, they should not suffer unduly, provided a reasonable day is chosen for the job.

There are a number of pour-on products now available which control ticks and they may prove to be more suitable for lambs, because they incur less stress than dipping and can be applied very quickly and easily even on the day of birth. The task could be carried out in several localised gathering pens situated in appropriate places on the hill. This would remove the need for large gatherings and substantially reduce the problem of mismothering.

The use of long-acting antibiotics to protect lambs which are to be turned out onto tick-infested hill ground has never been a practical or a particularly successful control measure. However, recent work has shown that the use of long-acting tetracyclines, together with dipping or the use of pour-ons, just before lambs are turned onto the hill with their dams, can substantially reduce losses from tick pyaemia. Further trials are needed to establish the best time to treat lambs with antibiotics. This is likely to vary from farm to farm, depending upon the timing of lambing, and from year to year, depending upon the estimated time of the tick rise. One factor which should be borne in mind is that if tetracyclines are used for prolonged periods or are repeated at intervals, they may completely clear the blood

393

of the rickettsia which cause tickborne fever. Thereafter, once the antibiotic has cleared from the system, the lamb will be completely susceptible to tickborne fever, since protection depends upon the parasite being constantly present in the animal (see above).

Coccidiosis

This is a disease which has become an increasingly important problem in parallel with the intensification of sheep systems over recent years.

The organisms responsible—the **coccidia**—are microscopic parasites composed of only a single cell, which are members of a group known as the **protozoa**. The form of the parasite which infects sheep—the **oocyst**—is found in the faeces of infected animals. Lambs can become infected immediately they are born from sucking their mothers, whose udders and teats are inevitably contaminated with faeces, or by nosing around amongst faeces on the pasture or bedding.

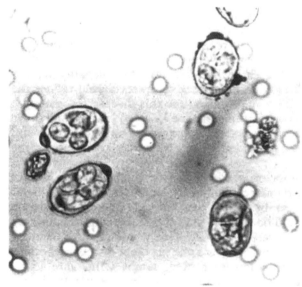

Plate 9.19 The large oval objects in this photo (taken down a light microscope) are coccidial oocysts. The small round objects are cryptosporidia. Taken from faeces of a lamb with diarrhoea.

Coccidiosis can affect all farm animal species and is probably most familiar to poultry farmers. However, the coccidia are almost invariably host-specific, that is to say, the coccidia which affect sheep do not cause disease in any of the other species and vice versa. So infected poultry do not pose any risk to sheep—a concern which is often expressed by farmers when they are first told their lambs have coccidiosis.

Most, if not all, sheep become infected with coccidia and usually with several different species of the parasite at the same time. Each different pecies causes damage to a different area of the intestine and whilst some produce severe damage, others appear to be relatively harmless. Two pecies in particular are considered the most serious in sheep, *Eimeria randallis* and *Eimeria ovinoidalis*. The coccidial oocysts are swallowed by the sheep and hatch in the gut, releasing active stages which invade the ells lining the gut. Here they undergo a complex process of multiplication vhich increases the parasite numbers enormously and causes severe damage o the intestine.

Coccidiosis is a disease of young lambs, older sheep having become mmune through previous contact with the parasite. Most outbreaks occur n lambs of one to two months of age and particularly in housed flocks. The disease may also occur in flocks which have been housed for a period nd are then turned out onto pasture, with cases appearing in lambs two or hree weeks after turnout. Coccidiosis may also strike in outdoor lambing locks, especially where high stocking rates are employed, which can lead o heavy faecal contamination of pasture, especially around feed and water roughs.

Source and weight of infection

Ewes provide the initial infection for lambs, since although they are immune, hey still produce small numbers of infectious oocysts in their dung. Around ambing in particular, the ewe's capacity to resist infection of any kind is onsiderably reduced. They may therefore put out relatively large numbers of coccidial oocysts, so 'seeding' the bedding or pasture for the lambs. It vill be clear why housed lambs are most at risk, since there will be a steady ouild-up of oocyst numbers in the confined area of the lambing shed, lead-ng to heavy contamination by the time lambing is in full swing.

Whether lambs succumb to the disease or not depends mainly on the number of infectious oocysts they swallow in the first few days of life. This irst infection does not normally produce any immediate symptoms, even hough the number of oocysts ingested may be high. However, because ambs have not experienced the infection previously, they have no immunity nd the parasite is able to multiply enormously in the lining of the gut. Around three weeks later, the parasite has completed its life cycle and very arge numbers of oocysts are shed in the faeces, which heavily contaminate he area. After two or three days these oocysts become infectious.

The teats and udders of ewes lying on sparse, wet, soiled bedding become heavily contaminated with oocysts, which are then swallowed by he sucking lambs. Lambs may also nibble at concentrates provided for the ewes or may be taking creep feed, either of which may be contaminated vith faeces. Water troughs may be at such a height that ewes or lambs may lung into them (especially as the bedding builds up), and this can provide nother source of infection.

Susceptible, young, housed lambs often show clinical signs of the disease t this time, due to the severe damage resulting from the multiplication of massive numbers of coccidia in the gut.

Build-up of immunity in lambs at pasture

The risks are somewhat reduced in outdoor lambing flocks. This is because the faeces are spread over a much wider area and lambs thus pick up fewer oocysts. This may allow them to build up a protective level of immunity to the disease over a period of weeks. Even though the number of oocysts is likely to increase during the weeks after lambing, they are less likely to reach overwhelming levels before the lambs become immune. Once lambs are immune, the coccidia cannot complete their life cycle in the gut so effectively. Therefore the number of oocysts in the faeces falls, so reducing the pasture contamination for later born lambs.

Depending upon the system of management of the flock, lambs can be expected to become immune from around six weeks of age. However, if lambs are protected from infection, for example, by medication (see below), this will defer immunity. Disease may then occur in older lambs of up to five or six months old.

Stress—in the form of a severe spell of cold, wet weather or an inadequate level of nutrition—may precipitate outbreaks of coccidiosis. Obviously the infection has to be present in the flock, but in well-fed and well-managed flocks, the severity of the disease may be reduced. Twins and triplets are generally more likely to succumb to coccidiosis and this may be as a consequence of their receiving less colostrum and less milk than comparable single lambs.

CLINICAL SIGNS

The first sign that coccidiosis may be affecting a flock is that lambs may not be growing as well as expected. Close observation will reveal a number of lambs with a tucked-up, open-fleeced appearance, and a few lambs may be dirty around the rear end due to a mild diarrhoea. The majority of lambs in the group will be affected to a greater or lesser degree. Lambs eventually lose their appetite and become weak and unthrifty. As the disease progresses, some lambs may become severely scoured, and there are often streaks of blood in the diarrhoea. Without treatment these animals may continue to scour for several weeks so they become severely dehydrated. In a bad outbreak, perhaps one in ten clinically affected lambs may die.

Whilst deaths represent the most obvious loss to the farmer from coccidiosis, by far the most costly aspect of the disease is the setback to the growth rate of affected lambs. This is because of the damage caused to the lining of the gut. Nutrients from food cannot be properly absorbed from the intestine into the bloodstream and thence converted into meat. Losses also accrue due to the cost of treatment for the lamb flock.

Diagnosis

Diagnosis of coccidiosis presents some difficulties for the veterinary surgeon. As mentioned earlier, most if not all sheep are infected with

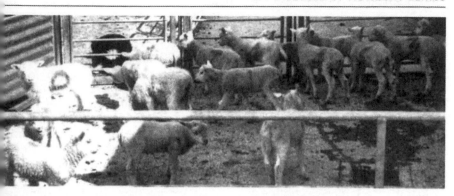

late 9.20   A group of Finn lambs with coccidiosis. Not all are scouring, but all
e infected. Note the generally poor condition. The aim should be to medicate
mbs during the period of risk to prevent clinical symptoms like this developing.

occidia and therefore an examination of faeces from lambs will invariably
now the presence of oocysts. Also, there are no hard and fast rules to say
hat particular number of oocysts in faeces is an index of serious disease.
ome lambs may be very ill from coccidiosis and yet have very low num-
ers of oocysts in their faeces; others may be perfectly fit and healthy, yet
e producing astronomical numbers of oocysts.

There are a number of other conditions which can be confused with
occidiosis. In housed flocks, lambs sucking well-fed, milky ewes and
ffered a creep feed with too high a protein content may scour and lose
eir bloom. At pasture, worms—particularly nematodirus—may produce
aths and symptoms very similar to coccidiosis in lambs of a comparable
e. Indeed, dual infections with nematodirus and coccidiosis are particu-
rly savage. Lambs turned out onto pastures recently treated with basic slag,
fore it has been washed in by rain, may be poisoned, with symptoms of
arrhoea and with occasional deaths.

If these and other possibilities are ruled out and a large proportion of
e lambs are scouring or losing condition and the veterinary laboratory
onfirms the presence (in faeces) of the strains of coccidia known to cause
vere disease, then coccidiosis is the probable cause. Any lambs dying
ould be presented for post-mortem examination. The results from this,
gether with the response to appropriate treatment, will further confirm
 deny the diagnosis. It is generally much easier for your veterinary
rgeon to be confident of a diagnosis on a flock basis rather than from the
sessment of individual sick animals.

REATMENT

reatment of coccidiosis can be a tedious and expensive business. It causes
onsiderable disruption, as it necessitates the medication of every lamb in

397

the flock, since even those showing no symptoms are likely to be infecte and contaminating their surroundings.

A number of products—such as the sulphonamides—are availabl for treatment. Some are administered by injection or by mouth, other in the feed or water supply. Usually, lambs need to be treated repeatedly either daily or every other day. Frequently, an 'on-off' treatment regim is employed, when medication is given for a few days, stopped for a few days, then repeated. This is designed to control the disease to the poin where damage by the parasite is minimised, whilst allowing some coccidi to remain, so ensuring that lambs will develop an immunity.

Following treatment, the flock should be moved to clean grazing s as to prevent lambs becoming reinfected before they are fully immune 'Clean' grazing is pasture which did not carry lambs clinically affecte with coccidiosis during the previous season. This is because oocysts ar capable of surviving for at least a year on pasture. Housed lambs should b moved to a clean area if possible. If this is impracticable, the original are should be liberally bedded with straw. Any sources of infection, such a contaminated troughs or water bowls, should be thoroughly cleaned using steam pressure hose. Farm disinfectants are of little use in killing coccidia oocysts. If feasible, the flock should be turned outside onto clean grazing after appropriate treatment, provided the weather is reasonable.

Lambs which have suffered a setback may benefit from the gradua introduction of some supplementary creep feed following treatment, t help their recovery and to try to prevent relapses occurring.

PREVENTION

Prevention is the obvious way to deal with this disease. If coccidiosi has once occurred in a flock under a particular management system, i is likely to occur again if the management has not been altered to dea with the problem. All sheep flocks become infected with coccidia, but no all flocks experience frank disease. This is due to the differing systems o management and their effect on the immunity of the lamb flock and the leve of coccidial challenge which confronts the lambs. It is essential to attemp to achieve a balance between these two factors.

With housed flocks, it is important that the stocking rate is such tha ewes have both adequate trough space and lying area. Coccidial oocyst need moisture to help them to mature and become infectious. Thus, ther should be adequate drainage and sufficient bedding supplied to ensure tha the litter remains dry. Feed and water troughs should be sited appropriately so that they are not easily contaminated by dung. Unless sheep are kept o slatted floors (which is unusual in the UK), then they have to lie in thei own faeces, so it is important to reduce contamination to a minimum.

Ideally, when lambs are born, they should be protected from contac with areas heavily contaminated with oocysts. This can be achieved t some degree by the above methods, but where the disease has occurre

398

n previous years it is probably wise to take extra precautions by way of preventive medication of either ewes or lambs or both. Your veterinary surgeon should advise you on whether it is necessary to medicate, on what product to use, on how to use it and on what other management factors are involved.

Medicating the ewes

Since most housed ewes are fed concentrates during the last six or eight weeks of pregnancy, it is possible to medicate the feed to reduce the output of oocysts by the ewes to a minimum, especially around lambing. If this is done lambs will be only lightly challenged in early life and this will give them an opportunity to build up a protective immunity without necessarily suffering too much of a setback. Decoquinate (Deccox, RMB) is available in a premix form for use with ewe rations or lamb creep (see later). Monensin sodium (Romensin, Elanco), whilst not licensed for sheep, can be used under veterinary prescription and has been shown to be effective in both ewes and lambs. It can be added to the ewe concentrate rations for a month or more before lambing. Monensin is somewhat unpalatable to sheep, and treated feed should be introduced gradually to ewes when late pregnancy feeding begins six or eight weeks before lambing. This should avoid the problem of ewes refusing their rations during the last month of pregnancy when to do so might precipitate twin lamb disease. The problem of unpalatability can be overcome to some extent by adding flavourings such as caramel or vanilla to the ewe rations. Some compounders offer this service at little or no extra cost.

Supplementation of ewe concentrates with monensin can continue for up to two months after lambing. This will cover the period around lambing and during early lactation, when oocyst numbers in ewe faeces would be expected to increase due to the ewe's immune system being less effective at this time.

Monensin is toxic if given at higher than the recommended dose. (It is also very toxic to horses and to other species should they accidentally consume the medicated feed.) Decoquinate is a safer and more palatable product. An added benefit of monensin is that it also gives a substantial measure of protection against toxoplasma abortion in ewes when fed during the mid and late pregnancy period and this is discussed in Chapter 5. Note that neither of the two products should be fed to ewes whose milk is to be used for human consumption.

Medicating the lambs

Lambs can also be medicated with either monensin or decoquinate, but this is only practicable when they are being offered creep feed. They may be treated for a month or longer, but it should be noted that the protection afforded by such treatment may interfere with the build-up of immunity. When medication is stopped, the lambs will be vulnerable should they be subjected to a heavy challenge. Lambs should therefore be moved to uncontaminated pasture following medication. The older the lambs, the less susceptible they tend to be. Strategic treatment, for example, with long-acting sulphona mides at three weekly intervals over the high risk period may also be employed.

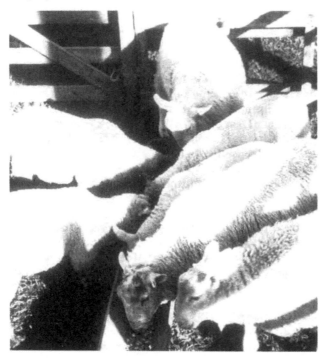

Plate 9.21 Where lambs are creep fed, a coccidiostat can be added.

Pulpy Kidney

Pulpy kidney is the popular, though somewhat misleading, name given to a fatal disease of sheep caused by a bacterium of the clostridial group—*Clostridium perfringens*—type D. Under certain circumstances this microorganism multiplies very rapidly in the small intestine and produces a potent toxin. The poison affects the brain and other organs, resulting in nervous symptoms and rapid death within only a few hours.

The disease may affect any age or class of sheep, but most commonly strikes young, thriving animals which are unprotected and which are suddenly moved onto better forage. There are certain times of year when the disease is most likely to occur and these often coincide with the availability of ample supplies of good-quality feed. However, pulpy kidney can occur at any time of the year and in any class of sheep, if the right conditions prevail.

Lambs up to three months of age are particularly vulnerable, even when sucking their dams. In the youngest lambs, a sudden flush of milk brought

400

n when ewes respond to lush spring grazing may be sufficient to bring on ie disease, especially in single lambs which are growing rapidly. In slightly lder lambs which are still sucking but are starting to graze themselves, the ombination of abundant milk plus lush grass may precipitate cases. Pulpy idney frequently occurs when lush growth follows a dry or frosty spell at ny time of the year.

In older lambs, the disease may occur when, for example, weaned lambs re moved onto aftermaths or onto stubble turnips or rape. Such lambs will ave been receiving progressively less and less milk from their dams as ie nutritional value of the pasture grass deteriorates during the summer. 'he sudden stress of weaning, coupled with movement onto abundant, lush orage, may produce conditions in the gut favourable for the multiplication f the bacteria responsible for pulpy kidney disease.

Ewes may also succumb when given sudden access to better-quality eed. In parts of the world besides the UK, the disease is sometimes referred) as 'overeating disease', and it is well recognised in the United States in eedlot sheep on ad lib cereal rations.

CLINICAL SIGNS

'linical signs of the disease are rarely observed, because death occurs very apidly once sufficient toxin has been produced in the intestine. Often, one r more of the best lambs in a flock will be found dead by the shepherd n his early morning round, followed by further deaths over the next few ays. If symptoms are seen, they are usually of a nervous character. Sheep iay be unsteady on their legs and excessively sensitive to the presence of ie shepherd and his dogs. They may fall over, be unable to rise and may ike fits. The head and neck may be drawn backwards and breathing is ften difficult. Sheep which survive for any length of time often develop iarrhoea, but few cases survive long enough to do so.

The disease is always fatal and treatment is of no avail, even if symptoms re observed early. The carcasses of sheep which have died from pulpy idney decompose very rapidly. Sudden deaths in any class of stock should lways be investigated and fresh carcasses taken to your veterinary surgeon r the local veterinary investigation centre for diagnosis. There are a number f causes of sudden death in sheep and it is important to obtain a correct iagnosis so that appropriate control and preventive measures can be taken.

CONTROL AND PREVENTION

Even in vaccinated flocks, occasional losses may occur from pulpy kidney r other clostridial diseases. No vaccine can ever provide one hundred per ent protection and an occasional ewe may miss being vaccinated, or a amb may suck insufficient colostrum to protect itself. In flocks with a ong lambing period, ewes which lamb last may have insufficient colostral antibody to protect their lambs up to the time when these are sold fat or ar themselves vaccinated.

If a flock is unvaccinated or inadequately vaccinated and sudden death occur amongst thriving lambs, it is very likely that pulpy kidney might b. the cause, and control measures will have to be taken promptly. Whils waiting for a diagnosis, the flock should be moved onto poorer grazing This should reduce the milk production of ewes and therefore set lamb back a little, but it should also reduce the number of deaths. Any mov back to better grazing must be made very gradually.

In unvaccinated flocks, all sheep are at risk, although deaths may b. occurring in only one class. In this situation, lambs will need immediat cover by means of antiserum, which contains ready-made antitoxin against pulpy kidney. This will give immediate, although only short-term protection for around three weeks. If lambs are to be fattened (but are stil very young) or ewe lambs are being kept as flock replacements, then the should receive an injection of a suitable combined clostridial vaccine at th same time as the antiserum, but on the other side of the body. A second dos of vaccine will have to be given four to six weeks after the first. Protectio will be complete only some two weeks after this second vaccination.

It will be clear, therefore, that lambs will still be at risk from the time tha the protection from antiserum wears off until protection from the vaccine i. complete—a period of around three to five weeks. If, after discussion with your veterinary surgeon, it is decided that there is an unacceptable risk o further deaths during this period, then one or two extra doses of antiserur may be given at two to three week intervals.

Ewes and rams in unvaccinated flocks should be started on a clostridia vaccination programme immediately.

Whilst vaccination is the only effective way to prevent pulpy kidney management factors which predispose to the disease should always be born in mind. If sheep are to be moved onto better forage or given any improve ment in diet, this should be done gradually wherever possible. It should b remembered that other problems may arise in similar circumstances to those which predispose to pulpy kidney—magnesium staggers in ewes around lambing, or pasteurella infections in ewes or lambs, for example.

Braxy

Braxy is one of the clostridial diseases responsible for sudden death ir lambs, hoggs and gimmers. It is caused by *Clostridium septicum*. Usuall the shepherd will simply find one or more of the better lambs in the flock lying apparently freshly dead on the first inspection of the day.

It is a relatively uncommon disease nowadays, but may still be encoun tered in unvaccinated or inadequately vaccinated hill and upland flocks ir the north and west of Britain. Clostridial organisms are found everywhere that sheep are found and the factors which predispose young sheep to braxy

402

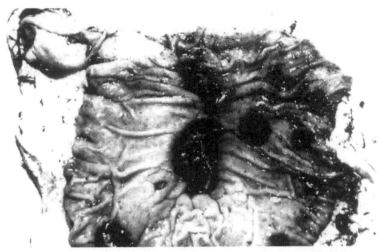

Plate 9.22 Ulcers (dark areas) in the stomach (abomasum) of a
sheep which died of braxy—a fairly rare condition in the UK
since the advent of clostridial vaccines.

re unclear. However, it is most likely to occur when, for example, hill
oggs are being folded over frosted rape or kale or are simply grazing older
ermanent pastures during frosty autumn and winter weather. The theory
s that the consumption of large amounts of frosted material devitalises the
ining of the abomasum (stomach) and allows the bacterium to multiply
apidly. It produces a potent poison or toxin, which rapidly kills the sheep.

Very occasionally a shepherd may see symptoms, with an affected sheep
anging back from the rest of the flock, grunting and grinding its teeth
nd in obvious pain. The abdomen may appear full and swollen. Affected
nimals rapidly collapse and their initial fever subsides to a hypothermia
mmediately before coma and death.

VACCINATION

On farms where the disease has been diagnosed in the past it is essential that
ll sheep, but particularly lambs, hoggs and gimmers, are fully protected
vith one of the multivalent (7 in 1) clostridial vaccines and that they are
given a booster braxy (or multivalent) vaccination in late summer or early
utumn, before the period of risk. Some shepherds, who consider that braxy
vaccination gives their sheep a 'setback', administer only a half-dose of the
vaccine. This is always unwise, since the sheep will then be inadequately
protected.

A sheltered grass layback should always be provided when sheep
re grazing roots, kale or rape. On sunny days, the risk can be reduced
by keeping sheep off the crop until the frost has thawed. However, there

are many days when the thaw never happens and unvaccinated flocks are then at considerable risk. Providing lambs have had at least two doses of a clostridial vaccine containing a braxy component at approximately 10 weeks and 18 weeks old, they should be adequately protected. Gimmers already on the vaccination programme should receive an early autumn braxy booster dose.

VACCINATION AGAINST THE CLOSTRIDIAL DISEASES

The clostridial group of bacteria are responsible for a long list of diseases in mammals (including man), and of all species sheep would appear to be particularly susceptible. The clostridial diseases affecting sheep are listed in the Quick Reference Chart at the end of this section and also at appropriate places in the text.

Because of the widespread distribution of clostridial bacteria on sheep farms throughout the world and because of the highly resistant nature of their encapsulated forms (spores) outside the body, eradication of any of all of these diseases is out of the question. These bacteria do not always produce disease, as they are present in the gut of healthy animals. Faeces contain clostridia which contaminate herbage and soil. The resistant spores may survive for many years and there is thus a constant risk of disease wherever livestock are kept.

The argument is sometimes put forward that if good husbandry is practised, then vaccination against the clostridial diseases should not be necessary. Whilst there is no doubt that the way a flock is managed may greatly influence the likelihood of disease, it is impossible for even the best-managed flocks to avoid all circumstances which are likely to put sheep at risk. **Vaccination against these killer diseases is therefore an essential part of sheep husbandry** and should not be considered an admission of failure. On the other hand because a flock is vaccinated it should not be assumed that management can be relaxed. Even the most efficient vaccine cannot be expected to give one hundred per cent protection in the face of overwhelming challenge. Good husbandry practice and vaccination must go hand in hand.

There is a temptation after a number of years with apparently no problems from clostridial diseases to assume that they have gone away and to stop vaccinating. This is most unwise, because the unvaccinated flock always runs an unacceptable level of risk. All sheep flocks, large or small, hill or lowland, should vaccinate and should continue to do so for as long as sheep are kept.

Choice of vaccine

The next question is which type of vaccine to use. There are dozens of clostridial vaccines available and a great many different combinations to choose from. Some protect against all the important clostridial diseases (i.e. '7 in 1') whilst others may cover against four or even only one disease (e.g. blackleg). Clostridial vaccines are inexpensive and there is very little difference in price between those giving full cover and those protecting against only one or two diseases. It is therefore recommended that for breeding stock (ewes and rams) and breeding replacements (ewe lambs, ram lambs and gimmers), full cover be given using a '7 in 1' type vaccine. For a few extra pence per sheep the flockmaster can have fully comprehensive cover. The death of even one good commercial breeding ewe could cost as much as 300–400 pre-lambing booster doses of vaccine.

Always read the vaccine manufacturer's instructions carefully. The old shepherd's tale about only half a dose of vaccine being necessary for protection against braxy, for example, is quite untrue. Such 'savings' leave the flock unprotected or inadequately protected, while the flock owner labours under the misapprehension that his sheep are safe.

Vaccination of adult ewes

Adult breeding ewes, already on a vaccination programme, will require an annual pre-lambing booster throughout their lives, to protect them and their lambs. This should be given about a month before lambing, where management allows, and it will ensure that a maximum amount of antibody transfers to colostrum to protect lambs. In flocks with prolonged lambings

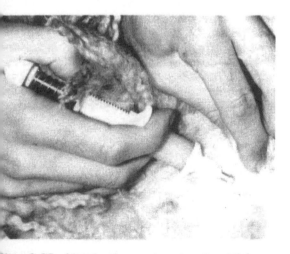

Plate 9.23   Vaccinating against the clostridial diseases. Choose a dry day and a clean area of fleece over the mid-neck region. The vaccine must be given under the skin. The plate to the right shows an automatic vaccinating gun. Change the needle frequently and take care not to touch the needle itself, only the plastic 'shoulder'.

(e.g. five weeks or more) this will mean vaccinating early, mid and late lambers on separate occasions at the appropriate times.

Heavily pregnant ewes should always be handled with extra care and the job should never be rushed. Whilst it is sensible to attempt to reduce the number of gatherings and handlings during pregnancy, it is equally important not to 'overload' ewes. If ewes are vaccinated, wormed, fluked, given a copper supplement, have their feet pared and are stood in a footbath, then they will be well and truly stressed. It would be no surprise to any reasonably informed person if there were to be a number of deaths amongst the flock over the following days and weeks. Indeed, if the flock was also inadequately fed, then the results of such treatment could be catastrophic.

It is not always practical to administer the pre-lambing clostridial booster at the ideal time. For example, on many hill farms, gathering is a major operation which can take several days. Many shepherds therefore delay vaccination until close to the start of lambing when ewes are being brought down off the tops into enclosures. By this time some ewes are almost due to lamb and there is insufficient time for the vaccination to boost antibody levels in colostrum to protect adequately the earliest born lambs. It must therefore be appreciated that these lambs are at risk. Should disease occur—for example, lamb dysentery—then the risk to later born lambs will also be increased because of contamination of the lambing area from scouring lambs.

Remember that on fluke infected farms, where there is a winter risk of black disease, a second annual booster will be necessary before the period of risk in autumn. Ministry fluke forecasts in the farming press and on radio and television are helpful in this regard.

Vaccines are now available which provide combined protection against pasteurellosis as well as the clostridial diseases. In some cases the vaccination programme timings may have to be altered slightly and the section on pasteurella in Chapter 10 should be referred to, particularly in regard to the protection of lambs. Your veterinary surgeon will guide you on the correct vaccination scheme for your flock's particular needs.

Protection for lambs

Newborn lambs must be protected passively by the ready-made antibodies from the colostrum of vaccinated ewes. Ewes should be given booster vaccinations, preferably three to six weeks before they are due to lamb. This ensures a high level of protective antibody in the ewe's bloodstream during the time when colostrum is being produced in the days immediately prior to lambing. The ewe is able to transfer large quantities of these antibodies into her colostrum to protect her newborn lambs, whilst at the same time retaining sufficient antibodies to protect herself. Lambs successfully sucking vaccinated ewes, which are in good body condition and have a plentiful supply of good-quality colostrum, should take in sufficient antibody to protect themselves against the important clostridial diseases of early life—lamb dysentery, tetanus and pulpy kidney—for up to three or four months.

If colostrum-protected lambs grow well and can be sold for slaughter before four months of age, they will not need to be protected by vaccination. If fattening or store lambs are to be retained for a longer period, they should be vaccinated against all the clostridial diseases or at least against those most likely to occur under the circumstances of a particular farm. Two doses of whichever vaccine is chosen will be necessary, given at least four to six weeks apart, for example, at 10 and 14 weeks of age. Lambs must not be vaccinated too early, otherwise the antibody from colostrum will interfere with the 'take' of the vaccine and lambs may be left inadequately protected. Follow the manufacturer's advice carefully.

Unprotected lambs

Lambs from unvaccinated ewes are a high-risk group, and vaccination should start in the first week of life. If the lambs are outdoors, choose the first reasonably dry day to give them their primary vaccination. A second injection of vaccine should be given four weeks later. Note that it is not until approximately a fortnight after the second vaccination (i.e. at around six or seven weeks of age) that levels of antibody are high enough to protect the lambs fully.

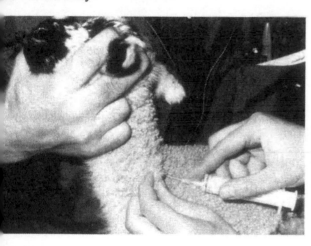

Plate 9.24 Injecting a lamb subcutaneously. Wherever there is a choice of route of administration with an injectable drug, this should be the route chosen. This would be suitable for injecting clostridial antiserum.

It is therefore necessary to protect these vulnerable lambs with ready-made antibodies, in the form of antiserum, immediately they are born and at the same time as their first vaccination. The antiserum and vaccine should be given using separate syringes and needles and on opposite sides of the body. The antiserum used must contain antibodies against lamb dysentery, tetanus and pulpy kidney at least.

The protection afforded by antiserum is good, but unfortunately short-lived—two to three weeks at most. As lambs are not fully protected by vaccination until at least six weeks of age, there is a period of risk between three and six weeks of age. This risk can be reduced by giving further doses of antiserum. However, it should be noted that repeated doses protect for shorter and shorter intervals and antiserum is also relatively expensive. It is obvious, therefore, that vaccination of ewes before lambing is the cheapest and most efficient method of controlling these diseases in young lambs.

Breeding replacements

Home-bred ewe lambs which are to be reared as replacements for the breeding flock should be started on a vaccination programme to protect them against all the clostridial diseases as soon as they are old enough. In the case of lambs from vaccinated ewes this would mean giving them their first or primary vaccination at around two to three months of age followed four to six weeks later, by a second injection. Gimmers or ewe lambs which are to be bred from will need a booster dose around the same time as the breeding ewes, that is, three to four weeks before lambing time.

Purchased animals

Any sheep purchased from a market or directly from another farm—such as ewe lambs or gimmers for breeding replacements, rams, ewes with lambs at foot or store lambs for fattening—should always be assumed to be unvaccinated. The only exception might be ewes which have a certificate, signed by a veterinary surgeon, stating when and with what they were vaccinated, such as is given in the Premium Sheep Health Scheme in Scotland. In all other cases sheep should be injected at the earliest opportunity with a primary dose of vaccine, followed four to six weeks later with a secondary dose.

Rams

Rams are often a neglected group, but it is essential that they are adequately protected. They should receive their primary and secondary vaccinations as ram lambs at around two to three months of age and six weeks later, respectively. They should be boosted annually at least a month before the mating period begins and the pre-tupping fertility examination is often a convenient time. However, as with ewes, it is unwise to overdo the number of vaccinations and medications which are carried out at any one time to avoid stressing animals unduly.

Redgut

In the spring and early summer months, occasional sudden deaths may occur in groups of weaned lambs on lush grazing. At post-mortem examination the abdominal contents are extremely red and when the small and large intestines are opened they are often full of blood (see Colour plate 25).

It is thought that rich pastures—such as those with a high clover content—speed up the process of digestion, so that part of the large intestine becomes abnormally swollen and changes its position in the abdomen. The tortion or 'twist' which results causes a blockage of some of the important blood vessels which serve the intestines, with the result that they haemorrhage into the gut.

Whilst the condition is seen most commonly in lambs, it may affect sheep of any age and is occasionally seen in cattle. As it occurs unexpectedly, there is little that can be done to prevent it. Sheep are unlikely to eat even top-quality hay when there is good grazing to be had. Limiting the amount of time spent on lush pasture—which is good husbandry practice—may reduce the risk.

Bloat

Bloat is an emergency condition of lambs and adult sheep which occurs when the gases which are produced continuously by the fermentation processes of the rumen cannot escape. The condition is less common in sheep than in cattle, possibly because sheep do not tend to graze such lush, heavily fertilised pastures and also because they are continuous grazers for the most part and are less likely to be turned out hungry onto a clover-rich sward.

Gas may not be able to escape from the rumen for a number of reasons. If an animal gets onto its back—such as fat ewes in autumn or heavily pregnant ewes in spring—then the liquid contents of the rumen cover the orifice through which the gases are belched up the oesophagus and out of the mouth. Sick sheep which lie on their side for a prolonged period may also 'blow-up'—hence such animals must always be propped up with bales. Should a sheep swallow a small piece of turnip or a tiny apple from the orchard, then the oesophagus may become blocked and prevent the gases from being belched up.

Certain plants, such as the clovers, may produce foaming agents in the rumen which trap the gas in tiny bubbles which then cannot escape. These foods also encourage rapid fermentation, so that gas is produced more quickly. Also, excess fatty acid production makes the rumen contents more acidic. The acid then acts on the bicarbonates in saliva (often produced to excess in bloat cases) to produce even more gas.

CLINICAL SIGNS

If bloated sheep are still on their feet when found, they may stand very stiffly with their legs wide apart. They may pant excessively and stagger about if moved. They urinate and attempt to dung frequently and young animals may bleat. A swelling will be seen in the left flank and also on the right side in advanced cases. Eventually animals will go down and, if not treated, will die fairly quickly. The pressure of the swollen rumen presses on the diaphragm, causing difficulty in breathing and finally suffocation and heart failure.

TREATMENT

Where it is a case of a ewe or ram getting over on its back, then simply stand the animal up and support if for a few minutes. It should 'burp' for some time and the swelling in the flank should gradually subside. If a badly bloated sheep is helped up and let go immediately, it will often stagger, lurch away and may go down again.

If frothy bloat is suspected, where the flock is grazing lush pasture or kale, get the flock off the dangerous area. There are a number of substances which will reduce surface tension and so release the gas trapped in the small bubbles. Linseed and other vegetable oils, or even cream, can be used. However, such liquids are difficult for bloated animals to swallow safely due to their smooth texture, and therefore drenching a 'blown' animal is fraught with danger, since the drench may go down the trachea and into the lungs with fatal results. Solid blocks of margarine about the size of a walnut can be pushed to the back of the mouth and often give relief at much less risk than liquids. It is essential to remain with the animal and to keep it on its feet and moving if possible.

If surface tension reducing agents do not work, or if the animal is very severely bloated and close to death, then more drastic emergency measures must be taken. It is unlikely that a proper instrument for the job (a trocar and canula) will be at hand, so a sharp pointed knife of 5 to 7.5 cm, preferably with a reasonably wide blade, will suffice. The knife should be thrust into the rumen, which lies on the **left** side as shown in Plates 9.25 and 9.26. The blade should then be twisted through 90 degrees to allow the gas to escape. In cases of frothy bloat this can be disappointing, as little gas may escape. However, a surface tension reducing oil, such as linseed, can be syringed directly into the rumen via the wound. For an adult ewe, 50 ml should suffice in most cases.

This is not an easy or pleasant thing to have to do and should only be undertaken in a real emergency. Rumen contents will inevitably escape into the abdominal cavity and this will cause peritonitis. The treated animal should be given antibiotics by injection on the advice of your veterinary surgeon.

It is occasionally possible to gag less severely affected animals and to pass a stomach tube. This is difficult in a struggling animal in great distress and the tube may go down the wrong way into the trachea. Sheep will cough violently if this happens. Even if the tube is passed successfully, it may block up with froth. If you are sure that the tube is in the right place, a vegetable oil can be poured down the tube and into the rumen. Keep a close eye on the patient and if the sheep is down it must be propped up.

PREVENTION

Prevention is difficult, since many of the methods advocated are impractical. Restricting grazing time or total avoidance of suspect or obviously

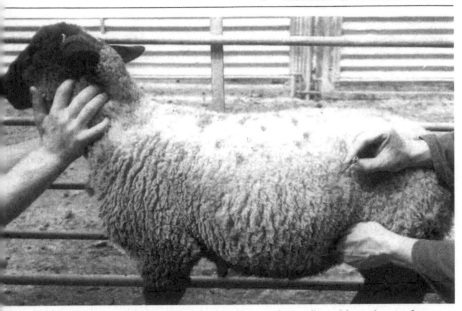

Plate 9.25   A long, wide-bore needle can be used to relieve bloat due to free gas in lambs. Note the position of the needle on left side of animal.

Plate 9.26   Trocar and canula for relief of bloat. The skin must be incised to allow insertion of the instrument.

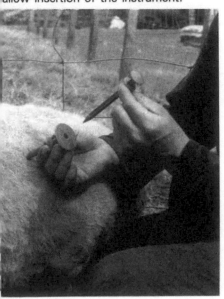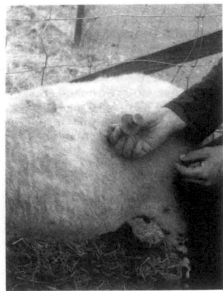

dangerous pastures is the safest approach. Sheep will rarely take hay when there is grass to eat. It is obviously sensible to avoid feeding anything of size or shape likely to stick in the throat or oesophagus.

Drunken Lamb Syndrome—Nephropathy

In the late spring and early summer months in the UK, a number of young lambs at grass—particularly on lowland farms, but also on upland and hill pastures—succumb to acute kidney failure. The disease is uncommon in lambs more than three months of age and may afflict lambs as young as a week, the majority of cases occurring in lambs from two to four weeks of age.

Nephropathy has been recorded for more than 30 years, but there seems to have been an increase in reported cases in recent years. The cause or causes remain unknown, but a toxic factor responsible for severe kidney damage and ultimately the death of affected lambs appears to be involved. It is known that certain bacteria produce such toxins, and one theory—as yet unproven—is that the clostridial bacterium which causes pulpy kidney disease might be a culprit. Pulpy kidney is a rapidly fatal disease with lambs rarely showing any symptoms of illness, but merely being found dead. Lambs with nephropathy, on the other hand, do show signs of illness often for some days before death. The theory is that the pulpy kidney organism—which is present wherever sheep are kept—may be able to multiply and produce its toxin to only a limited degree in the intestines of lambs which have received inadequate amounts of colostral protection from their dams. The amount of toxin produced may be insufficient to cause the sudden death associated with pulpy kidney, but sufficient to cause fatal kidney damage. It should be stressed that this is only a theory and that the toxin (if toxin it be) has yet to be identified.

An earlier theory was that the kidney damage was in some way associated with nematodirus worm infection in lambs, or with the use of anthelmintics. This would seem to be improbable, certainly in the younger affected lambs, which are unlikely to be picking up nematodirus infection and should not require worming much before six weeks of age.

CLINICAL SIGNS

The clinical signs of nephropathy vary somewhat in younger and older lambs. The common name for the condition—the drunken lamb syndrome—was coined because young affected lambs are very depressed, stop sucking, become very weak and stagger about as if drunk. Within a day or two they collapse, subside into a coma and die. Older lambs appear unthrifty and may scour, so that the shepherd may assume that there is a worm problem. However, treatment with anthelmintics brings about no improvement and although these older lambs may continue to suckle and appear reasonably bright, they eventually lose condition, collapse and die.

Incurable

Since the cause remains a mystery, no specific treatment can be advised and all remedies which have been tried have failed to effect a cure. This is not altogether surprising considering the degree of damage to the very enlarged kidneys as seen at post-mortem. Neither can any advice be given on prevention or control until more is known about the disease.

QUICK REFERENCE CHART Clostridial diseases of sheep

Disease	Animals affected	Symptoms	Notes
LAMB DYSENTRY (Cl. perfringens type B)	Lambs from a few days up to 3 weeks old.	Stomach pain—bloodstained diarrhoea—collapse—death	Often best lambs suckling ewes with plenty of milk.
PULPY KIDNEY (Cl. perfringens type D)	Especially lambs 6 weeks to a year old, but any age.	Unsteady—collapse—convulsions—death	Usually thriving lambs, especially after an abrupt change to better feed.
TETANUS (Cl. tetani)	Mainly suckling lambs, but any age.	Stiff—head back—difficulty feeding—falling over—convulsions—death	Especially after tailing and castration with rubber rings. Also from puncture wounds, e.g. at shearing.
STRUCK (Cl. perfringens type C)	Young adults of one to two years, occasionally lambs.	Abdominal pain—reluctant to move—convulsions—death	After a move to improved grazing in winter and spring. Restricted geographically, e.g. northern and western areas of Britain and Romney Marsh, Kent. Uncommon.
BRAXY (Cl. septicum)	Young sheep, e.g. hoggs.	Hang back—abdominal pain—collapse—coma—death	Frosted food in autumn and winter allows organisms to multiply in abomasum. Commonest on hill grazing and old permanent pastures in north and west of Britain. Uncommon.
BLACK DISEASE (Cl. oedematiens)	Adult sheep and older lambs.	Lag behind—lie down—breathing fast and noisy—rapid, quiet death	Follows liver damage, particularly from migrating young liver fluke in autumn and early winter. Less common after severe frosts.
BACILLARY HAEMOGLOBINUREA (Cl. haemolyticum)	Adult sheep.	Stop grazing—dark red urine—death	As for black disease. An uncommon condition in sheep.
BLACKLEG	Any age.	See appropriate text	Principally through contamination of wounds (e.g. castration and tailing, 'dirty' injection technique, shearing wounds). Also following bruising of tissues as after assistance at lambing (gangrenous metritis) or via head wounds in fighting rams ('big head').
GANGRENOUS METRITIS	Post lambing ewes.		
'BIG HEAD' or	Especially rams.		
MALIGNANT OEDEMA	Any age.		

(various clostridia, especially Cl. chauvoei, Cl. septicum and Cl. oedematiens)

10

PNEUMONIA AND OTHER RESPIRATORY DISEASES

Pneumonia is an inflammation of the lungs caused by infection with one or more of a number of microorganisms or other parasites. The disease is one of the most common to affect sheep and is responsible for enormous financial loss to the sheep industry in the UK and indeed worldwide. Pneumonia may result in sudden death or in a long, drawn-out illness. It may therefore be the cause of much suffering to affected animals.

The function of the lungs is to transfer vital oxygen from inhaled air into the bloodstream and thence to all tissues and to every cell in the body. Oxygen is, of course, essential for life and so when lung tissue is damaged or destroyed by an attack of pneumonia, then less oxygen can be transferred to the bloodstream. It is rather like a motor vehicle firing on fewer cylinders than are provided. Performance is reduced and the animal becomes a poor food converter and therefore unthrifty and uneconomic.

Whilst pneumonia is a common condition, not every animal that puffs and pants has pneumonia. Rapid breathing may be a symptom of warm weather or of any disease which raises the body temperature. Dead animals are frequently sent to the knacker or hunt kennels, where a 'diagnosis' of pneumonia is offered by the staff. Such advice is frequently wrong and misleading and as a general rule should be ignored.

Pneumonia is often the ultimate cause of death in animals suffering from many other illnesses. If an animal is so weak that it cannot get up and move around, it is at serious risk. If it remains lying on one side the blood tends to 'pool' in the underside of the lungs and the tissues become devitalised through lack of oxygen. Microorganisms capable of producing pneumonia—which are commonly found in the respiratory tract of nearly all healthy animals—may then attack the lung and produce a rapidly fatal pneumonia. However, in this chapter we shall deal with pneumonia as a primary problem and look at the most important causes of the disease in sheep in the UK.

It is sometimes assumed that pneumonia is only a problem of housed sheep, but it is also very common in sheep on lowland, upland and hill grazings. Sheep of all ages can be affected, although different causes may be involved in the various classes.

415

Whilst some of the causal agents—for example, maedi-visna virus—are uncommon amongst the general sheep population, others, such as pasteurella, are very widespread indeed and can be detected in a large proportion of healthy sheep. Yet all sheep do not succumb to the disease and this leads to the conclusion that there must be other factors at work which in some way compromise the animal. Such factors are called predisposing causes and they play an important role in pneumonia, as they do in many other diseases (see Chapter 1). Sudden changes in the weather may be sufficient to trigger an outbreak of disease. A sudden move from bare grazing to lush aftermath, or the crowding of a flock into an inadequately ventilated shed may precipitate cases of pneumonia. In many instances the precise mechanisms of the predisposing causes are unknown but the circumstantial evidence is sufficiently strong to warrant avoiding action. Before making any change in husbandry or before carrying out any routine task consider the possible consequences. Always attempt to minimise stress to the flock or to the individual animal.

Pasteurellosis

Pasteurellosis is by far the most common cause of pneumonia in sheep. It is the name given to diseases caused by the group of bacteria called pasteurella, named after the brilliant French bacteriologist Louis Pasteur, who worked on—amongst many other things—the vaccination of poultry against fowl cholera, which is caused by a member of the pasteurella group. The bacterium responsible for pneumonia and other diseases in sheep is called *Pasteurella haemolytica* and, as previously noted, can be found in the respiratory tract of the majority of sheep without necessarily causing disease.

This bacterium exists in two forms called A and T and each of these is further divided to give a total of some 15 different types. The T form of pasteurellosis does not produce a pneumonia, but a septicaemia (blood infection) of young sheep, and it will be described later in this section.

CLINICAL SIGNS

Pasteurellosis type A can occur at any time of year and in any age of sheep, but is most common in the spring and early summer. In very young lambs the infection tends to be overwhelming, causing sudden death without any symptoms of pneumonia. In older lambs and adult sheep a true pneumonia develops. Often the first sign of trouble in a flock is a dead animal found by the shepherd on the morning round. Further deaths may occur over the next few days and careful observation may identify other animals in the flock which are showing symptoms of distress. These will include animals apart from the main flock, which do not graze and whose breathing may be difficult and noisy. They may lie with the neck stretched out to help

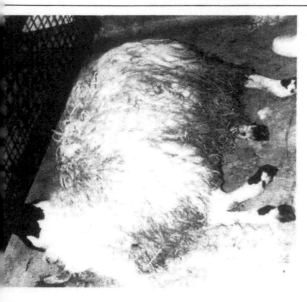

Plate 10.1   A young adult in the terminal stages of pasteurella pneumonia. Note how the head is thrown back due to difficulty in breathing. Animals in such a distressing condition should be humanely destroyed on the farm.

breathing and are usually very depressed (see Plate 10.1). Some may have a discharge from the nose and runny eyes. Animals which are near to death may froth at the mouth and often have great difficulty in breathing. They present a distressing sight. Such animals should be humanely destroyed and the carcass taken to the veterinary investigation laboratory so that a 'fresh' post-mortem can be carried out to arrive at an accurate diagnosis (see Colour plates 29 and 30).

TREATMENT

The farmer and his veterinary surgeon have some difficult decisions to make when a provisional diagnosis of pasteurellosis is made based on the recent movements of the flock and an examination of any sick animals. Should the flock have been moved recently—onto a lush silage aftermath, for example—then it may be prudent to move them back onto sparse keep and to reintroduce them to better grazing very gradually once the outbreak has subsided.

Drugs such as oxytetracycline are effective against pasteurella, but if the whole flock of ewes and lambs is brought in for treatment, with all the accompanying stress of gathering and mismothering, it is possible that further cases may be precipitated despite treatment. It may sometimes be more prudent to shepherd the flock closely, to draw out any animals which appear unwell with as little disruption of the flock as possible and to bring them close to home for treatment and observation. Since at least a week's treatment is necessary, long-acting antibiotics should be used to avoid unnecessary handling of the flock.

Animals which are very sick do not respond well to treatment. However, those which are detected early and nursed appropriately often make a good recovery following antibiotic and supportive treatment. Sick animals should be brought indoors if possible, or at least moved to a sheltered area. A temporary shelter outside can be constructed to protect them from wind and rain. If sheep are brought indoors, it is essential that they are put into a large, airy, clean and dry box, with generous straw bedding.

Clean, fresh water should be provided daily and, as many sick sheep will be off their food, they should be tempted with small amounts of fresh green material like cabbage leaves. Dry, dusty foods or mouldy hay should not be fed. No attempt should be made to drench sheep suffering from pneumonia, since the medicine is likely to go down the windpipe and kill the animal. Considerable patience and sympathy is needed to nurse animals back to health and they should not be released into the flock until they are fully fit and the weather agreeable.

If a nursing ewe is affected and her lambs are heavy enough, then they should be weaned. If an unweaned lamb is affected, its mother and any litter mates should be brought inside with it. Once the lamb is responding to treatment a supply of milk is likely to speed its recovery. Separating it from its mother and flock mates is likely to stress it further.

Animals which take a long time to recover and those which only partially recover are likely to have suffered considerable lung damage and are unlikely ever to thrive. Ewes, rams or ewe lambs in this category which were destined as flock replacements should not be retained for breeding but culled as soon as appropriate. Lambs so affected will take many weeks longer to finish and are unlikely to show a profit, so that early culling may sometimes be appropriate.

CONTROL AND PREVENTION

Prevention of pasteurella pneumonia depends first and foremost on attempting to avoid circumstances which may predispose to the disease. In flocks where the disease has caused only occasional deaths in the past, farmers may rely upon good husbandry practice to maintain a low level of disease. However, there is always a risk that a serious outbreak will occur if sheep are not vaccinated. In flocks where previous outbreaks have occurred or where shepherds wish to sleep more easily in their beds, then vaccination offers added security. Before discussing vaccination in detail, it is important to appreciate that on its own it is not sufficient. It thus remains important to be aware of the factors likely to make the flock vulnerable to disease.

Housing

Housing sheep may increase the likelihood of pasteurella and other pneumonias. Consider the possible stress put on the flock at the time of housing. Ewes in mid or late pregnancy are gathered and driven, penned up, foot bathed, condition scored, wormed, sorted into groups, kept in close proximity at high stocking rates and fed a different diet. In some cases they may also be sheared immediately after housing or a short time later. All these procedures are individually stressful and together they may tip the balance in favour of any disease-producing organisms present in the flock.

PI3 virus

A virus of sheep and cattle called *parainfluenza type 3* (PI3) is commonly present in a number of animals within a flock. On its own this normally produces a fairly mild disease, with symptoms which would usually go unnoticed by the shepherd. Under the special conditions of housing, the virus—which probably exists in carrier animals in the flock—tends to spread from sheep to sheep more easily than at pasture. This is because of the close proximity of animals and the considerable reduction in the movement of air in a building compared with outdoors.

Infection with this virus is known to increase the likelihood of pasteurella pneumonia and also to increase the severity of the disease. It is not difficult to imagine how a serious outbreak of pneumonia could occur in a flock under such adverse conditions. It therefore makes sense to attempt to minimise the risks by taking the precautions discussed in the section on housing and disease in Chapter 4.

Another pneumonia of sheep called jaagsiekte may also predispose them to pasteurella pneumonia, and this is discussed later in this chapter.

Transport

Sheep do not need to be housed to be stressed, however. Transportation is another hazardous operation, for similar reasons to those of housing. There are the added stresses of fear, discomfort and lack of food and water—often for considerable periods. Animals taken to market have the further disadvantage of being transported twice within a short time. They are also penned alongside sheep from other farms, carrying different microorganisms to which they may be totally susceptible, including those responsible for pneumonia.

A sudden improvement in feeding, such as when the flock is moved onto an aftermath, may precipitate an outbreak of pasteurella pneumonia. So too may a sudden change in the weather—particularly to warm, calm conditions.

Dipping

Many of the normal husbandry routines which have to be carried out on all farms may also present a risk. Dipping can be particularly stressful, especially if care is not taken to carry out the task properly. Problems can arise in several ways. Animals may be driven long distances in hot weather and plunged into a cold dipper without being allowed to stand in the shade and cool down beforehand. Others are dipped in inclement weather or roughly handled. The stress of the procedure can be sufficient to cause deaths and illness from pasteurella pneumonia. Occasionally sheep inhale the dip and die from pneumonia. 'Show' sheep are often dipped in phenolic dips. In this case the chemical is absorbed through the skin and if the concentration is too high this may produce a fatal pneumonia.

Other essential husbandry tasks such as castrating and tailing, worming and vaccinating, or indeed gathering and handling for any purpose, may precipitate an outbreak of pasteurella pneumonia. Every effort should, therefore, be taken to make all these procedures less stressful by careful advance planning and sympathetic handling.

VACCINATION AGAINST PASTEURELLA

In flocks where pasteurella pneumonia has been identified as a significant cause of loss in the past, your veterinary surgeon will probably recommend vaccination. Any vaccination programme should be tailor-made to suit your individual flock's requirements; otherwise inadequate or inappropriate cover may be provided. A few facts about pasteurella vaccines may help explain why it is not possible at present to guarantee full protection under all circumstances.

As explained earlier in this section, *Pasteurella haemolytica* exists in many different types (serotypes). Ideally, vaccines would provide cover against all of these types, but this has not proved possible to date. They do, however, contain the most important ones which are responsible for the majority of the outbreaks on farms within the UK and elsewhere.

What does all this mean to the farmer? It means that, at present, there is no way of ensuring 100% protection against pasteurella pneumonia. On the majority of farms, it is possible to give a very worthwhile level of protection, particularly where laboratory tests have shown that the pneumonia is caused by one of the serotypes present in the vaccine.

However, even if flocks are vaccinated, outbreaks may continue to occur for a number of reasons:

- Not all pneumonia is caused by pasteurella.
- Not all types of pasteurella are included in the vaccines at present and one of those missing may be causing disease in the flock—this can be confirmed only by laboratory diagnosis.
- Vaccination programmes may be inappropriately designed or incorrectly carried out.
- Management and/or climatic factors may be such as to present an overwhelming challenge of infection which swamps the protection afforded by the vaccine.

When so called 'breakdowns' do occur, they should be thoroughly investigated. Veterinary surgeons and pharmaceutical companies will treat complaints seriously and will attempt to determine if and why a product has failed to protect a flock adequately. It is therefore necessary to contact your veterinary surgeon immediately you suspect a problem and to submit fresh carcasses to the laboratory so that a diagnosis can be confirmed independently.

Ewes, gimmers and ewe hoggs—not forgetting the rams—should be protected initially with a primary course of two injections separated by a month to six weeks. Thereafter, annual boosters will be necessary. With breeding ewes this booster should be given in late pregnancy, preferably around four to six weeks before lambing is due. This will ensure that lambs which get adequate amounts of colostrum will be protected against type A pasteurellosis from birth until they are three or four weeks old.

Combined vaccine

Combined clostridial and pasteurella vaccines are available and because the timing of vaccinations against these diseases is similar, this method can represent a saving in cost and labour.

However, it must be remembered that whilst lambs will be protected against the clostridial diseases via colostrum from vaccinated ewes for up to three or four months, this is not so with pasteurella (see above). Lambs must therefore be protected from the time pasteurella immunity wanes until they are slaughtered, or until they join the adult vaccination programme. They must therefore be started on an active 'pasteurella only' vaccination scheme as early as possible.

Vaccines protecting against pasteurella only

Vaccines providing only pasteurella protection are available for use in flocks where the pasteurella risk is high and where additional booster doses are required. For instance, some hill farms experience deaths in ewes during the winter, especially where flocks are undernourished. It is essential to use a 'pasteurella only' vaccine in young lambs of just a few weeks of age, if they have sucked from vaccinated ewes. (Clostridial vaccination must **not** be carried out too early in life if the protective antibodies in colostrum are not to interfere with vaccination and vice versa. See notes on clostridial vaccination in Chapter 9.)

In vaccinated breeding flocks, the lambs should be given the first injection of a primary vaccination course against pasteurella only at around a fortnight old, followed by a second injection some three weeks later. This should protect them against *Pasteurella haemolytica* (type A) until either they are sold fat or—if they are to be kept as flock replacements—they are given a booster in late winter or early spring, in advance of the period of greatest risk (late spring to early summer).

If the ewe flock is not vaccinated against pasteurella, lambs are vulnerable from birth. Where the risk is appreciable this should be remedied before the next lambing period by vaccinating the ewe flock. In the meanwhile, lambs can be vaccinated at birth and as early as two weeks later with the second injection.

It should be remembered, however, that with so-called killed vaccines, such as those for pasteurella, it will take about two weeks for a protective level of immunity to build up following the second vaccination. This means that in vaccinated flocks, lambs are at risk from infection between four and seven weeks of age and in non-vaccinated flocks from birth to six weeks of age. There is little further that can be done about this. Pasteurella anti-serum—that is, ready-made antibodies for immediate protection, produced in the blood of another animal—is expensive and has not been shown to give satisfactory protection.

It always has to be borne in mind that in order to carry out all these various inoculations, the flock has to be gathered and animals individually handled, which is stressful in itself, particularly for ewes with lambs at foot. Careful planning can help avoid unnecessary handling by combining certain operations whenever it is safe to do so.

Unless bought-in animals have come from flocks on an official scheme which guarantees vaccination against the clostridial diseases and pasteurellosis (such as the Premium Sheep Health Scheme in Scotland), then it is always safer to assume that animals are unvaccinated and to start them on an appropriate scheme immediately. Remember that animals purchased from market, transported to a new farm and put on to good keep are prime candidates for pasteurellosis.

PI3 vaccination

Some veterinary surgeons may recommend the use of *parainfluenza type 3* virus vaccine in flocks where laboratory findings suggest that the virus may be playing an important role in predisposing a flock to pasteurella pneumonia. Whilst there is no evidence that PI3 vaccination prevents outbreaks of pasteurella pneumonia, work has shown that it may reduce the severity of the condition. Therefore under some circumstances it may make sense to vaccinate against PI3 virus as well as pasteurella.

Pasteurella T disease

Pasteurella haemolytica type T does not produce a pneumonia, but rather a septicaemia, which is an overwhelming infection that spreads to all parts of the body via the bloodstream. Older lambs and hoggs are the main victims, with the majority of cases occurring between early autumn and the turn of the year. It is a distinctly different disease from pneumonia, although outbreaks occur under similar circumstances and the two conditions can sometimes be confused.

The reason that outbreaks occur when they do is not understood. The typical pattern is for a number of sudden deaths to occur amongst a group of animals which have recently been moved onto improved feeding, such as lush autumn grazing, roots or forage crops, especially if the weather turns cold and wet, or if the sheep have been transported. Normally the outbreak is explosive, with a number of deaths occurring over a few days. Fatalities then peter out as the lambs or hoggs adapt to the better diet or because they are removed to poorer grazings in an attempt to control the outbreak.

CLINICAL SIGNS

It is unusual for sheep to show any signs of illness for long enough to be spotted by the shepherd. Those that do so will be lying down in great distress and will have difficulty breathing. Frothing at the mouth is a sign that death is imminent. As cases are so rarely seen, treatment is seldom attempted and is, in any case, likely to be of little or no avail.

CONTROL

As with pasteurella pneumonia it is difficult to decide what to do in the face of an outbreak. Discretion is probably the better part of valour. Rather than risk stressing sheep and precipitating further cases by gathering and injecting the whole flock with antibiotics, it is probably better to run them back onto some poorer grazing, leave them well alone and hope for the best. Reintroduction to the apparently offending crop must be done with great caution.

Just as with pasteurella pneumonia it is important to attempt to avoid situations which would appear to predispose to infection. Any introduction to better feeding must be done gradually, with limited access for short periods. Rather than simply allowing the flock to run back onto normal grazing, whilst on a rape break for example, they should be actively shepherded off the crop and the gate closed. Access to risky crops should be initially limited to an hour or two each day and then steadily increased daily until the sheep are acclimatised. If the weather turns bad, the risk appears to increase and some form of shelter close by is advantageous. Transportation, dipping and other stressful husbandry tasks all appear to increase the risks. Many are unavoidable, but forward planning may help to minimise handling and other disruptions.

Pasteurella vaccines are available which contain a T component, and if flocks are adequately vaccinated these should give some measure of protection.

Jaagsiekte

Jaagsiekte is the name given to a tumour of the lung of sheep, caused by a virus (retrovirus). The disease would appear to be relatively uncommon in Britain, but in Scotland there is a worrying level of infection which appears to be increasing. The reasons for these geographical differences in the distribution of the disease within the UK are unclear, but as the traffic in sheep is considerable, it is possible that jaagsiekte will eventually come to assume greater importance nationwide.

Jaagsiekte—otherwise known as sheep pulmonary adenomatosis or SPA—occurs in many other parts of the world. It derives its name from the Afrikaans for 'driving sickness' since it is most noticeable when sheep are being

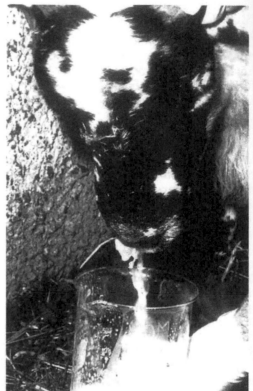

Plate 10.2 (*Below*) Scottish Halfbred ewes from a winter-housed flock showing clinical symptoms of jaagsiekte. Animals rapidly lose condition despite retaining their appetite.

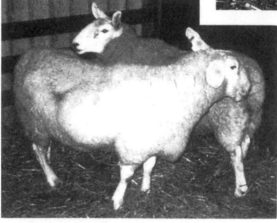

Plate 10.3 (*Above*) The wheelbarrow test for clinical diagnosis of jaagsiekte. Half a beakerful of lung fluid was collected from this ewe.

gathered or driven, affected animals tending to lag behind the rest of the flock. All breeds of sheep can become affected and although some appear to be more susceptible than others, this may be because of the predominance of a particular breed in an area, or because of particular sheep management systems.

424

CLINICAL SIGNS

Once a sheep becomes infected with the jaagsiekte virus it may be many months or years before any symptoms of disease become apparent, and the majority of cases are found in two or three year old animals. Affected sheep find it progressively more difficult to breathe as the tumour increases in size and takes over more and more of the vital lung tissue. In contrast to other forms of lung infection in sheep, jaagsiekte cases often remain relatively bright and alert and continue to eat until the final stages of the disease. The shepherd's suspicions that something is wrong may only be aroused when the flock is being gathered, when affected animals fall behind. On closer examination they are found to be breathing rapidly in an effort to get more oxygen through what little normal lung remains. Despite retaining their appetite, sheep will progressively lose condition (see Plate 10.2). In the terminal stages of the disease breathing is fast and shallow, even when the animal is resting.

Jaagsiekte is always fatal. Sheep may die from the effects of the tumour, or they may succumb to other infections—to pasteurella pneumonia in particular—as a result of being seriously compromised by the tumour. From the time the shepherd notices that the animal is unwell, it may be days, weeks or months before death occurs. No treatment will have any effect upon the tumour and this observation is helpful in deciding upon a diagnosis of jaagsiekte, since it is frequently confused with other chronic pneumonias which may respond to antibiotic treatment and are not necessarily fatal.

Another aid to diagnosis is to lift up the hind legs so that the sheep is held like a wheelbarrow. In well-established cases of jaagsiekte a variable amount of frothy fluid will flow from the tumour-affected lung down the nostrils. In some cases there is relatively little, but in others up to half a pint or more may be obtained (see Plate 10.3). A definite diagnosis can be arrived at only following post-mortem examination as there is no definitive diagnostic test available in the living animal.

In Scotland at least, jaagsiekte is recognised as an important predisposing cause of pasteurella pneumonia. In a number of flocks where pasteurella has been a problem and it has been controlled to a large extent by the use of vaccination programmes, cases of pneumonia have continued to occur. Some have been identified as jaagsiekte and it is suspected that in these flocks an underlying jaagsiekte infection has been partly responsible for the pasteurella problem. It is also possible that infection with jaagsiekte may predispose to maedi-visna.

CONTROL AND PREVENTION

Advice on the control of jaagsiekte presents some problems for a number of reasons. Scientists do not have a complete understanding of the virus or of how it is transmitted. As there is no diagnostic test to enable your veterinary surgeon to identify infected animals in the early stages of the

425

disease, the risk of spread of infection within the flock is increased, since infected animals may be discharging the virus into the environment. Also there is no treatment for the tumour and no vaccine available.

What is known is that the virus responsible for jaagsiekte is present in large quantities in the fluid which accumulates in the lung tumours of infected animals and that this fluid is thus a potential risk to other animals. For example, when an infected animal coughs, the fluid is distributed in aerosol form into the atmosphere and may then be inhaled by uninfected animals in close contact. For this reason jaagsiekte is thought to be more common in flocks which house ewes overwinter or for a period over lambing, although it also occurs in flocks at pasture.

It is therefore important to isolate any suspected cases immediately and, since the disease is always fatal, to have them slaughtered and a full post-mortem examination carried out. The lambs of infected ewes are probably at some risk because of close contact with their mothers. They should therefore be identified in some way for future reference. As far as is known, lambs are not infected in the womb and can be reared artificially away from their mothers, as is done in some countries for the control of maedi-visna. However, this method of control presents obvious practical problems for many flocks and has not been adequately evaluated in the field to date.

The disease is introduced into uninfected flocks through the purchase of infected animals. This may mean sheep of any age—lambs, hoggs, gimmers, ewes or rams—since although the clinical disease occurs principally in two and three year olds, it can also occur in younger or older sheep.

If it is not possible to keep a closed flock, it is obviously desirable to purchase replacements from flocks considered free from jaagsiekte. Unfortunately, at present it is not possible to identify such flocks. This problem is not likely to be solved until the advent of a diagnostic test for the disease.

In the meanwhile the State Veterinary Service offers a scheme—the Sheep and Goat Health Scheme—whose aim is to provide a pool of sheep flocks and goat herds of recognised health status. This is a monitoring scheme with various categories of membership. In Category I—the maedi-visna accreditation scheme—there are additional monitoring services which include jaagsiekte. This will involve (1) an annual clinical inspection of the flock and inspection of flock records, (2) two slaughterhouse inspections each year of the lungs of mature sheep and (3) an annual inspection of two to five year old animals intended for culling and sale. Whilst this will not guarantee a flock free from jaagsiekte, it should reduce the risk for purchasers. Should a diagnostic test eventually become available, then a much higher health status could be achieved.

Flock owners in the south and east of Scotland, where jaagsiekte is most prevalent, should always have this disease at the forefront of their minds. Wherever a pneumonia-like condition occurs in the flock it should be investigated and dealt with promptly. Sheep owners in other parts of the UK should always have the disease at the back of their minds.

Just as it is important to try to avoid purchasing infected animals, responsible flock owners should never knowingly sell, through a market or privately, any sheep they suspect to be infected. This, of course, applies to any infectious disease.

It should be noted that goats may also become infected with jaagsiekte, although it has been recorded only rarely.

Maedi-visna

Maedi-visna is a virus disease of sheep that has only recently been reported in the UK, although it has been recognised in many other parts of the world since the end of the last century. The name derives from two Icelandic words—maedi, meaning 'difficult breathing', and visna, meaning 'wasting'—the former referring to a progressive pneumonia and the latter to a nervous form of the disease. In some countries, such as the United States and Holland, a mastitis caused by the same virus has been reported and cases of arthritis have also arisen. Until very recently only the pneumonia—maedi—had been reported in the UK. However, at the time of going to press an outbreak of the full-blown disease has been reported, including the nervous symptoms, and this is a worrying—although predicted— turn of events.

The virus responsible for maedi-visna is from the same stable as the one which causes jaagsiekte. In common with that disease there is a long period from the time of infection to the onset of the clinical symptoms; it is uncommon for sick animals to be detected in a flock before they are four or five years old, even if they become infected as baby lambs.

There are probably two main ways in which the disease spreads within a flock once it has been introduced through the purchase of infected animals. The first, and probably the most important, is via the colostrum or milk of infected ewes, which contains the virus and therefore infects lambs when they suck (lambs are rarely, if ever, infected before birth). The second is via the aerosol droplets coughed or sneezed out by infected animals. This method of spread is likely to be much more important under intensive systems of management and particularly when the flock is housed over the whole winter, since the period of close contact is more prolonged. It has been observed in both Holland and the UK that if jaagsiekte is present in a flock, the rate of spread of maedi-visna, via secretions from the nose and mouth, is increased.

CLINICAL SIGNS

Symptoms of maedi pneumonia are vague initially, animals simply losing body condition. As the disease progresses, affected animals will lag behind the rest of the flock when driven and breathing will become more and more laboured. The disease may linger on for many months or even a year or more, until eventually sheep show great difficulty in breathing, even when lying down. The disease is invariably fatal and no treatment is available.

Often the extent of maedi-visna within a flock is underestimated, because affected ewes which lose body condition may be culled prematurely. This, of course, leads to increased ewe replacement costs and is a significant loss in flocks where the level of infection is high. Affected ewes also have a reduced lambing percentage. Diagnosis can be confirmed by blood sampling.

CONTROL

Control of maedi-visna in the UK is voluntary and the State Veterinary Service operates a Sheep and Goat Health Scheme which encompasses maedi-visna. Its aims are to provide a pool of sheep flocks and goat herds of recognised health status. The scheme for maedi-visna (category I membership) is based on identification, by blood sampling and slaughter, of infected animals and of all offspring which have sucked infected ewes. An official register is kept of flocks which attain accredited status.

The official scheme came into operation in 1982 and it is likely to have checked the spread of infection to a degree amongst pedigree 'exotic' breeds, whence the disease emanated through importations from continental Europe in the early 1970s. However, before the official scheme was implemented, the virus had already become disseminated amongst an indeterminate number of commercial flocks, through the purchase of sheep from infected pedigree flocks. Whilst accredited status will be of most interest to pedigree flock owners who wish to sell maedi-free stock, commercial sheep farmers who wish to do so may also join the scheme or otherwise consult their veterinary surgeon about alternative methods of control. The choice may depend to some extent upon the level of infection within the flock and the costs and convenience of the alternatives.

Dutch control methods

Two interesting alternative control schemes have been evaluated in Holland. One is based upon the fact that lambs are born free from maedi-visna and the other on the observation that young ewes are less likely to infect their lambs via colostrum and milk than are older ewes. In the first scheme, lambing takes place indoors and is closely shepherded 24 hours a day. All lambs are 'snatched' immediately they are born onto a clean plastic sheet and removed promptly from their mothers to a separate unit where they are fed artificially. For the first day lambs are given cow's colostrum and are subsequently fed ewe milk replacer, with hay and concentrates introduced at two weeks of age. After weaning, lambs are kept isolated from all other sheep and form the basis of a maedi-visna-free flock. Dutch experience has shown this to be a feasible, rapid and reliable method, but, it has to be said, a laborious and somewhat expensive one.

The second alternative consists of separating the youngest ewes in the flock—ewe lambs or gimmers—and lambing them in isolation from the rest of the mature flock. Lambs are suckled normally, but kept separate from the rest of the lamb flock post-weaning. In subsequent years, lambs out of young ewes are added to this group and it is possible to build up a flock with a very low incidence of maedi-visna in a comparatively short time and with a minimum of expense. If disease free status is then desired, this can follow by the normal method of blood testing and the slaughter of a reduced number of reactors. It should be pointed out that accredited status can only be achieved via the official Sheep and Goat Health Scheme, details of which can be obtained through your veterinary surgeon or local divisional veterinary officer of MAFF.

Views are sometimes expressed in the farming press and elsewhere about the wisdom of spending public money on the control of maedi-visna—often, it has to be said, by people with no training or experience in animal health or disease control. Whilst it is accepted that relatively few clinical cases have been identified in the UK to date, it would nevertheless seem reasonable to attempt to contain this disease in its infancy, rather than to have to deal with it when the infection in the national flock has reached a high level. The experience of other countries—particularly Iceland, where the disease assumed catastrophic proportions, albeit under more intensive husbandry conditions—suggests that a relatively small sum spent now may pay handsome dividends later. In the light of the most recent events referred to earlier, it would seem wise to consider reinforcing the present low-key measures in place for the control of this important disease.

CAPRINE ARTHRITIS ENCEPHALITIS (CAE)

This is a virus infection of goats which is distinct from, but closely similar to, the maedi-visna virus of sheep. In fact, the two infections cannot be distinguished from each other on a blood test, but only after subsequent laboratory tests. There have been some recent reports that this goat virus has been isolated from sheep and to that end the Sheep and Goat Health Scheme encompasses CAE. Goat colostrum is sometimes used to feed lambs, and whilst it is a good substitute for ewe colostrum, it should not be fed to sheep unless the goat herd is tested and free from CAE. Otherwise this technique could introduce the disease to a sheep flock. A recent report from New Zealand states that clinical disease has been diagnosed in lambs fed on goat colostrum containing the CAE virus.

Atypical Pneumonia

From time to time outbreaks of pneumonia occur in groups of older lambs and hoggs which cannot be slotted into any of the neat categories we have discussed so far in this chapter. Despite the fact that deaths are uncommon and symptoms are generally mild, these outbreaks often affect a large

429

proportion of the flock—up to a half in some cases—and are the cause of significant economic loss to the farmer.

These pneumonias are usually referred to as 'atypical' and usually affect sheep in their first year of life. The infection usually affects the lower forward areas of the lung and causes a chronic or long-standing disease. Deaths are uncommon, but the animals have a depressed appetite and a poor feed conversion and tend in consequence to take much longer to reach marketable weight.

Shepherds are often aware of coughing amongst a group of young sheep, particularly when they are settling down after being gathered, or in the quiet of an evening when a group of hoggs is on the rape or turnip break or resting in a sheep house. The majority of animals seem to be little affected, in that they continue to graze and do not show obvious signs of illness, apart perhaps from a little shortness of breath after exercise, or some discharge from the nose in a few cases.

Farmers and shepherds, therefore, often tend to ignore or overlook the situation. Even when it becomes obvious that lambs or hoggs are not thriving the problem is often put down to gut or lungworms, or to poorer-quality grazing. Whilst these may well play a role in some cases, the underlying pneumonia frequently goes unrecognised.

Outbreaks of this type of pneumonia are uncommon in extensively managed flocks and mainly affect lowland sheep, particularly where stocking rates are high or sheep are housed. The worst outbreaks often occur if groups of lambs or hoggs are bought from market or from various sources and are mixed. Under these circumstances a proportion of sheep may become sufficiently ill to require treatment and occasionally animals may die. This occurs particularly when *Pasteurella haemolytica* becomes involved in the outbreak. However, outbreaks may still occur without the introduction of 'foreign' animals. Home-bred lambs, housed or crowded onto a root-crop break for fattening, are subjected to close contact which aids the spread of the microorganisms which cause this disease and which are always present in a proportion of animals within a flock.

CAUSAL AGENTS

The most important microorganism involved in these atypical pneumonia outbreaks is called *Mycoplasma ovipneumoniae* and, as already intimated, *Pasteurella haemolytica* also plays an important role. It is possible that in some instances the initial damage may be due to a virus—parainfluenza type 3, which appears to affect the majority of young sheep in most flocks, once the protective effect of colostrum has waned.

These infections, particularly those due to mycoplasma, do not generally progress relentlessly to the point where the animal is really ill or its life is threatened, but they do produce sufficient damage to the lungs to stunt growth significantly. Appetite may be dulled and both feed conversion efficiency and daily bodyweight gain are adversely affected (see Colour plates 31 and 32).

TREATMENT AND CONTROL

Treatment of individual lambs or of hoggs which may be more seriously affected will involve the use of antibiotics and other supportive measures as prescribed by your veterinary surgeon. Such lambs should be separated from the flock and housed in a bright, airy box. It is seldom thought necessary or desirable to treat the whole flock with antibiotics, but management changes should be made to lessen the risks. Stocking rates should be reduced to minimise the chances of spread of infection from close contact. If animals are housed, the number per pen and per house should be reduced, if feasible. Any changes which can be made to improve the ventilation should be beneficial.

PREVENTION

Prevention of infection under intensive systems is difficult and the aim should be to reduce the risks to a minimum. Via the colostrum of their dams, lambs should be protected to a degree against the challenge from the specific organisms present on any individual farm. This protection will last for only a few weeks, however. Remember also that purchased animals may well be susceptible to the new population of microorganisms they will meet on your farm.

Heavy stocking rates should be avoided, especially where hoggs are being fattened on rape or swedes in a fairly confined area. Sheep should be provided with a reasonable area of 'run-back' grazing to avoid overcrowding and to provide shelter. If animals are purchased from different sources, they should be kept separately until they have settled down and fully recovered from the stresses of transportation, marketing, a fresh diet and a new environment. Occasionally—usually because of a previous history of pneumonia—antibiotics may be given to all purchased and home-bred animals if they are to be mixed. However, this is an undesirable and costly practice and should be avoided, where possible, by altering the management appropriately.

When animals are to be housed over the rearing or fattening period, the risk of pneumonia is much greater. Purchased sheep from different sources should be housed separately and preferably in a different air space. Where a separate building is not available, sheep from different sources should be kept in separate pens. The stocking rate in pens and the maximum number of animals per pen and in a given air space are crucially important factors. Apart from the close proximity of animals with the attendant risk of cross-infection by aerosol droplets, high concentrations of sheep in a building lead to a build-up of ammonia from urine, which is an irritant to the respiratory system. To prevent a build-up of ammonia in the atmosphere, reduce the

431

stocking rate and provide a generous supply of clean, dry and mould free straw bedding. Ventilation should provide a free flow of air above the animals without draughts at animal level. If these conditions are provided, there should be no build-up of foul air (see Plate 10.4).

There is no evidence that vaccination against *Pasteurella haemolytica* or parainfluenza type 3 virus provides any protection against atypical pneumonia.

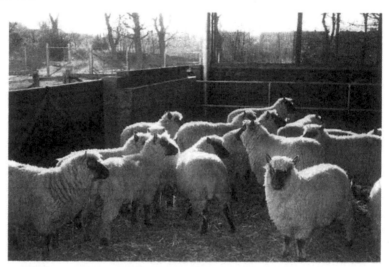

Plate 10.4   Clun Forest lambs (*above*) and Suffolk cross lambs (*below*) finishing indoors in comfortable, airy accommodation. Animals from different sources or of different ages should not be mixed and should never be overcrowded.

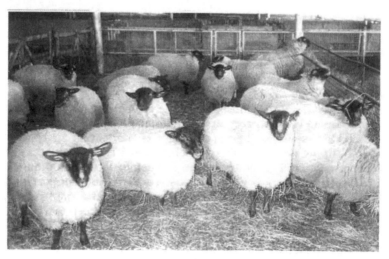

Lungworm

arasitic bronchitis, or lungworm, is principally a disease of young sheep
a their first grazing season and occurs during the late summer and autumn.
'he parasite most commonly responsible is a lungworm called *Dictyocaulus
laria*, which is closely related to the lungworm of cattle (husk). In the UK
t least, it is much less of a problem to sheep than its 'cousin' is to cattle.

IFE CYCLE

'he adult lungworms live in the main airways of the lung—the trachea and
ronchi—and may grow to a length of two or three inches (see Plate 10.5).
'he worms cause irritation which results in coughing, and the mucus coughed
p contains the eggs or larvae laid by the adult female worms which are
hen swallowed. Eggs which do not hatch into larvae in the air passages
o so in the gut, and thus only lungworm larvae are found in the faeces of
heep. These larvae are not immediately infectious to other sheep, but must
evelop during their first week of life on pasture—providing the weather is
easonably warm and moist—into infective, third stage larvae. These then
rawl out of the faeces and onto the herbage so that they can be devoured
y other sheep.

Once inside their new host the larvae burrow through the lining of
he small intestine and are carried, first by the lymph and then by the
loodstream, to the heart and thence to the lungs. This tortuous journey
akes around a week and during this time the larvae develop further into a

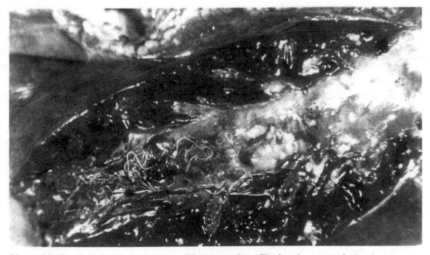

Plate 10.5   Adult lungworms—*Dictyocaulus filaria*—in one of the larger
air passages (a bronchus) of a sheep's lung.

433

fourth stage. From the tiny air sacs of the lungs the larvae migrate furthe and further up the respiratory tree until they reach the bronchi and trachea Here they mature to become fully grown adults within about a month o being swallowed by the sheep.

CLINICAL SIGNS

The journey of the larvae through the finest air passages of the lun; produces damage which causes the sheep to cough a little, but the wors effects are produced by the adult worms in the main airways, which ma become severely inflamed. Not all the eggs or larvae are coughed out an some may be breathed down into the deep recesses of the lung. This ma produce a severe reaction resulting in pneumonia. Sheep affected in thi way have a persistent cough and some difficulty in breathing and may los body condition. If the pneumonia is severe, death can occur.

Fortunately, however, the majority of cases of lungworm infection i sheep are relatively mild, Providing lambs are well fed and thriving an providing the stocking rate is reasonable (so as to avoid overwhelmin; challenge), they usually throw off the infection, becoming immune t further challenge in the process.

ANTHELMINTIC TREATMENT

Treatment of lungworm necessitates the use of appropriate anthelmintic which are effective against *Dictyocaulus filaria* as well as the gut worm: causing parasitic gastro-enteritis. The benzamidazoles and levamisole ar suitable, but it is uncommon for specific treatments to be necessary fo lungworm, since the regimes used for the control of gutworms also dea with lungworms.

If no adequate gutworm control regime is in operation, the risk of lung- worm increases. If infection occurs in this situation, a suitable anthelmintic should be used on all animals in the group. Lambs should then be moved to clean pasture and the dose of anthelmintic repeated three weeks later.

A number of other parasitic worms affect the respiratory system of sheep in the UK, and although they are very common, they are considered even less damaging than *Dictyocaulus filaria*. The two most often encountered at post-mortem are *Muellerius capillaris* and *Protostrongylus rufescens*. Both employ an intermediate host, either a snail or a slug, in their life cycle. The sheep must accidentally eat these in order to become infected and so complete the life cycle.

11

TRACE ELEMENTS, MINERALS, VITAMINS AND WATER

ESSENTIAL ELEMENTS

A large number of chemical elements are found in the sheep's body, some of which do not appear to have any particularly obvious function, whilst others play a vital role in maintaining health and productivity. The latter are referred to as essential **elements** and are usually divided into two groups, based on the amounts which are required by the animal. Thus, the **minerals** are needed in relatively large amounts, whilst the **trace elements** in only very small quantities or traces.

Normally these essential elements are needed on a daily basis and the requirements for each individual element have been carefully estimated for the different species of animals at different stages of growth and production. The body can often cope—for a short time at least—with small fluctuations in supply, but both deficiencies or excesses of these elements may have profound effects in the longer term.

DEPOTS

Some of these chemical elements are required by the animal on a regular daily basis because they are not stored in the body—sodium and potassium are examples. However, many of the minerals and trace elements are stored in various parts of the body for use as and when required. The liver, for example, is an important storage organ for many of the trace elements. The skeleton is a living and rapidly changing tissue which not only provides a scaffolding to support and protect the soft tissues and an anchor for tendons and muscles, but also acts as a reservoir for many of the minerals, such as calcium, phosphorous and magnesium. When levels of certain of these chemicals in the soft tissues become abnormally low, they can then be transferred from the skeleton to the muscles, liver, kidneys or to wherever they are required, by the transporting tissue—the blood. This process also acts in reverse, the blood transporting these substances from the gut and other tissues to the skeleton. This process is in a constant state of flux in an attempt to keep levels as near normal as possible at all times and in all tissues of the body.

435

The blood has requirements of its own for minerals and trace element and because it is the main transport medium and can so easily be sampled it is frequently used by veterinary surgeons to monitor the levels of these and other substances which it carries. The levels in blood may not always be the best indicator of a deficiency or excess of a particular mineral or trace element, however, and samples of other soft tissues, or of the skeleton itself, may be necessary. In these circumstances a plug of liver or kidney or a sample of bone can be obtained by a technique called biopsy, which necessitates the use of local or general anaesthesia.

DIET

The diet of an animal, whether it is grazing at pasture or receiving concentrate ration indoors, is a complex mixture of chemical substances comprising water, carbohydrates, fats, proteins, vitamins, minerals and trace elements. It is no simple matter for the farmer to provide a diet which is both palatable to the animal and ideally balanced to suit a particular class of stock so as to produce adequate growth or reproductive performance All the components of a ration interact with each other and many of the problems which arise due to deficiency (too little) or toxicity (too much of one or more chemical elements in the diet, arise from these interactions Some specific problems will be discussed in detail later in this chapter.

GRAZING

The sheep worldwide is predominantly a grazing animal. Under most systems of management in the UK lambing takes place in the spring, around the time when grass growth is anticipated. Apart from a period of six to eight weeks prior to lambing and perhaps for the first month of lactation when ewes receive concentrates to balance their basic diet of hay or silage grass provides the total ration of many flocks. If ewes are not housed during winter or over lambing, grass remains a significant part of the whole diet even when concentrates are provided. The quality of grazing is therefore of paramount importance to sheep at almost all times of the year and if no fresh grass, then conserved grass in the form of hay or silage.

Grass is a very variable crop. Its nutritional quality—including the content of minerals, trace elements and vitamins—will depend on a great number of factors. The type of land, the climate, season of year, manuring policy, seeds mixture, stage of growth, age of sward and grazing pressure are just some of these factors. With conserved grass crops the stage at which the crop is cut, the amount of weathering it receives, the method of harvesting and the conditions of storage will all influence the nutritional value of the crop.

When sheep are at pasture, it is very difficult (if not impossible) to estimate whether grazing is providing their requirements in terms of minerals and trace elements. In areas where deficiencies of one or more elements

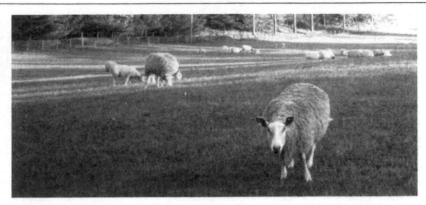

Plate 11.1   For most of the year sheep flocks in the UK depend on grazing or conserved grass—with its very variable mineral, trace element and vitamin analysis.

have been identified, that is a starting point from which the shortage can be rectified by one means or another. However, on many farms these facts are not known. It is probable that many grazings are inadequate in one or more of these important elements, at least at some stage during the year.

DIAGNOSIS OF DEFICIENCY

Where there is some suspicion that a deficiency (or a toxicity) exists, then some sophisticated detective work is required to confirm or refute the suspicion. This may involve the use of a number of different techniques which, although of limited value individually, may yield an answer collectively. An analysis of the mineral and trace element status of a representative sample of the herbage on offer may reveal that an element is in poor or inadequate supply. It will not reveal how available the element is to the animal once the food is digested. Similarly, the soil can be sampled for minerals and trace elements, but their availability to the plant will depend on many other factors.

Animals can be examined clinically and samples, such as blood, urine or faeces, can be taken for biochemical or other analyses. Animals which die or are destroyed may be examined at post-mortem. These examinations should give a clue as to whether or not there is a problem. Where information is available from a representative sample of the flock—say 10%— then it may be possible to say with some confidence that a deficiency exists.

However, only when the suspected deficiency is corrected and a positive response from the animals is obtained following treatment, can we be confident that the diagnosis was correct. This type of diagnosis by trial and error is a very valuable one in deficiency states. However, wherever possible, an untreated 'control' group should be included in such on-farm trials. This is necessary because some conditions will clear up spontaneously without treatment. This cannot be determined without including an untreated group grazing alongside the treated animals for comparison. An alternative method is to treat a small group first, before medicating the whole flock and observing the effects. This is often done in the case of suspected cobalt deficiency. Where the response is rapid, holding back treatment from the rest of the flock meanwhile is not likely to be too detrimental.

Diagnosis of mineral, trace element and vitamin deficiencies can often be confused with other conditions which may mimic the often vague clinical signs. For example, parasitic worm burdens or underfeeding may lead to unthriftiness reminiscent of that induced by the depressed appetite of cobalt deficiency. These conditions may, of course, exist at the same time. Treatment of a deficiency by supplementation may be largely wasted unless these other problems are corrected simultaneously.

Before embarking upon any treatment or control measures, an accurate diagnosis must be obtained. Implementing corrective measures when a suspected deficiency does not in fact exist may lead to poisoning—for example, both copper and selenium are highly toxic in excess.

CORRECTING DEFICIENCIES

The correction of existing deficiencies and their prevention in future may be attempted in a number of different ways. The farming system and methods of husbandry employed, the estimated economic importance of the deficiency and the particular element or elements involved are some of the factors which may influence the decision. It is unlikely that one method will be suitable for all farms and so any corrective measures must be chosen to suit the particular circumstances.

Correction can be attempted by indirect methods, such as the treatment of soil or herbage, but these are unlikely to be of any practical use under extensive conditions. Even under more favourable circumstances, this method may not be feasible. For example, the spraying of cobalt sulphate on highly alkaline or calcareous soils would be largely wasted since the uptake of cobalt by plants under such conditions is very poor. For this reason it is advisable to avoid liming prior to cobalt treatment.

Where sheep are receiving some portion of their ration as a concentrate feed, then some minerals and trace elements can be added to this—provided they are not excessively toxic, like copper. As long as the mix is appropriate and palatable and adequate trough space is available, this can be a good method for supplementing with a whole range of elements. Home-prepared rations should be thoroughly and carefully mixed and mineral and trace element analysis should be obtained from the manufacturer of compounded feeds. However, even this method cannot account for the slow or fussy eater or the animal which has a depressed appetite and fails to eat enough to satisfy its bodily requirements.

For most sheep systems, supplementation of the concentrate ration is only feasible for a few weeks each year and the problem remains of how best

o supplement sheep directly at pasture. This is, after all, the time when supplementation is most likely to be necessary. When sheep are indoors on concentrates plus hay or silage, the ration can be much more easily balanced
and controlled. Grazing is more likely to be inadequate in one way or another
and the minerals and trace elements in plant material generally are much less
readily available to the animal than they are in an inorganic supplement added
to a concentrate ration.

A bewildering range of products is available to the farmer—licks,
water dispensers, feed blocks and anthelmintics (wormers) laced with
various elements, injections of solutions or pastes, boluses made of soluble
glass or metal, gelatin capsules and free-access mineral and trace element
mixtures. The sales of such products are enormous and, like anthelmintics,
a large proportion of them are used incorrectly, inefficiently and even
dangerously.

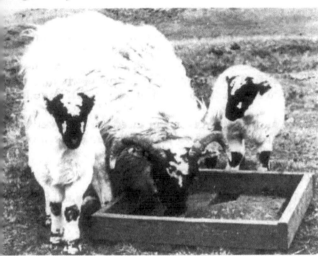

Plate 11.2   Scottish
Blackface ewe with
twin lambs eating a
feed block. This
breed is more
susceptible to copper
deficiency than, for
example, the Welsh
Mountain. Blocks and
concentrates contain
available copper.

Free-access products

As a generalisation, free-access products are not a satisfactory way of
providing essential elements. It is a fallacy that sheep will actively seek
out and eat the minerals or trace elements that are deficient in their diet.
The main reason why sheep (or cattle) eat free-access minerals is that they
like the taste of them! Most mixtures are purposely made palatable because
many of the minerals are unpalatable, magnesium being an example. Thus,
stock often tend to consume free-access minerals to excess, which is both
wasteful, costly and sometimes dangerous. Mineral licks are similarly
unsatisfactory since the vast majority of the lick is common salt, which
is highly palatable to stock and is therefore used as a carrier for the other
minerals. These proprietary products often contain minerals which are

439

being adequately supplied already from the grazings, or else they do not contain those which are deficient.

It is important to try to identify the needs of a particular flock on a particular farm and to supplement with minerals and trace elements as accurately as possible. The 'shot-gun' approach, as is so frequently advocated by the 'free-access' salesmen, is inappropriate. Before making any bulk purchases, always consult your veterinary surgeon about the most effective safe and cost-beneficial way of supplementing the flock feed. If you suspect that there may be a specific deficiency problem in your flock, then the initial outlay for a veterinary investigation with laboratory backup will cost very little and may save you ten-fold in unnecessary proprietary products. You are also more likely to control the problem (if indeed one exists) by the use of specific control measures rather than by the blunderbuss approach.

VITAMINS

Vitamins are essential organic chemicals required in very small amounts daily by both plants and animals for normal growth and health. It was not until this century that they were called—rather misleadingly—vital amines or vitamins. They were identified by letters of the alphabet before their complex chemical structures were elucidated and these are still commonly used.

Only vitamins which cause particular problems in sheep are discussed here. For further details, the reader is referred to texts on animal nutrition.

HYPOCALCAEMIA AND HYPOMAGNESAEMIA

The two important mineral deficiency disorders of the pregnant and lactating ewe—hypocalcaemia and hypomagnesaemia—are dealt with more appropriately in Chapter 6.

Swayback and Other Copper Deficiency Problems

In the UK the most commonly experienced clinical disorder of sheep related to a dietary deficiency of copper is swayback in lambs. However this obvious and distressing disease is probably only part of the story since less obvious, although probably more economically significant manifestations of copper deficiency are also likely to be at work in the flock.

Swayback takes its name from the incoordination shown by affected lambs, which causes them to sway about as they attempt to walk. This and the other symptoms of the disease described below are due to a lack of available copper in the diet of the pregnant ewe, which leads to defects of the nervous system of the developing lamb. This causes the congenital form of the disease—that is, lambs are born with the symptoms of swayback.

440

)ther lambs in the flock, although they may have had inadequate amounts
f copper during development, may be born apparently normal. However,
fter birth they may continue to receive inadequate supplies of copper in
ıe milk from their mothers or from any herbage they are also grazing. The
ffect of copper deficiency during late foetal life and immediately after birth
ıay lead to symptoms of swayback developing at a few weeks or months
f age—so-called **delayed swayback**.

It is also apparent from recent studies that other apparently healthy
ımbs in the flock may also be copper deficient, albeit not so severely as
ɔ produce nervous symptoms, but sufficiently to compromise their ability
ɔ resist the other diseases of early life and to inhibit their growth rate (see
ıter).

)IRECT AND INDIRECT COPPER DEFICIENCY

:opper deficiency may arise either because the soil and therefore the herbage
ɪn an area have a very low copper content, or because the copper present is
ɪnavailable to the grazing animal because of the presence of other chemical
lements which interfere with its availability. The most frequent offenders
ɪn this latter respect are **molybdenum**, **sulphur** and **iron**, but others such
ɪs zinc and lead may also give rise to problems. Where copper levels in
ɪe soil are marginal, sheep may run into difficulties, especially in the
ʋinter months when grazing is in short supply, because of the amount of
ɔil they ingest. This may occur because of close grazing or by soiling of
ɪe herbage through poaching, which increases the amount of inhibitory
ɪinerals ingested, particularly iron.

Under normal circumstances only about one-twentieth of the copper
ɪresent in the diet is absorbed through the lining of the gut into the blood-
tream and thence to all parts of the body where required. If high levels of
ɪnolybdenum or sulphur are present, this poor rate of absorption is roughly
ɪalved again. In the UK this molybdenum effect is most obvious on the
teart' pastures of Somerset, where severe symptoms of copper deficiency
ɔccur—predominantly in cattle—because of very high molybdenum levels
ɪn the soil.

MPROVED GRAZINGS

)ver the past few decades considerable acreages of hill and upland
ɪastures have been improved by drainage, ploughing and reseeding and
ɪy correcting the acidity (pH) of the soil by liming. This has resulted in
ɪ greatly increased level of production and has made much more viable
ɪnits of many hill farms which previously had little or no in-bye ground.
ɪowever, as with most benefits, there are some disadvantages and in this
:ase one is that the herbage on improved ground usually has a significantly
ɪeduced copper availability. Reseeding, often with a limited number of
ɪpecies, reduces the range of copper-rich grasses and other plant species

in the sward. Liming tends to increase the uptake of molybdenum from the soil by plants, so reducing copper availability to the grazing animal (see Colour plate 33).

Once understood, these problems can be corrected at a cost. If not appreciated, the losses from swayback and the less obvious forms of copper deficiency can be very substantial on farms depending on improved ground for grazing ewes during pregnancy, around lambing and during lactation.

COPPER IN FOODSTUFFS

Foodstuffs vary considerably in the amount of copper they contain and more importantly, on its availability to the animal once eaten. Fresh grass—especially lush, well-fertilised swards low in copper and rich in protein (and therefore also rich in sulphur)—often has much less available copper than conserved fodder. Hay, being made from mature swards with lower protein levels, contains less sulphur and thus more of its copper content is available to the sheep. It is also thought that molybdenum has less of an antagonistic effect on copper availability in hay than in fresh grass.

Silage

Silage is usually a reasonably good source of available copper, despite the fact that it is often made from lush, high-protein grass. However, the making of the silage is also important. There are a number of opportunities during the process when soil contamination can occur, and this should be reduced to a minimum since, as already mentioned, other minerals in the soil interfere with copper availability. If silage preservatives are used, it is probably better to avoid sulphuric acid because of its high sulphur content unless copper has been added to the product. Formaldehyde not only contains no sulphur, but also to some extent inactivates the sulphur already present in the herbage, so it is a better choice.

Root crops are generally low in available copper, although leafy brassicas, such as rape, kale and cabbage, have good levels of available copper as do cereals.

The housing of ewes overwinter, during the last third of pregnancy, may significantly reduce the risk of copper deficiency since they are generally fed a diet of hay, silage or straw, supplemented with a concentrate in the six to eight weeks before lambing. These feeds should supply sufficient available copper; hence ewes rarely need copper supplementation under these conditions.

Late pregnancy and lactation

During the last two months of pregnancy the lamb's nervous system is developing and the ewe's requirements for copper are increased dramatically. For example, a ewe carrying twins in late pregnancy requires roughly three times more copper than an empty, dry ewe. Once she starts milking er requirements double again. Colostrum from well-fed ewes usually ontains high levels of copper. However, levels in milk fall rapidly as actation proceeds, and if ewes are kept outdoors on sparse grazing—parcularly where copper levels are marginal to low and molybdenum and ulphur levels are high—then copper deficiency problems are a distinct ossibility. On very sparse grazing conditions during winter, ewes may eat p to one-tenth of their dry matter intake as soil, and as pointed out already, iis may seriously interfere with copper availability because of its high iron ontent. Therefore, concentrate feeding in late pregnancy not only makes ense in regard to protein and energy requirements, but is often essential) meet copper and other trace element and mineral requirements.

Not every farm suffers from frank disease due to copper deficiency in ie form of swayback in lambs. However, some flocks which have never xperienced the disease may still be suffering from sub-clinical copper eficiency. If cattle are kept on the farm, symptoms of stunted growth, couring and anaemia may be present without any symptoms being present 1 sheep on the same grazings. Such circumstances would warrant an ivestigation of the sheep flock, and careful recording of lamb performance iight show disappointing results.

Ireed and age effects

Iot all breeds of sheep are equally susceptible to copper deficiency. Scotsh Blackfaces and Swaledales, for example, are less efficient at absorbing opper from the diet and are therefore more likely to give birth to swayback ambs than some other breeds, such as the Welsh Mountain. Even within a ingle breed it is possible to identify individual animals which can absorb opper more or less efficiently than others; this appears to be a genetically iherited characteristic.

The age and status of an animal affect its ability to withstand copper eficiency. Lambs are more prone than mature ewes and on copper-deficient arms, older ewes which have become progressively depleted of their copper reserves over the years are more likely than younger ewes to produce wayback lambs.

orecasting the swayback risk

: is difficult to predict precisely where and when copper deficiency probems will arise. However, the Ministry of Agriculture, Fisheries and Food 1 the UK issues forecasts in the farming press and on radio and television of ie likelihood of the coming lambing season being a swayback year. These re given in time to allow flockmasters to take preventive action if the risk ; considered to be high.

These forecasts are based on a number of factors, including how evere a winter it has been, especially in terms of days of snow cover. n severe winters the risk is generally less, based on the assumption that lockmasters will have fed more concentrates in late pregnancy and that ill ewes are more likely to have been offered hay or feedblocks during prolonged periods of snow cover. In mild winters, fewer concentrates ar fed and more reliance is therefore placed on winter grazings, often with a accompanying increase in soil intake.

CLINICAL SIGNS OF SWAYBACK

Lambs which have suffered severe damage to the brain and spinal cor because of inadequate supplies of copper from their ewes during th last third of pregnancy (congenitally affected cases) may be born dead may succumb shortly after birth or may live long enough to show th well-recognised symptoms of swayback. Some lambs are small and weakl and display trembling movements of the head or grinding of the teeth an often react to their surroundings in a very sluggish manner.

The worst affected lambs are unable to stand up, even when helpe to do so (see Colour plate 35). Because they are unable to suckle they ver soon die, usually from hypothermia as a result of exposure or starvation It is believed that swayback lambs are, in any case, more prone to chilling because they appear less able to convert the brown fat supplies stored ir the body into energy. Most of these worst affected lambs live for only a few hours or, if they receive a little milk, for a few days at best.

Less severely affected lambs are able to get up with a little effort whe they are born. They are bright and alert and keen to suckle, but have difficulty in keeping up with their mothers, the exertion of doing so tending to exaggerate their problems. They stumble, stagger and sway about in ar effort to maintain their balance. The hind legs are usually worst affected and lambs may fall to one side and sit like a dog, supported on their forelegs

Lambs which are unable to keep up with their mothers may die or starvation. Others may succumb to diseases such as navel and joint-ill, since many are unable to suckle sufficient colostrum soon enough after birth to protect them adequately against infection. Some pull themselves along the ground so that the navel cord is dragged through the dirt and thus more likely to become infected.

Delayed swayback

As previously stated, a proportion of lambs born of copper deficient ewes are apparently normal at birth. However, because they continue to receive inadequate supplies of copper in the ewe's milk, the symptoms of swayback may show themselves any time up to, or even beyond, three months of age. This delayed form of swayback usually affects lambs gradually, although occasionally they may be struck down very suddenly. In the latter case lambs may appear to be perfectly normal one day but the following morning the shepherd may find them apparently blind and wandering aimlessly, or lying twitching or thrashing about before sinking into a coma and dying.

More commonly, however, the shepherd will notice something is wrong when some lambs fall behind the rest of the flock at gathering and exhibit a slight weakness in the hind limbs, often shown as a sudden sinking at the ock. Further exercise exaggerates the problem and the typical swaying movement soon becomes apparent. It is frequently the fastest growing and fittest looking lambs which are affected. Cases often appear after some husbandry task has been carried out, such as gathering for worming or vaccination, or for late castration and tailing—all stressful operations.

Apart from the worst affected, lambs may learn how to cope with their disability. Providing they can suckle or, if old enough, wean themselves, they can survive, although they take much longer to reach marketable weight and lack the finish of normal lambs. The ill-thrift of such lambs is reflected in the fleece, and the copper deficiency often affects the growth of the long bones of the body. If handled roughly the bones may be easily broken, since they are much finer and less robust, and fractures of the legs and ribs are not uncommon.

DIAGNOSIS

It is most important to have a correct diagnosis in cases where swayback is suspected since control and prevention will involve the administration of copper-containing drugs. Copper is poisonous if given in excess of requirements. Therefore, if the suspected problem is not swayback and copper is administered, it may lead to an outbreak of copper poisoning (see later).

A careful veterinary examination of affected animals will be necessary, as the symptoms of swayback can be confused with a number of other diseases. Any history of swayback in lambs or copper deficiency problems in cattle will help with a provisional diagnosis, but a definite diagnosis can only be reached after laboratory tests. Blood sampling a selection of sheep for copper, whilst a simple and practical approach, is less than perfect, and post-mortem material is very valuable in any copper investigation. Any lambs that die at any age, or any very sick lambs which are unlikely to recover and can be sacrificed for diagnostic purposes, should be presented for post-mortem in as fresh a state as possible. Examination of the brain and spinal cord is very valuable in diagnosis. Samples of liver and kidney from such casualties will give a much more accurate picture of the copper status of the flock than blood samples. (Liver samples can also be collected from the live animal by a technique called liver biopsy.) Herbage analysis for copper, molybdenum and sulphur may also be helpful in arriving at a diagnosis.

TREATMENT AND CONTROL

When cases of congenital swayback arise in a flock—that is, when lambs are born with the disease or develop symptoms very soon after birth—treatment of affected lambs is of no benefit, since the damage to the brain and spinal cord is irreversible. Severely affected lambs will eventually die and should be humanely destroyed. Mildly affected lambs may benefit from treatment and good nursing to prevent them from deteriorating further but this must be done with caution and only on the advice of a veterinar surgeon. The choice of copper product is important (see Quick Referenc Chart on pages 448–449). These cases may need help from the shepher initially, to see that they mother-up and receive adequate colostrum from their dams (or by stomach tube), so that they are protected from chillin and infectious disease. It is also helpful to keep the ewes and lambs indoor in bad weather, or in a small paddock near the farmstead in good weather until the lambs are strong enough to be able to follow their mothers.

Careful and time-consuming shepherding is essential to give lamb the best chance. It is inevitable in large flocks which have a moderate o severe outbreak that lambs may not receive sufficient attention from eithe their dams or the shepherd because of pressure of work. Many will peris sooner or later, either from starvation, chilling, predators or infectiou disease.

When congenital swayback cases occur in a flock, apparently norma lambs are also likely to be copper deficient to a degree. Your veterinar surgeon should be consulted and, if the diagnosis is confirmed, will prob ably advise that all lambs are copper treated (unless the flock is housed and that ewes yet to lamb should also be treated. This is likely to be mos successful with ewes which still have some weeks to go before lambing Similarly, where cases of delayed swayback occur in the flock, all lamb should be treated, plus any ewes yet to lamb.

In flocks where swayback or other copper deficiency problems have been encountered, the problems are likely to recur in future years unles radical management changes are implemented. The severity may vary perhaps occasional cases of swayback for a number of years, and then for no obviously apparent reason, there will be a serious outbreak with devastating effect. Preventive measures are essential in such circumstances but it must be emphasised that **a flock should not be treated with copper unless clinical, post-mortem and laboratory tests have confirmed that a deficiency exists.**

PREVENTION

Preventive measures for future years will consist of the copper treatment of ewes, either around tupping or, on more severely deficient farms, in mid pregnancy, for example at the time ewes are scanned for pregnancy diagnosis. Copper treatment should **not** be carried out at the same time as ewes are wormed with anthelmintics, since with some methods of treatment this can increase the risk of copper poisoning.

It is particularly important that when sheep, of whatever age or status, are receiving copper treatment, they **have access to only one source of copper**, be it directly by mouth or injection, or indirectly by the treatment of grazings with copper salts. Otherwise the risk of poisoning is real, particularly with housed sheep receiving concentrates. Feed should never e reduced or withdrawn during copper treatment, as this also increases the ısk of poisoning.

Mineral and trace element supplements, either for inclusion in concenate rations or for free-access, should not contain copper when intended ɔr sheep. This is a legal requirement.

One problem which arises in relation to copper deficiency is that mineral ıixtures for sheep often contain a high proportion of iron. Not only is ıis unnecessary (since there is usually ample iron in the herbage for the ⁼quirements of grazing animals), but it is positively harmful. Iron makes ɔpper unavailable and may induce a copper deficiency even where copper ⁼vels in the diet would otherwise be more than adequate. Excess iron is ɔmetimes added to mineral supplements as a sales gimmick to give them

(*text continues on page 450*)

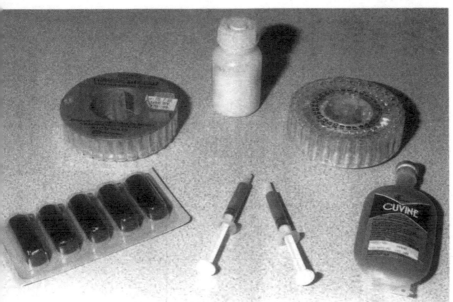

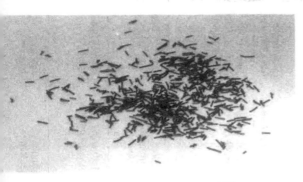

Plate 11.3   Above is a selection of products for the prevention (and treatment) of copper deficiency, including boluses, injectable suspension and paste, and copper sulphate crystals. To the left are copper oxide needles.

QUICK REFERENCE CHART

Some copper compounds for the treatment and prevention of deficiency disorders

Chemical name	Trade name (Manufacturer)	Given by	Manufacturer's recommended timing and treatment	Length of protection (Risk of poisoning)	Comments
Copper oxide needles	Copporal or Copprite (Beecham) Coppercaps (RMB)	Mouth	E at mating or in mid pregnancy L not under 5 weeks	Long (Low)	At present the most efficient, convenient and safe method of correcting deficiency. Capsules may rupture at dosing. Separate products for adults and lambs.
Copper methionate paste	Rycovet Coppa (Rycovet)	Injection s/c or i/m	E 10 weeks before lambing L see manufacturer's instructions	Long (Low)	Reaction (abscess) at site of s/c injection common. Ready-loaded syringe convenient.
Methionine copper complex	Copavet Injection (C-vet)	Injection s/c or i/m into brisket	E mid pregnancy L following laboratory diagnosis of deficiency	Long (Low)	Reaction (abscess) at site of s/c injection. Suspension must be shaken vigorously before use.
Copper heptonate	Cuvine (Rycovet)	Injection i/m in neck or shoulder	E 10 weeks before lambing L not suitable	Intermediate (Intermediate)	No problem with abscesses.

Chemical name	Trade name (Manufacturer)	Given by	Manufacturer's recommended timing and treatment	Length of protection (Risk of poisoning)	Comments
Copper complex	Cujec (Coopers Pitman-Moore)	Injection s/c only side of neck	E 6 to 8 weeks before lambing L over 6 weeks old where deficiency confirmed	Short (High)	Must not be given in conjunction with any other treatment.
Copper sulphate with cobalt chloride	'Copacobal' (C-Vet)	Mouth (after dilution)	E 12 and 8 weeks before lambing L no recommendations given	Short (High)	The need to be diluted increases risk of overdosage and poisoning.
Copper sulphate crystals	Chemist or agricultural merchant	Mouth (after dilution)	Consult your veterinary surgeon for dose and frequency.	Short (High)	Stock solution has to be made up and then diluted, with risk of overdosage and poisoning.

NOTES: A veterinary surgeon should **always** be consulted before any treatments are given.

Do not administer copper to any sheep which are housed for a prolonged period and fed on concentrates.

A short duration of action means that more frequent dosing will be necessary and that there is an increased risk of poisoning.

North Ronaldsay sheep should not be treated with any copper preparations.

Do not forget to treat rams where appropriate.

Key: E = ewes (rams)
L = lambs
s/c = under the skin
i/m = into the muscle

449

a rich brown colour, and farmers should be particularly suspicious of these and demand a full analysis (see Colour plate 34). Mineral and trace element mixtures and licks containing copper and intended for cattle should **never** be offered to sheep.

Copper products available for the treatment and prevention of deficiencies are given in the Quick Reference Chart.

COPPER DEFICIENCY AND SUSCEPTIBILITY TO DISEASE

Obvious clinical disease in the form of swayback in lambs is only part of the copper deficiency story on some farms. Recent collaborative work between the Moredun Research Institute (MRI) and the Institute for Animal Physiology and Genetics Research (formerly the Animal Breeding Research Organisation) in Edinburgh has shown that copper deficient lambs are frequently much less resistant to many common infectious diseases—such as pasteurella pneumonia or *E. coli* septicaemia—than lambs with normal copper levels.

In an experiment involving almost a thousand lambs grazing improved hill pastures, the death rate from birth to six months of age from all causes of infectious disease was twice as high in the low copper group as in the high copper group. The experiment showed very clearly how the combination of a genetically inherited characteristic (copper uptake from feedstuffs) can interact with an environmental change (improvement of hill ground, making copper less available) to produce circumstances which can have drastic effects on the survival of lambs. Also, it indicates that copper is not only important in the development of the nervous system, but that it may also play an important role in immunity to disease.

A third role for copper has also been established by the same group of workers. Again, on improved hill ground and using lambs of differing (genetically inherited) copper status, the growth rate up to six months of age was monitored. High copper status lambs were generally heavier and finished for slaughter earlier than low copper status lambs. However, if low copper lambs were supplemented by dosing with copper 'needles' (see Quick Reference Chart below), then the adverse effects of low copper status can be substantially reduced.

HIGH RISK FARMS

For hill and upland farmers grazing sheep on improved ground—or for other farms with low copper or high molybdenum status—the following important facts have emerged from recent experimental work:

- Improved ground is likely to have a low copper status.
- Pregnant ewes grazing improved ground are likely to produce copper deficient lambs with a high risk of swayback unless they are given copper supplementation during pregnancy.

- Apparently normal lambs (particularly Scottish Blackfaces and Swaledales) born out of ewes which have not been supplemented with copper during pregnancy are at risk of delayed swayback and are more likely to succumb to infectious disease.
- Lambs born out of copper-supplemented ewes and maintained on improved ground are likely to be protected from swayback, but may be unthrifty and show poor liveweight gain at pasture.
- Ewes producing swayback lambs are more likely to do so again in future 'swayback years' than other ewes in the flock.
- Rams also differ in their susceptibility or resistance to copper deficiency and this susceptibility is passed to their offspring.
- Breeding programmes based on the selection of ewes and rams of high copper status (through flock recording and laboratory tests) could, within only a few generations, improve the performance of a flock very significantly and permanently, even in the absence of copper supplementation.
- For fear of poisoning, care should be taken with the copper supplementation of lambs off improved ground where they are destined for fattening indoors on concentrates.
- Herbage copper availability may vary considerably.
- Even with reasonable herbage copper levels, the smallest increase in molybdenum will have a profound effect upon copper availability.
- Improved grazing which is high in molybdenum can be utilised more safely if it is conserved as silage or hay.
- Overliming should be avoided as it increases herbage molybdenum uptake.

Copper Poisoning

Of all the farm animal species, the sheep is particularly prone to copper poisoning and reported incidents increase year by year.

Sheep may be acutely poisoned when they receive a toxic dose of copper over a short period. This can happen when they are dosed with a rapidly absorbed form of copper (such as a solution of copper sulphate by mouth), either when the appropriate dose is exceeded or when the sheep were not copper deficient in the first place. Acute poisoning may occasionally occur following treatment with injectable copper compounds at the recommended rates.

A number of deaths within a day or two of the toxic dose may alert the shepherd to the possible cause. A post-mortem and laboratory examination of tissues will confirm or refute the diagnosis. Immediate treatment of all other at-risk sheep in the flock by your veterinary surgeon (using a solution of ammonium tetrathiomolybdate given subcutaneously) should counteract the effects of excess copper and reduce losses considerably.

451

Cumulative poisoning

Copper is a cumulative poison. Very small amounts taken into the body (usually by mouth) over a long period of weeks or months accumulate, principally in the liver. The sheep has a remarkable ability to store large amounts of copper in this way without ill effect, but should a 'crisis' occur, then massive amounts of copper are liberated from the liver into the bloodstream. This results in the rupture of red blood cells leading to a severe anaemia and jaundice which is rapidly fatal.

The predisposing causes of the 'crisis' which leads to the liberation of copper from the liver are not fully understood. It is thought that stressful situations, such as transportation, rough handling, the deprivation of food for even a short period, or a spell of bad weather, may, individually or together, precipitate an incident of copper poisoning.

Higher risk in housed sheep

Housed sheep are at special risk of copper poisoning. As mentioned above, hard foods such as hay and concentrates contain more available copper then fresh grass or root crops. Many concentrates contain quite high levels of copper, for example, more than 15 parts per million of dry matter. It is therefore prudent to make sure that concentrates and compound feeds for sheep are low in copper. When home mixes are prepared, it is important that the mineral, trace element and vitamin supplement contains no copper. Concentrates prepared for cattle may well have added copper, and pig rations often contain very high levels. These compounds should **never** be fed to sheep, even in a diluted form, since they are hazardous. Problems have arisen from time to time when sheep rations have been prepared

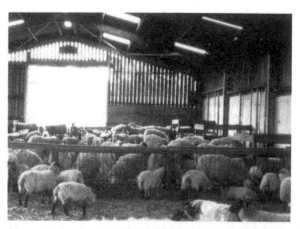
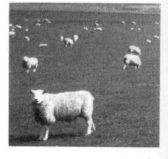

Plate 11.4 Housed sheep (*left*) are more prone to copper poisoning, especially breeds which are efficient at absorbing copper, such as the Texel, seen at pasture (*right*).

through mixers which have not been adequately 'flushed' after processing cattle or particularly pig rations. Free-access mineral and trace element mixtures or licks designed for cattle often contain copper and should **not** be offered to sheep.

Other sources of copper on the farm which may present a risk to sheep are listed below:

- copper sulphate for use in footbaths and for spraying areas of ground infested with the snail which transmits liver fluke
- copper-containing pesticides and fungicides such as are used in orchards, where sheep are grazed between the trees
- industrial copper waste, either dumped or as 'drift' from factories in rivers and streams
- slurry from pig units, or human sewage sludge spread on grassland and subsequently grazed by sheep
- poultry litter when spread on grassland or used as a component of sheep rations

Breed differences

Just as sheep breeds vary in their susceptibility to copper deficiency, so too do they differ in their susceptibility to copper poisoning, only in reverse. Scottish Blackfaces and Swaledales have a higher tolerance, whilst Suffolks and Texels (and their crosses) are extra-sensitive to copper poisoning. Great care must be taken with the latter breeds, especially when they are housed, to see that their diets are not too high in copper. Any copper treatments which are necessary must be accurately administered. North Ronaldsay sheep have become highly tolerant of copper deficiency through natural selection, by living predominantly on a diet of seaweed outside the seawall on the Orkney Island of Ronaldsay. They are consequently exceptionally prone to copper poisoning and should not be treated with copper products.

RULES FOR THE AVOIDANCE OF COPPER POISONING

- If copper deficiency is suspected, an accurate diagnosis must be obtained before any treatment or preventive measures are implemented.
- Use the safest and most effective product for correction of the deficiency and consult your veterinary surgeon regarding the appropriate dose rate for the different classes and weights of sheep.
- If a rapidly absorbed and therefore more risky copper preparation is to be used—such as copper sulphate by mouth or some of the injectable copper preparations—treat a small number of sheep first and before treating the rest of the flock wait for a week in case of any untoward effects.
- Handle sheep with extra care when treating them with copper and for a period afterwards.

- Do not administer anthelmintics for worm or fluke control at the same time as giving copper preparations, as this appears to make sheep more susceptible to poisoning.
- Avoid any period of food deprivation, however temporary, around the time of copper treatment.
- Make certain that **only one source of copper** is available.
- Feeds must be low in copper—**never** use feeds compounded for other species or which contain the by-products of other species (e.g. poultry litter).
- Avoid applying copper sulphate for snail control on pastures to be grazed by sheep. If it must be used, then a period of prolonged rainfall should elapse before sheep are released onto the grazing, although there is still likely to be an appreciable risk.
- Lock safely away all products containing copper.

Cobalt Pine—Vitamin B_{12} Deficiency

On pastures overlying particular soil types deficient in cobalt, or where the element is unavailable to plants because of the chemical nature of the soil, young ruminant animals fail to grow as expected. In cases of severe deficiency animals become anaemic and die if treatment is not provided. In the UK, for example, the granites and old red sandstones of the West Country are often deficient, whilst in other countries, such as Australia or the Americas, vast tracts of land are cobalt deficient.

Cobalt forms part of the molecule of vitamin B_{12} and it is a deficiency of this vitamin which is responsible for the unthriftiness or pine which occurs in animals grazing cobalt deficient pastures. Herbage does not contain any of the B vitamins and so the ruminant animal relies entirely upon the microorganisms which inhabit its rumen for the manufacture of these essential substances. Cobalt is therefore required continuously by the ruminant and young, rapidly growing animals, such as lambs on spring and summer grass, have especially high requirements. However, cobalt levels in the sward, which on some pastures may already be at a very low level, tend to fall even further as herbage growth accelerates. Supplies of cobalt are therefore at their lowest when the animal's requirements are at their highest.

Symptoms of deficiency begin to show in late summer and autumn in weaned lambs, once the rather meagre stores of vitamin B_{12} in the tissues have been exhausted. However, where ewes have been grazed on cobalt deficient pasture for some time, the level of vitamin B_{12} in colostrum will be low and lambs born to these ewes will start life with poor supplies. If such lambs continue to be raised on deficient ground, they may start to show symptoms somewhat earlier in the season.

The improvement of hill and upland grazings by drainage, ploughing and liming tends to make what cobalt there is less available. Reseeding replaces many natural species of grasses, which are relatively rich in cobalt, with a more restricted range of cobalt deficient species. Clovers, for example, contain more cobalt than grasses, so where high levels of fertiliser nitrogen are used, this may suppress the clover and further reduce cobalt availability. Under such circumstances, any attempt to increase the productivity of the flock—by increasing stocking density, for example—will only exacerbate the situation, unless cobalt is provided in one form or another (see below). A similar situation prevails with copper on improved ground and, indeed, these two trace elements are often deficient at the same time. This sometimes leads to a confusion over diagnosis in the absence of laboratory tests. Herbage analysis can sometimes be helpful in predicting the likelihood of deficiency problems, although levels may vary considerably from year to year.

CLINICAL SIGNS AND DIAGNOSIS OF PINE

The most obvious symptoms of cobalt deficiency are evident in lambs, especially when they should be growing well on lush spring and summer pastures. They gradually but progressively lose their appetite, because a deficiency of vitamin B_{12} allows the build up of toxic by-products of metabolism in the bloodstream. Growth rate declines initially and, as the deficiency progresses, there will be an actual loss of bodyweight, since vitamin B_{12} plays an important role in the utilisation of energy from the diet. Lambs become very dull and listless and may stop eating altogether, so that they waste or 'pine' away. They finally die of starvation, often in the midst of plenty. These worst affected animals show extreme pallor of the membranes of the mouth and eyes because of a severe anaemia.

A full post-mortem together with the clinical signs present in other lambs on the same grazings and perhaps a history of pine in previous years should suggest cobalt deficiency. This can then be confirmed by laboratory tests on blood, urine and also herbage. In situations where the deficiency is less severe, vague symptoms of unthriftiness may be overlooked, or put down to parasitism ('worms') or simply a shortage of grazing.

Probably the most reliable method for diagnosis of cobalt deficiency is to supply the element to a small number of lambs in the flock and watch for the rapid and dramatic effects. Cobalt is relatively non-toxic (unlike copper), so this is a safe technique and also sensible, especially since the presently available laboratory tests on blood are not always easy to interpret. Most lambs on a particular grazing will probably be deficient, even if only a proportion of the flock appears to show symptoms. Therefore the whole group should be treated once the diagnosis is confirmed.

Adult ewes may also be affected if the deficiency is severe enough, or continues for long enough. Clinical symptoms may not be obvious, but fertility may be adversely affected. As far as is known, these are secondary effects due to the generally poorer condition of the ewes. Poor conception rates and early foetal loss may lead to an extended lambing period, a lower lamb drop and a higher proportion of barren ewes than anticipated. In the UK at least, there would not appear to be any detrimental effect upon the lambs born from cobalt deficient ewes, apart from the fact that they will receive very little vitamin B_{12} from colostrum.

TREATMENT AND PREVENTION

Treatment of affected animals is always worthwhile and most animals will respond rapidly and dramatically. Lambs usually regain their appetite within a very short time, begin to lose their lacklustre appearance and start to put on weight once more. Severely affected animals close to death are unlikely to recover, however, and those with a significant anaemia will take much longer to respond to treatment. As the symptoms are due to a vitamin B_{12} deficiency, the most immediate response will be obtained by injecting the vitamin. (Giving vitamin B_{12} by mouth is not effective since it is only very poorly absorbed from the gut and into the tissues where it is needed.) This initial treatment will need to be followed up by providing cobalt, since in most cases animals will have to remain on the cobalt deficient grazings. (Frequent vitamin B_{12} injections would be a costly and impractical solution.)

Methods of providing cobalt

Cobalt must be given by mouth, since it is required by the microorganisms in the rumen which then incorporate it into the vitamin B_{12} molecule for use by the animal. Moreover, cobalt must be supplied continuously, albeit in very small quantities. Increasing the dose of cobalt in the hope that it will mean less frequent dosing is ineffective and animals will continue to be unthrifty.

There are a number of ways of providing cobalt and the choice will depend upon what is considered the most practical and economical solution for a particular flock. What is reasonable for a small 'hobby flock' may be totally inappropriate for an extensive flock which may take several days to gather and treat.

Dressing pastures

Probably the most obvious first consideration would be to correct the cobalt status of the grazings. This can be done by the use of cobalt sulphate, either as a spray (since it is soluble in water) or by incorporating it into regular fertilisers (such as superphosphate) at the manufacturing stage. The rate and frequency of application will depend on the degree of deficiency, the soil type (which may influence the uptake of cobalt by plants) and the climatic conditions. Since cobalt is a relatively expensive element and the cost fluctuates considerably, the final choice may depend on prevailing prices.

The amount of cobalt required is measured from ounces to a few pounds per hectare, applied every three or four years under most UK circumstances. The whole area need not be dressed, a third to a half being all that is necessary. These treated areas may become overgrazed, probably because the herbage is more palatable, rather than because the sheep 'know' they are deficient in cobalt. Cobalt also has some effect upon plant growth, and legumes in particular will respond.

Dosing

If pasture applications are unacceptable, the only other alternative is to supply cobalt by mouth as a preventative treatment. This can be done by dosing with cobalt sulphate solutions on a frequent and regular basis—for example, weekly or fortnightly—which is inexpensive in materials, but costly in labour and impractical on most farms with any significant number of sheep. A stock solution is made up by dissolving cobalt sulphate in water and then further diluting for use. A veterinary surgeon should be consulted regarding the dose rate, which will depend upon the bodyweight of the animal.

Wormers with added cobalt

Cobalt has been added to certain brands of anthelmintic in recent years. In theory, this seems reasonable, since anthelmintics are most frequently used during the grazing period when cobalt deficiency is most likely to occur. However, some flock owners attempt to operate 'clean' grazing systems, in which wormings are kept to a minimum and are certainly far too infrequent to protect against cobalt deficiency. Even where lambs do not have access to 'clean' grazing, it is debatable whether three-weekly dosing is sufficiently frequent to correct cobalt deficiency, although growth responses have been recorded. (Manufacturers of cobalt-containing wormers are presently being asked to present data to justify the claims made for such products.)

Free-access

Mineral and trace element supplements and licks offered on free-access do not invariably contain cobalt. Some cheaper products exclude it because of its high price, so farmers should check the analysis. In any event, because of the variability of intake, free-access is not a satisfactory method of supplying any element. Supplements are a valuable method for ensuring the correct mineral status of home mixed rations, but lambs are rarely fed concentrates during high-risk periods for cobalt deficiency.

It is also possible to add trace elements to piped water supplies, but this technique is more suitable for cattle than sheep and then only when there is only one source of water. Sheep do drink water, but when the weather is wet or the herbage lush, water intake is largely supplied from grazing and this method is therefore unreliable.

'Bullets' and boluses

The most practical alternative to supplying cobalt to animals in small amounts on a continuous basis is by the use of either so-called 'bullets' or slow-release glass boluses. Both these slowly dissolve in the reticulo-rumen and release cobalt on a continuous basis, which is the ideal situation for the rumen microorganisms' requirements.

The glass bolus products may also contain copper and selenium, both of which are toxic in excess. Therefore where cobalt is deficient but copper and selenium are not, this is an inappropriate form of treatment, particularly where lambs are due to be kept on and finished indoors on concentrates. (See section on copper poisoning.) If it is suspected that a combined copper, cobalt and selenium glass bolus has not been swallowed, or has been regurgitated, animals should on no account be given a second bolus because of the risk of poisoning by copper in particular. No other source of copper or selenium should be available to bolus-treated animals.

'Bullets' are probably the most appropriate method of treating and preventing cobalt deficiency. The bullet, which is made from cobalt oxide and iron grit, is very heavy, and when swallowed it sinks to the bottom of the reticulum or rumen and lodges there. Young lambs under six or eight weeks of age which are still sucking and do not yet have a fully functioning rumen should **not** be dosed, since the bullets may very quickly become coated with calcium phosphate, which prevents them dissolving. Treatment is uncomfortable and unnecessary at this early age. This coating effect occurs in some older animals too, but can be overcome, either by giving two bullets (which is unnecessarily expensive) or, better, by simultaneously administering a small steel bolt along with the bullet, so that the grinding action of one against the other prevents or chips away any coating.

A special dosing gun deposits the bullet in the oesophagus. The job should not be rushed and the sheep and lambs should be handled with care to avoid dosing injuries. Sheep should be allowed to stand quietly for a period after dosing and observed, as a few animals may regurgitate the bullet soon after dosing (also a possibility at a later date). Any animals in a treated group which appear to be thriving less well than their flockmates can be assumed to have lost their bullet and can be re-dosed, since cobalt poisoning is very unlikely.

In areas where copper deficiency occurs in tandem with cobalt, the iron component of the cobalt bullet may interfere with the uptake of copper by the animal, and an alternative treatment, such as the slow-release glass bolus, may be more appropriate to cover both deficiencies.

On cobalt deficient farms, ewe lambs which are to be retained for breeding should be given a cobalt bullet during the summer. There is some discussion over how long a period a bullet will protect sheep: on some farms a single bullet will last a lifetime, whereas on others, dosing may need to be repeated and veterinary guidance should be sought. If it is established that a farm or a particular grazing is deficient, then, unless pasture dressings are applied, the condition will remain. The lamb crop should therefore be dosed every year before the period of risk. Even though it is appreciated that the symptoms may be more serious in some years than others, there will always be some level of ill-thrift and treatment should always be economically beneficial.

There is a suggestion from recent research that cobalt-deficient animals may be more prone to other infections, in a similar way to sheep deficient in copper.

Selenium, Vitamin E and White Muscle Disease

White muscle disease (WMD) is a life-threatening muscular dystrophy which principally affects lambs and young sheep. It is sometimes referred to as stiff lamb disease because the symptoms in some lambs are similar to, and are often confused with, joint-ill. However, in white muscle disease the joints are normal and no infection is involved.

The condition is due to a deficiency of the trace element **selenium** and/or of **vitamin E**. These essential nutrients play a similar role in the body in protecting the muscles from the toxic effects of chemicals (peroxides) which accumulate in the body from natural foods or through muscular exercise.

Selenium (as part of an enzyme) detoxifies these harmful substances and vitamin E helps to prevent their formation in the first place. In the absence of either or both, the toxic peroxides will kill muscle cells. This causes stiffness when the muscles attached to the skeleton are involved and breathing difficulties when the muscles controlling breathing are involved. Sudden death may occur when the heart muscle is affected. The name 'white muscle disease' derives from the pale appearance of the affected muscles seen at post-mortem examination (see Colour plate 36).

Selenium status of feeds

It is only relatively recently that the widespread nature of selenium deficiency has been recognised. The amount of the trace element in herbage is a reflection of the selenium status of the soil it grows in. Selenium deficient soils, particularly acid soils in high rainfall areas, are also deficient in other trace elements, such as copper or cobalt.

Selenium levels in herbage are influenced by other constituents of the soil as well as by chemicals applied to it. For example, the application of superphosphate fertilisers containing sulphates may reduce the uptake of selenium from the soil by plants, or may reduce its availability to the animal, or a combination of both. On soils with adequate selenium status, this may have no detrimental effect, but where levels are already low, the use of such fertiliser may precipitate cases of white muscle disease.

Vitamin E status of feeds

Vitamin E levels in foodstuffs vary considerably depending on the type of plant, the stage of its growth and the method and efficiency of its preservation. Grass normally contains adequate levels of vitamin E, but lush spring grass may also contain high levels of polyunsaturated fatty acids (PUFA). When eaten by the animal, these PUFA are converted into the toxic peroxides referred to earlier, which damage muscles. Early spring

459

grazing is therefore a challenge to both selenium and vitamin E levels, and on farms where white muscle disease has occurred previously, the turnout onto spring grass should be gradual.

Forage crops such as rape and kale are a good source of vitamin E. So too is grass silage, but preservation with sulphuric acid may interfere with the availability of selenium. Both barn dried hay and field made hay which has had little or no rain contain good levels of vitamin E. However, poor-quality hay which has been badly weathered or has heated in the stack will have only low levels of vitamin E. Levels in straw are generally low, but feed-quality spring barley straw, for example, may contain higher levels of the vitamin than moderate or poor-quality hay. Cereals contain moderate levels of vitamin E, but treatment of moist grain with proprionic acid will destroy most of the vitamin E, as will alkali (e.g. ammonia) treatment of straw. Root crops such as swedes and turnips generally contain low levels of vitamin E. Scottish grown feeds generally tend to be low in both selenium and vitamin E.

Home grown feeds

Home grown rations can present a problem on farms where soil selenium levels are marginal or low. The crops grown on such farms will all contain inadequate levels of selenium and if conservation problems arise because of bad weather, then vitamin E levels may also be adversely affected. For example, on low selenium status farms, ewes fed medium to poor hay and a home grown barley-based ration during the last third of pregnancy are likely to be deficient in both selenium and vitamin E, and their lambs are likely either to be born dead, or to succumb to white muscle disease early in life.

CLINICAL SIGNS

Depending upon circumstances, white muscle disease can occur in lambs of any age. As just mentioned, if the ewe flock is selenium and/or vitamin E deficient during pregnancy, lambs may be born dead or very weakly and may die soon after birth from hypothermia, through being unable to get up and suckle. Others may die from heart failure. Some lambs may be born apparently normal, but then develop the disease during the first few weeks of life.

The clinical signs of white muscle disease vary very considerably and may be confused with a number of other conditions. The symptoms of trembling, stiffness when walking, preferring to lie down, having difficulty when getting up and flopping down again as soon as possible can easily be confused with joint-ill. Other lambs whose hind limbs are more severely affected may sway about and fall down, suggesting the possibility of swayback. Others may breathe in a rapid, shallow fashion, reminiscent of pneumonia. When the shoulder muscles are affected, lambs stand with their heads down and fore legs splayed apart, giving the appearance that the body is slung like a hammock between the shoulder blades. Stiff lambs can die of heart failure if both the skeletal and heart muscles are affected, and apparently healthy lambs may suddenly drop dead. In some flocks, only occasional lambs are affected, whilst in others an alarming proportion succumb in one way or another.

WMD in older sheep

Apart from problems around lambing time—which is when the majority of cases occur—older lambs or hoggs may succumb if they are fed a diet deficient in selenium and/or vitamin E. In Scotland, for example, swedes or turnips, which tend to be low in vitamin E, are a popular feed for fattening hoggs over winter. Where poor-quality hay or straw is offered to supplement the root crop, then the diet is likely to be deficient in both nutrients. Cases of white muscle disease may then arise, especially during a spell of severe weather, or when hoggs are stressed, by being gathered and transported, for example. Root-based diets are sometimes fed to ewes during pregnancy and on selenium deficient farms this may lead to white muscle disease in lambs, since, in the UK, the deficiency is rarely severe enough to produce clinical symptoms in adult sheep.

DIAGNOSIS AND TREATMENT

Your veterinary surgeon may make a provisional diagnosis of white muscle disease based on the symptoms shown by any affected lambs, the past history of similar problems on the farm and a post-mortem examination of any dead lambs. Any lambs showing symptoms may then be treated with selenium, or vitamin E, or a combination of both. Your veterinary surgeon is unlikely to advise the wholesale treatment of all lambs until the diagnosis has been confirmed by laboratory tests on blood samples from a random group of lambs, plus a microscopic examination of affected muscles from lambs which have died or were humanely destroyed.

Often the response to treatment will help to confirm the diagnosis and once this is established, all lambs in the flock should be treated with selenium and/or vitamin E products since they will all be deficient to some degree, even if not showing symptoms (see Quick Reference Chart). Gathering should be done as quietly as possible, since the stress and muscular exercise involved may precipitate further clinical cases.

Any affected lambs and their dams should be brought indoors and made comfortable. Treatment may need to be repeated if cases do not respond as well as expected, but this should only be done on veterinary advice.

PREVENTION OF WMD

On farms where selenium deficiency is established, the flock should be protected in future years by ensuring that adequate levels of selenium and of vitamin E are supplied to ewes during pregnancy to protect their lambs

461

(*text continues on page 464*)

QUICK REFERENCE CHART

Some products for the treatment and prevention of white muscle disease

Type of product	Trade name (Manufacturer)	Given by	Timing of treatment	Length of protection	Comments
Selenium in iron grit forming a heavy bullet	Permasel—S Selenium pellets (Coopers Pitman-Moore)	Mouth via balling gun	E before mid pregnancy L at weaning or before period of risk	Long—for a year or more	A steel 'grinder' given at the time of the bullet will prevent coating. Occasional bullets are 'lost'. Do not treat lambs under 2 months of age. Suitable for long-term protection of animals at pasture.
Selenium, cobalt and vitamins A, D₃ and E	Pardevit (Bayer)	Mouth as drench	E pre tupping and 3 weeks prior to lambing L 6 weeks of age or over—repeated at intervals of not less than one month	Short	Most suitable for treatment or short-term prevention, as repeated doses would be required.
Selenium as ready-to-use injectable paste	Rycovet Deposel (Rycovet)	Injection (under skin of the neck)	E first half of pregnancy L at weaning or before period of risk	Long—up to a year	Dose according to body weight. Safest form of injectable product. Some reaction at site of injection.
Selenium plus vitamin E	Dystosel (Intervet)	Injection (under skin of the neck or intramuscular)	E late pregnancy L at birth or before period of risk	Short—a few weeks	Frequent repeat doses of vitamin E necessary, so most suitable for treatment rather than prevention.

Type of product	Trade name (Manufacturer)	Given by	Timing of treatment	Length of protection	Comments
Selenium plus vitamin E	Vitenium injection (C-Vet)	Injection (under skin of the neck or intramuscular)	E late pregnancy L before period of risk	Short	Overdosage may lead to selenium poisoning so dosage, timing and frequency of treatment must be on veterinary advice.

NOTES: 1 Mineral and trace element mixtures for free access are not suitable for the correction of selenium deficiency (see text).

2 Where mineral and trace element supplements for mixing with home grown, cereal-based rations are to be used to correct selenium deficiency in the diet of pregnant ewes, they should be included at rates calculated on the whole rations (including roughage).

3 Anthelmintics containing selenium are an effective although often unsatisfactory method of dealing with deficiency since there is a danger of toxicity from frequent dosing. No other selenium products should be on offer. If clean grazing is available, sheep may not need to be wormed for prolonged periods and will therefore receive no selenium.

4 Addition of selenium tablets to water supply (e.g. Aquatrace) is not a suitable method for sheep.

5 The response to pasture applications of selenium salts (e.g. added to fertilisers) varies from farm to farm. They are better avoided because of the risk of poisoning.

6 Only one source of selenium should be supplied.

7 Withholding times for meat and milk should be strictly adhered to.

8 Numerous vitamin E products are available, but they are not suitable for the long-term correction of selenium deficiency.

NB: A veterinary surgeon should always confirm selenium deficiency and advise before any treatments are administered. All injectable selenium products require a veterinary prescription.

Key: E = ewes (rams)
L = lambs

463

in early life. It may also be necessary to treat lambs or young sheep in advance of periods of risk, such as when hoggs are to graze roots for a lengthy period.

Before implementing any preventive measures, it is vital to confirm the diagnosis of white muscle disease and to establish whether the condition is due to a deficiency of selenium, or vitamin E, or both. This can only be done after laboratory tests have been carried out. Selenium is highly toxic if given in excess and this could occur if an otherwise safe product were to be administered to sheep on a diet containing adequate levels of selenium.

There are a number of methods available for correcting deficiencies and a confusing number of products, some containing selenium alone, others with selenium plus vitamin E and others again with vitamin E alone. If the disease is to be treated, controlled or prevented successfully and safely, the correct choice of method and product for a particular flock's circumstances is critical and veterinary advice is essential.

Examples of some products containing selenium available for sheep are given in the Quick Reference Chart.

In other parts of the world, such as Australia and New Zealand, selenium deficiency appears to cause unthriftiness in young growing stock and infertility in ewes, both of which respond to selenium treatment, but not to treatment with vitamin E. Research workers in Scotland have obtained a response to selenium supplementation in unthrifty sheep and there are reports that sheep with a low selenium status are not able to mount a full antibody response when challenged by infection.

Selenium Poisoning

Selenium poisoning in grazing animals caused by soils rich in the element does not occur in the UK, whereas in other parts of the world, such as Eire, Australia and the United States, an excess of selenium in the herbage leads to disorders like alkali disease and blind staggers.

Poisoning does, however, occur in the UK due to the following:

- treating with selenium when a deficiency does not exist
- providing more than one source of the element, such as could occur by dosing with selenium pellets ('bullets') whilst at the same time supplying selenium in a mineral mixture on free-access or in the concentrate ration
- giving an overdose of selenium by injection, by drench or in the diet

The symptoms depend upon the degree of poisoning. In the most severe cases, such as a hefty overdose, animals become blind, get up and down and kick at their flank due to severe abdominal pain. They may also press their heads against the wall, grind their teeth and drool saliva. Some develop difficulty in breathing and eventually become paralysed. Death occurs soon after the appearance of these distressing symptoms.

In less severe cases, sheep become very dejected, lose their appetite and therefore body condition, develop a lameness and, if not treated, may die of starvation. Blood sampling will help to confirm the diagnosis.

TREATMENT

Any free-access minerals or diets containing selenium should be removed immediately. If animals can be encouraged to eat, then a high protein ration will minimise the effects of selenium poisoning and your veterinary surgeon may prescribe additional treatments. However, there is no specific cure and whilst mild cases and those which have not yet begun to show signs may be saved, others showing more severe symptoms are unlikely to survive.

Once any of the products for the treatment of deficiency have been administered, the damage cannot easily be reversed and it will be appreciated why it is so important to be sure that a selenium deficiency exists before treatment is applied.

Iodine Deficiency and Goitre

There is a gland in the neck, the thyroid, which produces the hormone **thyroxine**. Thyroxine contains iodine and controls or coordinates the rate at which many of the bodily functions proceed. It is the body's own metabolic stimulant and if it is deficient, then the animal is sluggish, growth rate slows down, reproductive efficiency is impaired and milk production is reduced. Unborn and newborn lambs are most susceptible to thyroxine deficiency and this is manifest by abortion or the birth of stillborn or small, listless and weakly lambs.

Thyroxine deficiency may occur because the soils—and therefore the plants—in an area are deficient in iodine. The best-known example of this in the UK is in Derbyshire. Both livestock and the human population once suffered from goitre—an enlargement of the thyroid gland in response to

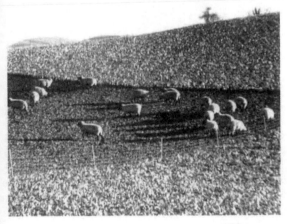

Plate 11.5 Lambs folded on rape. Iodine deficiency (goitre) is a risk where rape, kale or cabbage is fed to excess.

465

iodine deficiency—until the cause was identified and corrected. In humans this was known as 'Derbyshire neck' and small amounts of iodine are now added to common salt to counteract the problem.

Thyroxine deficiency may also occur in sheep (and cattle) when they graze on certain plants which contain substances (goitrogens) which prevent the uptake of iodine by the thyroid gland (see Colour plate 37). Kale, rape and cabbage are the most common offenders in the UK. Other goitrogens are found in soya, linseed, groundnut and peas. These crops or seeds should never be fed in excess to any class of sheep, particularly ewes in late pregnancy because of the effect upon foetal lambs. Cereals have a low iodine content, which may exacerbate the situation if ewes are also grazing a brassica crop.

TREATMENT AND PREVENTION

Lambs born with goitre may be treated with iodine preparations such as potassium iodide (a few drops daily in water). Seriously affected lambs, especially those which are mentally retarded, may not respond to any treatment.

Obviously it is preferable to aim at prevention. In iodine deficient areas, ewe diets should be supplemented by adding iodised salt to the concentrate ration in late pregnancy. Alternatively, ewes can be individually dosed with potassium iodine during the fourth and fifth months of pregnancy.

Fishmeal is rich in iodine and is in any case an excellent ingredient for concentrate rations fed in late pregnancy. Lowland ewes should receive about 75 g and hill ewes 50 g per day, or else the concentrate should comprise around 10% fishmeal. Even at the relatively high cost, it is good value for money.

Where seaweed is available it may be incorporated into the ration as it is also rich in iodine. Iodised licks can be used but are a much less effective way of supplying the element.

Deformities of the Skeleton

There are a number of conditions affecting the bones of sheep which are due to some form of malnutrition. Young, growing sheep are most commonly affected, but adults may also suffer.

Some problems arise from dietary imbalances between calcium and phosphorous. Others may be due to a straightforward deficiency of either or both of these minerals, or of vitamin D. Protein is also essential for normal bone development, but protein cannot be utilised without an adequate energy supply. Therefore semi-starvation can predispose animals to defects of the skeleton. Anything which indirectly affects the uptake of hese essential nutrients from the gut, such as diarrhoea, will worsen the situation.

Bones may become fragile or brittle and therefore more vulnerable to fracture. They may soften and become distorted, as in rickets of young sheep or osteomalacia of older sheep, or they may be of normal consistency but stunted. The symptoms displayed by affected sheep will depend upon their age and the nature of the deficiency or dietary imbalance.

It is important to appreciate that any deformity of the bones represents a relatively advanced stage of an underlying condition which has probably been causing ill-thrift and reduced productivity for some time. These problems usually affect the flock rather than individual animals.

Rickets

Rickets is a condition which affects sheep in their first year of life. It is less common than it used to be, probably because of better feeding generally. However, cases still occur, especially in animals which are growing fast. In the UK the condition arises most frequently because of a deficiency of vitamin D, although phosphorous deficiency may also be a factor.

Most foods contain low levels of vitamin D, especially moderate- or poor-quality hays which saw little sunshine in the making. Vitamin D is manufactured in the skin when it is subjected to ultra-violet rays from the sun. Ruminants depend upon this source to a substantial degree to make up for deficiencies in their diet. As the winter days are shorter and the sun shines less strongly, this is the time when deficiencies tend to occur most frequently. Animals kept indoors in buildings which do not allow in much light are at greater risk. Ram lambs being prepared for show and sale, which are kept indoors for prolonged periods and fed heavily for rapid growth, are particularly vulnerable. The thick woolly fleece prevents sheep from getting as much sun on their skin as cattle do, and shorn sheep generally have higher vitamin D levels in their tissues.

Spring grass, especially when heavily fertilised and growing rapidly, is not without risk either. This is thought to be due to its high carotene content which has some anti-vitamin D activity—that is, it destroys the vitamin in the gut. Therefore, fast-growing lambs sucking their mothers' milk (which is low in vitamin D) and eating lush spring and early summer grass, may also succumb to rickets, although less commonly than do housed animals.

CLINICAL SIGNS

Affected animals may have been lacklustre and performing less well than expected for some time before any lameness or bone deformities are noticed. If they are at grass, worms may be blamed, and even light parasitic infestations may exacerbate the situation by hindering the uptake of calcium, phosphorous, vitamin D and protein from the gut.

In rickets, the bones are inadequately mineralised and therefore are considerably weaker than normal. The long bones in the limbs are unable to bear the weight of the body and so become distorted. The front legs are usually worst affected, since they bear substantially more weight than the hind limbs. They tend to curve outwards and forwards, particularly at the knee, and the feet may splay outwards or turn in. The joints may also be swollen.

Rickets is a painful condition and affected sheep are usually lame and reluctant to move. They often spend a lot of time lying down. They may resent being handled and should be treated with great respect. Despite the weakness of the bones, fractures are relatively uncommon. Since it is painful to walk, affected sheep tend to graze less and since vitamin D deficiency itself reduces appetite, sheep may lose condition rapidly.

TREATMENT AND PREVENTION

Animals must be removed from the offending pasture, or, if housed, the diet must be adjusted. An analysis for calcium, phosphorous and vitamin D will confirm or refute the diagnosis and this may help to identify where the deficiency lies. Any other disease or deficiency which may add to the problem, such as worms or copper deficiency, should be treated simultaneously. Individual treatment with vitamin D is usually necessary and this is best provided by injection in the first instance. Animals usually make a good recovery over a number of weeks, and although severely affected animals may remain deformed, the bones should strengthen as they become mineralised.

The condition can be prevented by checking the mineral and vitamin status of the diet to be fed. This is particularly so when animals are expected to perform above average. Injections of vitamin D can be given at strategic times over the winter period to housed animals or others thought to be at risk. Professional advice should be sought since it is most important **not to overdose with vitamin D** as toxicity may result.

Double Scalp

Double scalp or 'scappie' is now an uncommon condition, but is still occasionally seen in hoggs on the poorer winter grazings of northern Britain. The flat bones of the skull between the eyes often become parchment thin. When pressure is applied, it is sometimes possible to feel the underlying bones of the frontal sinuses—hence the name double scalp. In fact, the whole skeleton is affected, but the thinning is most obvious in the flat bones.

Whilst the mineral and vitamin D status of the flock may well be inadequate, this is often because the sheep are semi-starved. Affected animals are usually in poor bodily condition and noticeably thin and

ight when handled. Trace element deficiencies and parasitism may further
xacerbate the problem.

If animals are kept on poor grazings they must be supplemented
vith good hay and trough or block feeding as appropriate. Once the
pring arrives the condition of the animals will improve, but they never
ully recover and will remain stunted. It is not necessarily helpful to feed
ree-access minerals, since what is required is a balanced diet rather than
a haphazard approach.

Shepherds in days gone by believed that by fracturing the thin bones
between the eyes they could cure the condition. To that end they would
use the handle of a pocket knife or, in the worst affected cases, simply use
heir knuckles to inflict the injury. There is not, and never was, any truth
in this old wives' tale, and shepherds were more likely to produce brain
haemorrhage and death than cure the hoggs! Any apparent improvement
vould only be due to an improvement in feeding and a result of a change
of pasture.

Open Mouth

This is a condition affecting hoggs during the late winter months. Like
double scalp it is seen on poorer land when sheep are not provided with
supplementary feed. The whole skeleton is affected, but the jaw bones,
become especially thin and soft. Since the lower jaw in particular is used
to tear at the grazing, it becomes bent downwards because of a weakness
of the mandibular joint at the angle of the jaw. This means that the teeth
in the lower jaw cannot meet with the dental pad in the upper jaw—hence
the name 'open mouth'. In some cases there may be a gap of an inch or
more between the upper and lower jaws.

This serious defect means that sheep cannot eat, so that they rapidly lose
weight. If the condition is not diagnosed, then some members of the flock
may die of starvation. Animals which have badly deformed jaws should therefore be destroyed on humane grounds. The rest of the flock should be removed
to better pastures and/or offered good-quality hay and a properly balanced
concentrate mixture. (Obviously, feed blocks are totally unsuitable, since
affected sheep cannot eat them.) Their progress should be carefully monitored over the following weeks and months.

Prevention is achieved by providing animals with a balanced diet in
adequate amount.

Osteomalacia

This is a condition of older ewes on hill or marginal grazings and is the
equivalent of rickets in lambs or hoggs. Its colloquial name is cruban.

It is due to an imbalance or deficiency of calcium and phosphorous and is most common in lactating ewes which are producing plenty of milk and doing their lambs well. The effect of this deficiency is to demineralise the bones so that they become thin and fragile. In some flocks, as many as a fifth of the ewes may be clinically affected and the rest are likely to be on a knife edge.

Affected ewes become stiff and lame and continually shift their weight from foot to foot. They eventually become unwilling to move and spend a lot of time lying down. Consequently they lose weight, their milk supply dries up and their lambs suffer.

Injections of vitamin D will improve the uptake of calcium and phosphorous from the gut as an immediate treatment for clinically affected ewes. The whole flock must be moved to better pastures and given a balanced supplementary concentrate until they have fully recovered. The bone deformities often persist, however.

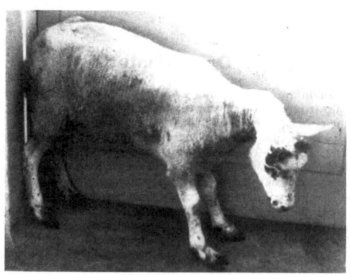

Plate 11.6   An unusual skeletal deformity.

Urolithiasis or Urinary Calculi

This is a distressing and troublesome condition affecting young rams, particularly castrated lambs which have been fed on rations comprising a high proportion of concentrates for some weeks. It is therefore most commonly encountered in housed sheep, but creep-fed lambs at pasture may also suffer.

The problem arises because tiny crystals—usually magnesium ammonium phosphate—form in the urine under certain dietary and other conditions. In most cases the crystals are like grains of sand which are carried along in the flow of urine and tend to sludge up and block the narrow tube (the urethra) which carries urine from the bladder and along the penis to the exterior. The crystals, or calculi, tend to lodge either at the sharp 'S' bend in the penis called the sigmoid flexure (which straightens out during erection) or at the tip of the penis in the very narrowest part of the urethra, the vermiform appendage or 'worm' (see Colour plates 38, 39 and 40).

The consequence of the blockage is that urine dams back, causing the bladder to distend enormously until eventually, after several days, the pressure causes either the urethra or the bladder to rupture. Urine is then forced between the tissues in the former case, or it floods into the body cavity in the latter. Urine is a waste product containing toxic substances, which will eventually cause the death of the lamb when absorbed into the bloodstream this way.

CLINICAL SIGNS

As can be imagined, the consequences of these events on the affected lamb are most unpleasant. Lambs become very restless and spend long periods tail wagging and crouching whilst attempting to pass urine. Sometimes the sheer force of straining plus the back pressure of urine may cause a drop of blood or urine to seep past and stain the hairs around the prepuce. Lambs soon stop eating and drinking, but the formation of urine continues nevertheless. As the discomfort and pain increase, lambs isolate themselves from the group and kick at their abdomen which becomes visibly swollen due to the enormous size of the bladder. Lambs detected at this advanced stage should be handled with great caution for fear of rupturing the bladder before any treatment can be instigated.

If the bladder ruptures, the lamb gains only temporary relief since it soon becomes very lethargic and sick due to the toxic effects of the urine (uraemia). The great majority of lambs die without treatment, and if rupture occurs, treatment is not possible. Carcasses of lambs slaughtered in the terminal stages of the condition are always unfit for human consumption.

TREATMENT AND PREVENTION

Shepherds who have experienced the condition in the flock previously will be on the lookout for cases and should recognise them early on so that the veterinary surgeon is given a reasonable chance of instigating successful treatment. Various methods are available, including surgery to amputate the penis or to divert it so that the ram lamb can urinate from a position similar to that in the female. Most medical treatments, such as the use of muscle relaxants, give only temporary relief despite changes in diet. In the worst cases lambs should be humanely destroyed to avoid further suffering.

When a case occurs in a group of lambs it is inevitable that others will have calculi or will be at risk. Avoiding action must be taken immediately.

471

In the short term this means reducing the proportion of concentrates in the ration and encouraging lambs to drink water (see below).

Calculi are formed when there is an excessive amount of phosphorus in the urine, especially when the urine is concentrated, perhaps because of inadequate water intake. This situation arises most frequently where concentrates make up more than about three-quarters of the ration and where the ratio of calcium to phosphorus in the diet is incorrect. As a guide there should be roughly two parts of calcium to one part of phosphorous in the diet and the ratio should not fall below one to one. Having the correct proportion of these two minerals in the ration causes more phosphorus to be excreted in the dung, so reducing the amount excreted in urine, which in turn reduces the risk of calculi formation. Neither magnesium nor phosphorous should be added to concentrate diets for lambs. Extra calcium in the diet is well tolerated by sheep, so where rations are unbalanced they can be counterbalanced by adding ground limestone.

Water intake

Water intake plays an important role in the occurrence of this condition. If water intake is restricted—for example, because the troughs are too high for lambs to reach easily, or the water is contaminated with faeces because the trough is too low—then the urine becomes more concentrated and crystal formation more likely. Therefore, from the first week of life, fresh clean water should be provided. A running water system (e.g. in cut-away drain pipes) is preferred by sheep and is less likely to freeze in winter.

Water intake can be increased by ensuring that the compound ration contains roughly 3% of common salt. Less than this proportion is unlikely to influence the amount of water drunk and much more will probably reduce food intake. Salt should not be added to the water supply, since lambs find it unpalatable and so will actually drink less.

Supplying a small amount of high-quality hay for lambs will indirectly help prevent urolithiasis by encouraging salivation and rumination, which in turn cause more phosphorus to be excreted in the dung and less in the urine. It also helps to prepare those lambs which are to be turned out onto grass for final fattening to cope with the changeover.

Females and entire males

Calculi may also form in the urine of female lambs, but because of their different anatomy and because the urethra is wider in ewe lambs obstruction is very unlikely ever to occur. Entire ram lambs are also less prone to urolithiasis. The male hormone testosterone, which is produced in the testicles, is responsible for the maturing of the penis. When penis maturation occurs at a normal rate, the urethra correspondingly grows and widens so that the risk of blockage is reduced. In castrates, however, the supply of testosterone is cut off, the penis remains infantile and the urethra narrow, thus increasing the likelihood of blockage should calculi form in the urine. Lambs castrated within the first month of life are most at risk, and

nce the majority of lambs in the UK are elastrated with rubber rings during
e first week of life, there is good reason to consider carefully whether it
necessary or desirable to castrate lambs which are to be artificially reared
r fattened for slaughter in intensively housed conditions on predominantly
oncentrate rations.

reed differences

reeds of sheep and individuals within the same breed differ in their
usceptibility to calculi formation. For example, Texels tend to absorb more
hosphorous from the diet and to have higher blood and urine phosphorus
evels than Suffolks and are therefore more at risk from urolithiasis on
ntensive fattening regimes. Some breeds drink more water and so produce
ore diluted urine than others and are therefore at less risk—Scottish
lackfaces, for example.

Because of the distressing symptoms and unsatisfactory treatment of
rolithiasis, it is obvious that every effort should be made to adjust the
nanagement of intensively fed lambs as described above, so as to reduce
r prevent its occurrence.

Cerebro-cortical Necrosis (CCN)

his condition (for which there is no short, simple name) is one of
he commonest nervous diseases of sheep. It may affect animals of any
ge, but is particularly common in growing lambs, especially on lowland
arms. It occurs quite unexpectedly and under widely differing management
ituations. Often only one or two animals in a group are affected, but
occasionally a small outbreak may occur.

The brain damage which occurs is caused because of a deficiency of
he B vitamin called **thiamine**. However, sheep do not need any of the B
itamins in the food they eat once they become ruminants, that is, after they
re a couple of months old. This is because the microorganisms which live
n the rumen manufacture all the B vitamins the animal needs from the raw
naterials supplied in the diet.

In CCN, the deficiency of thiamine arises because of the presence of sub-
tances called **thiaminases**, which destroy the thiamine produced by the
nicroorganisms. These substances can be detected in excessive amounts in
he rumen liquor and the faeces of sheep suffering from CCN. They are
robably present in low concentration at all times, but under particular
circumstances—which are not understood—they may be produced to excess.
'or example, it is thought that when the level of fibre in the diet is low
nd the level of volatile fatty acids in the rumen falls as a consequence, then
ertain groups of bacteria which are known to produce vitamin B 'destroyers'
nay be present in excessive numbers.

It is also known that certain drugs, notably the anthelmintics (wormers), may precipitate cases of CCN under certain unknown circumstances, pre sumably by altering the population of microorganisms in the rumen. (Th anti-coccidial drug, amprolium, has been shown to do this in cattle, but is not known if it has the same effect in sheep.) Antibiotics, especiall if given by mouth, may alter the rumen population, but it is uncommc (and contraindicated) to give antibiotics to ruminating animals by th route. It has also been suggested that certain plant species—for exampl the ryegrasses—may harbour bacteria which produce thiaminases, but th is unproven. It is often difficult or impossible to identify what factors hav been responsible when cases of CCN arise in a flock and therefore virtuall impossible to predict when it might occur.

CLINICAL SIGNS

Although CCN may be a cause of sudden death, most affected animal will show symptoms before death. Whilst affected lambs may be in goo condition, it sometimes appears on closer examination that the group a a whole are lacklustre and some lambs may be scouring. Affected lamb wander aimlessly away from the flock and within a short time (a day or so they appear to be blind, carrying the head aloft. Some may circle, whils others may stand with their feet well apart and refuse to move for fear c falling. Others may press their heads against a solid object, as if they had severe headache—which they probably have. Any sudden noise or activit may precipitate a convulsion and lambs may collapse and perform paddlin movements with their limbs whilst the head is thrown well back. Despit treatment, most animals die within a day or so of collapsing.

These varied symptoms may be confused with a number of other disease affecting the nervous system, such as 'gid', listeriosis, louping ill or pulp kidney, so that a post-mortem examination of the brain will be necessary t confirm the diagnosis. Your veterinary surgeon may take blood and faece samples for laboratory examination from affected animals and others in th flock.

TREATMENT

Unfortunately, the condition does not seem to respond to treatment witl thiamine (or multivitamins containing thiamine) as well as in cattle, whicl frequently make a spectacular and rapid recovery from a quite advancec stage of the disease. If thiamine is administered and the animal makes a good and permanent recovery, this helps to confirm the diagnosis. It is alsc sensible to observe the rest of the flock carefully for other early cases so that prompt treatment can be given.

Bring any affected animals indoors and make them comfortable. If they are unable to support themselves, prop them up on their brisket with a wal of straw bales. More severely affected sheep will need good nursing—in cluding the provision of fresh, clean water and some palatable food wher ey begin to recover. Blind animals may be slow to regain their sight and ome may become permanently blind.

Move the flock onto some rough grazing to encourage better rumen rmentation. Except in very small flocks or with particularly valuable nimals, it is rarely cost-effective to treat the whole flock with thiamine. nly when the disease is fully understood will it be possible to give more pecific advice on the prevention of CCN.

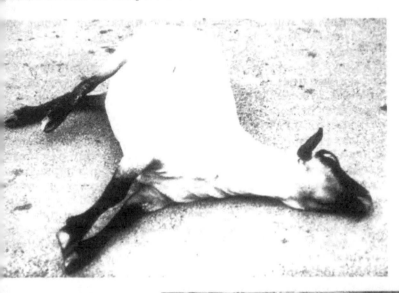

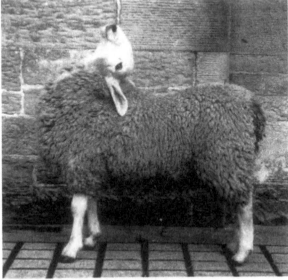

Plate 11.7   Adult ewe (above) and ewe lamb (right) with cerebro-cortical necrosis (CCN).

Water

Sheep obtain their water from three sources. Water is present in all foods but the amount varies considerably, depending on the type of food: concentrate containing very little, grass considerably more and turnips being largely water. Water is also formed from chemical reactions within the body, and it is drunk voluntarily by sheep. The old wives' tale that sheep do not drink water blatant nonsense and, as with all other livestock, fresh, clean, wholesome water must be available to all classes of sheep at all times.

Non-pregnant/non-lactating sheep in moist, humid conditions, where evaporation is low, will obtain most of their water requirements from succulent herbage and from dew falling on the sward. However, in dry windy conditions of low humidity and high evaporation, sheep will drink considerable amounts of water—in the region of 2 to 3 kg for every kilo gram of dry matter consumed.

Ewes in late pregnancy and during lactation have the highest requirement for water of any class of sheep. Their needs depend not only on climate but on the amount of dry matter consumed. For example, in mid pregnancy a ewe will require around 3 kg (6 to 7 pints) of water for every kg of dry matter eaten, and in the last month of pregnancy more than 4 kg (over gallon) of water for every kg of dry matter intake in the total diet.

Ewes' needs in lactation are about the same as in mid-pregnancy, that is around 3 kg water for every kg dry matter consumed. As the lactation progresses in most spring lambing flocks, lush spring grass provides a fair proportion of the water requirements, and ewes therefore drink less than they would in mid pregnancy. Ewes deprived of an adequate supply of water during lactation will produce less milk and will suffer from a depressed appetite, further reducing milk yield. This will have disastrous effects on the growth rate of lambs.

12

INTERNAL PARASITES

A parasite is any living organism (plant or animal) which lives inside or on the surface of another organism (the host) and from which it gains its food supply. Parasites do not benefit their host in any way and in many cases are injurious. Strictly speaking, all organisms which cause disease in animals are parasites, including viruses, bacteria, protozoa, fungi and others. In veterinary terms, the word 'parasite' has become much more restricted and generally taken to indicate the internal parasites (tapeworms, fluke and roundworms) and the external or skin parasites (ticks, lice, keds, etc).

The aim of this and the following chapter is to give a full account of the parasites of sheep, so that farmers and shepherds may be able to control these unwelcome parasites more effectively and thereby substantially improve the profitability of the flock and the welfare of the animals.

ROUNDWORMS

The roundworms which parasitise sheep belong to a large group called the **nematodes**, most of which are free-living in the soil and quite harmless. Some nematodes parasitise plants and others parasitise animals, including all farm animals and pet species.

The roundworms which cause disease in sheep are generally very small, being mostly less than one centimetre long and only the thickness of a hair. *Haemonchus contortus*, or barber's pole worm, is an exception in that it can easily be seen by the naked eye in stomach contents. It is relatively uncommon in the UK, except in parts of southern England, but it is one of the most important worms affecting sheep in the southern hemisphere. (In contrast, one ascarid roundworm of the pig may reach well over a foot in length and the thickness of a pencil!)

There are numerous species of roundworms which affect sheep but only relatively few cause serious problems. The ones we are concerned with in this chapter live in the gut, the different species of worms inhabiting different sites. Several species may affect a sheep at the same time, but at any particular season of the year one or another would normally be the dominant species responsible for any clinical disease symptoms seen. Lungworms are also roundworms but these are discussed in the chapter on pneumonia.

477

LIFE CYCLE OF ROUNDWORMS

In order to predict when problems are likely to occur and in order t implement effective control measures, it is necessary to understand the li cycle of these parasites. To all intents and purposes the life cycles of th different species are very similar, with the exception of the nematodiru species which will be described separately.

Both male and female roundworms are present in the gut and here the mate. The females then begin to lay eggs in enormous numbers, which pas out onto the pasture in the dung. Since sheep may be parasitised by man thousands of egg-laying female worms in even a moderate infestation, it i not surprising that the daily output of dung from one affected sheep ma contain many millions of roundworm eggs.

Worm eggs cannot infect sheep directly, but have to go through process of development to become **infective third stage larvae.** Thi process is entirely dependent upon the weather, since it is essential tha there is adequate moisture and warmth. Providing these conditions ar met, the eggs hatch and first stage larvae emerge, which then feed upo bacteria found in the dung. These larvae shed their skins to become secon stage larvae, which again feed in the dung. Neither first nor second stag larvae are capable of infecting sheep and if swallowed they are simpl digested and destroyed. Also, they are not very tough and are vulnerabl to adverse weather conditions. Many larvae therefore perish before they ca undergo the final moult to become the infective third stage larvae.

When conditions are suitable, these infective larvae wriggle up into th sward in the thin film of moisture on the blades of grass (see Colour plate 41) Once swallowed by a grazing lamb, the larvae burrow into the mucous mem brane of either the stomach or small intestine, depending upon the type o worm involved. Within approximately a week the third stage larvae will hav

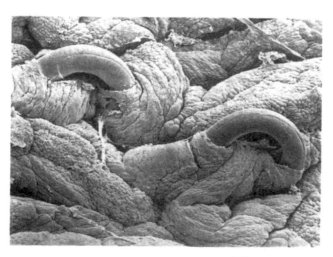

Plate 12.1
A roundworm
(*Trichostrongylus
vitrinus*) burrowing
through the surface
layers of the gut of a
lamb. This photograph
was taken down the
scanning electron
microscope at 300
magnifications. The
worm is only the
thickness of a hair and
less than a centimetre
long (see Plate 12.2).

478

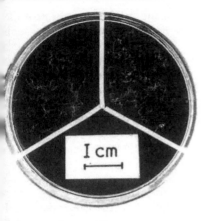

I cm

Plate 12.2   Adult forms of two of the important gut worms of sheep: ostertagia to the left, trichostrongylus to the right. These specimens were recovered at post-mortem and washed so that they can be more easily seen. Note how small and thin they are: then observe the damage they can do as seen by the electron microscope pictures in this chapter.

become immature adult worms which then return to the surface of the gut. Within another week males and females will have mated and the whole cycle will begin again, with females laying eggs and further contaminating the pastures.

Infection on pastures

If eggs are deposited on pasture at an unsuitable time of year for development—for instance, in late autumn in the UK, when it becomes too cold, or during a very dry, hot spell in June—then most of these eggs will eventually perish. Most eggs develop during the late spring, summer and early autumn, the speed of development increasing as the conditions of moisture and warmth become optimal in July and August. It may take as long as three months for eggs deposited in early spring to develop into infective larvae, but less than three weeks for those deposited in a warm, moist spell in July to do so.

This last apparently uninteresting fact is crucially important, since it means that an accumulation of worm eggs will all be developing at differing rates depending upon the weather conditions and upon when they were deposited. The effect of this is that by mid summer, countless millions of infective larvae will be lying in wait for the unsuspecting lambs. This massive challenge is more than sufficient to cause serious clinical illness and even death.

One other feature of infective larvae which is of considerable importance is that they are extremely tough and resistant to a wide variation of climatic conditions, largely because of the protective sheath they retain at their moult. For example, they can withstand many consecutive days of freezing or of hot, dry, desiccating conditions down in the bottom of the sward or in the soil itself. So, whilst many infective larvae which are not eaten by sheep inevitably perish, a significant proportion will always survive right through the winter time, so carrying over infection from one season to another on the pasture. As soon as the ambient temperatures reach around

479

10°C (50°F) these larvae will become active in the sward and so provide the earliest source of infection for any ewes or lambs moved onto such contaminated pastures.

Before discussing the main periods of risk of worm infestation and how to minimise the risks by strategic control measures, we will first consider how these worms cause damage to the sheep, what the clinical signs of infection are and how to treat affected animals. A thumbnail sketch of digestion in ruminants is given to provide a clearer understanding of how worm damage is inflicted.

DIGESTION IN RUMINANTS

The main function of the gut of an animal is to digest food and transfer the nutrients so released into the bloodstream so that they can be transported to every cell in the body. In the case of ruminants, such as the sheep, the process begins in the reticulum and rumen where food is first deposited after swallowing. The rumen is a vast muscular organ which contracts and relaxes in a rhythmic fashion in order to mix the food with the rumen liquor, which contains astronomical numbers of bacteria and protozoa. In ruminants, these friendly microorganisms actually perform the first stage of digestion, which is a continuous fermentation process.

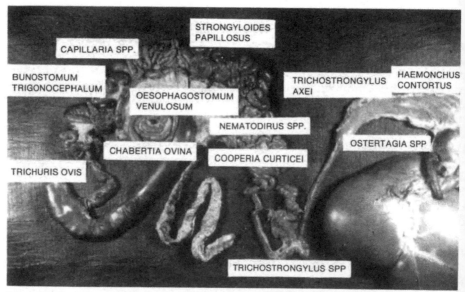

Plate 12.3 The digestive tract of the young ruminant sheep showing where individual roundworm species live in the gut. No worms inhabit the rumen or reticulum (bottom right). The abomasum or true stomach is at top right (above the reticulo-rumen). The small and large intestines are partially unravelled (left). The rectum is at centre bottom!

After a prolonged period of continuous grazing, sheep will lie down and relax. During these relaxation periods—which may occupy up to a third of each day (and night)—they ruminate or 'chew the cud'. During rumination the sheep contentedly chews and rechews small quantities of food which are brought back into the mouth from the rumen by a process known as regurgitation. The small parcels of regurgitated food are first squeezed in the mouth and the liquor swallowed. After about 50 to 60 chewing movements the food is then reswallowed and after a pause of a few seconds another wad of food is propelled from the rumen up the oesophagus, with some considerable force, so that it lands neatly in the mouth. The whole process is then repeated over and over again in order to reduce the food to a fine consistency so that the fermentation process is more efficient.

As in all fermentations, large quantities of gas are produced—mainly methane—which is continually belched up in a most discreet manner. (The quantities of methane which accumulate in a cow with 'bloat' are enormous. One unfortunate, newly qualified veterinary surgeon in Holland some years ago, who was treating such a case, was keen to demonstrate to his farmer client that the gas was, in fact, methane. He foolishly set alight to the stream of gas issuing from the cannula he had inserted into the rumen through the side of the cow. The bazooka-like flame which ensued quickly set fire to some fodder and reduced the entire farm to ashes!)

Fermentation produces large quantities of fatty acids which are an important energy source for ruminants. These are largely absorbed through the wall of the rumen and so into the bloodstream. The proteins in the food are broken down by the microorganisms into their individual amino acid components. The microorganisms divide, incorporating these amino acids into their own proteins. The microorganisms are then themselves digested and broken down in the abomasum (or 'true' stomach) and in the intestine. So, the sheep feeds the microorganisms and they in turn feed the sheep. This interesting process allows ruminants to make use of cellulose and other complex carbohydrates which form a large proportion of the grazing animal's diet. Single stomached animals like man and the pig cannot do this.

Parasitic Gastro-enteritis (PGE)

Roundworm parasites do not inhabit the reticulum, rumen or omasum, but only the abomasum and intestines. Of the important roundworm species in sheep, ostertagia, haemonchus and trichostrongylus (*T. axei*) are found in the stomach, whilst nematodirus and other trichostrongylus species inhabit the intestines. The presence of large numbers of developing worm larvae in the stomach lining causes a gastritis which destroys the cells which produce the gastric juices and enzymes which carry out the initial digestion

481

process. Worms in the intestine cause an enteritis which seriously reduce the efficiency of digestion and the absorption of nutrients. Hence a collectiv name is given to gut roundworm damage—parasitic gastro-enteritis o PGE.

Protein loss

The consequences of roundworm damage, whether produced by adul worms living on the surface of the gut wall or by larvae burrowing into o developing in the wall of the gut, are therefore considerable. The exten of the damage will depend upon the number of worms present, the specie: of worm and the age, health and nutritional status of the animal. In heav infections the inner lining of the gut is severely damaged by the worm: and sloughs off. Blood proteins are then able to 'leak' back into the gu and are lost, either in the faeces or urine. This means that both energy an protein are diverted away from vital processes such as meat, milk and woo production in order to repair the damaged gut and to maintain the level o protein in the circulating blood. The carcasses of parasitised sheep therefor contain less protein (per unit weight) than worm-free sheep.

Diarrhoea

Another essential function of the gut is to regulate the water and mineral balance of the body, and worms seriously interfere with this process also.

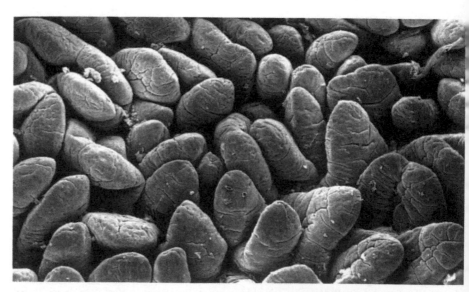

Plate 12.4 The lining of the small intestine of a normal worm-free lamb as seen via the scanning electron microscope magnified 40 times. The villi increase the surface area of the gut enormously. Compare this normal gut with the worm-damaged gut in Plate 12.5.

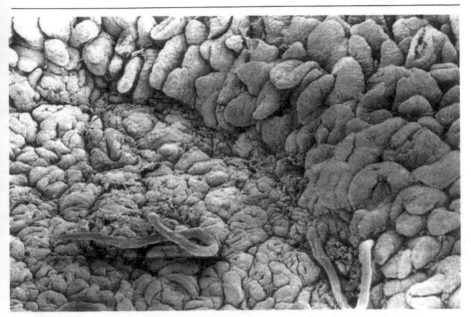

Plate 12.5   Parasitic gastro-enteritis damage in the small intestine of lambs, seen via the scanning electron microscope. In the top plate (magnified 26 times) note the severe stunting of the villi where the worms are, as compared with the relatively early damage on the right of the picture. In the bottom plate (magnified 40 times) a heavy worm burden has completely destroyed the structure of the intestine.

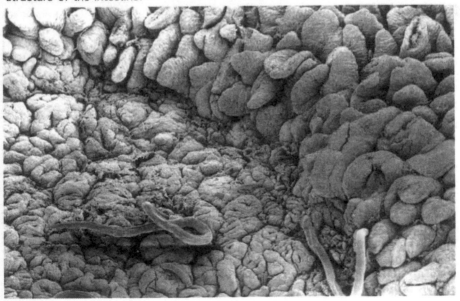

The upset in water balance leads to diarrhoea and dehydration with consequent loss of weight. The mineral imbalance means that the skeleton is improperly mineralised, which further contributes to the stunted growth. Parasitised carcasses are also 'wet' since they contain more water and the worst cases will be condemned at meat inspection.

Roundworm infections always reduce appetite. Even in light infections, food intake may be reduced by 10 to 20% and by considerably more in severe cases. The problem is added to by the fact that food conversion efficiency is also considerably reduced.

Where infections are relatively light (sub-clinical), no obvious clinical signs such as diarrhoea may be present. However, close examination of a group of affected lambs will reveal a reduction in weight gain, poor food conversion, lower growth rates, poorer fleece quality and, at slaughter, adverse changes in carcass composition. In adult suckling ewes, even a mild infestation will reduce milk yield.

These vague signs may be mistaken for undernutrition. Indeed, if lambs are underfed, particularly where protein levels are low, then the symptoms of parasitism will be exaggerated. There is also a growing body of evidence to show that these animals are more prone to other infections and less able to fight them off. This is understandable, since both protein and energy are essential to the proper functioning of the immune system which helps the animal fight off infection.

If the intake of infective larvae is light and lambs are well fed, they will gradually build up an immunity with increasing age. However, there will always be some reduction in growth rate. With medium intakes of worm larvae, the flock as a whole may be 'poor doers', but there may still be no diarrhoea. In heavy infestations, diarrhoea, dehydration and even death may follow. The appearance of scouring in a flock of 'wormy' lambs can be compared to the oil warning indicator glowing red on the car dashboard—it is not so much a signal that the oil is low, but that damage has probably already occurred and a big bill can be anticipated.

CLINICAL SIGNS OF PGE

Symptoms vary somewhat depending upon which worm or worms are present. As mentioned earlier, disease at different seasons of the year may be caused by different worms. The following is a description of the most common summer worm problem in lambs caused most frequently by a worm called *Ostertagia circumcincta*.

The first sign of mild infection may simply be that lambs are performing disappointingly. Their fleeces have a dry and lacklustre appearance. A number of them may show signs of diarrhoea. If a diagnosis is not made and prompt treatment applied to the whole flock, then the situation will deteriorate rapidly, with more and more lambs beginning to scour and lose condition.

Lambs quickly become dehydrated through the loss of fluid in the diarrhoea and when handled are very tight-skinned and light weight. The scour is often watery and profuse and the dirty hindquarters attract blowflies to lay their eggs, which may lead to maggot strike. (Even in recently dipped sheep, strike may occur because of the gross contamination of the fleece.) In severe infestations some lambs may die before, or despite, treatment. Scouring lambs which are treated and 'dry up' nevertheless suffer a severe check from which they never fully recover. Such lambs are rarely if ever profitable.

Diagnosis of PGE

Worms are so common a problem that it may seem unimportant to discuss diagnosis. However, confusion can arise over other conditions with similar symptoms during the grazing season, such as cobalt pine or coccidiosis. Also, worms can occur in a flock where control measures are being applied incorrectly through a misunderstanding of the pattern of disease in a flock.

Obviously if clinical signs of scouring appear in lambs during the summer grazing season, then worms must be a strong possibility, especially on farms which do not practise appropriate control measures. However, as with making any diagnosis, the history is of vital importance. The age of the sheep involved, the season of the year, the type of pasture—whether 'clean' or 'dirty'—and the timing of any worm dosings are all important information.

Any dead or moribund lambs should be submitted for post-mortem, since a full examination should yield valuable information regarding the rest of the flock. It is frequently a waste of time for the farmer or shepherd to take random dung samples into the veterinary surgery for worm egg counts without first discussing the best animals to sample. Worm egg counts are used to provide evidence that there are adult egg-laying female worms present in the gut of the sheep and also to give an estimate of the burden of adult worms likely to be present. However, they can sometimes be misleading and need careful interpretation. For example, clinical symptoms may be due to hatching larvae and there may be few adults present in the gut and therefore few worm eggs in the dung. Also, with *Ostertagia circumcincta* the magnitude of the worm egg output is not necessarily related to the size of the worm burden.

If the history and clinical signs strongly suggest roundworm infection, response to treatment with an anthelmintic may be used as an aid to diagnosis. Where lambs have been scouring they should dry up within a day or two of worming, providing they are moved to clean, worm-free grazing to prevent reinfection. The damage to the gut is often considerable and may take many weeks to heal, so that recovery is generally slow.

If there is no response to anthelmintic treatment the diagnosis may be incorrect, or another infection that also makes lambs scour may be present in the flock at the same time as worms. Coccidiosis is probably the commonest example.

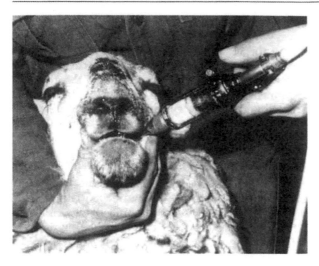

Plate 12.6 Animals which are dosed with anthelmintics should always be moved to clean grazing if possible. If they must remain on dirty ground, they will become reinfected and therefore require frequent dosing.

TREATMENT OF CLINICAL PARASITIC GASTRO-ENTERITIS

Where a proportion of the lamb flock is scouring and worms are diagnosed, then the whole flock must be dosed with an anthelmintic, not just those affected. It must be appreciated that whilst a dose of one of the modern drugs will kill around '99% of all known worms', sheep will become re-infected within a day or so if they remain on the same pasture or are moved to other dirty grazings. If possible, always **worm and move to clean ground.**

Many of the wormers available are ovicidal, which means they will also kill worm eggs present in the gut contents. Since it takes a few hours for the drug to act, it is best to keep dosed sheep (but not pregnant ewes) in the handling pens or in a building for four or five hours after dosing. In this way very few eggs should survive to contaminate the clean grazing.

Any severely affected animals—for example, very thin, dehydrated lambs with a profuse diarrhoea—must be pulled out from the group and brought close to home or housed if possible. These sheep will need careful nursing if they are to make a reasonable recovery. Provide them with some good-quality hay and a supply of fresh water. These animals will be dehydrated, and since this is what kills many wormy sheep, they must be treated with oral electrolyte solutions.

Great care should always be taken when treating severely debilitated animals with any drugs. Although most wormers have a reasonable safety margin, sick animals should be weighed before dosing so that they are not overdosed. Dehydrated lambs may weigh considerably less than their flock mates which have not begun to scour.

Remember that having to treat animals for the clinical disease is an admission of failure, since it means that control measures have been unsuccessful. Anthelmintics are most effectively used as part of a worm control programme, about which more detailed notes are given later in this chapter.

THE CONTROL OF PARASITIC GASTRO-ENTERITIS

There is no time of year when the shepherd can afford to completely forget about worms in one class of sheep or another. Nevertheless, there are certain seasons of the year or particular circumstances which create a high risk. These arise largely because of the life cycle of the parasites, the weather and the husbandry systems under which the sheep are kept. Remembering that it is pasture which carries the infective worm larvae, it is important to understand how and when grazings become infected under any particular management regime. Only then is it possible to take appropriate control measures.

Worm infections in ewes

Although the healthy, well-fed ewe has a fair degree of immunity to worm infestation through previous challenge in the first year of life, she nevertheless plays a most important role in contaminating pastures which will be grazed by her own lambs.

Ewes grazing contaminated pasture in the autumn—that is, during the tupping and early pregnancy period in spring lambing flocks—will pick up infective larvae. However, at this time of year the majority of larvae do not develop into adult worms inside the sheep. Instead they burrow into the wall of the gut and remain there to undergo a form of hibernation as 'arrested' larvae. They do this in the best interests of parasitism. If they were to develop into egg-laying females, most of the eggs deposited on the pastures would perish during the winter months. By 'arresting', they can keep warm and cosy inside the ewe until the spring, when conditions on the pasture are more suitable for development of the worm eggs.

THE SPRING OR PERIPARTURIENT RISE IN WORM EGG OUTPUT

Coincidentally, changes take place in ewes during late pregnancy and well into lactation which, in spring lambing flocks particularly, further assist the parasites in their development. Hormonal changes, particularly those associated with milk production, have a depressive effect upon the ewe's immune system. This relaxation of immunity allows the arrested larvae to hatch en masse and develop into adults. Additionally, the female worms, being less inhibited by the ewe's immune system, lay more eggs than they would during the rest of the year. In consequence, ewes contaminate pastures very heavily with worm eggs—particularly with those of the stomach worm (*Ostertagia circumcincta*). This is known as the spring or the periparturient rise, since it occurs just before, during and after lambing. Eggs deposited by the ewes at this time develop into infective larvae over

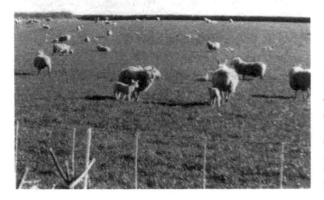

Plate 12.7 Scottish Halfbred ewes and lambs turned out onto clean grazing in February in Dorset. Ewes must be dosed before turnout to prevent them contaminating the grazings for their lambs.

the following weeks and are therefore the main source of infection for the lambs once they begin to graze.

Although it has already been stated that adult ewes have a considerable immunity to roundworms, there is nevertheless good evidence to suggest that because of the relaxation of immunity around the time of the spring rise, the parasites may produce sufficient damage in the ewe to reduce milk yield significantly. We have therefore established two very good reasons why ewes must be dosed with an anthelmintic around this time.

Effect of worming on lambing percentage in housed ewes

Before deciding exactly when is the best time to treat the ewe flock for worms, there is some other evidence which should be considered, particularly in relation to flocks housed over the winter period. Trials carried out at Rosemaund Experimental Husbandry Farm in Herefordshire showed that if ewes mated in October and housed in late December or early January were given a dose of one particular anthelmintic—levamisole—some ten days after housing, there was an improvement in lambing percentage. Approximately nine more live lambs were born to every 100 ewes put to the rams, as compared with untreated ewes. Moreover, the birth weights of the lambs from the anthelmintic treated ewes were the same as those from the untreated ewes.

This beneficial effect may be due, in part, to clearing the ewes of all roundworm parasites, thereby increasing appetite and improving feed conversion rate. It may also be partly due to a stimulatory effect upon the ewe's immune system, which is known to be an additional feature of this particular drug. Whatever the mechanisms involved, these results—obtained over some four years of trials—cannot be ignored when such a significant benefit in increased lambing rate is involved.

It is interesting to note that the ewes on trial (Welsh halfbreds and Mules) already had a very respectable lambing percentage (180%) in the

488

years before anthelmintic dosing was initiated. They were in good body condition and showed no outward signs of suffering from parasitism. Nevertheless, they obviously benefited significantly from treatment. (Increases in milk yield have also been demonstrated in adult dairy cows following anthelmintic treatment on some, although not all, farms.) Providing the benefits more than cover the costs—as they would appear to do in the case of housed ewes—it would seem to make good sense to dose the ewes at this time. In practice there is no extra cost involved. Ewes will not pick up any worms in-house and in any case they must be wormed before turnout onto clean ground with their lambs. They can therefore be treated shortly after housing, with the dual benefits of a possible improvement in lambing percentage and an increase in milk production. It also means one less task for the busy shepherd at lambing time, since they will not require worming again before turnout, providing they have not been allowed out to graze by day.

Worming ewes at lambing time

Ewes which remain at pasture throughout pregnancy and are brought indoors for only a few days over the lambing period can be wormed at any convenient time before they are turned out. Ewes which are brought into a lambing paddock and perhaps confined in a strawed lambing pen for only 24 or 48 hours should be wormed in the lambing pen. If they are wormed whilst in the lambing paddock, they will become reinfected, since these small fields are usually heavily contaminated.

It is most important to select the correct anthelmintic for this dosing before turnout. The product must be effective against adult worms, larvae and inhibited or arrested larvae, so that ewes are cleared of all stages of worms. If the chosen product also kills worm eggs, as many do, then all to the good.

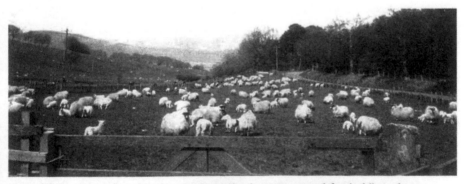

Plate 12.8 A small paddock next to gathering pens used for holding sheep. These and lambing paddocks around the steading are always likely to be heavily contaminated with parasites through regular use and high stocking rates. Even if animals are held in such areas for only a short time, they will become contaminated.

Other winter worm problems

Worm problems do not disappear with the end of the summer grazing season. A large percentage of the larvae picked up off the pastures from late autumn onwards do not develop into adult females but burrow into the tissues of the gut and hibernate as 'arrested' larvae. These may remain dormant right throughout the winter period, but should a sheep become stressed, perhaps because of inadequate feeding or severe weather conditions, the animal's immune system can become temporarily depressed. This allows arrested larvae to hatch, a process which can cause very considerable gut damage. Occasionally the hatch is massive, leading to severe loss of condition and even death. All age groups of sheep can be affected, from ewe hoggs to adult rams.

'Black scour'

A steady build-up of adult trichostrongylus worms may cause extensive gut damage, producing the profuse, dark and evil-smelling diarrhoea which gives the condition its colloquial name of 'black scour'. Twin bearing hill ewes in late pregnancy on an inadequate diet are particularly prone. Store lambs or hoggs grazing on kale, rape or swedes are also at risk, especially when no adequate lay-back or shelter is provided and the weather turns nasty. However, either trichostongylus worms or *Ostertagia circumcincta* (the brown stomach worm) may cause unthriftiness and occasional diarrhoea in any class of sheep, whether housed or at grass.

Obviously, husbandry practices likely to precipitate such outbreaks should be avoided, but worming in the late autumn, early winter, or soon after housing with an anthelmintic capable of killing arrested larvae will largely prevent such problems. Hoggs travelling away to wintering pastures should always be dosed before they go and immediately on their return, before they

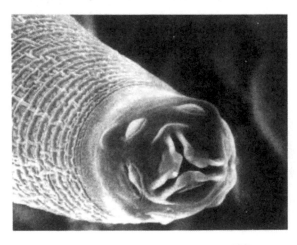

Plate 12.9 The head end of the gut worm *Trichostrongylus vitrinus* magnified 1,000 times (scanning electron microscope). This is the worm that causes 'black scour' during the winter months.

are turned out onto the grazings. This should also apply to any purchased sheep, such as ewe-lamb replacements and rams.

Barber's pole worm

Whilst *Haemonchus contortus* (the barber's pole worm) can cause acute anaemia in lambs in the summer time, it may also cause a chronic, wasting anaemia during the winter and early spring in adult ewes or hoggs. In this case it is the adult worms which cause the damage through their particularly savage blood-sucking activities. A late autumn dose with an anthelmintic active against arrested larvae should prevent this problem.

CLEAN GRAZING SYSTEMS

The value of clean grazing cannot be overemphasized. Lambs which have access to pastures carrying very low worm burdens grow faster and are ready for slaughter significantly earlier than those grazing worm contaminated ground, providing there is no other underlying problem, such as a trace element deficiency.

When worms are kept under control, stocking rates can be increased without the inevitable depression in lamb growth and performance that is always seen on dirty grazings, despite regular worming. Considerable savings are made through the minimum use of anthelmintics. There is also the added benefit of fewer handlings for dosing, which is especially important for ewes with lambs at foot, to avoid mismothering problems. Scouring should be reduced, so minimising the risk of fly strike, and there will be the added benefit of a clean fleece at shearing.

Before describing how a clean grazing policy can be put into effect, it is necessary first to define what is meant by 'clean' and 'dirty' grazing in relation to parasitic gastro-enteritis.

Clean pastures

Completely clean and uncontaminated pasture is very uncommon. Even a sward which is ploughed and reseeded may become contaminated with nematodirus infective larvae which have burrowed back to the surface. However, for all practical purposes, the level of contamination on clean grazing will be so low as to pose no threat to young susceptible lambs grazing it, either before or after weaning. In other words it is as safe as can be practically achieved under most commercial farming circumstances.

Examples of clean grazings are the following:

- pastures which have not been grazed at all, such as new leys following cereals or some other arable crop
- pastures which have been grazed but where the level of infection has subsided to very low levels, such as

—grass which has not carried sheep for 12 months

491

—aftermaths—from July onwards—which have not carried sheep since the previous autumn

—grazings—from July onwards—which have carried cattle since the previous spring, but have not carried sheep since the previous autumn

—areas which were used solely for the conservation of hay or silage during the previous season

—aftermaths which were not grazed by sheep before being shut up

Not-so-clean pastures

In between clean and dirty, the level of contamination on pastures varies greatly, but all carry some degree of risk. If they are grazed by young, susceptible animals, the egg-laying females which develop from the infective larvae picked up by the lambs will lay eggs in huge numbers and heavily contaminate the pastures. As the season progresses and the weather improves, the whole worm life cycle speeds up considerably, so that by mid summer, what began as a lightly infected pasture may have become deadly dangerous.

Examples of grazings which would present an acceptable risk would be as follows:

- fields which have carried only dosed adult ewes during the previous autumn
- previously clean aftermaths which have carried only dosed weaned lambs since July
- pastures grazed only by cattle since the previous July—although these carry the risk of *Nematodirus battus* infection

These examples are not exhaustive and advice should be sought if there is any doubt about the safety of particular grazings.

Whole farm strategies designed to provide clean grazing

A number of 'systems' have been devised to accommodate different farming situations. These systems are based on the principle of providing **clean grazing for clean sheep**. Where both sheep and cattle are farmed, the area designated to them can either be divided into two roughly equal areas, one for each species, or into three areas, the third being used for conservation.

Where no hay or silage crop is taken from the stocked area of the farm—perhaps because of the problems of harvesting on difficult ground— then the area grazed by cattle one year will be grazed by sheep the next and so on. One problem with this very simple alternate grazing system is that there is no clean grazing for weaned lambs—unless they can be moved to clean aftermaths elsewhere on the farm. Another problem is the risk of *Nematodirus battus* being perpetuated on the grazings, as is explained later in the discussion of that parasite. This is especially risky where young dairy calves are the alternate grazers.

Rutter ring system

It is always preferable to include conservation in a clean grazing rotation if at all possible, as this largely overcomes the nematodirus problem at the same time as providing clean aftermath for weaned lambs. The most successful strategy for this was developed by Bill Rutter, formerly of the East of Scotland College of Agriculture in Edinburgh. In this system, the order of things is important: sheep should follow cattle and conservation should follow sheep.

Lambs are dosed at weaning and moved back onto clean hay or silage aftermaths, while the ewes remain on the same sheep area all season. The following season, ewes and lambs graze the cattle area of the previous grazing season. Grass for hay or silage is grown on the previous season's cattle grazings, while cattle graze over last year's conservation area, which carried dosed weaned lambs in the second half of the season. This pattern can be used either on permanent pasture or on a three year ley system where conservation is undertaken.

Adaptations are necessary, for example, where leys are left down for longer or shorter periods, where there are no cattle on the farm or where the proportions of cattle to sheep are widely disproportionate in terms of livestock units.

Mixed grazing

The grazing of cattle alongside sheep on the same pastures is unsatisfactory in terms of controlling parasitic gastro-enteritis and can engender a false sense of security. Whilst cattle will certainly consume and destroy a proportion of the sheep worms on a pasture and vice-versa, the sheep will nevertheless consume more than sufficient sheep worm larvae to become infected and so contaminate the pastures to a considerable degree, despite the dilution factor. Whilst it is often satisfactory from a sward management point of view to mix the species, these pastures should be considered risky or even dangerous for sheep.

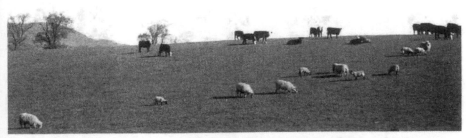

Plate 12.10   Mixed grazing of cattle and sheep does not control worms.

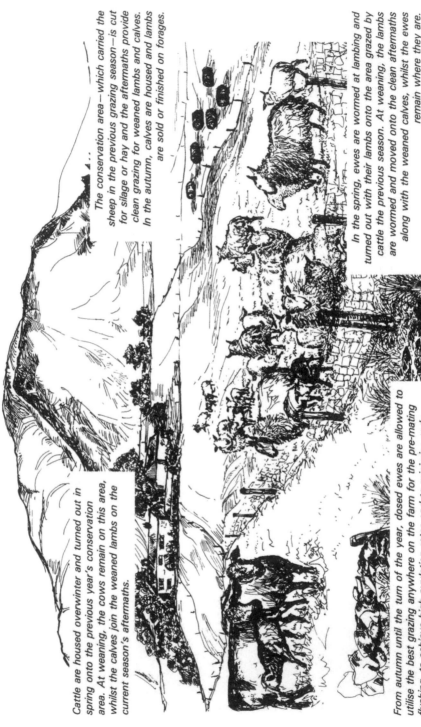

The conservation area—which carried the sheep in the previous grazing season—is cut for silage or hay and the aftermaths provide clean grazing for weaned lambs and calves. In the autumn, calves are housed and lambs are sold or finished on forages.

In the spring, ewes are wormed at lambing and turned out with their lambs onto the area grazed by cattle the previous season. At weaning, the lambs are wormed and moved onto the clean aftermaths along with the weaned calves, whilst the ewes remain where they are.

Cattle are housed overwinter and turned out in spring onto the previous year's conservation area. At weaning, the cows remain on this area, whilst the calves join the weaned lambs on the current season's aftermaths.

From autumn until the turn of the year, dosed ewes are allowed to utilise the best grazing anywhere on the farm for the pre-mating flushing, to achieve high ovulation rates and to minimise early embryo losses.

494

Figure 12.1   Rutter ring system for upland beef and sheep enterprises (spring lambing).

Dirty pastures

Dirty grazings are those which are contaminated with significant numbers of worm eggs, infective larvae or both. They are especially dangerous to lambs and hoggs during their first grazing season. Any pastures grazed by sheep—especially lambs or undosed ewes—during the previous or current grazing season are potentially dangerous. Infective larvae can survive over-winter on pastures and even if these swards are not grazed from the turn of the year, they will remain a source of infection—albeit a diminishing one—until June. By that time most over-wintered larvae will have died off and a dirty pasture will have become a relatively safe one.

Worm control on lowland farms

The dosing of the ewe has been discussed already and it will be assumed that ewes housed over the whole winter period will be dosed 10 days after housing and therefore will not require dosing again at turnout with their lambs at foot.

Ewes housed for only a short time over the lambing period, or those which lamb in an outside yard or lambing paddock, should be dosed immediately before turnout wherever they are going on the farm. This will eliminate the spring rise in worm egg output and so prevent the contamination of clean pastures for lambs. Also, by reducing the worm burden of the ewe, milk production may be significantly increased, perhaps by as much as 15 or 20% in well-fed ewes.

There is often insufficient grass growth for ewes and lambs to go straight out of the lambing area and onto the clean fields where they will remain up to weaning. Also, because of the spread of lambing, it takes time for sufficient ewes to lamb to stock these fields fully. Frequently, therefore, some ewes and lambs are put out to graze for a week or two onto whatever grass is available. Not all of this will be clean and indeed some may be decidedly dirty. This need not be too great a problem provided that when grass growth does take off, the ewes are dosed again before being moved onto the clean ground.

Whilst this system reduces the quantity of supplementary feed needed for ewes in early lactation, it does delay the shutting up of fields for hay and silage and also may delay cattle turnout. However, whilst moving ewes and lambs directly to their clean grazing after lambing overcomes these problems, it does increase the need for supplementary feeding and may cause poaching and overgrazing of new leys, so reducing future stock carrying capacity.

Providing the ewes have been adequately trough fed to encourage high milk production, lambs under three weeks of age on dirty pastures will not be grazing sufficiently to warrant dosing. However, any lambs older than this must be dosed along with their mothers before going onto the clean grazing. It is always highly desirable to get lambs onto clean ground before they begin consuming grass to any significant extent. Worm-free ewes and lambs moving onto clean grazing should keep the pasture contamination at a very low level, so that dosing should not be necessary until weaning.

If for any reason lambs on clean grazings fail to thrive or even begin to scour, then it is probably sensible to have faeces samples from a proportion of the lambs checked for worm eggs. If there is a worm problem, then the whole lamb flock should be dosed and the reason for the breakdown investigated. If there is no evidence of a worm infestation, or if lambs are dosed but do not respond to treatment, then further investigation will be required in order to arrive at a diagnosis. Coccidiosis is always high on the list of suspects in these circumstances.

Turning ewes and lambs out onto dirty grazing

What can be done if there is no clean grazing available at lambing, so that ewes and lambs have to be turned out onto contaminated ground? The first thing to appreciate is that the rule about keeping pasture contamination to a minimum still holds and ewes must be dosed at turnout. However, the ewes will reinfect themselves by picking up infective larvae which have survived over the winter. Because the ewes' immune defences are low at this time, these larvae will be able to establish an infection. The female worms which develop will lay eggs and the ewe's faeces will then further contaminate the ground for the lambs.

DOSING EWES If this is allowed to continue unchecked, then the new contamination contributed by the ewes—added to that already present in the

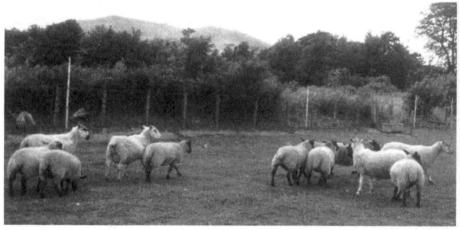

Plate 12.11   East of Scotland College of Agriculture greyface ewes with Suffolk cross twin lambs grazing a 2 cm high sward (tetraploid perennial ryegrass plus clover S184) during the drought of July 1989. Lambs were growing at 330 gm per day at a stocking rate of six ewes plus twin lambs per acre on pasture contaminated with worms from the previous year. This could not be achieved without regular three week dosing with a broad spectrum anthelmintic. Note the clean, unsoiled rear ends of the lambs.

form of over-wintered larvae—will build up to very dangerous levels for the lambs by June, July or August. The period of greatest risk will largely depend upon the prevailing weather conditions. Therefore ewes must be dosed regularly whilst on the contaminated grazings and at short enough intervals to prevent the female worms reaching the egg-laying stage. This means dosing ewes at three week intervals until their immune defences have sufficiently recovered to prevent the development of infective larvae picked up off the pasture. Generally, if ewes are dosed at turnout and at three weeks and six weeks after turnout, then this should be sufficient, providing they are in good condition and well fed.

DOSING LAMBS   Lambs sucking ewes with an ample milk supply will not take in substantial amounts of grass or infective larvae much before they are four or five weeks old and therefore will not need to be dosed up to that age. However, as soon as they begin to ingest significant numbers of infective larvae, then they must be dosed at intervals of three weeks for as long as they are grazing dirty ground. In practice, this means they will probably receive their first dose of anthelmintic when the ewes have their last—that is, at around six weeks of age (see Plate 12.11).

In a few restricted areas in the south of England, where *Haemonchus contortus* is a problem, dosing may be given less frequently—for example, every four weeks—in an attempt to reduce the risk of anthelmintic resistance. This is a compromise, since lambs will suffer some setback due to worm damage, even if they do not actually reach the stage of scouring.

Obviously, since lambing takes place over a number of weeks, the lambs on a particular grazing may not all be the same age. As a general rule when dosing a flock, it is better to dose some lambs when they are less than six weeks of age rather than leave older lambs undosed and so risk serious damage. This is particularly important when *Nematodirus battus* is a risk. Dosing every three weeks should continue until weaning in flocks on contaminated grazings. This regime has been shown to increase the weight gain of lambs and to reduce the proportion which fail to reach marketable weight and which subsequently have to be stored overwinter.

Lambs sucking ewes which are not milking well will tend to begin grazing earlier than those getting plenty of milk. They will therefore become infected earlier and, because they are less well nourished, will also tend to suffer more severely from worm damage than better fed lambs.

Nematodirus Infection in Lambs

Nematodirus battus, which is of great importance in lambs in the UK, has a different life cycle from the other roundworms and therefore will be described separately. If avoiding action is not taken, it can cause explosive outbreaks of disease and death in young grazing lambs which can have a disastrous effect on the profitability of the flock.

Adult female nematodirus worms lay their eggs in the sheep's gut and,

497

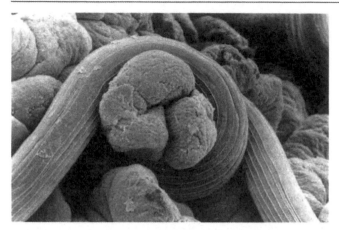

Plate 12.12 A nematodirus worm hanging on to the surface of the small intestine by coiling around the villi (scanning electron microscope at 250 magnifications). This worm is less than 1 cm long and only the thickness of a hair.

as with all other roundworms, the eggs pass out in the faeces and onto the pasture. However, unlike those of other worms, these eggs take a very long time to develop, and the larval stages remain inside the eggshell rather than living free in the sward. Eggs dropped on the pasture in early summer will have reached the third infective larval stage only by autumn at the earliest. Rather than hatch at this time, when the temperatures have dropped, the majority of infective larvae remain protected inside the eggshell for the whole of the winter. In this protected form the larvae are very resistant to even the harshest weather conditions; indeed, they can survive for at least two years and probably longer. They can even survive ploughing, some larvae burrowing up through the soil when conditions are suitable.

The nematodirus hatch

Before hatching can occur, the larvae require the stimulus of a cold snap in the weather followed by a mean 24 hour temperature of around 10°C (50°F). These conditions may occur as early as February or March in the south, or not until much later, perhaps April, May or even June in a very late northern spring. Because the conditions are fairly exact, it is possible to predict mathematically when hatching is likely to occur by examining meteorological data for the various regions of the country. These forecasts are published in the farming press and announced on radio and television and are a great help, especially to farmers who do not have clean grazing available for lambs.

Whilst the infective larvae are well protected inside the eggshell, they become more vulnerable after hatching and gradually die off if not eaten by lambs. From the time young lambs begin grazing to a significant extent, they are very vulnerable to infection. However, once they reach three or four months of age they are beginning to become resistant and by the time they are six months old this resistance is quite strong. Therefore, the timing of the nematodirus hatch in relation to when lambing occurs in the flock is very significant. For example, if spring arrives early and the nematodirus eggs hatch long before the lambs begin to graze, then the great bulk of infective larvae will have perished before they have the chance to infect the lambs. With spring lambing flocks, the most dangerous situation is when spring arrives late—as it so frequently does in northern Britain—so that young, vulnerable lambs of six or eight weeks old are grazing when the hatch occurs.

Because all the larvae overwinter inside the egg and hatch simultaneously, they are often present in massive numbers on the sward. This ensures that all lambs grazing a contaminated field receive an overwhelming dose of larvae simultaneously. There is no gradual build-up of infection as occurs with the other roundworms. Outbreaks of disease—which are most common in May and June—are often explosive in nature. The whole of the lamb flock may begin scouring at around the same time and in the most severe outbreaks the first sign of trouble may be a number of sudden deaths. In some outbreaks a third or more of the lambs die.

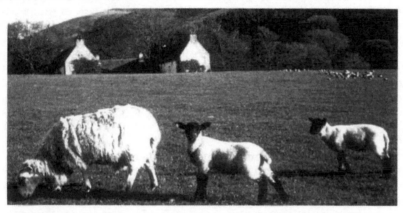

Plate 12.13 Lambs grazing pastures used by lambs during the previous season are at risk from nematodirus infection and must be dosed routinely during the danger period.

Clinical signs

The damage is done, not by the adult worms, but by the huge numbers of infective larvae burrowing into the lining of the gut simultaneously. This causes the lambs much pain and the symptoms of nematodirus reflect this—lambs often standing with their heads down, ears drooped, belly tucked up and most reluctant to move. There is often a sudden and severe diarrhoea, but because lambs stop eating, they pass very little other than a slimy mucus. The sunken eyes and tight skin indicate a severe dehydration which makes lambs very thirsty, so that they tend to congregate around a watering place. The author has seen a lamb so weak and in so much pain that it toppled over into a stream in the effort to get a drink. In the worst cases death is very rapid, whilst other lambs may take several days to die.

Diagnosis and treatment

Post-mortem examination of lambs which die, or are humanely destroyed some time after the acute stage of the disease, may reveal huge numbers of adult worms in the small intestine (estimates of over 50,000 are not uncommon), but, as stated earlier, it is the burrowing larvae which do the damage. Therefore, in the early stages of an acute and explosive outbreak an examination of the faeces for worm eggs may reveal nothing, since the larvae may not have developed into egg-laying adult females.

In an outbreak, treatment with an appropriate anthelmintic must be prompt, but despite this, lambs may continue to die over the following days. The worst affected lambs will need very careful nursing, but recovery is always painfully slow and always incomplete. In the worst outbreaks, the lamb flock is decimated and a dismal sight to behold.

The nematodirus season quite frequently coincides with the coccidiosis season and this is really bad news for lambs. If an outbreak of nematodirus follows one of coccidiosis, then the death rate may rise substantially, and if the two diseases occur simultaneously in a flock, the death rate may even double. If treatment for one or the other disease does not bring about a response, this double infection may be the reason. Where either of these conditions is suspected it is always wise to seek professional advice.

Prevention and control

Prevention of nematodirus hinges upon providing grazing for lambs which was not grazed by lambs during the nematodirus season of the previous year and if possible the year before that also. The safest grazings are new leys following the plough. Land grazed in the previous year by adult ewes will not pose a nematodirus risk, since ewes are solidly immune to this parasite, carry no adult nematodirus worms and therefore do not contaminate pastures with eggs. They do of course harbour other roundworms.

If clean (nematodirus-free) grazing is not available, then lambs must be protected from this potentially disastrous disease by dosing with a suitable anthelmintic every three weeks during the high risk period. Lambs grazing contaminated pastures should in any case be dosed at three weekly intervals from six weeks of age until weaning. However, where nematodirus is a risk—and the official forecasts are of assistance here—then the first dose may need to be given to lambs of less than six weeks old. This is because the high risk period may extend from the end of April or early May through into June. Also, the challenge is heavy and comes all at once. Even young lambs which have just begun grazing properly may therefore take in a heavy infection. Since it is the burrowing larvae which cause the damage they may become ill very quickly. This may mean one extra three week dosing during the season, but the cost and inconvenience are as nothing compared to an outbreak.

500

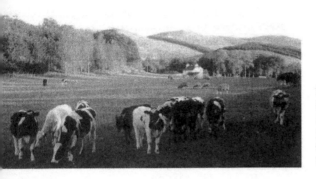

Plate 12.14   Calves can become infected with nematodirus and infect pastures for lambs grazing the following season.

Problems with *Nematodirus battus* control in alternate grazing systems

As explained elsewhere in this chapter, some considerable measure of control of parasitic gastro-enteritis can be obtained by grazing cattle in one season and sheep in the next because the worms affecting cattle do not generally infect sheep and vice versa. One known exception to this rule is nematodirus. This was not fully appreciated until relatively recently when outbreaks were observed in lambs on alternate grazing systems. Indeed, it is possible that this worm has 'adapted' to the husbandry changes taken in an attempt to control it and this may be the reason why breakdowns were not identified before now.

It is known that young calves—particularly dairy calves—can become infected with *Nematodirus battus* after grazing pastures where larvae have been deposited by lambs grazing during the previous season. The adult female worms lay eggs which are then passed out in the calf faeces. Although there may be relatively few eggs in every gram of faeces as compared to a full-blown infection in lambs, the calves nevertheless contaminate the ground sufficiently to be a danger to lambs the following season.

Even if the number of larvae present is not sufficient to cause obvious clinical disease after one year, lambs—being more susceptible than calves—will multiply up the parasite numbers enormously during the first year. Since a significant proportion of infective larvae will survive overwinter, pasture burdens will soon increase to disease-producing proportions.

A recent report has described severe *Nematodirus battus* disease in dairy calves within a month of turnout onto pastures heavily contaminated by lambs the previous season. A number of calves died despite treatment. This possibility will have to be considered in future.

Because adult cattle are strongly immune to nematodirus, there is less risk of a breakdown where suckler beef cows and their calves are the alternate grazers. The cows 'mop up' a significant proportion of the infective larvae which are then digested and destroyed. Spring born suckler calves graze less than their weaned dairy counterparts and since they are still sucking their mother's milk over the danger period they rarely become heavily infected. Older calves and yearlings are usually resistant to nematodirus infection through earlier contact and so pose little threat.

It should be noted that one cattle worm—*Cooperia onchophora*—can infect sheep sub-clinically and so may become a problem for calves on an alternate grazing system.

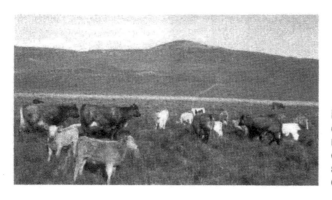

Plate 12.15 Beef calves present less of a risk from nematodirus on alternate grazing systems than do dairy calves.

Autumn nematodirus infection

Nematodirus battus is generally a spring infection of lambs. In recent years, however, outbreaks have been recorded in the late summer and autumn. For an outbreak to occur it is necessary for susceptible lambs to graze heavily contaminated pastures. Because more farmers are rearing lambs under clean grazing systems, some lambs are reaching the first autumn of their life having encountered only a relatively insignificant or non-existent challenge from nematodirus. These older lambs therefore have little if any immunity and may be very susceptible to a heavy challenge from this worm. It is thought that a proportion of nematodirus eggs contaminating pastures in spring may hatch in the autumn, rather than overwintering as the majority do. In addition, some infective larvae which hatched in the spring will have survived. Therefore, if older susceptible lambs are moved onto these contaminated pastures, clinical disease may occur.

To complicate things further, there is another nematodirus worm (*N. filicollis*) which may produce disease in the autumn. It is therefore possible that both worms establish an autumn-to-autumn transmission on some farms, possibly in response to modern husbandry systems. Operators of clean grazing systems must therefore be aware of the possibility of autumn disease. Many hill and upland farmers who have little or no clean grazing available may attempt to finish lambs on grazings which have carried lambs year after year. Autumn nematodirus has been observed on such farms and dosing lambs every three weeks has been found necessary during August and September.

PLANNING CLEAN GRAZING FOR PGE CONTROL FOR NEXT SEASON

Just before weaning is the time to decide on which areas of the farm are to be allocated as clean grazing for ewes, lambs and other classes of young sheep for the following year. (In a mixed enterprise this will also mean doing the same planning for cattle, since both species will benefit from an integrated clean grazing policy.) Pastures which have only carried cattle during the current season, direct reseeds, undersown cereals and leys used for conservation of hay or silage are all suitable as clean grazing for sheep next season. However, they must not be grazed in the second half of the current season by any group of susceptible young sheep, such as weaned lambs or ewe lamb replacements. Even if these classes of sheep are dosed before being moved, their poorer resistance to worm infections (as compared to adult sheep) would inevitably compromise the status of the clean grazings and so introduce an element of risk.

These clean grazings are valuable as an autumn bite for cattle and are particularly useful for flushing ewes prior to tupping and during the early pregnancy period. Providing they are not liable to poaching, these swards need to be grazed down if they are to be fully productive the following season. Grazing with non-lactating ewes (whose immunity to worms should be largely restored) is acceptable, with the important proviso that immediately before being moved onto the grazings they are wormed with a broad spectrum anthelmintic. It is more than likely that many of these ewes will have been grazing contaminated ground, possibly at heavy stocking rates, ever since they were weaned, so it is important that they are completely cleared of all adult worms and larvae.

This pre-flushing dosing will ensure that ewes obtain maximum benefit from autumn grass in terms of ovulation and conception rates. It is also a much safer time to worm ewes than during the early pregnancy period, when any unnecessary handling or medication should be avoided if at all possible. Spring lambing ewes which are overwintered indoors should be dosed shortly after housing, during mid pregnancy when treatment is safer. It is essential to use an anthelmintic which is safe for pregnant ewes. Ewes which remain at pasture throughout pregnancy may also benefit from a mid pregnancy worming dose but this is not always essential, since they will be dosed at turnout after lambing.

Worm control in lambs after weaning

It is to be hoped that on most sheep farms, there will be some clean grazing for lambs after weaning, such as hay or silage aftermaths which have been shut up since February at the latest. If not, then the prospects of getting most of the lambs away to slaughter before grass growth and feeding value decline are poor. Whether lambs have been grazing clean or dirty ground before weaning, they must be wormed immediately before a move to clean—or not so clean—ground. If the ewes are removed at weaning

503

and the lambs stay for a few days on the original grazing to settle down, then dosing should be delayed until the move. An exception is where lambs are grazing contaminated ground and have to remain there for some time, when the regular three week dosings should continue. Whenever possible any dosing should be timed to coincide with a move or vice versa.

Lambs which can be weaned, wormed and moved to clean grazing should not require any further anthelmintic treatment before they are marketed. Providing grassland management is of a high standard and there are no other underlying disease problems or deficiencies, these lambs should fatten several weeks ahead of lambs which do not have access to clean grazing. Further economic gains are made through the purchase of minimal amounts of anthelmintic and the savings in labour through not having to gather and dose.

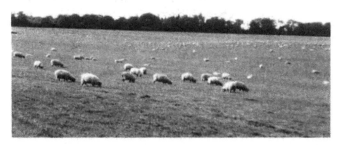

Plate 12.16 Weaned and dosed lambs which are moved onto clean, worm-free aftermaths such as this should need no further anthelmintic before they are slaughtered off grass.

If no clean grazing is available for weaned lambs, they must continue to be dosed at three week intervals until they are marketed—remembering, of course, to allow the recommended withdrawal period before slaughter, as indicated on the product pack or data sheet. A much larger proportion of these lambs will fail to reach marketable weight whilst at grass and will need to be stored overwinter—which may be a less profitable enterprise. After weaning lambs eat more grass than when they were supplementing their diet with milk from the ewe and they therefore take in more infective larvae. Where control measures are inadequate from lambing onwards, heavy pasture contamination will occur by mid summer, just in time for the freshly weaned lambs. This will produce a severe check in growth rate and in many cases serious clinical disease with some deaths.

It is important to appreciate that frequent three week anthelmintic treatments do not prevent the massive intakes of larvae which occur continuously. Even though larvae may be cleared out every three weeks, the damage they do is considerable, despite the absence of outward signs such as scouring. Lambs subjected to only moderate intakes of infective larvae may take up to six weeks longer to achieve marketable weight as compared with comparable worm free lambs. Also, parasitised lambs produce inferior carcasses, especially in terms of protein content. Their fleeces weigh considerably less and the quality of the wool is reduced.

Additionally, they are continuously pumping out enormous numbers of worm eggs onto the pastures, so perpetuating the problem for future seasons.

PGE control in rams

Rams are not thought to suffer any lapse in their immunity to disease as ewes do around the lambing period. Nevertheless they must be dosed in much the same way as ewes, since they may also contaminate grazings intended for lambs. Rams require flushing before mating and if they are to be grazed over ground intended as clean grazing for next season, they should be wormed before they are moved. Otherwise they may be dosed at any time up to about three weeks before they are to join the ewes and a good time is when they are being assessed for reproductive soundness. Before rams move to pastures-new, consider whether their presence will compromise lambs in the future. If the answer is yes or maybe, then dose them before the move.

PGE control in hill sheep

Because of the extensive conditions and the gathering difficulties often encountered on hill farms, it is seldom possible to implement such precise worm control measures as are possible on lowland or upland farms and a compromise often has to be reached.

The first thing to be clear about is that hill sheep—rams, ewes and lambs—may all suffer from parasitic gastro-enteritis. This has not always been appreciated, the argument being made that since hill grazings are so extensive, the infection levels are probably so light as to be negligible. However, whilst the sparsely grazed and roughest areas may be only lightly infected, other areas—notably where the pickings are sweet and where sheep tend to congregate—may become very heavily contaminated. It is now widely accepted that control measures are necessary. On improved ground and in-bye fields which are used in much the same way as lowland pastures, similar rules apply, except that the timings may need some adjustment because of weather conditions or the later lambing.

It has been shown that hill ewes respond well to treatment with anthelmintics which rid them of both adult worms and inhibited or arrested larvae, especially when food supplies are scarce. (Black scour has already been discussed.) Ewes will respond to a worm treatment in the last third of pregnancy by making better use of available food and producing more milk. This dose is often given at the same time as a fluke treatment, perhaps as a combination product on fluky farms. Care must be taken not to overload ewes with treatments very close to lambing, especially in bad weather or when food supplies are limited.

If dosed ewes are returned to the hill after lambing, they will become reinfected. Therefore worming must be repeated and this is most conveniently done at the next gathering, which is usually at the marking of the lambs.

In flocks where ewes are accustomed to block feeding, anthelmintic-medicated blocks can be substituted for regular ones during late pregnancy and early lactation, but only where ewes are retained in hill enclosures. Medicated blocks are a waste of money on extensive grazings and may engender a false sense of security. There is always a tremendous variation in intake of blocks, and young ewes especially are unlikely to get much of a look in, or indeed to show much interest. Therefore the pre- and post-lambing wormings mentioned above should be retained, despite the provision of wormer blocks.

Where ewes are scanned for lamb numbers and twin bearing ewes are retained on in-bye pastures to lamb, they can be treated as lowland ewes and wormed before being moved to the fertilised fields immediately after lambing. If all ewes are brought down to in-bye enclosures for lambing, then the ewes with singles can be wormed before returning them to the hill. Ewe hoggs which have been in-wintered and which were dosed at housing will not require a repeat dosing before returning to the hill.

Hill lambs may suffer from nematodirus, although generally less commonly than lowland lambs. Past experience of the disease on the farm, together with official forecast information, will help in deciding whether lambs will have to be gathered and dosed during May and June. Hill lambs should always be dosed at weaning and where possible moved to clean grazings. If lambs are retained for fattening or as breeding replacements, they must be dosed through the autumn and winter as described for lowland flocks.

All hill breeding stock—rams as well as ewes—should be wormed before tupping. This is best done in October so that they can make the best possible use of the better grazings provided for flushing.

Anthelmintics (Wormers)

Anthelmintics are drugs which will remove internal parasites. The compounds described here are active primarily against the roundworms of the gut, although some also possess activity against lungworms, tapeworms and liver fluke. One group (the avermectins) is also active against a number of external parasites. Drugs which are used to treat liver fluke are dealt with in the relevant part of the text.

There is a bewildering range of products available—more than 80 to choose from for the sheep farmer alone. It has been estimated that possibly up to half of all anthelmintics sold are used incorrectly. Not only does this represent a waste of resources amounting to tens of millions of pounds sterling annually, but it also means that some sheep are still suffering from roundworm infections unnecessarily.

GENERAL COMMENTS ON WORMERS

- The choice of anthelmintic will first of all depend upon a correct diagnosis of the problem—not all diarrhoeas in grazing lambs are due to roundworms.
- Different species of worms may be active at different seasons of the year. For example, it is most important to destroy arrested ostertagia larvae in ewes at housing or before turnout after lambing. Whilst most of the modern anthelmintics will destroy adult worms and larvae in the lumen of the gut (free amongst the ingesta or on the gut surface), only about half are capable of killing arrested larvae deep in the tissues of the gut wall.
- The method of administering the anthelmintic may be important for different reasons on different farms. For example, on hill farms where gathering may be difficult at certain times, medicated feed blocks may be used for convenience even though they are a less effective method of treatment.
- Because of the possibility of anthelmintic resistance occurring, it is often wise to alternate the group of anthelmintic used each year (see later).
- There is a considerable variation in the time that meat or milk must be withheld for human consumption following anthelmintic treatment and this may dictate the choice of product, particularly in the case of milking flocks.
- On a limited number of occasions throughout the year, combination products, which are effective against both worms and fluke, may be used. However, some of these products contain inappropriate mixtures or dosages of drugs.
- The class of animal to be treated is important. For example, certain products may damage or kill the foetus (teratogenic) and therefore cannot be used at any time during pregnancy. Parbendazole is one such.
- Most modern anthelmintics have a reasonable safety margin, but some may be risky in very sick animals, especially if the dose is not measured accurately.
- A number of anthelmintics for sheep contain trace elements such as cobalt and selenium. Single doses of cobalt in a wormer are often an unsatisfactory method of control, since the element is required continuously on a daily basis and there are better ways of providing it. Selenium levels in some products are adequate and may protect against deficiency if the wormings are given frequently enough, but on clean grazing systems this would be unnecessary and selenium would have to be provided separately (see Chapter 11).

Treatments during pregnancy—a warning

Late pregnancy is a particularly stressful time for ewes, as explained elsewhere in this book. In recent years a number of farmers have reported that heavily pregnant ewes have received a setback following the pre-lambing gathering to give them their various medications. In some flocks a significant number of deaths have been reported. In the majority of cases, ewes have received a number of treatments at the same time. For example, a clostridial and a pasteurella booster vaccination, a copper injection, a drench for worms and another for fluke, plus perhaps having their feet pared and being stood in a footbath. These combined treatments and manipulations put a heavy burden on an already hard-working liver and may tip the balance, resulting in pregnancy toxaemia or the downer ewe syndrome. Always consult your veterinary surgeon before using any combination of treatments, especially during pregnancy.

ANTHELMINTIC GROUPINGS

Whilst there are many modern anthelmintics available, they all belong to one of only three or four major groups of chemicals. These are described briefly below, mainly for guidance when deciding on a change of anthelmintic in an attempt to avoid resistance problems. The chemical names are long and almost unpronounceable, and to list all the trade names would be tedious and very soon out of date. Remember that when alternating drugs on an annual basis you must choose the new drug from a different **group** of chemicals. Your veterinary surgeon will have full details of all individual products.

Benzimidazoles

Thiabendazole revolutionised the wormer market when it was introduced in the early 1960s. It has now largely been overtaken by even more effective benzimidazole chemicals, which constitute the largest group of anthelmintics. Whilst most have a wide safety margin, a number cannot be used in pregnant sheep. Because they are all insoluble compounds, they are formulated as drenches ('white drenches'), pastes or in-feed preparations.

Most benzimidazoles are very effective against both adult and larval worms, but some do not kill the arrested larvae and this is particularly important at certain times of the year. Some are also effective against tapeworms and liver fluke, but the dose rate may need to be increased in order to kill liver fluke. One member of the group (triclabendazole) is different from the rest in that it is highly effective against liver fluke but has no activity against roundworms of the gut.

Although these chemicals are given by mouth, the active ingredient gets into the bloodstream and reaches all parts of the gut via the circulation. Being relatively insoluble substances, this is a lengthy process and the active ingredient is cleared from the blood only very slowly—hence they have long withholding times for meat and milk. They act by depriving the parasites of their food supply so that the worms starve to death.

Imidazothiazoles

Levamisole is the only chemical available for sheep in the imidazothiazole group, and it acts by paralysing the worms, which are then digested by the sheep. Levamisole acts rapidly and is cleared from the body quickly, so that withdrawal periods for meat and milk for human consumption are short. Partly because of this rapid action the risks of toxicity from careless overdosing are slightly increased, so that greater care is needed in estimating the weight of animals, especially if they are stressed or in poor body condition. Levamisole is effective against lungworms but not against liver fluke.

Avermectins

Avermectins are the latest group of anthelmintics to be introduced, and at present there is only one chemical available for sheep—ivermectin. It is highly effective against all stages of all the important roundworms of sheep (including lungworm), but has no activity against roundworm eggs, liver flukes or tapeworms. Of particular interest is its action against certain ectoparasites, such as the nasal bot maggot in sheep and warbles in cattle.

Like levamisole, ivermectin causes a paralysis of the parasites, which are then dislodged and excreted. It has a good safety margin, but a fairly long withdrawal period for meat and it must not be used in milking flocks.

CORRECT USE OF ANTHELMINTICS

All medicinal products, including anthelmintics, have to go through rigorous testing procedures, including efficacy trials designed to determine whether the product will do all that the pharmaceutical company says it will. (This does not apply to black market products, of course, of which there are always a number, including anthelmintics.) Therefore when you buy a well-known brand name from a reputable company, you can be sure that it will do what it is supposed to do—providing it is used correctly. However, these products are frequently misused and this often leads to disappointing results.

Diagnosis

It is important to know what is wrong with an animal or flock before applying any treatment, and making a wrong or incomplete diagnosis is common in the case of worms. For example, lambs suffering from cobalt deficiency may also be carrying a heavy worm burden. Treating them for worms will certainly help, but will not cure the underlying deficiency. Therefore if anthelmintic treatment does not bring about the expected result, the diagnosis must be questioned first of all.

Another common mistake is to choose the wrong drug for a particular situation. When ewes are to be treated after lambing and before turnout onto clean grazing, it is imperative that the product used is active against the inhibited larvae of ostertagia and other worms.

Worm and move

Probably the commonest mistake of all is to treat sheep and then leave them where they are or move them to other contaminated grazings. Anthelmintics given as a single dose (as opposed to 'pulse-release' products, which are not as yet available for sheep) will kill only parasites present in the animal at the time of dosing. Once the product is cleared from the body, sheep may become reinfected immediately. Lambs may show symptoms of worms again within a couple of weeks of dosing if they are grazing heavily infected ground in mid summer. Dosed animals must always be moved to clean grazing within a few hours of treatment.

Correct dosage

It is important to treat animals with the correct dose of anthelmintic and it is equally as important not to underdose as not to overdose. Underdosing may result in the selection of a population of worms partially resistant to the anthelmintic.

Despite the fact that most anthelmintics have a reasonable margin of safety, overdosing may still lead to toxicity. This is especially the case with sick or pregnant animals, or with those in poor body condition through undernutrition or old age. Such animals should always be weighed accurately in order to calculate the correct dose. It is similarly wise to weigh a selection of any group of animals to be dosed. Providing the weights are all reasonably close, then it is usually safe to dose the whole group at the rate calculated for the top-weight animals. However, the manufacturer's instructions should always be followed in this regard.

Even if the intention is to dose animals with the correct amount of the chemical, this can be confounded by other factors. Drenching guns and automatic syringes may be set wrongly or inaccurately calibrated. Damaged or worn equipment may leak so that the barrel does not fill completely. Attempting to dose sheep too quickly may also lead to improper filling and underdosing. If the dose of a drug is relatively small, any error becomes more significant.

With drugs formulated as suspensions—that is, where the active ingredient is insoluble and settles at the bottom of the container—it is most important to invert the container frequently. This is especially so after the product has been standing for some considerable time. If the active chemical is not properly mixed, some animals will be underdosed and others dangerously overdosed. (Shaking containers vigorously produces air bubbles which cause inaccuracies in dosage and thus should be avoided.)

Mixing

Never combine products which are not formulated together by a manufacturer. For example, it is dangerous to mix a wormer and a fluke treatment to make up your own combination product. It can be equally dangerous to dose animals with two such products separately, but on the same occasion. Indeed, never treat any animal with more than one product at the same time before checking with your veterinary surgeon that it is safe to do so.

Only use products specially formulated for sheep. Most importantly— always use the correct route of administration. The author has seen the serious results of injecting a product intended as an oral drench in cattle.

Human risks

It is worth remembering that anthelmintics are potent chemicals and may pose a risk to the operator if proper precautions are not taken. Smokers and nail biters are at greatest risk, since the hands are frequently put to the mouth.

Handling for worming

Above all, worming should be done carefully, not like an olympic event to see how many can be treated in a morning. It is a most important task and worth doing well. Accidents happen in the best organised circles, but in careless hands the most horrific injuries can occur, sometimes resulting in the death or humane destruction of the animal. For example, a drenching gun can damage the throat, trachea or oesophagus, the anthelmintic being deposited in the surrounding tissues and causing much pain and eventually death. (See Colour plate 42.)

The animal should be restrained gently but firmly. Hold the head straight with the body and tilt it slightly upwards, but not too far, so as to avoid choking. Insert the nozzle carefully into the side of the mouth, but only as far as the back of the mouth. Allow the animal time to settle down if it struggles and gently squeeze the anthelmintic into the mouth. Squirting it in may cause the sheep to choke so that the drug goes down the windpipe and into the lungs with fatal results. Allow the sheep time to swallow, at the same time keeping its mouth closed before releasing it. If the drug is not deposited at the back of the mouth, some or most of it may be spat out. If dosing in a pen, mark sheep so as to avoid double dosing or missing any.

In-feed formulations

Wormers are also supplied as in-feed formulations or in medicated blocks. The problem with these products is that it is impossible to ensure that animals receive the correct dose. Sheep will get either too much, too little or none at all. Attempting to identify shy feeders for separate treatment is usually impractical, especially with hill ewes. Medicated blocks are suitable only for animals well accustomed to eating them and in relatively small enclosures on the hill. In general they are an unsatisfactory method of worming sheep, but may be better than nothing under difficult circumstances. All other non-medicated feed must be removed whilst these products are being used.

RESISTANCE TO ANTHELMINTICS

Resistance is deemed to have occurred when parasites which are normally susceptible to a particular anthelmintic are able to survive the recommended dose or even a much higher one. When resistance occurs it usually does so across a whole group of anthelmintics, such as the benzimidazoles. This is because all the anthelmintics in a group have a similar chemical structure and mode of action on the parasites. In some cases cross-resistance may occur, so that parasites become resistant to more than one group of anthelmintics.

Anthelmintic resistance is an inherited characteristic of the parasite, so that the resistance is passed on to future generations of the worms. This means that the parasites which survive treatment may become dominant on the pastures and therefore in the sheep which become infected. The result is that the choice of drugs for treatment is reduced. Should a particular parasite become resistant to all the groups of anthelmintics, then the disease it produces will become untreatable. Obviously, this is a serious situation.

A number of factors may predispose to resistance. These include very frequent dosing (e.g. more often than every three weeks) and under-dosing. Purchased sheep may introduce resistant worms, which eventually dominate on the pastures. Ironically, if resistant worms develop in a clean grazing system, they may very soon pose a problem. When sheep are dosed and moved to clean ground, the resistant worms will be virtually the only worms on that pasture. Susceptible grazing lambs may then become populated by worms resistant to one or more groups of anthelmintics. Nevertheless, it still makes very good sense to provide as much clean grazing as possible so as to limit the need for anthelmintics.

Whilst resistance is worrying, it must be put into perspective in the UK, where up to the present it is fairly rare. Some farms in southern England—especially in the Home Counties—appear to have a problem with resistance in *Haemonchus contortus*. This particularly damaging worm appears to have become more common in the south, possibly because of a change in weather conditions in recent years. In other isolated incidents, resistance has been recorded with ostertagia in areas where haemonchus is absent.

In other parts of the world the problem is a very real one. This applies particularly to the sheep rearing areas of the southern hemisphere, such as Australia, New Zealand, South America and South Africa. Here, *Haemonchus contortus* is the major parasite and it is particularly adept at developing resistance. Also, in many of the worst affected areas, the grazing season is often very long due to the favourable climatic conditions, so that sheep tend to be dosed very frequently and for much of the year.

Avoiding anthelmintic resistance

The risk of inducing resistance can be reduced by ensuring that sheep are dosed accurately and that clean grazing is provided wherever possible, so reducing the frequency of dosing. Another wise precaution is to alternate

512

the group of anthelmintics annually. For example, if the benzimidazoles are used one year, ivermectin could be used the next year and levamisole the following one.

Frequent dosing does increase the likelihood of resistance developing, but where no clean grazing is available for lambs, there is really little alternative to three week dosing, apart perhaps from drastically reducing stocking rates to totally uneconomic levels. Whilst it is important to be aware of the possibility of resistance and to take avoiding action where possible, it would be unwise and neglectful to the diseased lambs to fail to implement proper control measures just because resistance might occur at some indeterminate time in the future. On a number of farms where regular three week dosing of lambs has been employed for a number of years, careful monitoring has shown no evidence of resistance to any of the anthelmintics by any of the worm species present.

New groups of anthelmintics with a completely different mode of action are developed very rarely, not least because of the enormous development costs involved. At present there are no alternatives to anthelmintics for the control of sheep worms, although the new biotechnologies may some day make vaccines a possibility.

IMPORTANT FEATURES OF PARASITIC GASTRO-ENTERITIS

- Parasitic gastro-enteritis is always a **flock problem** rather than a problem of a few individual scouring lambs.
- Sheep do not transmit roundworm infestations to each other directly, but through the **contamination of pastures**.
- Roundworms do not multiply inside the sheep's gut.
- Sheep suffer most severely from roundworm infection during their first year of life.
- Adult sheep attain varying degrees of immunity to infection through exposure to worms in younger life. Worms are therefore unable to establish heavy infections in healthy, well-fed ewes and rams. However, adults (and especially ewes in late pregnancy and during lactation) do play an important role in contaminating the grazings for the lambs.
- Ewes do not pass any protective immunity against worms to their lambs via colostrum.
- With a few notable exceptions, the parasitic roundworms of sheep do not infect cattle and vice versa.
- It is not possible to see most species of adult roundworms in the dung of sheep, since they are far too small to be seen easily with the naked eye. (Tapeworm segments can be seen—see later.)
- Symptoms of roundworm infection in the lamb flock, such as diarrhoea, soiled fleeces, weight loss or simply disappointing growth rates, mean that control measures have failed, you have already lost a lot of money and you are about to lose considerably more.

- Even on the best managed farms, anthelmintics will play a crucial role in roundworm control. However, the aim should always be to use them in a preventive manner, through pre-planned strategic dosing regimes, rather than in a haphazard way when lambs become ill.
- Aim to identify the high risk periods under the particular management system on your farm and take avoiding action.
- Eradication of roundworms from a farm is a forlorn hope, but a high degree of control is achievable, even with heavy stocking rates.
- The most cost-effective and efficient way to combat roundworm infection is to plan to provide **clean grazings** for lambs in their first season at grass. To reduce pasture contamination, never move any sheep of any age onto clean grazings without first treating them with an anthelmintic.
- Always consider carefully the consequences **before** moving any group of sheep from one grazing to another, since your actions may have far-reaching effects.

TAPEWORMS

Tapeworms are so called, because they are flat and ribbon-like. The adult forms of these unappealing creatures live in the small intestine of their final (definitive) host, anchored to the gut wall by means of either a sucker or a set of hooks at the head end. The body of the worm is composed of a series of segments which 'float' free in the lumen or cavity of the gut. They are bathed in the gut contents and since they have no gut of their own, they simply absorb nutrients—kindly supplied by their host—through their cuticle or skin. Generally speaking the adult stage of the tapeworm does little damage, since it simply 'hangs on' and takes a little of what is going.

Tapeworms grow continuously, new segments budding off from the head end of the worm. Each segment carries its own set of both male and female sexual organs so that segments can fertilise themselves or—if they are feeling more sociable—each other. Fertilised segments fill with eggs and as new segments grow from the head end of the worm, the egg-filled segments mature and are shed from the tail end and pass out onto the pasture in the host animals' faeces.

The eggs liberated when the segments disintegrate must be eaten by another species of animal called the intermediate host. After liberation from the egg, each embryo undergoes development, usually in the body cavity of the intermediate host, to produce one or more heads or scoleces. Each of these scoleces is then capable of infecting a final host animal and growing into an adult tapeworm—providing they are devoured by the appropriate species of final host. As this is a bit of a hit and miss affair with some species of tapeworm, it is often a good time to step in with control measures.

Anthelmintics can be used to clear some adult tapeworms from their final

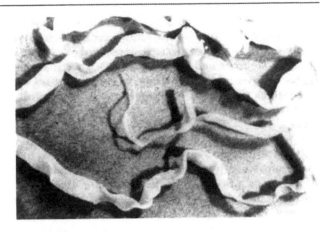

Plate 12.17   A tapeworm from a lamb. These unappealing creatures do relatively little harm despite the fact that they may reach several metres in length. The head end which anchors to the gut is the narrow section in the centre of the photo and the ripe tail end segments are at top left.

hosts, but unless the whole of the worm is removed, in particular the head end, fresh segments will grow and become a new worm.

The sheep can act as a final host for some tapeworms and as an intermediate host for others. Only one—an intermediate form which causes a nervous disease called gid or sturdy—is of any real significance to sheep in the UK. One other intermediate stage in sheep—the hydatid cyst—is of interest because it is of great public health concern.

Moniezia—the Milkworm

Moniezia is the only adult tapeworm of any interest in sheep, not because of any damage it causes, but rather because it is somewhat obvious and shepherds and sheep farmers tend to worry about it, probably unnecessarily.

The adult tapeworms live in the small intestine of young lambs during the summer months of May, June and July, particularly when lambs are grazing but still sucking their dams—hence the name 'milkworm'. They may grow to a length of 4 or 5 metres and as lambs may be infected with several tapeworms at the same time, segments may be very obvious in the faeces. Ribbons of segments may occasionally be seen twirling in the breeze as lambs run along behind their mothers. However, despite the fact that at slaughter it may be possible to collect literally a bucketful of these from the guts of only two or three heavily parasitised lambs, they apparently do little harm. Moniezia do not parasitise older resistant sheep and generally live for only a few months in lambs.

The ripe segments disintegrate on the pastures, liberating the eggs. For further development the eggs must be eaten by an intermediate host, in this case a particular small pasture mite (orabatid) of which there are literally millions on every hectare of grazing land. Only a small percentage of these mites become infected, but this is sufficient to carry over the infection from year to year. This is because the intermediate stage (a cysticercoid) which develops in the body cavity of the mite can survive for many months, certainly over the winter period. Mites crawl up the herbage in warm, moist, summer weather and so are eaten by sheep. In lambs, the infective stages of the tapeworm are liberated when the mites are digested. They attach themselves to the gut wall and develop into adult tapeworms. Within less than two months of infection the lambs are shedding ripe segments in their faeces.

Providing they are getting plenty of milk and good grazing, lambs are unlikely to suffer to any significant degree from moniezia, despite the heavy infections sometimes encountered. Occasionally, clinical symptoms such as ill thrift or a pot-bellied appearance are ascribed to tapeworm damage, but these are more likely to be the effect of other problems such as roundworms or trace element deficiencies.

It is rarely, if ever, necessary to dose lambs specifically for tapeworms. A number of anthelmintics which are used routinely for the control of parasitic gastro-enteritis, such as albendazole, fenbendazole and oxfendazole, are also effective against the moniezia tapeworms. If lambs are on land grazed by lambs during the previous season they will need to be dosed for nematodirus and if an appropriate wormer is used, it will control both parasites simultaneously.

Sheep as the intermediate hosts of tapeworms

There are a number of adult tapeworms which live in the gut of the dog but which have their intermediate stage—a bladderworm—in sheep. Dogs—the final hosts—become infected by eating the carcasses of infected sheep which contain bladderworms. Sheep in their turn become infected through grazing pastures contaminated with dog faeces containing the ripe segments of the adult tapeworms.

Gid or Sturdy

This is a nervous disease of sheep and, less commonly, of other herbivores. It is caused by the bladderworm stage of a tapeworm of the dog called *Taenia multiceps*.

Dogs become infected by eating sheep's heads which contain the bladderworm stage, *Coenurus cerebralis*. Sheepdogs and other farm and sporting dogs which are allowed access to sheep carcasses left unburied are at risk. Hounds fed raw or improperly cooked sheep's heads from the kennel knackery are a particular hazard to sheep, especially as large numbers of hounds traipse over grazing land defaecating at will. Indeed, any area where sporting or working dogs congregate will pose a risk to grazing sheep.

The embryo forms of the tapeworm which escape from the disintegrating segments in dog faeces contaminate the area and are then picked up by sheep during grazing. Once inside the sheep, they burrow through the wall

516

of the gut and into small blood vessels, whence they are transported to all parts of the body. However, unfortunately for the sheep, they are only able to develop in nervous tissue and particularly the brain. Here they grow over a period of several months into a cyst filled with fluid which may reach the size of a golf ball in some cases. Each of these cysts contains scores of scoleces or tapeworm heads, which can develop into adult tapeworms only if they are eaten by a dog. (See Colour plates 43 & 44.)

CLINICAL SIGNS OF GID

On rare occasions lambs pick up a very large number of infectious tapeworm embryos from a heavily infected area. This may produce severe nervous signs of depression, aimless wandering, blindness and convulsions, which can kill the lamb within a few days. Unless a thorough post-mortem is carried out, including a detailed examination of the brain, these cases will go undiagnosed, as most of them probably do. Some may survive only to become more typical gid cases, whilst others may recover completely.

More commonly, however, the symptoms of gid develop gradually and are due entirely to the pressure exerted on the surrounding brain tissue by the slow growing cyst. At first the signs are vague, affected sheep becoming dull and losing weight through not eating. Later, as the cyst grows, the symptoms which develop will depend upon where the cyst is located in the

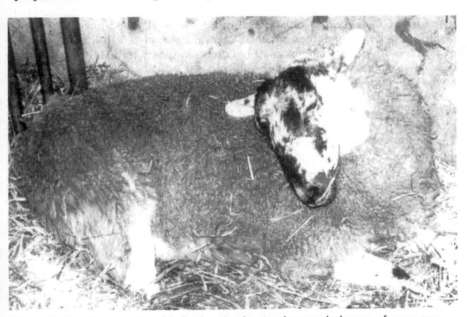

Plate 12.18   A ewe with gid. Such animals stand a good chance of recovery following surgical removal of the cyst.

brain (or rarely the spinal cord) and they will therefore vary somewhat with each case.

The head may be held abnormally high or to one side. Sometimes it is rested on the ground or on some other handy object. Vision is frequently affected, some animals becoming blind, usually in one eye. This generally indicates that the cyst is located on the side of the brain opposite the blind eye. A proportion of sheep may circle, and the feet of suspect animals brought indoors may get entangled with straw bedding.

Some sheep become very excitable, stumbling and falling or rearing up and lunging forward uncontrollably. In a proportion of sheep the bones of the skull become softened and thin due to the pressure from the cyst, especially when it lies near the surface of the brain as is often the case.

The symptoms gradually worsen as the cyst continues to grow and if not treated sheep will eventually go down, become comatose and die. Some sheep may die within days of the first symptoms, whilst others may take weeks to do so. Obviously, this should not be allowed to happen, because your veterinary surgeon will be able to treat a fair proportion of cases by removing the cyst surgically and with a good chance of recovery. The proportion which cannot be treated can be slaughtered and, providing they pass meat inspection on all other counts, will be safe for human consumption.

Diagnosis and treatment

Before any treatment is possible, a diagnosis must be arrived at. Gid can be confused with a number of other nervous diseases such as louping ill, listeriosis, CCN, scrapie and several more. Generally, gid occurs in only a single animal, although there may be several cases on a farm over a number of years, so that the shepherd will become familiar with the symptoms and be able to spot them early. The majority of cases occur in older lambs, hoggs or young ewes. It is relatively uncommon in older ewes or rams.

From the behaviour of the sheep and clinical tests, your veterinary surgeon can usually determine where the cyst is located. Providing surgical removal is possible, around four out of five cases may recover completely. The wound will take some weeks to heal over, since some bone has to be removed. The patient should be kept indoors to recover in clean, comfortable surroundings and offered tasty food with fresh water available. Remember that any sheep which cannot stand should be supported with bales to prevent bloat. Most surgical cases will be up and about and more or less back to normal within a week or ten days.

CONTROL OF GID

The life cycle of the parasite must be broken and this is best done by making sure that dogs do not get access to sheep's brains by disposing of carcasses as quickly as possible—as is required in law! Sheep's heads should **not** be fed to dogs. If sheep's offal of any kind is fed to dogs, then it must be

thoroughly cooked. This means keeping it on the boil for at least one hour, preferably longer.

Dogs should be treated every two months with an anthelmintic which is capable of killing and removing the whole length of these tapeworms, particularly the head end from which they grow.

A number of other dog tapeworms have their bladderworm stage in the sheep. Although they generally cause no clinical disease and therefore go unnoticed, they do contribute to the condemnation of sheep offal at slaughter. Regular worming of dogs will reduce these losses to a minimum. Hunt kennels have a particular duty to observe the above measures, so that hounds do not contaminate the grazings over which they hunt. Farmers are well advised to take a strict view of stray dogs and are entitled to request that anyone who seeks permission to walk their dogs across farmland have them regularly treated for tapeworms. The preparation used must be one which has been specially formulated for dogs. **On no account should wormers designed for any other species, such as sheep or cattle, ever be used on dogs**.

Hydatid Disease

This disease presents a public health problem and is mentioned in this book because both sheepdogs and sporting dogs play a role in its life cycle. Neither dogs nor sheep suffer any obvious clinical disease as a result of hydatid infection, but the disease in man is most unpleasant. It is difficult to treat and may prove fatal in some cases. In Tasmania and New Zealand, where there is a much higher incidence of the disease than in the UK, legislation requires the licensing and compulsory treatment of dogs at regular intervals because of the risk of hydatid disease to the human population.

The adult tapeworm, which is called *Echinococcus granulosus*, lives in the small intestine of the dog. It is very small by tapeworm standards, being only about half a centimetre in length and therefore very difficult to see in dog faeces. Dogs may harbour many hundreds of these tiny tapeworms with no obvious ill effects. However, their faeces will contain thousands of eggs in the ripe tapeworm segments, and these eggs are a source of infection for sheep and for the human population.

Sheep—the intermediate hosts—become infected by grazing pastures contaminated by infected dogs. The intermediate stage, called a **hydatid cyst**, will grow in any part of the body, but most frequently in the lungs and liver (see Colour plate 48). These cysts, which may grow to a large size, contain vast numbers of daughter cysts and scoleces or tapeworm heads. These scoleces do not die immediately the sheep dies and so any dogs scavenging carcasses may become infected by eating the infected organs.

519

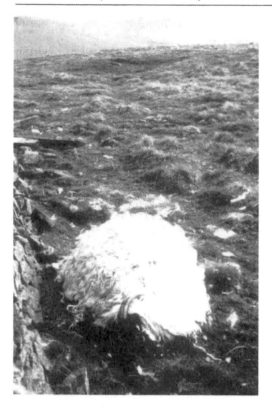

Plate 12.19 Sheep carcasses should be buried or otherwise responsibly disposed of promptly as they may be a source of viral, bacterial and parasitic disease. Dogs must be denied access to carcasses.

HUMAN INFECTION

Humans become infected by accidentally swallowing tapeworm eggs from the faeces of infected dogs. Even stroking infected dogs can lead to infection from dried faeces on the coat. Because children tend to play more with dogs and are less aware of the need for simple hygiene precautions, they are at particular risk. Farm children are even more at risk because of the higher incidence of echinococcus infection in sheepdogs. They should be discouraged from cuddling dogs near their faces and reminded about washing their hands immediately after handling dogs, or indeed any other pet animals. Humans cannot become infected with hydatid by eating lamb or mutton.

Until relatively recently the treatment of hydatid disease in humans was usually surgical and was not always successful. More recently, albendazole—a benzimidazole anthelmintic—has shown considerable promise as a medical treatment, even in relatively serious cases. However, prevention of human infection is obviously highly desirable.

Some areas of the UK have an above average infection rate in both sheep and dogs, which results in a higher incidence in the human population.

These areas generally have heavy densities of both sheep and sheepdogs and also a high proportion of rough hill grazings where dead sheep are less easily seen and disposed of.

In one such area in south Powys, Wales, a control scheme was put into operation to try to reduce the incidence of the disease. In one valley, more than half of all dogs tested were infected with adult echinococcus tapeworms, and a very large proportion of the sheep were infected with the intermediate hydatid cyst stage. At the time the scheme was introduced the infection rate in the human population of the area was around one case for every 2,000 inhabitants, which is unacceptably high. The simple expedient of dosing all dogs regularly with an anthelmintic effective against the echinococcus tapeworm dramatically reduced the infection in the dog population, and therefore also in the sheep and human populations.

CONTROL IN DOGS

Control of hydatid disease is obviously important because of its public health considerations. The same rules as for the control of gid also apply here. Farm and sporting dogs should be treated every two months with an anthelmintic effective against echinococcus. Dogs should never be fed any raw meat, and cooking should mean boiling for at least an hour. The carcasses of dead sheep should be buried or incinerated as soon as possible.

LIVER FLUKES

The Common Liver Fluke—*Fasciola hepatica*

Fasciola hepatica is a flat, leaf-like worm (trematode) which lives in the liver of various mammals, including sheep and cattle, where it causes severe damage. It has a worldwide distribution, and in the UK, liver fluke disease occurs most commonly and most severely in the western livestock areas, which are particularly wet during the late spring, summer and autumn periods. The extent of the disease varies from year to year, being largely dependent upon the pattern of rainfall in an area. However, in the west there is almost always a sufficient level of infection on pastures to make liver fluke one of the most widespread and economically important diseases in British agriculture.

LIFE CYCLE OF *FASCIOLA HEPATICA*

The intermediate host

The life cycle of the liver fluke is complex and involves not only cattle and sheep (the final hosts), but also a small and humble **mud snail**, called

Lymnaea truncatula—the intermediate host. The life cycle cannot be completed without the intermediate stage in the snail and it will be appreciated that if there are no suitable snail habitats on the farm, liver fluke will not occur there.

SNAIL TERRITORY The mud snail, as its name suggests, requires the soil to be saturated with a little free-standing water on the surface. Very acid soils, such as the peaty deposits which occur on many hill farms in the UK, are generally unsuitable, snails preferring only a slightly acid soil. Many upland pastures which would not normally support a mud snail population become ideal breeding grounds following improvement by liming to correct high acidity. Other suitable conditions are those that occur on poorly drained and rushy land on the edges of slow running open ditches and streams, areas

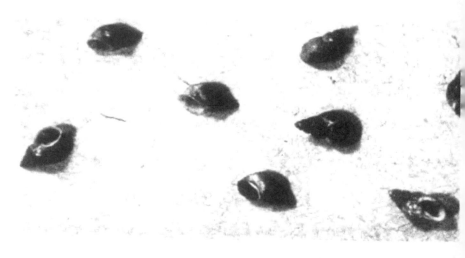

Plate 12.20 The mud snail (*Limnea truncatula*)—the intermediate host of the liver fluke—and its territory.

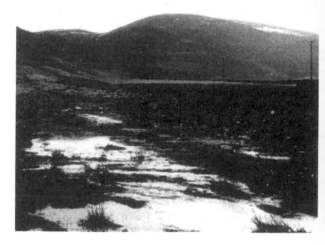

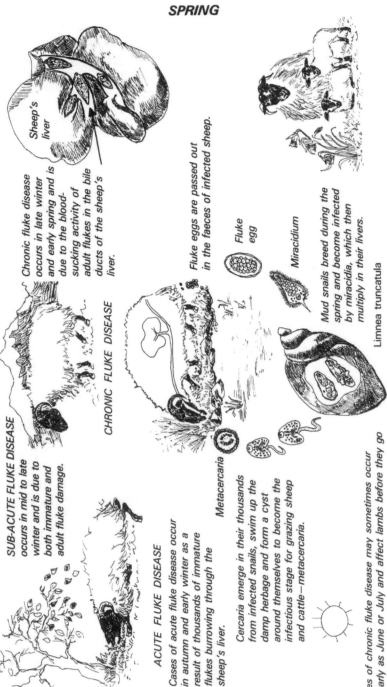

SPRING

WINTER

SUMMER

AUTUMN

Sheep's liver

Chronic fluke disease occurs in late winter and early spring and is due to the blood-sucking activity of adult flukes in the bile ducts of the sheep's liver.

Fluke eggs are passed out in the faeces of infected sheep.

Fluke egg

Miracidium

Mud snails breed during the spring and become infected by miracidia, which then multiply in their livers.

Limnea truncatula

SUB-ACUTE FLUKE DISEASE occurs in mid to late winter and is due to both immature and adult fluke damage.

CHRONIC FLUKE DISEASE

Metacercaria

ACUTE FLUKE DISEASE

Cases of acute fluke disease occur in autumn and early winter as a result of thousands of immature flukes burrowing through the sheep's liver.

Cercaria emerge in their thousands from infected snails, swim up the damp herbage and form a cyst around themselves to become the infectious stage for grazing sheep and cattle—metacercaria.

Cases of chronic fluke disease may sometimes occur as early as June or July and affect lambs before they go for slaughter.

Figure 12.2   The life cycle of the liver fluke—Fasciola hepatica—and the diseases it causes.

523

below broken drains, tractor wheel ruts where water accumulates, area. poached by livestock (such as around drinking troughs and the headwaters o streams), plus anywhere else where water is stagnant or slow running.

SNAIL BREEDING SEASON The snail is very small, being only about 5 t 6 mm in length. Under suitably warm, moist conditions it can breed ver effectively, a single female being capable of producing many hundreds o eggs in a season. With perhaps several hundred snails in every square mete of suitable habitat, it is not difficult to appreciate that the mud snail popula tion is rarely a limiting factor in the spread of liver fluke disease, excep in particularly unfavourable weather conditions.

The breeding season begins when the temperature rises above about 10°C (50°F) and snails which have hibernated in the mud overwinter become active, grow and reproduce rapidly. Eggs are laid in the spring and sum mer, and new generations of snails appear from these eggs from May onwards with a peak around August. Normally, only a few snails die over winter, and even if control measures are taken to kill them by spraying, a few snails will remain and these can quickly repopulate a habitat with sufficient numbers to pose a serious fluke risk to both cattle and sheep. Generally speaking, a moderate snail population, which is not too over crowded, produces the greatest risk.

Infection of the snail

Snails become infected with an intermediate stage of the liver fluke. The adult flukes lay eggs in the bile ducts of the liver of sheep, cattle and other mammals. These eggs are passed out of the gut and onto pasture in the faeces. If the weather is warm and wet (similar to that necessary for snail activity), the eggs become washed out of the dung and develop over a few weeks into a small larval stage called a **miracidium**. This is a very vulner able creature which must swim around to find and penetrate the soft under belly of a mud snail within a very few hours or else it will perish. Needless to say, the vast majority do perish, because in most circumstances the dung of cattle and sheep is deposited on areas unsuitable for snails.

When a miracidium infects a snail it penetrates its liver, where it spends anywhere from six to ten weeks. During this time it multiplies itself several hundred times to become the next stage, called a **cercaria**. These are minute, tadpole-like creatures which leave the snail and attach themselves to the herbage. They then immediately shed their tails and form a tough outer shell or cyst as protection from the elements. These resistant stages, called **metacercariae**, can survive for many months, including the whole winter period. This stage is infectious to sheep and cattle—and also to other mammals such as horses, deer, rabbits and even humans. To become infected an animal must graze contaminated herbage, and humans occasionally are infected through eating wild watercress. (Eating snails or any of the other stages of the fluke will not cause liver fluke disease in mammals.) There may be as many as 2,000 metacercariae on a kilogram of dried herbage from an infected snail habitat.

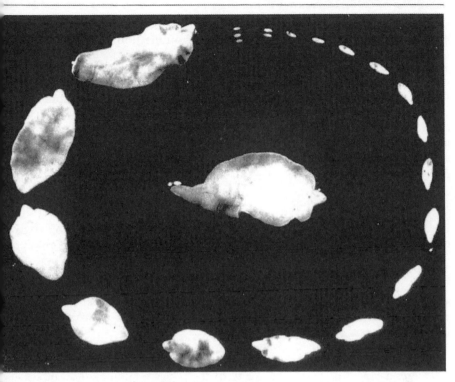

Plate 12.21   Preserved liver fluke. The tiny flukes at top cause acute disease as they wander through the liver in their thousands. The adult flukes (centre) cause chronic disease through sucking blood in the bile ducts.

Infection of the sheep

Once eaten by the sheep, the cyst surrounding the metacercaria dissolves in the gut, releasing the immature fluke which proceeds to burrow its way through the gut wall. From there, it traverses the body cavity in search of the liver. It then burrows into the liver and wanders through its substance for many weeks, eating voraciously as it does so. When a great many metacercaria invade the liver all at once, it becomes seriously damaged (see Colour plate 47).

As they grow, the young flukes enter the tubes which transport the bile—the bile ducts. Here they attach themselves to the walls by means of a sucker and feed on blood which they suck from small blood vessels (see Colour plate 46). Eventually they become mature liver flukes ready to begin laying eggs and thus start the whole life cycle over again. It takes up to three months or more from the time a sheep eats metacercariae to the point where mature flukes are laying eggs in the bile ducts.

Each liver fluke has its own set of male and female reproductive organs so they can be quite independent sexually, and one fluke can produce a million eggs or more during its lifetime. Because flukes provoke very little immune reaction in sheep, there is no limiting factor on the number that can invade the liver and sheep may accumulate flukes from year to year if not treated with anthelmintics. Flukes picked up early in the sheep's life may remain with it for life. It is not uncommon to find two or three hundred mature flukes in the bile ducts of a sheep's liver at slaughter or post-mortem.

(In cattle, the presence of flukes in the liver stimulates the body to attempt to limit the infection by thickening and calcifying the walls of the bile ducts. In consequence, flukes will not normally persist for more than a year or eighteen months, and although reinfection can occur, it is usually not as damaging as in sheep.)

ACUTE FLUKE DISEASE

Liver fluke may affect sheep in a number of ways and with varying degrees of severity. The symptoms are largely dependent on the level of challenge (weight of infection) and the length of time they are subjected to it. If sheep eat massive numbers of metacercariae, the damage to the liver may produce severe haemorrhage and death. Sometimes death occurs very suddenly in sheep in perfectly good condition. Termed acute liver fluke disease, this form is seen only in sheep and the diagnosis can be confirmed only at post-mortem examination.

When deaths from acute fluke disease occur, an examination of the rest of the flock will probably reveal other very weak and anaemic animals. Affected sheep often resent handling of the abdomen and should be treated very carefully, since the liver may be so severely 'shot-up' that it is easily ruptured. Occasionally animals may even bleed to death internally before the shepherd's very eyes. Post-mortem examination will reveal a very

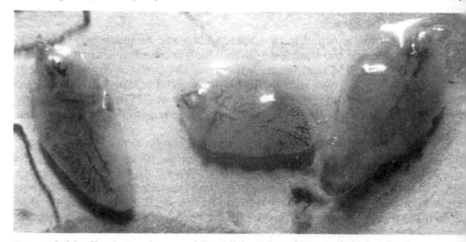

Plate 12.22 Fresh specimens of liver fluke taken from a sheep's bile ducts. Their digestive tracts filled with sheep's blood can be seen clearly.

enlarged liver with much blood. Thousands of immature flukes (only 5 mm long) may be collected from such a sheep's liver. There may be no fluke eggs in the faeces, since the disease is caused by immature flukes which do not, of course, lay eggs.

Acute fluke incidents are most likely to occur after a wet summer, particularly if there have been three wet months in a row. (As a generalisation, the more wet months in succession, the more severe the outbreaks will be. A 'wet' month is one in which rainfall exceeds evaporation, so that the soil is continuously saturated.) Such summers are relatively uncommon, so serious acute fluke epidemics are fortunately rare. However, as local conditions can vary considerably, individual farms in high rainfall areas may experience outbreaks more frequently than other farms only a few miles distant.

The first cases of acute fluke will appear roughly six weeks after the infection is picked up off the pasture. Outbreaks are most frequent in the autumn and early winter, coinciding with early and mid pregnancy, which may lead to the loss of early embryos or foetuses. The liver fluke forecasts issued by the Ministry of Agriculture via the media are very helpful in deciding upon the control and preventive measures necessary to avoid serious loss. As outbreaks can occur at any time of year, any sudden deaths on a flukey farm should be treated with suspicion and a full investigation carried out.

Treatment of acute fluke disease

If acute fluke disease is confirmed, the flock should be carefully gathered and treated with an anthelmintic which is particularly effective against immature forms of fluke (such as triclabendazole) and then moved immediately to fluke-free pasture if at all possible. Otherwise they will need repeated dosings at three week intervals, since the metacercarial infection will remain a danger for many months. Ewes which have suffered severe liver damage may die despite treatment.

Black disease

Diagnosis of death from acute fluke disease may be confused with a clostridial disease usually (although not exclusively) associated with acute fluke infection—namely black disease, which is caused by a bacterium called *Clostridium oedematiens*—type B. This can be determined only by laboratory examination. On farms where the disease has occurred previously, the resistant spores of the microorganism will be found in the soil and also in the livers of normal healthy sheep. Clinical disease appears to be triggered by the migration of the immature liver fluke through the liver substance, which stimulates the bacterium to multiply and produce a toxin which kills the sheep—if the liver flukes do not do it first!

Sheep with black disease are rarely seen alive, the animal usually being found apparently asleep, but in fact dead. Very occasionally a sheep may be seen in a state of collapse or standing stock-still before collapsing.

Death follows quietly and swiftly. Flocks should be given a '7 in 1' type clostridial vaccine and an additional booster in late summer on farms which are at particular risk. Control of liver fluke will further reduce the risk.

SUB-ACUTE FLUKE DISEASE

In years of heavy fluke challenge—sometimes following an outbreak of acute fluke where treatment has been given only once and the flock has had to remain on flukey ground—a less dramatic although equally devastating form of the disease may occur. Sub-acute fluke tends to affect the whole flock during mid and late winter (slightly later than the acute disease) and is due to sheep picking up a heavy infection over a prolonged period. In most flocks this tends to coincide with mid to late pregnancy. As the disease causes unthriftiness in the flock and pulls ewes down in body condition, it often has serious implications for the unborn lamb as well as the ewe.

If ewe deaths occur, post-mortem examination will reveal damage to the liver substance from wandering immature flukes and also from blood-sucking adult flukes in the bile ducts. Fluke eggs will be present in the faeces. Treatment with a suitable anthelmintic should be aimed at both immature and adult flukes. Sheep should be moved to fluke-free grazing or dosed every three weeks if this is not possible.

CHRONIC FLUKE DISEASE

By far the most common and economically significant form of the disease is chronic fluke. It is very widespread, especially in western areas of Britain and on flukey farms it occurs every year to a greater or lesser degree, depending on the previous summer's weather. It is caused principally by the blood-sucking activity of adult flukes in the bile ducts, which causes anaemia and therefore unthriftiness, weight loss and death, depending upon how many flukes are present and how well the flock is fed.

Chronic fluke usually occurs later in the year than the acute or sub-acute forms and is therefore seen in late winter and early spring. However, in some seasons, weather conditions may lead to a late hatch of snails in autumn, and these may become infected from miracidia hatched out of fluke eggs deposited by sheep and cattle in late summer and early autumn. Because cold weather then intervenes, the snails hibernate overwinter, so halting development of the fluke. Hatching of cercariae from the snails does not then occur until the following spring. Sheep may pick up infective metacercariae at this time and show symptoms of chronic liver fluke as early as June or July. Even lambs being fattened off grass may be infected and a high proportion of their livers may be condemned at slaughter.

When there is no late generation of snails to infect, the fluke eggs which are deposited and hatch in the late summer and autumn perish. Eggs put out in the dung by stock during the winter months do not hatch, but remain dormant until the following spring, when the weather once more becomes suitable for hatching and for snail activity. This is one way that infection is carried over from one year to another. The other is due to the fact that adult flukes can live for many years in untreated sheep which then deposit eggs, so continually contaminating pastures.

Clinical signs of chronic fluke disease

Chronically affected animals lose body condition progressively due to the anaemia and loss of appetite. The fleece is dry and open and the wool clip from affected flocks is significantly reduced. The anaemia causes dropsy or oedema, which shows as a swelling below the jaw in severely affected animals, known as 'bottle jaw' or 'watery poke'. The eyes are watery and the membranes of the eye, mouth and vulva are very pale instead of being a fresh pink colour.

Post-mortem inspection of fluke-affected animals, which die from either chronic fluke or some other condition such as pneumonia, will reveal adult flukes in the bile ducts of the liver. A thorough search will reveal scores or even hundreds of them in the thickened bile ducts of a shrunken liver. The body cavity is often full of fluid (ascites) and all tissues appear pale and bloodless because of the anaemia.

Chronic fluke disease coincides with late pregnancy and early lactation in many flocks. A reduction of appetite and loss of condition in late pregnancy increases the risk of pregnancy toxaemia and may also affect the weight of lambs at birth. If the condition remains untreated, the milk

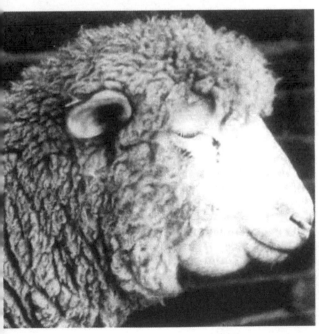

Plate 12.23 'Bottle jaw' or 'watery poke'—a symptom of severe chronic fluke disease. This symptom is less common in sheep than in cattle.

529

yield of ewes will be significantly reduced. Even though a flush of spring grass may appear to improve the condition of ewes, this is only temporary and they will continue to lose condition in the midst of plenty. Lambs especially multiples, will suffer because of the lethargy of affected ewes at lambing time and from their lack of milk. If the fluke burden is heavy and the feeding poor, a number of ewes may die around lambing and during the first weeks of lactation—stressful times for the ewe, even under normal circumstances.

It is a feature of liver fluke disease that a high proportion of the flock is generally infected. Therefore, above average lamb losses and a high proportion of orphans and of slow growing lambs are often features in flocks where preventive measures are not implemented.

Diagnosis of chronic fluke

The diagnosis of liver fluke in a flock or on a farm is most important. Whilst no deaths may be attributable to the condition in most seasons, it may nevertheless be grumbling away in the background, causing very significant economic loss. When any deaths occur on fluke-infested farms, for whatever reason, particularly in adult sheep and cattle, the livers should be checked for the presence of flukes or fluke damage.

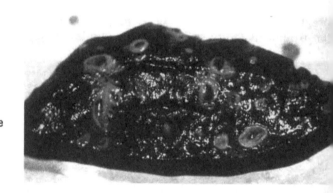

Plate 12.24 The cut surface of a sheep's liver affected by chronic fluke. Note the thickened bile ducts caused by the blood sucking of the adult flukes.

If there is any doubt about whether a farm is infected, fresh faeces samples should be taken, preferably during the winter, from at least a dozen ewes in poor condition which have not been treated with a flukicide for some considerable time. Any cattle on the farm should also be sampled. Your veterinary surgeon will be able to tell you whether fluke eggs are present. If they are (in whatever numbers), this is significant and control measures will be necessary every year. If no fluke eggs are found, further faeces samples plus blood samples (from which the condition of the liver can be determined) should be taken. Flukes do not lay eggs continuously, so negative samples do not necessarily mean the disease is not present. Another useful check is to get feedback from the abattoir on the condition of the livers of ewes and lambs sent for slaughter.

CONTROL OF LIVER FLUKE

There are a number of ways of tackling liver fluke. These may be aimed at controlling the snail population, at keeping stock off infected areas of the farm or at controlling the damage done to sheep by the strategic use of flukicidal anthelmintics, or a combination of these measures.

Environmental control

As already stated, the snail has very particular environmental requirements. As with many infectious agents it is often possible to control the disease by interrupting the life cycle at a vital stage. Snail numbers can be fairly effectively reduced by drainage of their habitats in the early spring, which diminishes the snail population quite dramatically. However, whilst many snails die, a few will always survive by becoming dormant. If conditions then change, such as in a very wet season, or if the drainage breaks down, then even if a handful of snails is left they can repopulate an area very quickly. It is often difficult or impossible to drain certain areas really effectively, or indeed to identify all areas which will support snails and are therefore in need of draining.

Obviously on many flukey farms where there are large areas of mud snail habitat, plus many smaller ones, drainage may well be too expensive and impractical a method of control. On farms with just an odd wet corner it may be much more cost-effective to fence off these small patches, which in any case are often populated by less productive and less palatable species of herbage. Streams and open ditches present real problems, because stock tend to trample the edges when coming to drink and heavy rains cause erosion, so that the rate of flow slows down, pools form, rushes grow and they become ideal snail habitats. Maintenance of ditches is expensive, as is fencing them off.

Molluscicides

Chemicals which kill snails—molluscicides—are expensive if large areas need to be sprayed, but may be worth considering for smaller areas. It should be appreciated that spraying is unlikely to kill all the snails and, yet again, the few remaining may rapidly repopulate the area. These chemicals are very potent and are toxic to fish, to livestock and even to the operators spraying an area if they are not used responsibly. Expert advice should be sought to identify likely snail habitats and to advise on the timing and application of molluscicides and on the likely cost-benefit of the exercise.

Except on a small proportion of farms, the use of molluscicides, fencing and drainage is very unlikely to eliminate the snail. Therefore the risk of fluke is still present, although it may be much reduced. Keeping susceptible stock off flukey grazing during periods of highest risk—apart from being very inconvenient and often totally impractical—does not eliminate the risk, since some snail habitats may be overlooked and stock may still become infected at other times of the year.

Anthelmintics

On most fluke-infested farms, therefore, shepherds have to resort to treating stock with flukicidal anthelmintics, since the presence of even light infections can significantly reduce productivity. Regular dosing of stock also reduces the contamination of snail habitats with fluke eggs, so reducing the risk of infecting snails. A combination of strategic dosing with anthelmintics, together with one or more of the other controls mentioned above for reducing snail populations, can therefore lead to a very significant degree of control. The secret lies in finding the most suitable combination of any particular farm.

There are some important points in regard to the use of anthelmintics. It is most important to choose the correct drug. Some are more effective against immature flukes and are therefore more suitable when acute fluke is a risk. Others are most effective against adult flukes in the bile ducts and so are ideal for the treatment of chronic fluke. Rarely is a product highly effective against both immatures and adults. There are a bewildering number of products available, but your veterinary surgeon will guide you. Beware particularly of combined fluke and worm products: there are few times of the year when such products are suitable, and even then they do not always contain the best combination of drugs.

The correct dose rate is important, since overdosing can be toxic and underdosing will fail to kill all the flukes. It is often worth weighing a representative sample of sheep, particularly where there is a mixture of ages of stock being dosed. Do remember that it is most important to include all susceptible species on the farm—sheep, cattle, goats and deer.

TIMING OF TREATMENTS The use of anthelmintics to cure animals in the face of an outbreak of disease has already been discussed. Here we are concerned with the control of liver fluke, the aim being to prevent heavy infections of both sheep and snails. With regard to timing, the fluke forecasts are of great benefit, but beware of local conditions. Farms in high rainfall areas are at particular risk from heavy infections and will almost certainly need to treat more frequently. On farms where there are normally only moderate fluke infections, or in dry years, treatment once during the spring in late April or early May, with a product particularly effective against adult flukes, will reduce pasture contamination for snails during the summer period. This in turn will reduce the weight of infection for stock during the late summer and autumn. Second and third doses are required in autumn (October) and winter (January). On high risk farms and in very wet years this programme may need to be augmented by further doses six weeks after each of the above mentioned timings, namely in June, November and February.

Treatment programmes of this type aim to reduce the overall weight of infection on a farm. Whilst anthelmintic treatments alone are unlikely to eliminate fluke disease entirely, they can reduce it to manageable levels so that the benefits can be seen in extra productivity. Whilst it may be more appealing to use only control measures against the snail, such methods are

532

unlikely to eliminate the need for anthelmintics. Therefore, a carefully planned anthelmintic programme can be beneficial in the long and the short term. After all, very large quantities of flukicides can be purchased for the price of a contract to drain ten hectares of land.

The Lesser Liver Fluke—*Dicrocoelium dendriticum*

In the Western Isles of Scotland, stock may become infected with the only other type of liver fluke which occurs in Britain. It is smaller than *Fasciola hepatica* and is called *Dicrocoelium dendriticum*. Its life cycle is even more complicated than that of the common liver fluke, in that it has two intermediate hosts. The first is a land snail (one of various species), which eats the eggs of the fluke off pasture and at a later date expels an intermediate stage in the form of a 'slime ball'. The slime ball is eaten in turn by a formica ant—the second intermediate host. The ants are eaten by sheep, which then become infected by the fluke.

Dicrocoelium dendriticium causes much less damage than the common fluke, which is fortunate, since the majority of available anthelmintics are ineffective against it, unless they are used at high doses, when there is a risk of toxicity.

OTHER FLUKE INFECTIONS WORLDWIDE

There are a number of other important flukes found in parts of the world other than the UK, such as the giant liver fluke (*Fasciola gigantica*), which occurs in Africa and Asia, and the blood flukes which inhabit the blood vessels of domestic animals and humans causing the disease known as schistosomiasis. The reader is referred to the standard textbooks on parasitology for further detail.

13
THE SKIN PARASITES OF SHEEP

The external parasites or ectoparasites live on or in the skin of sheep and their presence on an animal is usually referred to as an **infestation** rather than an infection. Some parasites such as keds do little or no harm to their host. Others cause serious damage or irritation, and lice and the mites responsible for sheep scab are examples. Others cause little damage directly, but transmit infections and so indirectly cause serious disease or death; the sheep tick is an example.

Mites, lice and keds are obliged to spend their whole life on the host sheep and hence are called obligate parasites. Other species like cattle, pigs and horses may also become infested with lice or mites, but broadly speaking, the lice or mites which infest sheep will not affect other species and vice versa. As with most generalisations this is not strictly true, in that cross-infection may occur between different farm animal species, but the infestations are usually light and short-lived.

Control of mites, lice and keds should, in theory at least, be relatively straightforward, since they cannot survive for long away from their natural host or on another species. Therefore, if they can be eliminated from all sheep in the flock and providing no bought-in sheep are introduced into the flock without being dipped or otherwise treated, these infestations can be eradicated from the flock. However, as we have seen in the UK in recent years with sheep scab, eradication of a disease from the national flock presents real problems because of the difficulty of ensuring that every sheep in every flock is properly dipped at the appropriate time.

The other external parasites—ticks, blowflies and headflies—are not obliged to spend their whole life on the sheep, nor are they obliged to feed only off sheep if other host species are available, domestic or wild. Ticks usually feed off sheep because there are plenty of them around, but they can make do equally well on cattle, deer, hares, grouse or other warm-blooded vertebrates when sheep are unavailable.

535

Ticks

Ticks play a very important part in the life of sheep, not particularly because of the damage they cause to the sheep directly, but because of the important diseases they transmit when they suck the sheep's blood. These diseases—louping ill, tickborne fever and tick pyaemia—are discussed in Chapter 9. In this chapter, the life cycle of the tick, its relationship with its principal host, the sheep, and the general measures used in its control will be dealt with.

Hill and upland sheep account for a large proportion of the UK national flock, and the tick is of profound importance to the sheep economy of the less-favoured areas. With the likely changes in British agriculture in the foreseeable future, it is improbable that much of the rough terrain which is the habitat of the tick will be reclaimed. Indeed, it it more likely that previously reclaimed land will revert to the rough, or become afforested. Whatever happens, the tick is likely to remain an important parasite of sheep.

LIFE CYCLE OF THE TICK

The only tick of importance to sheep in the UK is *Ixodes ricinus*. It is called a **three host tick**, because during the three years of its life it must find a warm-blooded animal from which to take a blood meal on three separate occasions at approximately yearly intervals. The first two feeds are necessary to allow the immature stages—larvae and nymphs—to grow and shed their outer skin and develop into nymphs and adults respectively. The blood meal also provides sufficient stored energy for them to find a host for another meal the following year. In the case of the adult female the blood meal provides nutrient for the production and laying of several hundreds or even thousands of eggs before she finally dies.

The adult female tick is mated frequently by the male whilst she is firmly attached to the host sheep and in the process of feeding. (Males and females are too scattered to find each other on the ground.) The female tick drops off the host when she has finished feeding and rests for some weeks, protected from drying out by the high humidity in the decaying vegetation close to the soil. She lays her eggs in very large numbers, because the wastage from egg to mature adult is enormous due to predators, frost, desiccation, exhaustion of energy supplies whilst trying to find a host and many other causes.

THE TICK 'RISE'

Ticks are active only when the weather warms up in the spring and they can leave the protection of the thick vegetation where they spend most of their life in a resting state. In order to find a host from which to take a blood meal, they must climb to the tip of the herbage and await a passing animal. This is called **questing** and is rather a hit and miss affair (see Plate 13.3). If unsuccessful, the tick will descend into the protection of the herbage to prevent drying out in the wind or sun. It will keep trying until it finally finds a meal or runs out of energy and perishes. Thus, few ticks remain active during the summer months except in some upland regions of the north where the weather only warms to the threshold for tick activity in late May. Here, ticks may be active during June, July and August.

These periods of tick activity are often referred to as the tick 'rise'. In the wetter, warmer western areas of Britain there is often a second period of tick activity in the autumn due to a small, separate population of ticks which do not digest their blood meals until the following summer.

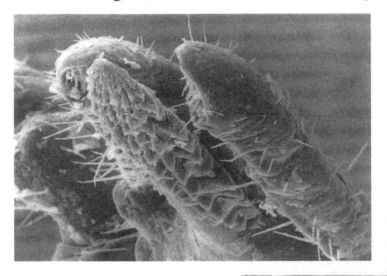

Plate 13.1   (*Above*) The mouth parts of the tick (magnified 260 times by the scanning electron microscope). The object in the centre with the backward pointing barbs is the hypostome which is thrust through the skin and enables the tick to both draw blood and hang onto the sheep.

Plate 13.2   Tick with its mouth parts embedded in the skin of its host.

537

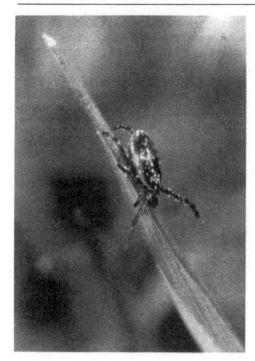

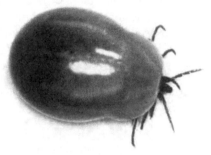

Plate 13.3 (*Left*) When weather conditions improve in the spring, ticks begin 'questing'. This female has climbed up the herbage and is waiting (with open arms) for a passing sheep to latch onto for its once-a-year feed of blood. (Male ticks do not take a blood meal.)

Plate 13.4 (*Above*) An adult female tick (*Ixodes ricinus*) in the engorged state after spending several days feeding on sheep's blood.

Active ticks cling on to the passing host sheep wherever they can, but attach primarily to the head and legs or bare areas of skin on the underside. Adult ticks move about the sheep and often migrate to the neck (usually the only woolly area they penetrate), between the forelegs and the chest wall (axillae) and the groin. Second year ticks—nymphs—travel shorter distances than adults and first year ticks—larvae or 'seed ticks'—stay wherever they can hang on and so are usually found on the legs, lips and ears, often in very large numbers. On infested sheep there will usually be representatives of all three stages, with nymphs outnumbering adults and larvae outnumbering nymphs by many times.

ADULT HOSTS

Adult ticks will usually be found on the larger mammals, especially sheep, but also cattle, deer, and hares. The sheep flock in most situations provides blood meals for perhaps more than 95% of adult ticks. This means that the intensity of sheep stocking largely governs the prevalence of ticks. Systematic control of ticks on sheep may thus have a profound effect upon the tick population (see below).

Once they have clung onto their host using their claws, the ticks select a feeding site, cut into the skin with their sharp jaws and then bury their special barbed mouth parts into the skin, which anchors them very securely.

They drink from the pool of blood and tissue fluids which forms around their mouthparts. Adult female ticks take one or two millilitres of blood and this may take them up to ten days or a fortnight. Nymphs and larvae take relatively less blood and engorge themselves in less than a week. Only when the tick is fully engorged will it retract its mouth parts and drop off.

The ticks fall off their host and crawl down into the mat of vegetation where they will take some time to perform the next stage of their development. In the case of larvae, this is to moult (cast their outer skin) and develop into nymphs. In the case of nymphs, this means becoming an adult. The immature stages remain inactive in their protective environment for a variable period, usually until the next spring or autumn, depending upon which population they belong to. At this time they again feed and, if successful, move on to the next stage of development. Spring feeding ticks will not quest again until after they are subjected to a cold shock in winter.

Adult female ticks rest for some weeks after feeding and then take about a month to lay their eggs, which they deposit deep in the vegetation in any suitable nook or cranny. Her work done, the female then promptly dies. How quickly the eggs hatch into larvae will depend particularly on the weather—the colder it is, the longer the delay before hatching. In any event, the larvae lie low and do not look for a meal until almost a year after the eggs were laid.

In her lifetime on a heavily tick-infested hill, a ewe may provide a blood meal for many thousands of ticks—even up to a million! Despite this, the loss of blood is rarely a problem, since the immature stages—which make up the vast majority of the population—take only minute quantities of blood.

TICK CONTROL

Various methods for controlling the tick population are available, none of which is totally effective. As ticks depend on the cover from a thick protective mat of vegetation for their survival away from a host, one of the most successful methods of controlling them is to alter the habitat by land improvement. Methods like drainage, reseeding and stocking with cattle all help to remove the rough mat. Such reclaimed land can no longer support a tick population. Land improvements, which are expensive, have depended heavily on grants in the past and have been used primarily to increase the output of farms rather than to control the tick.

It is important to appreciate that sheep brought down off infested hill grazings at a time of tick activity will carry ticks with them. Once the ticks have finished feeding they will drop off but will not survive for long because there is too little protection from desiccation. However, those ticks which drop off in rough corners or along uncultivated headlands may survive and lead to unexpected outbreaks of tickborne disease in subsequent years. It is obviously important to dip sheep or to apply pour-on products before such a move. (These methods are discussed later in this chapter and also in Chapter 9 in relation to the control of tickborne disease.)

Blowfly Strike

Blowfly strike (myiasis) was the cause of untold misery and death in sheep flocks before the advent of dipping. Hill shepherds would spend much of the summer searching out wretched sheep which had been 'struck' and had crawled away to find shelter. Sheep could be literally eaten alive by successive waves of maggots.

There is no doubt that the development of insecticidal dips with a lengthy residual action in the fleece was one of the most significant contributions that scientists have ever made to the livestock industry worldwide and especially to sheep farming in the UK. Early products such as dieldrin, which were particularly effective and long-lasting, have had to be replaced because of the problem of accumulating residues. The new generation of safer chemicals is a boon to sheep farmers and few could farm without them.

Although a number of flies can cause strike in sheep, in the UK the most important by far is the **greenbottle** (*Lucilia sericata*), which generally prefers to lay its eggs on living sheep rather than carrion. It is attracted by the smell of decomposing matter which contains liquid protein upon which it feeds and amongst which it lays a batch of around a hundred eggs. Adult flies will live for roughly a month and during that time will lay up to two or three thousand eggs in a number of different sites.

Sheep are most commonly struck around the rear end where the wool becomes soiled by faeces and urine (breech strike). Animals suffering from scour (diarrhoea) or ewes which have not been crutched are more susceptible. Castration and tailing wounds, clipping wounds, dog bites, head wounds on fighting rams, indeed any open wound will attract flies (wound strike), particularly if infected by bacteria as is often the case.

Strike may also occur on any part of the body where the fleece has become soiled or infected with bacteria (body strike) (see Plate 13.5). For example, if a sheep has footrot and the fleece over the chest wall becomes contaminated from the infected foot when the sheep lies down, this will attract blowflies. Infected feet themselves smell attractive to flies, of course, and frequently become struck (see Plate 13.6). Rain-soaked wool which becomes infected by the microorganisms causing fleece rot may also attract blowflies.

MAGGOTS

The eggs, once laid in such unattractive surroundings, hatch within a few hours or days. The emerging larvae or maggots are very active and secrete enzymes which liquefy the skin and flesh of the sheep upon which they are

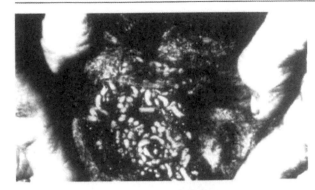

Plate 13.5   (*Left*) Fly strike on a body wound. The greenbottle fly (*Lucilia sericata*) lays its eggs in the wound. When the maggots hatch they feed voraciously on the tissues.

Plate 13.6   (*Below*) Fly strike in a case of footrot.

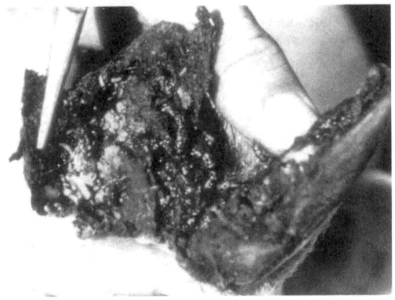

feeding. Flies whose larvae can do this are called primary flies. There are others—secondary flies—which lay their eggs on wounds already made by primary flies and their larvae simply make matters worse by extending the wound.

Larvae feed for a variable period of time depending upon the availability of food and competition from other maggots. They undergo two moults before maturing to full-blown maggots within one to three weeks. The mature maggots, which measure up to one and a half centimetres in length, crawl off the sheep and pupate in the soil. In suitable weather conditions in the summer it takes less than a week for the fly to emerge, but often it is two or three weeks. With flies possibly laying thousands of eggs, it is easy to see why the population of blowflies increases so rapidly under warm, thundery summer conditions.

Plate 13.7 Close-up of maggots in a wound.

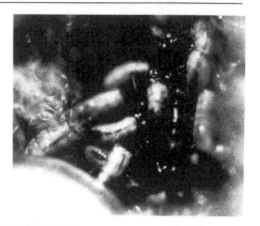

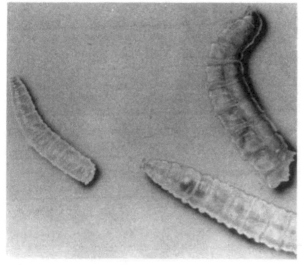

Plate 13.8 High magnification of maggots removed from the scene of the crime.

CLINICAL SIGNS

Sheep which have been struck are obviously tormented. They spend less and less time grazing and more and more time lip-smacking, tail wagging, rubbing the affected area and nibbling the struck areas they can reach. They very rapidly lose body condition when they are badly affected. If the condition goes unrecognised and secondary strike occurs, the wounds can become very extensive, and bacterial infection may lead to serious complications, even death from toxaemia and septicaemia. In hill areas, sheep may hide away amongst dense bracken, which itself harbours flies, so that secondary strike is inevitable. They are often so ill that they will not respond to the presence of the shepherd or the dog and may go unnoticed at gatherings.

Careful examination of sheep will reveal the damage—often smelt before it is found—and of course sheep may be struck in more than one place. The damage caused by the maggots produces liquids which mat the wool fibres together and once this is gently parted the extent of the damage will be seen. The wound is often a mass of writhing maggots feeding voraciously on the flesh of the sheep and the smell from the wound is appalling. If maggots are disturbed they may retreat into the fleece and care should be taken to avoid this.

TREATMENT

Treatment of blowfly strike should aim to kill all maggots present, prevent the possibility of further fly strike and assist the wound to heal. Badly affected sheep should be brought near the steading as they will need close attention for some days.

The wool should be carefully clipped away from around the wound and surrounding area. A suitably **mild**, but effective insecticidal cream with healing properties should be applied, first to the clean surrounding skin and then to the wound itself. This will cause considerable resentment in the maggots, which will attempt to leave the area but should not be allowed to escape into the fleece. In severe wounds, maggots are embedded deep in the flesh and are difficult to extract. The cream should be packed into the wound and the process repeated until all maggots are removed and the wound is clean.

On no account should neat dip, disinfectant or antiseptic be applied to strike wounds. These substances are very toxic in concentrated form and will be absorbed from the wound into the body and may produce toxicity. They will also kill healthy tissue, damage normal skin and cause much pain and lasting discomfort. Even correctly diluted dip is totally unsuitable for application to raw wounds. Suitable insecticidal powders are available, but creams are preferable.

Mild cases should heal quickly with correct treatment. In severe cases it is always best to consult a veterinary surgeon or to destroy the wretched animal. If one sheep has been struck it is likely that others will also have been attacked. Special attention should be paid to high risk sheep, such as those with soiled back ends. In groups of lambs, for example, scouring may be due to worms, and anthelmintic treatment indicated. Meanwhile if the weather is such that fly activity is likely to remain high, the flock should be dipped.

PREVENTION

In attempting to prevent blowfly strike it is necessary to avoid situations which will attract flies during the period of risk, which is usually from May to September. Whilst it may be wise to dock the tails of lambs to prevent excessive soiling, in so doing a wound is inflicted which itself could attract flies. The task must therefore be done hygienically and the wound encouraged to heal well before the onset of fly activity. No other technique which leaves an open wound should be carried out during the fly season if at all possible. Wounds inflicted at clipping should be protected with suitable fly repellent preparations.

Crutching of both ewes and lambs prior to the risk period is an essential husbandry task. This consists of clipping the wool off the breech and from around the tail. This helps prevent soiling of the back end if scouring occurs.

Blowflies tend to be found in largest numbers where there is some cover for them to shade themselves. Woodland, scrub and bracken covered hillsides harbour many times more flies than open ground. Whilst it is obviously impractical to suggest always keeping sheep away from such areas, it would nevertheless be unwise to graze a group of scouring lambs adjacent to a forest at the height of the fly season.

The most effective way of protecting sheep at the present is by dipping. This must be carried out before the period of risk and should be repeated as conditions dictate and depending upon the period of residual effect of the dip used.

In the early part of the season before sheep have been clipped it will be particularly important to immerse sheep for at least a full minute—and probably a minute and a half in heavily fleeced breeds—so as to ensure that the dip thoroughly saturates the whole fleece. The length of time a dip will protect depends upon the chemical used and the amount of insecticide which is retained in the fleece. Apart from thorough soaking, it is essential to maintain the strength of the dip by regular topping up during the procedure in the recommended manner (see Appendix 7).

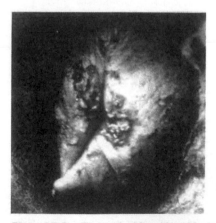
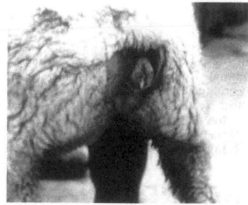

Plate 13.9 Short docking like this is now illegal. This ewe has an inflammation of the vulva which is vulnerable to fly strike, especially as she does not have a tail with which to swat the flies.

Headfly

Headfly disease is a condition of horned or partially horned sheep, particularly in northern Britain. The headfly—also known as the hornfly or forest fly—causes worry and the development of extensive open wounds on the head. Apart from head damage, an increase in the number of cases of eye infections and mastitis has been noted in flocks where the problem is serious. It may also be implicated in cases of infection of the vulva and vagina of ewes.

The fly responsible—*Hydrotaea irritans*—causes worry in a number of species because of its habit of feeding on various body secretions. In cattle it is thought to transmit the microorganism responsible for New Forest disease by feeding on the secretions of the eye, and it also transmits various bacteria which cause summer mastitis in cattle by feeding on the secretions of damaged teats. It has also been implicated in the spread of myxomatosis in rabbits.

Headfly disease appears to be limited to areas of northern England and southern Scotland, although isolated outbreaks have been recorded elsewhere and the fly itself has a wide distribution in Britain. The reason for this restriction to the Border areas is unknown, but is thought to be

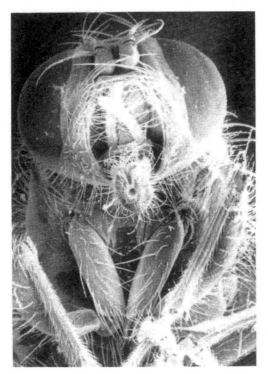

Plate 13.10 The headfly (*Hydrotea irritans*) magnified 45 times (scanning electron microscope). The head and thorax only are shown.

Plate 13.11 Headflies feeding around the base of the horn of a young sheep. (See also colour plates 49 and 50.) This damage is intensely irritating to the sheep.

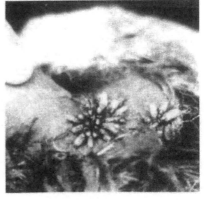

545

due in part to the presence of large flocks of susceptible horned sheep and ever-increasing afforestation.

Horned breeds such as the Swaledale and Scottish Blackface and partially horned breeds like the Cheviot and the Hexham (Bluefaced) Leicester are particularly susceptible. So also are sheep with hair rather than wool on the head. Large flocks appear to have a higher incidence of the disease than small flocks.

LIFE CYCLE OF THE HEADFLY

The flies shelter at night and for most of the day on trees around the perimeter of woods and forests. They require a diet of animal protein before they can lay their eggs, which they do only once a year towards the end of the summer. They deposit the eggs in pasture soil adjacent to woodland, especially near or under dung pats. The larvae which emerge a week or so later feed on insects or dung beetle larvae until the autumn. They rest in the soil overwinter and then resume feeding in the spring, pupate and emerge as adult flies around June or July.

Flies choose warm, humid, windless days to feed on livestock and they take a meal for around 20 minutes every few days. They are present in enormous numbers when conditions are suitable and counts of around 200,000 active flies per hectare have been recorded—hundreds of times more than blowfly numbers. The flies can travel long distances—up to two miles—and have a long life of up to two months.

CLINICAL SIGNS AND TREATMENT

Headflies attack livestock in swarms and feed on the secretions of the nose and eyes. In sheep they also attack the soft spongy tissue where skin and horn join and where there is often a break in the skin oozing with serum (see Colour plates 49 and 50). The flies do not bite, but have a harsh rasping action. Their presence in large numbers is extremely irritating to the sheep. They rub their heads on any available object and scratch at their heads with their hind feet, causing further damage. This attracts more swarms of headflies which extend the wounds. If blowflies are active at the time, they may be attracted to the wound and lay their eggs, thus leading to maggot strike. The wounds may be very extensive and disfiguring in severe cases.

Treatment of individually affected sheep will depend on the severity of the case. Extreme cases should be temporarily housed and may need treatment with a suitable antibiotic to treat or prevent bacterial infection of the wound. Soothing antiseptic creams or powders containing an insecticide may be applied to the wound and the surrounding area. As with blowfly strike, dip, disinfectant or antiseptic solutions should **not** be used on the wound.

PREVENTION

Prevention of headfly necessitates applying a suitably effective insecticide, with a prolonged residual action, before the fly season begins in June. The ideal insecticide would have a strong repellent and a rapid 'knock-down' effect together with a prolonged action. As the majority of headflies feed on cattle, even where sheep are grazing alongside, preventive measures aimed only at sheep are unlikely to reduce the number of flies present to any significant extent.

Summer dipping against blowfly strike will not prevent headfly. (Dieldrin, considered by many farmers to have been effective before it was banned, had in fact no effect on headfly.) The most effective group of insecticides available at present is the **synthetic pyrethroids**, some of which are available as spot-ons. Most have a residual effect of at least a month and are quick and easy to apply to the head—between the horns—as sheep pass through a race. They may be used safely on sheep which have just been dipped, which saves an extra gathering. The manufacturer's directions should be read carefully, since a withdrawal period before sale for human consumption is usually required.

Lambs may be more susceptible to headfly attack than ewes since the horns are softer and are growing fast. Ram lambs of the horned breeds may need more frequent preventive treatment. Lambs may be safely treated at the same time as they are being wormed. Additional weight gains of around 2 kg over the summer grazing period have been recorded in protected lambs compared with untreated lambs in the same flock. Trials using plastic tags impregnated with a synthetic pyrethroid (cypermethrin) tied between the horns of ewes have shown that a good degree of protection can be afforded, not only to the treated ewes but also to the untreated lambs grazing alongside them. However in areas where flies are abundant, like fields adjacent to woodland, lambs with horns should also be treated, especially after weaning when they appear to become more prone to attack. Rams, whether horned or hornless, often fight and should always be treated in areas where headfly attack is expected.

However effective an insecticide is at knocking down flies, it does not prevent flies approaching sheep or even beginning to feed. Worry may still be a problem in some areas despite preventive treatment. Small flocks may be housed but this is not a practical proposition under most systems. However, it may be sensible to graze flocks of horned sheep in pastures well away from woodland or forest from July to September.

Other preventive treatments which have largely been superseded include the use of headcaps and Stockholm tar. The latter may itself cause irritation or scalding of the skin and cannot be recommended in view of the more effective and safer modern products.

If the problem is particularly severe, consideration may be given to changing to a cross breed, or other non-horned or woolly headed breed. A cross between the Derbyshire Gritstone and a polled Scottish Blackface

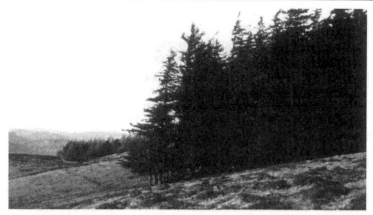

Plate 13.12   Headflies shelter for most of the day around the edge of plantations such as this.

at the Redesdale EHF has produced ewes which are virtually hornless and rams with much-reduced horn growth. Whilst this approach would mean a long-term and costly investment, it may be worthy of consideration on farms with a serious headfly problem.

Attempts have been made to spray the edges of woodlands with insecticides. The number of flies may be significantly reduced, but because of the huge numbers of flies the problem of attack remains. Fencing off a 20 metre strip adjacent to forest land may reduce the attack frequency, but it will not totally alleviate the problem, since the headfly can travel up to two miles, and fencing is, of course, very expensive.

Nostril Fly

Nostril fly or nasal bot is a relatively uncommon condition of sheep in the UK, but does occur in south-west England and occasionally elsewhere. It is a very common problem in other parts of the world, where the fly may even strike humans—particularly shepherds—in the eye, nose or mouth, often with unpleasant results.

The fly—*Oestrus ovis*—is a grey-brown colour and just over a centimetre in length. Flies are active in the warm summer months and cause much alarm amongst sheep when they strike. The fly belongs to the same family as the warble fly of cattle and both have a similar effect on their host when they attack. The female fly does not alight on the sheep, but hovers and strikes, depositing larvae (rather than eggs) around the nostrils. She will strike a number of sheep over the summer season, depositing a total of several hundred larvae.

LIFE CYCLE

Using large mouth hooks and spines along the body, the larvae crawl up the nostrils causing considerable irritation. A nasal discharge develops in response to the irritation and the larvae feed on this material. As they grow and moult they progress up into the sinuses. Here they continue to feed on the secretions produced due to their presence and the mature larvae may reach 3 centimetres in length. A dozen or more mature larvae may be present in a sheep, and the damage and irritation they cause can result in considerable loss of body condition and occasionally more serious symptoms. The mature larvae are sneezed out of the nostrils onto the ground where they burrow into the soil and pupate. After several weeks or months they emerge as adult flies. Following mating the females produce eggs which develop into larvae ready to be deposited around the nostrils of sheep. The whole life cycle of the fly may take only two months in warm climates, but usually takes considerably longer in temperate climates such as in Britain, where the larvae may remain in the warmth and comfort of the nostrils and sinuses for many months.

CLINICAL SIGNS

When the sheep are being attacked by flies they show considerable alarm. They rub their noses on the ground or against each other and run about shaking their heads and stamping their feet. When there are large numbers of flies about, the continual annoyance may lead to loss of body condition through interference with grazing.

The presence of the larvae crawling up the nostrils produces considerable irritation, and sheep may have characteristic fits of sneezing. The nasal discharge can cause difficulty in breathing and may be confused with pneumonia. Some larvae may crawl into the sinuses and grow too large to get back out, with the result that they die there. Larvae may even cause damage to the brain, producing nervous symptoms such as circling, high stepping and incoordination, which may be confused with gid (an alternative name for the nostril fly is false gid).

TREATMENT

Treatment presents some problems, since killing the larvae means that they remain in the sinuses and may produce severe symptoms when they die en masse. If treatment is thought necessary, it should be carried out in the autumn when the larvae are relatively small so that there will be less dead material to cause problems. The anthelmintic ivermectin (Ivomec, MSD) is highly effective at killing the larvae. So too is the fluke treatment, rafoxamide (Flukanide injection, MSD). It may be that treatment is considered more of a risk than allowing the larvae to develop and be sneezed out.

Prevention is difficult also, because available insecticides do not have a long enough residual effect to protect for a whole season. In Britain the problem is uncommon and is more likely to be an interesting incident rather than to present a flock problem requiring preventive measures.

Sheep Scab

Sheep scab or psoroptic mange is a contagious disease caused by a mite—*Psoroptes communis ovis*—which feeds off the skin of sheep. It is a notifiable disease and its presence or suspicion of it in a flock must be notified to the Ministry of Agriculture or to the police without delay.

The disease was eradicated from Britain in 1952 after almost 50 years of compulsory dipping. Double dipping was introduced during the First World War and after the Second World War the persistent organochlorine compounds were used at a single dipping. Unfortunately the disease was reintroduced by an importation of sheep in 1973 and this has necessitated the resumption of compulsory dipping under the Sheep Scab Order of 1977.

CLINICAL SIGNS

The mite causes intense irritation of the sheep, which react by rubbing against any convenient object such as fence posts, gates, walls or pen divisions. If none of these is available, they rub against other sheep, so spreading the disease. They scratch themselves with their feet or nibble at the fleece, often leaving tell-tale strands of wool between their teeth.

In the early stages of the condition the wool has a dirty, rubbed appearance and this, together with the obvious signs of irritation, should make the

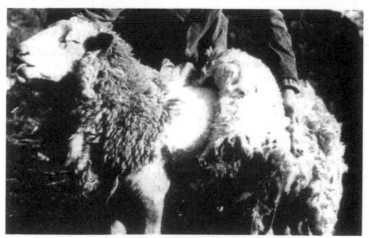

Plate 13.13 Sheep scab or psoroptic mange. Note the nibbling reflex due to the intense irritation.

shepherd suspicious of sheep scab. The activity of the mites feeding off the skin causes blood serum (which is straw coloured) to ooze out and dry to form crusty scabs. If the fleece is parted over an affected area it may look as if brown sugar has been sprinkled amongst the wool. The mites are particularly active at the edges of these scabs and can sometimes be seen by the naked eye, the adult mites being half a millimetre in length. Diagnosis of sheep scab is made by microscopic examination of scrapings from the edge of scabs.

When being examined in this way, the sheep will often extend its neck, throw its head back and make nibbling and lip smacking movements. The activity of the mites together with the self-inflicted damage causes the fleece to fall out, first over the shoulders, chest and flanks and then, if the condition is not treated, eventually over the whole body. This process can take three to four months, during which time the sheep becomes emaciated through not eating.

As the condition progresses the animal becomes more and more alarmed by noise and when handled may fall over or take fits. In any untreated outbreak there will always be a number of deaths from starvation, secondary bacterial infection of the skin or other diseases (such as pneumonia), brought on when the animal's resistance is low because of undernourishment. Animals in poor body condition are likely to be more seriously affected by sheep scab than well-nourished sheep in good body condition.

The mites spend their whole life on the sheep. If they are rubbed off onto fence posts or pen divisions they may survive for a week or two, but will eventually die due to lack of food and desiccation. Sheep coming into contact with mites on posts and gates may become infested and this is thought to be an important indirect method of spread of the disease. However, the most important method of spread is from sheep to sheep by direct contact (contagion).

SEASONALITY OF SHEEP SCAB

Sheep scab is an all year round disease and this is important to remember, despite the fact that the majority of outbreaks occur during the winter months of October to March. Mites are more active and the females are thought to lay more eggs in winter, because conditions in the fleece are most suitable. This is especially so in housed sheep. In summer, when the fleece tends to dry out more, the mites feed less, become less active and lay fewer eggs, especially on shorn sheep. However, they are ever present and tend to congregate on certain areas of the body such as in the groin, between the fore legs and body (axilla), inside the ears, in a small fold of skin below the eye, in between the cleats of the hoof, in the wrinkled skin of the scrotum of rams and at the base of the horns. If conditions are suitable, outbreaks can and do occur during the summer months.

During the winter, the female mite lays a few eggs every three or four days, totalling around a hundred eggs in her six week life. The eggs are laid at the edge of the scabs or at the base of adjacent wool fibres. They hatch in two or three days into larvae and undergo a further two moults to nymph and adult. Females—which generally outnumber males—then moult again and proceed to lay eggs. The whole cycle takes less than a fortnight, so it can be seen how, from an initial infection of only a few mites, enormous numbers accumulate in a very few weeks.

Infection builds up in a flock slowly but relentlessly. A third of the flock may become infected from the introduction of even a single infected animal. The control of the disease through compulsory dipping is hampered by the considerable movement of sheep within the country. Also, on extensive hill farms it is difficult to gather 100% of the flock, and if infected animals are present, they will tend to shelter in bracken or other cover and can easily be missed. Boundary fences on high ground are often breached and there may be mixing of sheep, as on common grazings.

(Other species, such as cattle, do not become infected with sheep scab, but they do have their own less serious forms of mite infestation.)

Costs of the disease

Losses to flock owners from sheep scab include those from ill thrift, wool loss and death, plus the not unsubstantial costs of dipping. Nationally, the eradication scheme costs a great deal of money, but to allow the disease to go uncontrolled would cost considerably more. In the days before compulsory eradication, around 3,000 new flock outbreaks would be confirmed annually and today there are many more sheep in the national flock.

CONTROL OF SHEEP SCAB

The compulsory dipping regulations in the UK are announced each spring and in 1989 were reduced from double to single dipping. The timings of these dippings have been and will continue to be altered as the situation demands. Inevitably, problems arise when legislation is enforced upon such a diverse industry. Gathering and dipping is a stressful business for sheep. In some flocks it will coincide with the mating period and may therefore adversely affect flock fertility. Nevertheless, there is some leeway in the timing of the compulsory dipping and it would be well worthwhile for shepherds to discuss scheduling with their veterinary surgeons.

It is essential that all flock owners comply with the regulations and ensure that **all** sheep are dipped thoroughly. Any suspicion of infection such as loss of fleece or rubbing and scratching, should be investigated—winter or summer. **If there is any doubt, the matter should be reported.** The Ministry would much prefer to investigate a false alarm rather than allow an outbreak to go undiagnosed. It should be remembered that sheep can be infested by more than one external parasite at the same time, e.g. sheep scab and lice, so diagnosis of lice would not preclude scab.

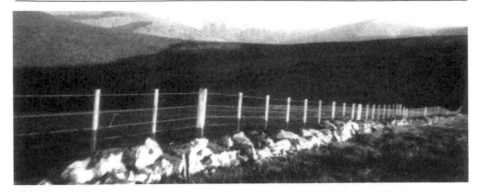

Plate 13.14 A sound boundary fence between two hill farms replaces a broken-down stone dyke. Security is important in disease control and makes gathering in extensive areas more efficient—for example, for scab dipping.

Plate 13.15 Sheep with scab may take cover and be overlooked at gathering.

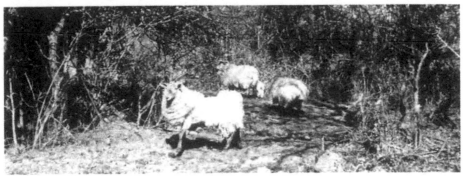

Remember also that under the present UK regulations, local authorities must receive at least three clear days' notice of your intention to dip. The dip used must be one drawn from the MAFF list of approved dips for the control of sheep scab and at the present time this will mean formulations containing either diazinon or propetamphos.

Foot Scab

Foot scab is another mange infestation of sheep caused by the mite called *Chorioptes ovis*. It causes a crusty irritation of the mainly hairy parts of the lower limbs (including between the cleats), around the eye, on the brisket and on the scrotum of rams. It is treated by dipping or by the use of sprays or powders containing a suitable ectoparasiticide. Whilst foot scab is not a notifiable disease, it is important to differentiate the condition from sheep scab.

Sarcoptic Mange

Sarcoptic mange is a notifiable disease in sheep and is caused by a mite called *Sarcoptes scabiei* var. *ovis*. It has not been present in the UK for some years. The mite affects the hairy areas of the face and legs. Control would be governed by legislation if the condition were to be reintroduced into the country.

Harvest or Forage Mites

Harvest or forage mites (*Trombicula autumnalis*) live in the soil or grassland or cereal crops. Their larvae, which are very small, attack all species, including humans, causing intense irritation. Sheep are usually attacked around the face and a dermatitis may develop. Forage infested with mites may cause problems in housed sheep—especially if winter shorn—but otherwise the parasite is of little importance in the UK. In other parts of the world, however, related species transmit important diseases, such as scrub typhus in man.

Lice

Lice or louse infestation (pediculosis) is a common contagious disease of sheep. Like scab, lice are more noticeable in the winter months, but are present all year round. They are small wingless insects and there are a number of different lice which infest sheep, the most common being *Damalinia ovis*. The adults are visible to the naked eye, being brown in colour and up to 2 mm long. They are not so easy to see on the sheep except in heavy infestations, and a lock of wool from an affected area of fleece should be examined in good light using a magnifying glass.

The female lice attach their eggs (nits) to wool fibres and in about ten days they hatch to become nymphs. Two to three weeks and several moults later, the nymphs become adults.

Lice feed on debris on the surface of the skin and their scavenging produces intense irritation. In an effort to relieve the irritation, sheep rub and bite the wool, breaking the fibres and damaging the fleece. The faeces of the lice also foul the fleece. Sheep in poor body condition appear to be more prone to heavy infestations and may lose even more weight through interference with feeding.

Sheep become affected by direct contact with infested sheep and also indirectly by rubbing against posts and gates where lice have been rubbed off by affected sheep. Lice can live only a few days off the sheep, and whilst they may attach themselves to species other than the sheep—including humans—they do not stay long. All farm species have lice, but they are very specific to a particular species. For example, pig lice will not infest cattle and cattle lice will not infest sheep or pigs. The loss to the farmer results from damage to the fleece, loss of body condition and the need for treatment.

Because of its contagious nature, louse infestation spreads most rapidly when sheep are in close contact, such as when gathered or housed. All ages of sheep can become infested, but hoggs appear to be most often affected.

It will be apparent that the symptoms of louse infestation are very similar to those of sheep scab, and this should always be borne in mind. Animals

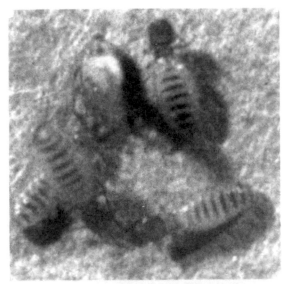

Plate 13.16   Close-up of a louse. 'Lousy' sheep are most commonly found in winter, especially amongst housed animals.

Plate 13.17   Lice on a sheep's face.

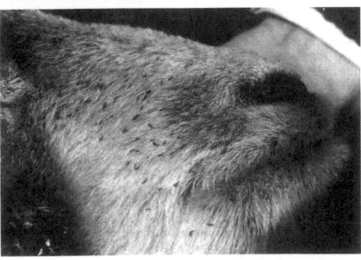

may harbour both parasites at once. If in doubt inform the police, the Ministry of Agriculture's veterinary department or consult your veterinary surgeon.

Control of lice is most effectively done by thorough dipping. The compulsory dipping for sheep scab in the UK should control lice adequately, providing the dips used have a sufficient residual effect to kill eggs, as they hatch up to two weeks after being laid. The fleece must be thoroughly soaked by the dip.

Suitable 'spot-on' and 'pour-on' products are much more convenient and less stressful than dipping, but take up to a month or longer to clear the sheep of all lice. This is because these products spread slowly over the complete surface of the skin, as they are carried in the fleece grease. They do have a long residual effect, however, which keeps sheep clear for several months. This method is particularly useful for treating sheep immediately before housing or when infestations occur in housed or heavily pregnant sheep. These products can also be used to treat sheep which are to be moved to an area or a sheep shed which has recently been vacated by infested sheep. Such accommodation should preferably be left empty of sheep for at least a fortnight.

Face lice (*Linognathus ovillus*) and **foot lice** (*Linognathus pedalis*) are blood-sucking lice but are uncommon in Britain because they are very well controlled by modern dips. Occasionally, heavy infestations occur which may lead to loss of body condition or even anaemia through excessive blood loss.

Ked

The sheep ked is a dark brown, leathery, wingless insect about half a centimetre long, called *Melophagus ovinus* (see Colour plate 51). It is a blood sucker which spends its whole life on the sheep. Heavy infestations cause irritation which makes the sheep rub and nibble, thus damaging the fleece. Ked faeces also stain and downgrade the fleece and may cause scoring of the hides. The symptoms are similar to those of lice and sheep scab. Although the ked is easy to identify, remember that sheep can be infested with keds, lice and sheep scab at the same time.

Sheep become infested directly from other infested sheep. Thick fleeced breeds are said to be more likely to pass on keds, since the insects tend to move to the surface of the fleece. The female ked 'glues' her single larva to the wool, the larva immediately pupates for about a month and then it emerges as an adult. The adult immediately mates and the females carry the developing larvae for roughly ten days. The whole life cycle takes around five or six weeks. Females live for about five months and deposit around a dozen larvae during that time.

Many adult keds and pupae attached to the wool are removed at shearing—some onto the shearers! Although the pupae are able to hatch and the females to survive for a week or so, they will eventually perish unless they can find a sheep (their only host) to feed off. The chances of this are fairly remote, so shearing itself provides some measure of control. Numbers of keds on sheep rise during the autumn and the heaviest infestations occur in winter, when symptoms are likely to be most noticeable.

Control measures for the more important ectoparasites such as ticks, blowflies and sheep scab are also effective against keds—especially the late autumn dip for scab which is currently in force. The residual effects of modern dips keep sheep clear of keds for months.

Control of the Skin Parasites of Sheep

Control measures have been discussed under the individual disease headings, but a few general remarks may be helpful in the overall planning of control measures in flocks.

DIPPING

At the time of writing, compulsory dipping of sheep for the control of sheep scab mite is in force in the UK and so this is a starting point for all flocks. Only two compounds are approved for scab control—**diazinon** and **propetamphos**—and these chemicals are sold under a variety of different trade names for the control of both scab and other external parasites.

These compounds must be applied by **plunge dipping**, since this is the only method which, if carried out correctly, will allow thorough penetration of the fleece. A single dipping in either diazinon or propetamphos will ensure eradication of sheep scab mites and give at least one month's protection against reinfection.

The sheep scab mite is an obligate parasite—that is, it spends its whole life on the sheep and cannot survive for long away from the sheep. The same is true of lice and keds. Control of scab, therefore, will also control lice and keds which are present on the sheep at the compulsory dipping periods, whenever they happen to be.

Keds are highly sensitive to parasiticides and because of the compulsory dipping in recent years, the ked could almost be regarded as an endangered species. Lice, however, are far from endangered and to some extent this is a reflection of the inefficient way dipping is carried out on many farms. It is small wonder that sheep scab—a much more resistant parasite than lice or keds—is proving such a difficult disease to eradicate.

Ticks, blowflies and headflies—parasites which spend only a short period of their life on the sheep and which can complete their life cycles in the absence of sheep—are much more difficult to control. Application of parasiticide must be timed to precede the period of risk and must have a sufficiently long residual effect (or else be reapplied) to protect for as long as these parasites are likely to be a problem. The compulsory dippings for

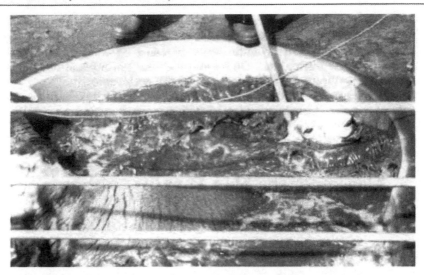

Plate 13.18 It is vital that plunge dipping is carried out correctly, efficiently and safely.

scab are not so helpful with these pests, since either the timing is inappropriate or the method ineffective.

For example, it is necessary to dip for ticks in the spring rather than the summer and autumn, and dipping is inappropriate for headfly control. Whilst the late summer sheep scab dipping will assist with blowfly strike, it may be a bit late in the day since the greenbottles have usually been at work in the early summer, so that specific control measures should be taken prior to the period of risk.

Traditionally a dipping for blowfly is carried out three or four weeks after clipping, when there has been a sufficient regrowth of fleece to hold on to or 'strip' the insecticide from the dip. However, in many areas and seasons it will be necessary to dip before clipping. Where a spring dip for ticks is necessary, this will normally control blowfly until shearing if an appropriate dip is used.

Dipping has been carried out for the control of the skin parasites of sheep for almost two centuries. It is often considered a tedious, run-of-the-mill task, and this may explain why it is often done so inefficiently. Almost all the reported problems which arise—be they complaints about the product's lack of efficacy or disease or injury caused to sheep or shepherd—can be put down to incorrect technique. There is simply no point in dipping sheep unless the job is carried out correctly, since it is a waste of time and money and leaves the flock owner with the false impression that his sheep are parasite free and fully protected.

See Appendix 7 for step-by-step notes on dipping techniques.

IMPORTANT NOTE—SHEEPDOGS Sheepdogs should **never** be put into the dip bath or treated with pour-ons or spot-ons in any way, shape or form. These substances are toxic and may make dogs ill or even cause death. If a dog should fall into the dipper, dry it thoroughly by dabbing with a towel. Put it into a well-ventilated place on a comfortable bed and keep a close eye on it. Should it become ill, contact your veterinary surgeon immediately. Sheepdogs are valuable friends—don't take risks with them.

'TOPPING UP' 'Topping up' or replenishing of dip baths is one of the areas where most mistakes are made. Manufacturers generally advocate that initially the dip be made up stronger than necessary to kill the parasite to be controlled. This is to allow for gradual dilution as dipping progresses. The active chemical ingredient (parasiticide) of the dip is actively retained by the fleece. This is called **stripping**, and has the effect of gradually reducing the concentration and therefore the activity of the dip. The whole point of dipping is, of course, this retention of parasiticide in the fleece: the chemicals dissolve in the wool lanolin and creep down the fibres as they grow.

Manufacturers usually advise that once the depth of the dip bath has fallen to a certain level—usually to around four-fifths of the original total capacity—the bath should be topped up. This stage has been carefully calculated so that there is still an adequate amount of parasiticide remaining in the dip immediately before topping up is recommended. The topping up concentration is always higher than the original bath-full, because it has to increase the strength of the remaining dip in the bath which has become considerably diluted. Automatic topping up devices are now available which should ensure correct dip concentrations throughout the dipping.

MIXING CHEMICALS A number of additional chemicals can be added to dip washes and these include bacteriostats (see below) and fungicides. However, on no account should any other chemicals be added to a dip unless on the manufacturer's specific recommendations. Dip concentrates are extremely toxic substances and mixtures could react together with serious consequences to the operator or the sheep.

Post-dipping Lameness

This is a serious disease which can cripple or kill sheep. It is a consequence of dipping sheep in a bath of dip which is heavily contaminated with the bacterium *Erysipelothrix rhusiopathiae*. This microorganism is common in soil and sheep faeces and can multiply very rapidly in dip washes which have become contaminated and especially in warm weather.

Old-fashioned dips contained high concentrations of phenols, which are bacteriostats and therefore prevented the multiplication of bacteria. It is not possible to include these bacteriostats in a sufficiently high concentration to be effective in many modern concentrated dips, and they must therefore be added separately to the diluted wash in the dipper. Many manufacturers supply separate sachets of bacteriostats which are compatible with their particular dip. For the reasons mentioned above, never add your own chemicals. Bacteriostats should be added when the bath is freshly made up at the recommended rate.

A dip should not be used for a second day if at all possible. If this is unavoidable, then bacteriostats must be added at the rate recommended by the manufacturer for overnight storage of dip. **Never ever use dip after two days' dipping.** The dip is bound to be heavily soiled and apart from the risk of erysipelas infection, fly strike is more likely after dipping in dirty dip. Also, modern dips are less stable than the older, more persistent chemicals and they will not retain sufficient activity in the dipper for more than two days in most cases.

CLINICAL SIGNS

Post-dipping lameness occurs within a few days of dipping and can be dramatic. The most common finding is for a number of animals to become very lame. The bacteria gain entry via any small cuts or abrasions on the skin and cause an inflammation of the tissues underneath the skin. The whole of the lower limb and foot is usually affected and feels hot when handled. In some cases more than one, or even all, of the limbs are affected and animals may lie down and stop grazing. It can be an alarming sight to see three-quarters of the flock crippled, as sometimes happens. Occasionally there may be damage on other parts of the body (see Colour plate 63).

A veterinary surgeon should be called promptly to diagnose and deal with the outbreak. Correct treatment for a sufficiently long period is essential if a satisfactory rate of cure is to be achieved and relapses prevented. The

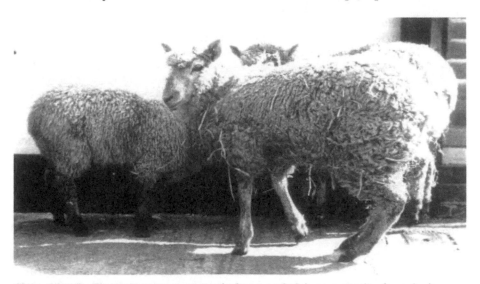

Plate 13.19 These sheep are severely lame and sick as a result of erysipelas infection from contaminated dip.

bacteria may get into the bloodstream and cause blood poisoning, which may cause some deaths. In others which do not respond to treatment the bacteria may eventually invade the joints and produce an arthritis.

The cost in terms of deaths, non-productive crippled sheep, drug treatments and labour can be substantially more than that of discarding a bath-full of dip and starting with fresh for each new day.

HUMAN INFECTION RISK   It should be mentioned that if an outbreak has occurred, any dip solution remaining in the bath and any sludge left after draining the bath will be heavily contaminated with bacteria, and the bath should be thoroughly cleaned out and rinsed. Care should be taken by shepherds handling any of this material, since the erysipelas bacteria can infect humans. This normally occurs on the hands or arms. An area of skin becomes very itchy, swollen, hot and painful and eventually turns purple with death of the tissues involved—this is called an **erysipeloid** (see Colour plate 52). The local glands (lymph nodes) become swollen and in some cases arthritis of the joints in the hand or wrist may occur. Prompt medical treatment is essential.

POUR-ONS AND SPOT-ONS

Pour-ons and spot-ons are now available with the advent of a new group of parasiticides, the **synthetic pyrethroids**. These compounds are applied in small quantities as a concentrated liquid at a particular spot, such as the head for headfly control, or in a stripe down the back for tick control. They act by being slowly carried across the surface of the skin in the sebum—a greasy secretion of glands in the skin. Cypermethrin, for example, combines with the sebum and is therefore less likely to be washed out by rain. Neither is it absorbed into the body and so, providing it is applied to milking sheep immediately after milking, the milk from the following milking will not need to be discarded. Always read the manufacturer's instructions on withdrawal periods, however, as individual products differ.

The pour-on and spot-on type products are quick and easy to apply and generally have a long residual effect. They are suitable for the treatment of lice, ticks and headfly, but as yet none is approved for sheep scab control. Neither are they sufficiently effective for controlling blowfly strike.

This method of application is particularly suitable for treating pregnant ewes for the control of lice prior to housing in mid to late pregnancy when dipping could predispose to pregnancy toxaemia. Mismothering can be a problem when dipping lambs for tick control in spring, and pour-on products are a useful and efficient alternative with a good residual action. The liquid should be poured on the top of the lamb's head and along its back, but avoiding the tailhead, since this could confuse ewes, which sniff this area as a means of identifying their lambs.

The synthetic pyrethroids in spot-on form are being used in other parts of the world, such as Australia, in automated systems which identify sheep with an electronic 'eye' as they run through a race and 'spot' them as they pass. These systems can treat at the rate of 2,500 sheep per hour.

561

RESISTANCE

Resistance to parasiticides is a growing problem in certain countries of the world, particularly where sheep or cattle have to be dipped very frequently—sometimes every few days. To date in the UK, however, there have been very few instances of resistance to either the organophosphorus compounds or the synthetic pyrethroids. Resistance to a product is more likely to occur with frequent use, and particularly if the concentration is not high enough to kill all parasites. Those surviving parasites tend to produce offspring more likely to develop resistance.

QUICK REFERENCE CHART

Important skin parasites of sheep in the UK

Disease/parasite	Main symptoms	Season/conditions	Control
Tick (*Ixodes ricinus*)	Occasionally tick-worry (lambs). Tickborne diseases (louping ill, tickborne fever and tick pyaemia) are the main risks.	Spring (all areas) and autumn (western Britain).	Dips, pour-ons, sprays. Land improvement.
Blowfly strike (myiasis) (e.g. *Lucilia sericata* – greenbottle)	Stop feeding, agitated, rubbing, lip-smacking, seeking cover, foul-smelling wound with maggots, loss of condition, death in severe cases.	Summer (fly season), especially in hot, humid weather.	Dipping or spraying just before risk period. Worm and scour control, crutching and dagging.
Headfly (broken-head) (*Hydrotaea irritans*)	Especially horned breeds. Irritation leads to self-inflicted damage (broken-heads), further fly damage, large wounds around base of horn. Blowfly strike may occur.	Summer (fly season), especially in woodland areas in northern England and central and southern Scotland.	Pour-ons, spot-ons or impregnated tags before risk period.
Sheep scab (mite) (*Psoroptes ovis*)	Severe irritation, rubbing, nibbling. Loss of body condition. Affects especially shoulders, chest, flanks. Matted, moist, scabby wounds with wool loss.	All year round – most noticeable in winter.	NOTIFIABLE DISEASE. At present, compulsory single dipping is required by law using scab-approved dip.
Lice (pediculosis) (*damalinia*, biting lice; *linognathus*, sucking lice)	Loss of fleece through rubbing and nibbling due to irritation. Loss of condition in heavy infestations.	All year round – most noticeable in winter and especially in housed sheep.	Dipping, pour-ons and spot-ons.
Ked (*Melophagus ovinus*)	Irritation and spoiling of the fleece.	All year round – especially noticeable in winter.	Dipping, spraying, etc.

14

MISCELLANEOUS SKIN, EYE AND GUM CONDITIONS

Mycotic Dermatitis

Mycotic dermatitis or lumpy wool disease is an extremely common bacterial condition of the skin and fleece of sheep in the UK. It is, in most cases, a mild condition which is often missed or ignored by farmers. Nevertheless, it causes damage and downgrading of the fleece and therefore represents a loss of income.

The bacterium responsible is called *Dermatophilus congolensis*, and it causes infections in many other species besides sheep, including man. The disease may spread directly from sheep to sheep or from cattle to sheep, or indirectly from rubbing against infected woodwork or other contaminated objects. It is possible that insects may play a part in its spread also.

CLINICAL SIGNS

Whilst infections may be present at any time of year, the bacteria are most active in wet conditions when the fleece is saturated and the skin is denatured and less able to resist invasion. The bacteria cause an inflammation of the skin, and the blood serum which oozes into the fleece dries and forms yellow-brown crusts, most obvious at shearing. Because the disease in the UK usually causes little itchiness or discomfort to sheep, it may be noticed only at clipping, even though a large proportion of the flock is infected. Several layers of crustiness may be seen in the fleece, indicating repeated infections, often in short succession. (See Colour plate 55.)

The infection affects both the woolly and hairy areas of the body. In adult sheep it is usually found along the back and sides of the body and around the neck, that is, in woolly areas. In rams it may be seen on the scrotum if it is covered in wool. In lambs it most commonly occurs on the hair-covered areas of the head, particularly on the nose and ears and on the lower limbs around the top of the hoof. It should be noted that the orf virus is frequently found in these affected areas along with the dermatophilus bacteria, and care should be taken in handling cases since both organisms, particularly orf, may cause infections in humans.

565

The infections above the hoof in lambs often become very swollen and painful and bleed when damaged. Because of the appearance, this is referred to as **strawberry footrot**, which is discussed more fully in the chapter on lameness and also in the section on orf. In some of the more serious cases the wool becomes very moist and matted over the affected area and this may attract blowflies and lead to maggot strike.

Other bacteria of the same group (dermatophilus) may cause green or yellow staining of the fleece, as in **canary stain** which downgrades the wool. The inclusion of bacteriostats in dips may prevent this type of infection, which is sometimes referred to as **wool** or **fleece rot.**

CONTROL

Eradication of this infection in a flock is not possible because of the widespread nature of the bacteria in both sheep and other species. Control is based on the use of **mycotic dips**—which may be necessary on an annual basis on some farms. These usually contain the salts of zinc or aluminium which immobilise the spores of the bacteria. The dipping may need to be repeated in six or eight weeks for adult sheep, but this is rarely necessary in lambs. In small flocks, the fleeces can be treated with powdered alum, but this is laborious and impractical in large flocks.

Individual animals which are badly affected should have the fleece clipped away from the affected area and powdered alum applied. Your veterinary surgeon may recommend an injection of penicillin and streptomycin for serious cases.

Ringworm

Ringworm is an uncommon disease in sheep and is usually caused by a fungus called *Trichophyton verrucosum*. It is thought to occur through contact with cattle or, more likely, indirectly from troughs, posts and pen divisions infected with spores from infected cattle or other species. The infection does not normally 'take' well in healthy sheep. It also clears up more quickly than in cattle, suggesting that the sheep is not a natural host for the disease. Sheep in poor body condition or suffering from some other debilitating condition are likely to be more seriously affected, as is often the case with skin conditions.

The disease is important nevertheless, since the scabby, crusty areas on the ears, face and along the back are similar to sheep scab and should always be thoroughly investigated to rule out this possibility. Affected animals should be kept apart from the flock until the infection has disappeared of its own accord—usually after a month or six weeks—or after treatment with griseofulvin, **which should not, however, be used in pregnant ewes**. Remember, too, that ringworm can be transmitted to humans

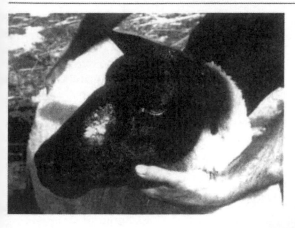

Plate 14.1   The crusty white lesions forward of the eye in the Suffolk ewe (*left*) and ram (*below*) and also on the poll of the ram are ringworm.

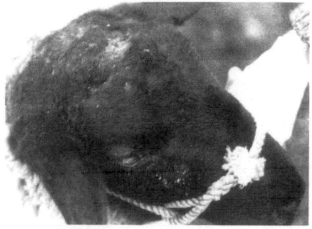

from animals and can cause disfiguring scars, especially in children. (See Colour plate 53.)

Facial Dermatitis

This disease, otherwise known as **staphylococcal dermatitis,** or **facial** or **periorbital eczema**, is an increasingly common condition of sheep in the UK. (See Colour plate 64).

It is caused by a very common bacterium, *Staphylococcus aureus*, which causes a number of large abscesses on the face. These are commonly found around the eye, but also on the forehead and on the poll around the base of the horns, especially if there has been any damage through fighting.

567

Large areas of the head can be involved and when up to half the ewe flock is infected, as sometimes occurs, it can be a most startling and distressing sight.

An outbreak can continue for several months and, despite treatment, individual animals heal only slowly and are left with unsightly scars. Severely affected animals may be depressed and lose some body condition, but the majority appear surprisingly little affected considering the extent of the damage. Occasionally, however, the eye itself may become involved, which can lead to a permanent loss of sight or even the loss or surgical removal of the eyeball in especially bad cases, but fortunately this is rare.

TREATMENT AND PREVENTION

Treatment of individual sheep consists of the injection of long-acting antibiotics, which shorten the course of the disease, so hopefully reducing the spread within the flock.

The disease occurs principally in trough fed sheep so that ewes being fed concentrates in late pregnancy, store lambs or fattening hoggs are most commonly affected. Outbreaks are usually most severe when inadequate trough space is available. A particularly severe outbreak occurred in a flock which was winter sheared to allow for an increase in stocking rate in the sheep house. Totally inadequate trough space led to jostling and fighting amongst ewes when concentrate rations were fed, and this caused damage to the ewes' faces, which became infected. The disease spread alarmingly through the majority of the flock. When such an outbreak occurs, it is helpful to segregate affected sheep from the rest of the flock. Trough space should thereby be increased automatically for the ewes remaining and this combination should limit the spread of the disease.

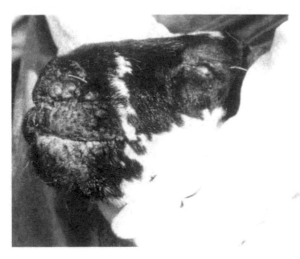

Plate 14.2
A staphylococcal infection of the muzzle.

Photosensitisation

This condition, which is sometimes known as **yellowses**, is primarily a condition of young sheep. It is caused by the action of sunlight on the skin when certain photodynamic chemicals are present in the bloodstream. These are able to absorb more energy from the sun's rays than is normal, and this causes damage to the skin. The effects are most noticeable on non-woolly areas of white skin. In breeds such as the Scottish Blackface there is often a clear line of demarcation between the unaffected black skin and the photosensitised white skin. The condition arises in late spring and early summer when lambs start to take in appreciable amounts of herbage, some of which contains substances which are photodynamic. For example, St John's wort, which is common on many moorland pastures worldwide, contains the photodynamic substance hyperacin.

Photosensitisation may occur indirectly, because some plant poisons, fungal toxins and certain drugs (used as treatments for other ailments) cause liver damage. This interferes with the excretion of photodynamic substances present in the body, which are normally rendered harmless by the liver. The most common of these is **phylloerythrin**, which is present in the blood of all herbivores since it is produced from the breakdown of chlorophyll, the green pigment found in grass and all green plants.

One of New Zealand's most important sheep diseases—facial eczema— is caused in this way by a fungal toxin which proliferates in pasture litter. Whilst deaths are uncommon, outbreaks of the disease cause severe production losses through reductions in wool growth and growth rates and from poor reproductive performance. A similar condition has been reported from the United States, parts of South America and occasionally the UK.

SYMPTOMS

Regardless of the reason for these harmful substances circulating in the blood, the symptoms are similar. The head region is most commonly affected in sheep, especially the thin, unprotected skin of the ears, eyelids and lips, and any painful swelling can be made worse by the animal rubbing itself in an attempt to alleviate the discomfort. The damage causes oozing of fluid from the skin which dries to form a yellowish crusty scab. The skin dries out and cracks like parchment. Dead skin may drop off, and this can lead to the loss of part of the ear in some lambs. Secondary infection by bacteria or even blowfly strike may occur in some cases.

Symptoms can begin within only a few hours of exposure to direct sunlight, which need not be intense. Animals may become quite distressed, cease grazing and seek shelter. Occasionally they may be temporarily blinded and cases have been recorded of lambs stumbling and drowning in water courses as a result. Most affected lambs fail to thrive for many weeks as a result of the poisoning, especially those in which the liver damage is

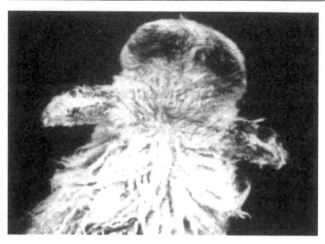

Plate 14.3
'Yellowses' or
photosensitisation in a
lamb. Note the
crustiness of the
ears—parts of which
may drop off in some
cases.

severe enough to result in jaundice. The condition generally occurs in individual animals, although there may be minor outbreaks involving a number of animals over a short period. Except where the problem arises each year—as it may do on hill farms in association with St John's wort—it is often difficult or impossible to identify the offending plant or toxin. Indeed, many of the causative agents have never been identified.

TREATMENT AND PREVENTION

Bearing in mind that the condition is most common in hill flocks in the UK, treatment presents some problems. Affected animals should be brought indoors out of the sun to minimise the damage. Moving the flock to shelter from the sun—for example, adjacent to woodland—may increase the risk of blowfly or headfly worry.

In badly affected cases your veterinary surgeon may prescribe drugs to alleviate the discomfort and antibiotics can be given by injection to minimise the risk of secondary bacterial infection. Pour-on insecticides—**not** directly on the wounds—will protect against maggot strike. Some insecticides are available in creams which can be applied to the damaged skin to prevent drying and cracking.

In lowland flocks where grazing of a particular paddock is unavoidable, housing during the day with grazing at night has been used until the main period of risk is over (by July). In affected Scottish Blackface hill flocks, it has been suggested that ewe lambs to be retained for the breeding flock should be selected with predominantly black faces. This would also apply when purchasing rams. Susceptibility to facial eczema is a heritable trait, and flockmasters in New Zealand are having some success in breeding animals which are more resistant to the disease.

Orf

Orf, or **contagious pustular dermatitis,** is a painful, unsightly and disfiguring disease of sheep (and goats) which causes much distress to affected ewes and lambs. It is also a cause of considerable economic loss to the farmer through occasional deaths, ill thrift and from the costs incurred in the treatment of individual cases and in flock preventive measures.

The disease is caused by a virus which grows in the surface layers of the skin and in the mucous membrane of the mouth, nose and elsewhere. Non-woolly areas of the skin are primarily affected. The virus penetrates through small abrasions in the skin, such as are caused by nosing amongst thistles, brambles and hedgerows or against troughs or feeders. Even very minor damage to skin may allow the virus to enter.

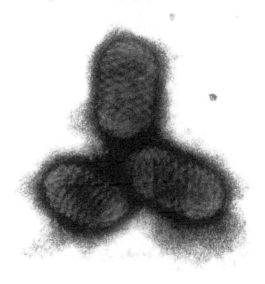

Plate 14.4   The orf virus magnified 50,000 times by the transmission electron microscope.

CLINICAL SIGNS

Once in the skin, the virus multiplies and causes small spots and pustules which rapidly increase in size and merge together. These become damaged, bleed and scab over, often forming wart-like clusters which may hang like a bunch of grapes in the most severe cases. (See Colour plate 58.) These orf wounds frequently become secondarily infected by bacteria, sometimes with serious consequences. Occasionally, the wounds may attract blowflies with resultant maggot strike.

571

Lambs and young sheep are especially susceptible, but ewes are fre quently affected on the udder and teats (see Colour plate 59). Occasionall orf may cause a genital infection on the vulva of ewes and on the sheat of rams. The sores may make the rams reluctant to work and delay mating so extending the lambing period.

Whilst the disease may occur at any time of year, there are two peaks o infection, the first in young sucking lambs and their ewes and the secon in older lambs in the late summer.

In ewes and lambs

Sucking lambs become affected on the face, particularly on the lips an around the nostrils. Serious outbreaks may occur in artificially fed lamb because of the shared teats on automatic feeders. Orf may produce lesion inside the mouth, on the tongue, in the throat and occasionally it ma extend down into the oesophagus and stomach or, rarely, even into th lungs (see Colour plate 60). Ewes pick up the infection on the udder from their infected lambs as they suck. Lesions frequently become secondaril infected with bacteria, which may lead to serious mastitis with loss of th affected half and subsequent culling of the ewe. Deaths occur from case of mastitis which began as orf infections.

These orf lesions are painful to both ewes and lambs. Lambs with sor mouths are disinclined to suck and ewes with sore teats may not allow thei lambs to feed. The consequence is that many lambs become hungry and ma attempt to feed from other ewes, so spreading the infection further. Unles alternative feeding arrangements are made, some of these lambs may suffe a severe setback. Lambs undernourished in this way are more prone to othe diseases such as pneumonia, and deaths may occur from these secondary infections.

In weaned lambs

In older, weaned lambs the problem often starts on the lower parts o the limbs or feet. Lambs grazing late season, stemmy grass, undersow stubbles or root crops may scratch their legs and feet on the sharp plan stems and this is sufficient to allow the virus to get into the skin an multiply. The lips and nose may also become infected because of lamb nibbling at their affected limbs. Dry weather often precipitates an outbreak.

The infection on the limbs may become damaged and bleed. This i often referred to as **strawberry footrot** because of its appearance. (There i some confusion as to whether this condition is due to orf virus or begins a lumpy wool disease caused by the bacterium *Dermatophilus congolensis* Both microorganisms may be identified in these leg lesions, but it is unclea which initiates the damage.) Lambs should be growing fast at this time and orf infection may seriously interfere with feed intake and lead to a setback in growth rate with consequential economic loss. (See Colour plate 61.)

TREATMENT

Treatment of orf is particularly unrewarding since, being a virus disease, it is not susceptible to antibiotics. A number of proprietary products claim to be able to effect a cure, but there is no evidence to support these claims. Within a few weeks the disease will clear up on its own and all that can reasonably be done is to aim to reduce the risk of secondary bacterial infection with the use of topical antibiotic creams, powders or aerosols. In serious cases antibiotics may be necessary by injection.

Treatment of individuals is very time-consuming and, in large flocks with a high proportion of lambs infected, may be reserved for the worst cases. Separation of affected lambs may reduce the rate of spread, but early cases will be missed and the outbreak will continue and may even be prolonged. In smaller flocks, separation of orf cases for treatment makes good sense.

If the scabs are so bad that they interfere with feeding, affected lambs should be fed artificially to tide them over until the infection heals. Baby lambs can be fed milk by stomach tube.

Ewes which are affected on the teats or udder should receive special attention, since bacterial infection can lead to serious mastitis and even the death of the ewe. In the worst cases the lambs should be removed from their mothers and fed artificially. (They should **not** be fostered onto a 'clean' ewe, since she may become infected.) Intramammary antibiotics can be used to try to prevent mastitis. If mastitis has already occurred, antibiotics by injection will be necessary. In many of these cases the half will be lost and it will be a matter of saving the ewe to sell her as a cull once she has fully recovered.

PREVENTION AND CONTROL

In order to prevent or control orf it is necessary to know something of the way the disease is spread. The virus is a fairly tough one. Under the correct conditions it can survive for months or possibly years away from the sheep. Virus stored on the roof of Moredun Research Institute in Edinburgh overwinter survived for six months in scabs from orf lesions, provided a cover prevented rain from soaking the scabs. Even after a harsh Scottish winter with temperatures below minus 7°C, the virus recovered from the scabs was still capable of causing infection. The virus in scabs unprotected from the rain did not survive.

It is unlikely, therefore, that scabs dropping from affected sheep onto pasture would survive to infect lambs the following spring or summer. However, the virus is very likely to remain viable for considerable periods in scabs which have dropped off infected housed sheep. It will also survive on troughs, pen divisions and walls where lambs have rubbed their infected faces. In this way the infection can survive from year to year.

Another important and largely unrecognised method by which orf virus may be perpetuated within a flock, or introduced into a flock, is

573

through a chronic form of the disease. In some animals—for example, in some fine skinned rams—dry, crusty growths appear on the poll or on the face, especially where they have damaged their heads by fighting. These growths may persist for many months or they may die back for a period and then reappear. Orf virus capable of producing typical infections has been isolated from a number of these cases. Many of these growths probably go unrecognised as orf, but they may represent an important reservoir of infection. (See Colour plate 62.)

Prevention of orf presents the farmer and his vet with some very difficult decisions. In flocks where the disease has never been identified, every effort should be made to keep infection out by maintaining a closed flock. If animals have to be bought in, it is important to examine them carefully for any evidence of the disease and to enquire of the vendor whether there is any history of disease in the flock. Never knowingly purchase affected animals, or apparently unaffected sheep from a known infected flock, especially when your own flock is free from infection.

Vaccination

It is most important to appreciate that **orf vaccine should not be used in any flock where the disease has never been known to occur**. The reason for this is that the only vaccine available is made from live virus isolated from the ground-up scabs of 'modified' orf infections. The virus is treated in such a way as to prevent it from causing serious disease, but allowing it to produce a mild form of orf. This mild form of the disease should confer sufficient short-term immunity to help the vaccinated sheep resist the worst ravages of a natural infection. The vaccine does not prevent sheep becoming infected with the natural virus, but it should reduce the degree of damage and shorten the course of the infection, both in individual animals and also in the flock as a whole.

Unfortunately, the vaccine presently available does not produce a strong and long-lasting immunity, probably because the natural disease does not produce a good immunity either. Lambs affected with orf can become affected again as gimmers, or as ewes suckling lambs.

Neither the vaccine nor the natural infection stimulates the production of high levels of protective antibodies against orf in the colostrum of ewes. It is possible, however, that antibodies present in colostrum and milk may inhibit the formation of orf lesions around the mouth where the milk comes directly into contact with the skin. This local effect could only be expected to give partial protection to baby lambs and for only a short time. The low level of antibody in milk will decline quite rapidly, leaving lambs totally vulnerable once more.

Where an outbreak of orf has occurred in a flock and it is possible to isolate affected lambs, the vaccine can be used on the lambs not as yet affected. This may reduce the severity of any new cases and it may also shorten the course of infection in a flock. However, if the disease is already well established, this approach may not work. Where the disease has proved a problem in previous years and is likely to occur again, as in flocks housed over lambing, for example, vaccination may be considered. Ewes can be scarified some two months before lambing. This allows the scab which should form at the site of vaccination to develop and drop off before the lambs are born. It is strongly recommended that **vaccinated ewes be moved to a fresh area to lamb**, so that the lambs will have no contact with the infectious scabs which fall off. If this is not possible, liberal straw bedding should be provided in an attempt to bury the scabs.

Ewes are best vaccinated on the smooth, clean skin inside the elbow, between the fore leg and chest wall. The groin should not be used, because if scabs have not dropped off before the lambs are born, they may become infected when they go in to find a teat to suck. If the skin under the tail is used, scabs may become infected from soiling with faeces.

Newborn lambs, having little or no protection from colostrum, may be vaccinated if the risk of infection is considered to be high from the experience of previous years. It is important to point out that vaccinated lambs may sometimes spread the vaccine-type orf to the udders of their dams when sucking. Some veterinary surgeons may therefore advise the use of the vaccine only in the case of an outbreak. As already noted, artificially fed lambs are often badly affected, especially if they are reared in the same pens year after year and if disinfection of pens and feeders is inadequate. These lambs often share a common automatic feeder and constantly swap teats, so that every lamb in the group can become affected. Stockworkers attending to such lambs should take care not to spread infection from pen to pen, either on their hands or boots or on shared utensils. These lambs also present a high risk of human infection because of the close attention they receive.

Purchased sheep which are to join an infected flock may be vaccinated since there is a high risk of infection, especially if they are from an unaffected flock.

Rams and ewes with infections of the penis or vulva thought to be due to the orf virus should **not** be vaccinated. If infections of this type have occurred previously, rams should be checked at a pre-mating examination and not be used if infection is suspected. If the condition occurs during mating, an attempt can be made to identify affected sheep and isolate them. However, this is not always successful.

Vaccination should, if possible, be carried out some two months before the expected period of risk. As mentioned earlier, the vaccine is made from living modified orf virus and is presented in vials with a scratching attachment with which to scarify or abrade the skin. This allows the virus to get into the skin where it multiplies and produces a mild form of the disease. The task should be done hygienically, but **on no account should the skin be swabbed with spirit or disinfectant before vaccination**, as this would destroy the virus and hence prevent the vaccine from 'taking'. Follow the manufacturer's instructions to the letter and always use fresh vaccine which has been stored appropriately. Protective gloves should be worn when administering the vaccine, as the live virus is infectious to humans.

A vaccination scab normally forms within a week of vaccination and it is as well to check a number of sheep from the group to see that they have 'taken'. If a fair proportion have not done so, then the whole flock should be checked and all those which have not responded should be revaccinated with a fresh batch of vaccine.

The vaccine, being a living virus, has a very short life of around 10 days. It is important to place orders with your veterinary surgeon in good time, as the vaccine has to be specially ordered and will have to be used on the first suitable opportunity after delivery. Never use out-of-date vaccine or vials which have been part used on a previous occasion, even though they may still be in date. The scab normally drops off within a month of vaccination and reasonable protection should persist for some months. Remember that vaccine may not always prevent sheep from becoming infected, but it may reduce the severity and duration of the disease.

Freshly vaccinated or naturally infected sheep with active lesions and scabs should not be marketed or sold directly to another farm, as this will spread the disease to other flocks.

Disinfection

Disinfection of premises where outbreaks have occurred is important. The virus is susceptible to many disinfectants, but the house or pens must be very thoroughly cleaned beforehand to remove all dung; otherwise many of the disinfectants will be rendered useless. Woodwork should receive special attention. Jeyes fluid is effective in a reasonably strong solution, as is dairy hypochlorite, but the latter does not work if any straw or dung is present. Iodophores and formaldehyde are effective, but are expensive and hazardous respectively. **These products should never be used on animals.**

Human infection

Orf is a zoonosis, that is, it can be spread from animals to humans. The virus causes a painful sore, usually on the hands, arms or face, which may take many weeks to heal (see Colour plate 54). Most cases in humans are uncomplicated, but a small proportion of patients have a very painful arm and may be quite ill. Very occasionally a patient may require a spell in hospital. The condition can be unpleasant in children, and they should never be allowed to handle affected lambs.

Both the natural infection and the vaccine can affect humans. Rubber gloves should be worn when administering the vaccine or when handling infected lambs or contaminated equipment such as automatic feeders. Hands should be washed **immediately** after handling affected animals, but the nailbrush should **not** be used, to avoid damaging the skin. A suitably mild disinfectant for use on the hands can be applied after washing. Smokers and nail biters should take extra care not to infect themselves around the mouth.

'Cruels'

'Cruels' is caused by the same bacterium (*Actinobacillus lignieresii*) that is responsible for wooden tongue in cattle. The organism is found on the skin and in the gut of normal healthy animals and is also present in soil and dung. It rarely causes problems, but will invade wounds or abrasions of the skin. It most commonly affects rams which have been fighting, producing large, unpleasant abscesses full of thick, plastic, greenish pus (see Colour plate 65).

The abscesses usually form on the head and face, including the lips and cheeks. They may 'track' through the soft tissues and discharge to the surface, further contaminating the skin and infecting other minor wounds. Occasionally, abscesses may also form in the lungs and the lymphatic glands which drain lymph from infected areas. Animals eventually die if they are not treated satisfactorily.

Treatment consists of antibiotic injections (e.g. dihydostreptomycin) twice daily for several days. Sometimes your veterinary surgeon may have to drain the larger abscesses. Little can be done to prevent the disease, but if rams have been fighting, wounds should be cleaned up and dressed with a suitable antibiotic ointment or powder.

Sheep Pox

This is a notifiable disease—indeed, the first disease ever to be made notifiable in the UK. It was eradicated in 1866 and although it is unlikely to occur again it is theoretically possible since it is widespread in many areas of the world. As the name implies, the disease is caused by a pox virus, related to the viruses causing mild diseases such as chicken pox in man or cow pox in cattle and severe diseases, such as smallpox in man, now fortunately eradicated worldwide.

Sheep pox is a very contagious, severe and frequently fatal disease, which may affect sheep of any age but which is most severe in lambs and young sheep. Affected animals run a high fever 41.5°C (107°F) and become weak and depressed. They have difficulty in breathing and may have a discharge from the nose and eyes. Raised circular lesions may be found on the face or all over the body in the most severe cases. These ooze serum and eventually scab over and leave a scar. It is unlikely to be confused with other skin conditions, such as orf, because the animals are so very ill and the death rate is very high.

Any suspicion of the disease by the owner or person looking after the sheep must be reported to the police or to the Divisional Veterinary Officer, MAFF (see Appendix 5).

Pinkeye

Pinkeye, otherwise known as heather or snow blindness, is an infectious and contagious disease of sheep. It may occur at any time of year and in sheep of any age. It is caused by any one of a number of different micro-organisms and its proper name is **ovine keratoconjunctivitis**. The micro-organisms most commonly associated with pinkeye are *Chlamydia psittaci ovis* (the same organism which causes enzootic abortion in ewes) and *Mycoplasma conjunctivae*.

The disease tends to occur as an outbreak in a flock, with the majority of animals becoming affected. Spread occurs by direct contact, and consequently pinkeye is most common under intensive conditions with high stocking rates and especially with housed sheep. Close contact at feeding—especially if inadequate trough space is provided, so that sheep rub against each other's faces—is thought to be the most important method of spread. It is often a serious cause of loss in feedlot lambs in the United States and elsewhere, where very large numbers of lambs share the same building, especially if they are overcrowded and the ventilation is poor. Whilst it is possible that flies or other insects may transfer the disease from sheep to sheep (in the same way they spread New Forest eye in cattle), this has not yet been proved.

Infection may be brought into a flock via purchased sheep in the first instance, but in many affected flocks the organisms persist in carrier animals, so perpetuating the infection from year to year. Clean sheep brought into an already infected flock are very likely to become infected.

CLINICAL SIGNS

Whichever microorganism is responsible, the symptoms are similar. Affected animals blink repeatedly and have an aversion to bright sunlight, and tears stain the face. A closer examination shows the membranes of the eye are red and inflamed—pinkeye—and the condition is obviously painful. In most cases these relatively mild symptoms progress no further and the majority clear up, with or without treatment, in a week to 10 days. If both eyes are affected at different stages of the disease, recovery may take a little longer. (See Colour plate 66.)

Occasionally, however, a few cases progress to a more serious stage, with a thick discharge and some damage to the surface of the eye which may lead to partial, although usually temporary, blindness. These more serious cases may persist for several weeks despite treatment, but the majority recover full vision. Pinkeye tends to spread most rapidly in young susceptible sheep but the more serious cases are generally found in adult animals. (See Colour plate 67.)

TREATMENT

Treatment is a tedious and expensive business if all affected animals are to be dealt with, so that often only the most severely affected ones are treated. It is necessary to apply an appropriate antibiotic, such as tetracycline, or some other drug, such as ethidium bromide, once daily for three or four days. Ointments are preferable to powders, since the latter may be more irritant to an already inflamed eye. Your veterinary surgeon should advise initially on the most suitable treatment under the particular circumstances of your flock and may decide to administer antibiotics by injection under the conjunctiva of the eye, to reduce the number of treatments and therefore gatherings. (This method should never be attempted by lay persons.)

Serious cases should be drawn out of the flock and made comfortable in a clean, airy box or in a paddock close to the steading, so they can be attended to more frequently. Some may be partially or totally blind and not able to find the trough or hayrack and may lose considerable body condition as a consequence. If this occurs to ewes in the later stages of pregnancy it may predispose them to twin lamb disease, with serious consequences.

A proportion of animals, although apparently normal, will harbour the microorganisms responsible for pinkeye and become carriers. Since the immunity to these infections is generally poor, further outbreaks may be seen in the same group of sheep within weeks or months and may recur repeatedly in the flock over a number of years.

CONTROL AND PREVENTION

Control and prevention depend upon reducing the risk of spread, since it is unrealistic to attempt to eradicate the disease in view of the carrier state

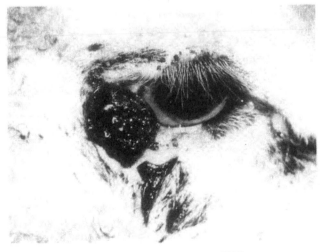

Plate 14.5   An eyelid tumour on a young sheep.

of some sheep and the wide distribution of many of the microorganisms thought to be responsible.

Overcrowding should be avoided, especially in housed sheep. Adequate trough space should be provided to reduce the risk of direct contact spreading infection at feeding times. Purchased sheep should be kept apart from the main flock for a quarantine period, and if there is a risk to them from the home flock, they can be treated with an ointment to try to prevent infection. Sooner or later, however, they are likely to become infected.

Whilst pinkeye is not a spectacular disease it can—like New Forest eye in cattle—be a niggling source of financial loss to the farmer and a painful irritation to the sheep. Losses are due to reduced weight gain in lambs or hoggs, early foetal loss in ewes, occasional deaths (e.g. from pregnancy toxaemia) and the not inconsiderable expense of treatment, of which labour costs are the major component.

Broken Mouth

Broken mouth is the name given to a bacterial infection of the gums (gingivitis) which, over a period of months or years, leads to the loss of incisor (lower front) teeth. It is a very common condition, with more than two-thirds of all ewes slaughtered showing some degree of it. In the UK it is probably the most important reason for culling sheep before the end of their productive life. Indeed, some farmers of hill and upland farms affected by this disease feel obliged to cull ewes after only two or three lamb crops, as they consider affected ewes to be less able to cope with the tough grazing conditions.

The disease is less of a problem on lowland farms, inasmuch as the grazing conditions are easier. Therefore, affected ewes are better able to maintain an acceptable body condition, possibly by grazing for longer than full mouthed sheep or by putting on extra condition at times of year when grazing is not a limiting factor. Some hill farmers, who have adequate in-bye fields or improved grazings, faced with the considerable replacement costs and the significantly lower price obtained for broken mouthed cull ewes, are keeping affected ewes on and feeding them preferentially on the lower pastures. This has been shown to be cost-effective on some farms, but a proportion of ewes carrying twins still tend to produce lighter, more vulnerable lambs.

Although broken mouth is very common, occurring in all areas of the UK and in most other sheep producing countries of the world, not all farms are affected. Those that do experience the disease may suffer very differing levels of infection. On some farms only one ewe in twenty is affected, whilst on others it may be as many as two out of every three. The disease most commonly affects ewes three years of age or older, although the infection which is responsible for the tooth loss may have been established long before this age. Recent investigations have suggested that one particular group of bacteria may be present in broken mouth flocks, but this work is at an early stage.

Probably every shepherd, farmer and veterinary surgeon has his or her own theory as to the reason for broken mouth. However, the factors which make individual sheep or flocks more or less susceptible to broken mouth remain unknown.

CLINICAL SIGNS

All sheep have a mixed population of bacteria affecting the gums. In broken mouth flocks the gums of affected sheep become swollen and red and often bleed. As the infection worsens, pus may form in the gap between the gums and the teeth. Gradually, over a period of months or years, the gums recede, so that the tooth crown (the portion showing above the gums) appears longer, giving a peg-like appearance. The bacteria eventually creep down to infect and destroy the strong ligament which attaches the tooth to the jaw. Bacteria may also infect the jaw bone itself. This process gradually loosens the teeth in their sockets so that they eventually fall out. The teeth will be lost more rapidly if sheep graze hard foods, such as feed blocks or swedes, but it must be stressed that these foods are not responsible for causing broken mouth initially. The speed of tooth loss varies greatly, from around one year to three years. The period also differs widely from farm to farm. (See Colour plates 68 to 70.)

TREATMENT AND PREVENTION

There is no treatment for broken mouth. Flockowners can attempt to prolong the active life of ewes by avoiding circumstances which it is thought hasten the loss of teeth once the disease has loosened them in their sockets. Therefore, older hill ewes can be brought down to easier territory where grazing is more available and softer on the mouth. Roots and feed blocks can be avoided.

Any management changes made in an attempt to prevent the disease have failed. It is unlikely that such changes would have much effect in the short term, because of the long-term nature of broken mouth. Even if the causal factors are eventually established, it is likely that an avoiding strategy of many years would be necessary to make any impact.

Splints

Meanwhile, efforts have been made to prolong the useful life of ewes in broken mouthed flocks by splinting the teeth of sheep considered at risk, using stainless steel bands which fit over the full set of teeth, or what remains of them. The idea is to apply the splints to three and four year old ewes before tooth loss occurs, so that there is a good anchorage for the splint and the dental cement which holds it in place. The improved models work satisfactorily and most remain in place for one or more years. However,

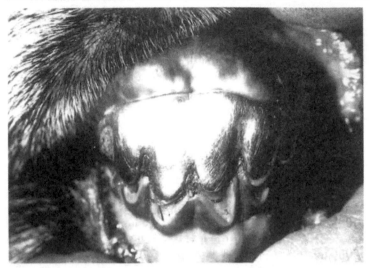

Plate 14.6   An early prototype ewe tooth splint (*above*) and a later model (*below*). Splints are applied around all remaining incisors. Note the gum erosion and swelling in both these cases.

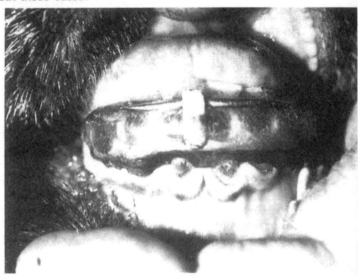

the technique has had only limited uptake, probably because it is fairly costly and the economics appear difficult to justify. (See Plate 14.6.)

Tooth grinding and trimming

More recently, a new approach, originating in Australia, has been used on a number of farms in the UK. The theory is that shortening the length of the incisor teeth will reduce or delay tooth loss and thereby prolong the useful life of the sheep. Two methods have been employed, one of which is merely a less severe form of the other.

So-called tooth grinding—the more severe Australian technique—consists of shearing off the entire crown of the incisor teeth to the level of the gums, using an electric grinder running at 11,000 rpm. A special gag is used to protect the tongue, lips and cheeks during cutting. It is claimed that if the procedure is used on three or four year old ewes, it will improve bite, 'firm up' the teeth, reduce grazing time by increasing the efficiency of biting, prolong the active life of ewes and improve performance overall. However, these claims have been made in the absence of any objective research. Work at the Animal and Grassland Research Institute some years ago showed that in the first 24 hours following tooth grinding, animals grazed for 30% less time than sheep which were not subjected to the procedure; that five days later the treated sheep spent the same time grazing as they did before treatment, but that their biting rate was still reduced that treated sheep spent the same time as non-treated sheep in chewing and ruminating; and that they showed no significant differences in either body weight or tooth loss.

Australian workers who were concerned that the technique was being widely used without any evidence that it was of any benefit asked for moratorium until some objective assessment was made. Their research showed that there were no positive effects in terms of wool growth, lamb weaning percentage or lamb growth rate. They also showed that the

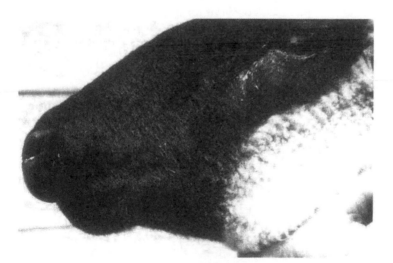

Plate 14.7 'Parrot mouth' in a Suffolk. The incisors will tend to close behind the dental pad. ('Sow mouth' occurs when the lower jaw extends beyond the upper jaw.)

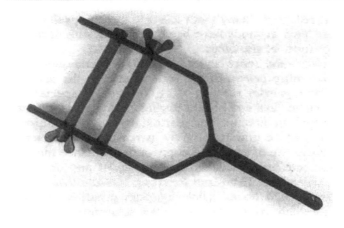

Plate 14.8 Mouth gag for sheep. This can be used to examine the mouth and cheek teeth.

procedure caused the sheep pain, but that the level of pain was no greater than for many other routine husbandry procedures. In the majority of sheep, the grinding exposed the tooth pulp (where the nerves and blood vessels lie) in one or more teeth. These workers concluded that because of the lack of any objectively demonstrated benefits—either to individual sheep or to flock productivity generally—it was difficult to justify inflicting the pain associated with the procedure.

The results from an investigation carried out on a Scottish hill farm suggested that this method may have been beneficial on that particular farm when used on ewes before any dental problems were apparent. The technique did not, however, prevent early tooth loss in ewes which already had incorrect mouths. Further work (under Home Office authority) will be necessary under a variety of husbandry situations before sufficient evidence can be collected to evaluate the method properly.

Bite correction

Bite correction is the term applied to a less severe trimming of the incisor teeth, using an electric grinder at 5,500 rpm, to give the crown of the incisor teeth an even and correctly angled surface in order to restore a correct bite. In this case the crowns are not reduced to gum level. No claims have been made of improved body condition or immediate increase in productivity, but it is postulated that it will improve longevity, although this has yet to be demonstrated.

The incisor pulp is a very sensitive structure, well supplied with nerves, and the pulp cavity comes very close to the tip of the tooth. In either of these techniques the pulp may be either exposed or damaged by the heat generated by the grinder disc. It is not surprising that the procedure is painful therefore, but we should not fall into the trap of assuming that sheep's teeth are necessarily the same as human teeth, because there are subtle differences. Reducing the length of the teeth may indeed delay tooth loss by reducing the turning forces applied during grazing. However, the claim that grinding actually 'firms up' the tooth in the socket is entirely unfounded and most unlikely. Damage from broken mouth infection is likely to proceed uninterrupted and tooth loss is likely to continue despite the use of either of these techniques.

There are also fears that, despite Australian findings to the contrary, exposure or damage to the pulp may lead to infection or other long-term problems. Research at the Moredun Institute is in progress on this aspect. Work is also in progress at a number of centres to evaluate the welfare aspects of these controversial techniques and to attempt to assess objectively the various claims which have been made.

In the meanwhile a number of organisations and societies, including the welfare lobby, have, quite reasonably, expressed the view that any technique which causes pain—however transient—should not be used unchecked on farms throughout the UK. The government, after consulting parties on both sides of the argument, have **banned both procedures** until the findings of the research become available. At the time of going to press, this ban is still in force. In the current welfare climate, it is unlikely that the severe Australian mutilation—for that is undoubtedly what it is—will ever be approved. However, should the research show that the less severe method of bite correction has long-term benefit in flocks affected by broken mouth and the welfare aspects are put into proper perspective, then the ban may be lifted. This milder technique may yet become an acceptable one in the hands of suitably trained personnel.

An argument put forward by some proponents of bite correction is that not to use the technique presents a welfare issue in itself. This is argued on

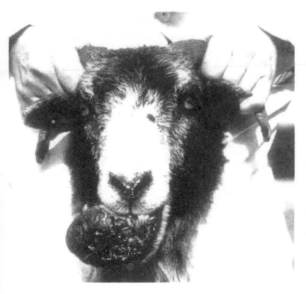

Plate 14.9 Osteosarcoma in an old ewe. Tumours are relatively rare in farm animals, partly because they do not have a long life. This distressing neglected case should never have been allowed to progress to this stage.

the grounds that sheep are being left to suffer the pain of broken mouth, when a technique is available to alleviate the problem. However, it is surely right and proper to thoroughly research the technique before advocating yet another painful routine husbandry procedure, only to discover later that the proposed benefits are unfounded.

CHEEK TEETH

Disease of the cheek teeth is relatively common although less often diagnosed because of the difficulty of examination. In some flocks the condition is as important as or more so than broken mouth (see Colour plate 71).

Sheep with abnormal cheek teeth cannot chew their food adequately and consequently may develop digestive upsets. This may predispose them to other conditions, such as twin lamb disease in late pregnancy, or it may mean that they give birth to small lambs and produce insufficient milk to feed them adequately.

The cheek teeth of thin sheep should be examined by feeling along the outside of the face for any hard bony tissue which should not be there, or for an abnormally smooth outline to the face which may indicate the presence of impacted food between the teeth and the cheek. Alternatively a gag may be used and a torch shone into the mouth. (Do not attempt to feel the cheek teeth since it is all too easy to lose a finger!) Affected sheep often have a foul breath (due to the impacted rotting food) and may drool green rumen liquor when attempting to chew the cud.

There is no satisfactory treatment and very thin ewes should be culled. As the cause is unknown there are no preventive measures, although it would be prudent not to retain breeding stock from ewes or rams with abnormalities of the teeth.

15

FOOT LAMENESS

Lameness is one of the most important welfare problems of sheep worldwide. Whilst most shepherds spend a considerable proportion of their time treating lame animals, or attempting to control or prevent the infectious forms of foot lameness, others look upon it as a necessary evil. A change of attitude is clearly desirable in the latter case.

Lameness can never be totally eliminated because fractures, sprains, puncture wounds and the like will always occur from time to time in every flock. However, many of the infectious causes of lameness—and footrot in particular—could be controlled much more effectively than at present by using already available techniques, chemicals, drugs and vaccines in a more concerted manner.

Apart from much unnecessary suffering, lameness results in not inconsiderable economic loss to the sheep farmer. Sheep worldwide are predominantly grazing animals, and anything which interferes with their ability to range freely for food is bound to affect their productivity, whether it be through a loss of body condition, poor growth rates, a reduction in wool yield, poor milk production, or disappointing reproductive performance.

Some forms of lameness have been dealt with where appropriate elsewhere in the book—for instance, joint-ill in Chapter 9 and post-dipping lameness in Chapter 13—and this chapter concentrates on foot lameness. It should be borne in mind that apparent lameness or abnormal gait may be associated with other diseases—ewes with acute mastitis and lambs with louping ill or swayback being examples.

Footrot

It is important to stress at the outset that footrot is an **infectious disease**, spread from sheep to sheep via **pasture or bedding** contaminated with bacteria from the feet of infected animals. It should always be viewed as a **flock problem** rather than simply one of the individual animal. Footrot may be present in individual animals at any time of the year, but the disease does not spread within the flock unless certain climatic and other factors are favourable for transmission. In some parts of the world, such as certain areas of Australia, the predictable climatic changes permit reasonably

587

accurate forecasting of outbreaks. However, in the UK the unpredictable climate makes forecasting very difficult. Nevertheless, there are periods of the year when the disease is more likely to be a problem and it is helpful to know when these periods are in considering treatment, control or eradication measures.

The bacteria causing footrot

Footrot is caused by two different bacteria. The first, *Fusobacterium necrophorum*, is found wherever sheep are found. It survives for very long periods and under all weather conditions, in the feet of sheep, in soil, on pasture and in bedding. It is also associated with other farmed animals such as cattle, goats and deer and its eradication is quite out of the question. This bacterium attacks the skin between the cleats or digits of the foot and causes an inflammation called interdigital dermatitis. The bacterium may

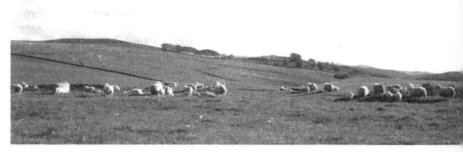

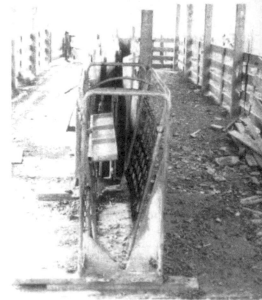

Plate 15.1 Footrot is an infectious bacterial disease. Pasture, bedding and handling areas which become contaminated with the bacteria act as a source of infection for clean sheep.

cause lameness on its own account and is a common cause of scald or scad (see later in this chapter).

True footrot requires the intervention of a second microorganism, *Bacteroides nodosus*, of which there are many different strains. Some cause a virulent form of footrot, whilst others are less invasive and are termed intermediate or benign—although the latter term is somewhat misleading, since the damage they cause may still produce considerable pain and obvious lameness. *B. nodosus* can invade the foot only if the skin has already been damaged by *F. necrophorum* and so cannot produce footrot on its own. Whilst the bacterium can survive in an infected sheep's foot for months or years in the absence of effective treatment, it cannot survive away from the foot—on pasture, bedding or in the soil—for more than about 10 days. Therefore it is possible, although difficult, to eradicate this bacterium from a flock.

THE SPREAD OF FOOTROT

A number of factors increase the likelihood of footrot appearing or flaring up in a flock. Obviously *Bacteroides nodosus* must be present in the feet of sheep on the farm. In a previously footrot-free flock, this means the introduction of infected sheep, such as purchased replacement females or rams, or the purchase of infected cattle, goats or deer. The straying of a neighbour's infected animals onto your land (or yours onto his!) may also do the trick. All purchases should therefore be kept separate from the home flock for at least a month. They should be examined carefully for footrot, any cases treated, the whole batch footbathed and then re-examined two weeks later. They should not be allowed to join the flock until all infection is cured. The home flock should be kept away from the area grazed by the bought-in sheep for at least 10 days after the purchased animals have been moved off the area.

Footrot is principally a disease of lowland flocks and particularly intensively stocked sheep units. The disease is relatively uncommon on the hill, since the stocking rates are lower and the risk of sheep encountering ground infected with footrot is much less likely. Also, *F. necrophorum* does not survive well on the acid conditions of many hill soils.

Predisposing factors

The chances of sheep becoming infected with footrot are increased under certain weather conditions. Wet conditions underfoot—which prevail for a large proportion of the year in the UK, especially in the west and north—tend to denature the skin between the claws of the foot, and this adversely affects the natural ability of the skin to resist infection. However, probably the most important factor in temperate climates such as the UK is **temperature**. Once the thermometer reaches around 10°C (50°F) and providing the conditions are sufficiently damp, the chance of *B. nodosus* surviving for long enough on pasture to spread from sheep to sheep is greatly increased, and if there are a significant number of sheep harbouring *B. nodosus* in footrot lesions, there may be an explosive outbreak.

HOUSING Housed sheep are particularly at risk, since whatever the time of year, conditions underfoot indoors are always more likely to favour the spread of infection. Again, providing there is at least one infected foot in a group of housed sheep, the disease will almost inevitably spread. It is therefore most important to clear up any infection well before sheep are housed; otherwise very frequent treatment will be necessary throughout the housed period.

CLINICAL SIGNS AND EXAMINING FEET

It is important to appreciate that not all lameness is due to footrot. Indeed, where severe lameness suddenly occurs in a number of animals in the flock, the possibility of foot and mouth (a notifiable disease) should always be considered. Also, not every sheep affected with footrot will be lame and it is therefore necessary to inspect every foot of every sheep in the flock in order to identify all infected animals. This is important when implementing control or eradication measures. There may be three times as many sheep with footrot in the flock as there are obviously lame sheep.

The mildest form of lameness may show merely as an exaggerated nod of the head when walking, and when such sheep are gathered they may not be detectable. Animals in more severe pain may hobble when walking and stop frequently to hold a foot up off the ground. Others, especially those with more than one affected foot, may spend a lot of time grazing on their knees, crouching or lying down. When they are moved on they may be very reluctant to do so, stopping frequently, puffing and panting due to the pain.

Sheep should be tipped up so that the feet can be thoroughly examined. A semi-stiff brush should be used to remove gross dirt and the feet should be washed with water if necessary. The earliest sign of infection is a reddening of the skin between the cleats, which also appears moist and is painful when touched. This is due to *F. necrophorum* and is often referred to as scald. Strictly speaking, scald is any inflammation of the skin between the cleats, from whatever cause, but in this context it is considered an early stage of footrot. The damage done allows *B. nodosus* to invade the foot. Together these organisms then cause much more serious damage.

As mentioned earlier, *B. nodosus* exists in several (at least 10) different strains or types and these vary in the degree of destruction they inflict upon affected feet. The so-called benign strains 'eat' away at the soft horn at the bulb of the heel, causing a certain amount of under-running and separation, but do not usually progress further. This form of footrot usually responds well to treatment by footbathing alone.

The more severe or virulent forms of *B. nodosus* cause more extensive damage and under-running of the hard horn covering the sole, hoof wall and toe. If the flaps of separated horn are lifted up or clipped off, a greyish, cheesy material with an unpleasant and characteristic smell is revealed (see

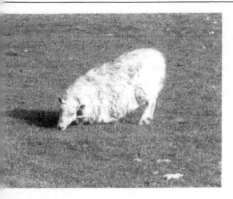

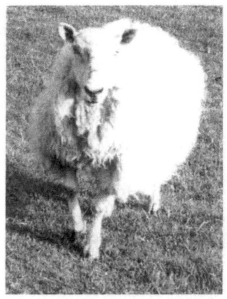

Plate 15.2   This greyface ewe on its knees (*above*) is not evaluating the quality of the sward! She is severely lame due to footrot in the right front foot (*right*). As a consequence she was not milking well and her twin lambs were poor doers.

Colour plates 72 to 74). Eventually, with or without treatment, horn will regrow to cover and protect the delicate tissues inside the foot. However, this tends to happen in a very haphazard way and the shape of the foot may become deformed.

Some particularly susceptible sheep may be affected with footrot on many occasions throughout their lives, in the same or in different feet, and each time the deformity becomes more extreme. These animals, which may carry the infection for long periods—months or even years—are a constant source of infection to the rest of the flock and should be ruthlessly culled.

Diagnosis of footrot can usually be made satisfactorily by moderate paring and by a careful visual examination of the feet, with the important exception of the cases which are in the early incubation stage, when no obvious damage can be seen, even by very experienced people.

Consequences of footrot

If footrot is neglected, the consequences can be serious, both for the individual animal and for the flock as a whole. Footrot in rams may discourage them from working, especially if the hind feet are affected, since they put much weight on them when mounting and thrusting. If the disease is severe and of long standing, it may pull the rams down in condition and this may adversely affect their fertility. Autumn is a common time for outbreaks of footrot in the UK, and in most flocks this coincides with mating and the early pregnancy period. If ewes lose condition at this time, it can have a profoundly adverse effect upon the lambing percentage and barren rate. In late pregnancy, footrot may prevent ewes from getting their fair share of

591

feed, especially of concentrates at the trough. This check in food intake may precipitate cases of twin lamb disease and also lead to the birth of underweight lambs with poorer survival chances.

At lambing time, especially in housed sheep, contamination of the lambing pens with *F. necrophorum* from footrot cases increases the risk of navel-ill and liver abscesses in lambs. Also, lame ewes are likely to produce less colostrum and milk and to mother their lambs less effectively, further increasing the risks to the newborn from hypothermia and disease.

In summer weather, neglected cases of footrot may be struck by blowflies (see Plate 13.6). When such sheep lie down, maggots may crawl into the fleece, causing further damage.

TREATMENT

Treatment of footrot cases must be prompt and effective, so as to cure the sheep as quickly as possible, not only for their own sakes but also to reduce the risk of spread to the rest of the flock. There are many ways of tackling the disease and the methods of choice will depend on a number of factors such as the time of year, severity of cases, ability of staff, suitability of handling facilities and size of the flock. There is no one simple method of treatment or control, so a combination of the available techniques must be employed. Control strategies will be dealt with later, after a consideration of the various treatment methods available.

It must be stressed that **all treatment methods are much less effective if applied during warm, wet weather conditions which favour the spread of infection.** Therefore, whilst it is often necessary to treat individual animals, or to control spread by footbathing during these periods, it is far more effective to attack the disease in the flock during non-transmission periods.

Paring

Paring consists of cutting away areas of under-run hoof horn which have become separated from the delicate underlying tissues. Flaps of loose horn may rub against the soft tissue underneath and stimulate excessive growth causing raw, bleeding, protruding areas known as **granulomas or 'proudflesh'**. Often very painful, these have to be removed surgically by a veterinary surgeon and take a long time to heal. Paring is also necessary for the diagnosis of footrot, especially in sheep which are not lame. Only by removing the separated horn can the shepherd find any hidden pockets of infection which may otherwise go unnoticed.

However, the main purpose of paring is to expose the infected tissues to the fresh air. This aids healing considerably, because neither of the bacteria responsible for footrot can survive in the presence of oxygen. Healing will take place more quickly following paring in dry weather, when the feet are kept clean and free from mud. If footbathing follows paring, then the removal of superfluous horn also allows better penetration by the chemicals in the footbath to the areas where the bacteria are hidden away beneath under-run horn.

Trimming feet is much easier when the horn is soft. If a foot-wash bath is available, sheep can be allowed to stand in water (preferably running water) for an hour or so before paring, to soften up the horn. Clean feet make it easier to see what you are doing and also help prevent soiling of the footbath.

Only skilled, careful and patient operators should be employed to pare sheep's feet, since great damage can be done by carelessness, callousness

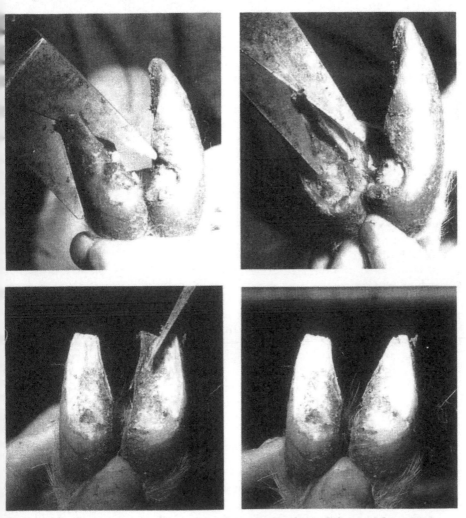

Plate 15.3   Four stages in the paring of overgrown horn. It is most important not to cause bleeding, especially when trimming the toe. Sufficient hoof wall must be left to bear weight and so protect the sole.

or ignorance. It is a time-consuming, tedious and backbreaking task and operator comfort is thus essential. The tools required are a pair of heavy duty foot shears, a footknife and a small hand rasp of the 'Surform' type, all of which should be sharp. The task is best done on a concrete or wooden area.

Remember that footrot is an infectious disease and in going through a flock it is inevitable that the operator will spread infection from 'dirty' (infected) to 'clean' (uninfected) sheep if precautions are not taken. Shed off obviously lame or infected animals and deal with them last. Whilst it is not so easy to work wearing rubber gloves, they are more easily cleaned after dealing with an infected foot and they also help to keep the objectionable smell off the operator's hands. Do not wipe a contaminated knife on the fleece, as the smell may attract flies in summer which can lead to fly strike. Between sheep, stand the implements in 10% zinc sulphate solution to kill any bacteria. Rinse with clean water, dry and grease them after a day's use.

Whilst all this may seem pernickety, there is hardly any point in doing a second-rate job and possibly spreading infection, when the object of the exercise is to clear it up. As a precaution, sheep should always be effectively footbathed after paring to prevent cross-contamination.

Shears should be used to cut only thick and easily accessible under-run or overgrown horn. The knife should be used with a 'wristy' movement against the ball of the thumb, and the horn should be shaved away, little by little, until all under-run horn is removed. **Do not over-pare and avoid causing any bleeding**. Infected feet are already painful and a bleeding wound on the foot is almost certain to become infected. This may lead to further problems such as 'proudflesh' or a foot abscess. A great deal of pain is inflicted and damage done by careless and overzealous footparing. If very extensive paring is necessary, the job should be done in two or more stages, with a week or so in between. The rasp can be used to shape the foot finally, but a sufficient amount of wall horn should be left to contact the ground and so protect the sole from bruising.

If a sheep has two or more badly affected feet, only one should be thoroughly pared and the others merely 'tidied-up'; otherwise the poor animal will be in considerably more pain than before treatment. Badly affected animals should be clearly marked and, wherever possible, kept apart from the main flock, preferably near the steading so they can be easily re-examined and re-treated. Consider the use of antibiotics by injection for the worst cases (see later).

Once the task is completed the clippings of infected horn should be swept up and burned and the whole area washed down and disinfected where possible. Earth-floor pens can never be adequately cleaned and it should be borne in mind that the area is likely to be infected for many weeks if infected clippings have been left lying around. Where straw is readily available it can be spread liberally in the pens before bringing in the sheep. This should reduce the risks and in muddy pens reduce the contamination of the footbath with mud.

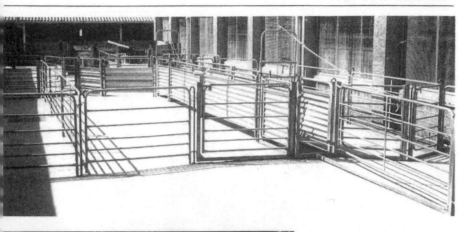

Plate 15.4   Sheep handling areas are best concreted for ease of cleaning. Hard-core is second best. Earth floors are unsatisfactory. Remember that footrot can be spread in dirty handling pens.

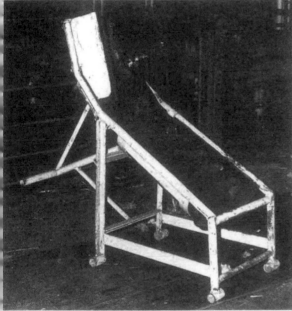

Plate 15.5   A sheep cradle. The animal is reversed up to the cradle, which tips back with the weight. Note the wooden board beneath to catch all the infected foot parings, which should be gathered up and disposed of.

Footbathing

Footbathing is a time-honoured method used for both treatment and control of footrot. It is frequently carried out in a slipshod manner at inappropriate times and is, in many cases, largely a waste of time and money. However, when it is carried out effectively it can be a very valuable technique, especially following careful paring. It is likely to remain one of the shepherd's chief weapons against footrot.

Paring the feet as described above is carried out to allow oxygen and footbathing chemicals to reach and refresh the parts they otherwise

595

(*text continues on page 598*)

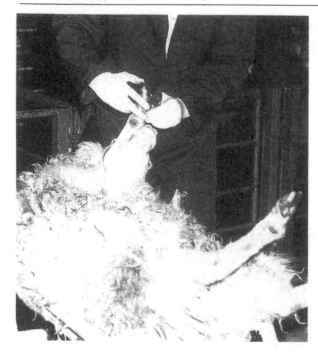

Plate 15.6 Foot examination. When examining large numbers of sheep, it is easier on the operator (and the sheep) not to have to struggle with the patients. Note the rubber gloves which keep the hands clean and can be washed to prevent the spread of infections.

Plate 15.8 Firstly, shears are used to remove bulky, overgrown horn.

Plate 15.7 A footrot case with overgrown horn.

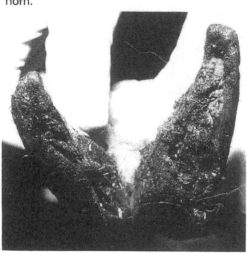

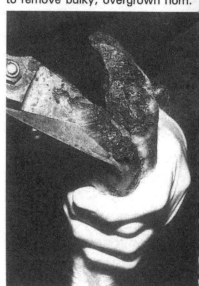

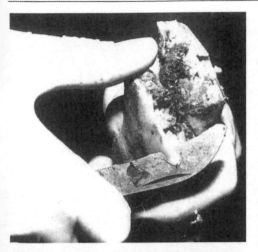

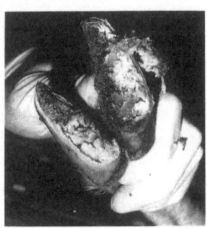

Plate 15.9   (*Left*) A sharp knife is used to cut the soft horn to shape. Note the cheesy dead material.

Plate 15.10   (*Above*) Note how the wall of the hoof has been left a little above the level of the sole to take some of the pressure off the delicate sole underneath. All cheesy material should be removed and destroyed.

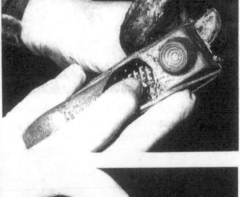

Plate 15.11   (*Left*) A rasp can be used to shape the foot if necessary, especially if it is very hard—for example, after formalin footbathing.

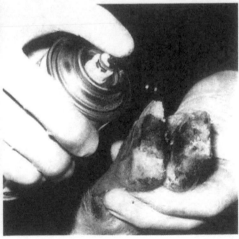

Plate 15.12   (*Left*) Sheep individually treated with antibiotic aerosol should *not* be footbathed.

wouldn't reach! However, it takes some time for the chemicals in the foot-bath to penetrate all parts of infected and often deformed feet. It is unlikely that the chemicals will penetrate every tiny nook and cranny unless some wetting or penetrating agent is added (see below). Sheep must therefore be allowed to remain in the footbath for a sufficient length of time, depending on the chemical used and the condition of the feet.

The chemicals used must kill the bacteria responsible for footrot quickly and effectively without damaging the skin or other delicate tissues of the foot. Chemicals such as formalin do not work properly if the footbath is full of mud or dung and therefore the feet should be as clean as possible before footbathing. Because the chemicals are likely to do a much better job if they

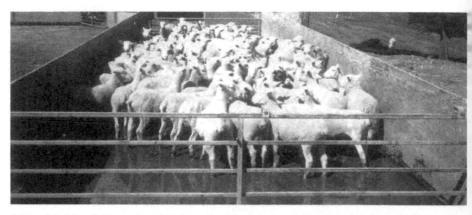

Plate 15.13 A large stand-in type footbath, containing zinc sulphate, adjacent to the handling pens for a large ewe flock in the eastern United States. Zinc sulphate may foam (*below*) and make sheep reluctant to enter the bath.

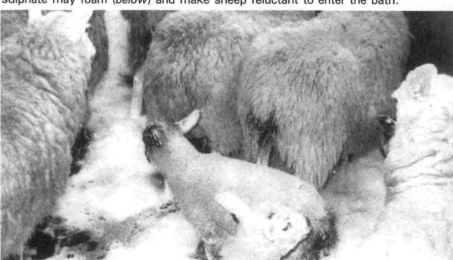

remain in contact with the foot for some time, it is best to allow the sheep to stand on concrete for up to an hour after footbathing. They should then go back to **dry pasture** so that the chemicals are not immediately washed out of the feet by water on the herbage. As stated earlier, footbathing will be most effective during weather which does not allow spread of the disease.

The job should not be rushed, since a 'hop, skip and jump' through the footbath is largely a waste of time and money. The chemical will have no chance of penetrating to the seat of infection, especially in cases where there is any under-running of horn. The fact that sheep may hold up a foot after running through formalin does not necessarily mean that the chemical has done some good, but simply makes the point that formalin stings in the slightest wound, or that the solution is too strong and is damaging the skin between the cleats.

The design of the footbath should be such that sheep are compelled to have all four feet in the chemical, since they may hold a painful foot out of the solution. Sheep which have been individually treated—for example, with an antibiotic spray—should not be run through the footbath, as this will nullify the treatment. Otherwise, all sheep in the flock should be footbathed.

The use of a portable footbath when moving sheep from field to field has a number of limitations. It is rarely possible to arrange for the feet to be clean before footbathing and it is usually impractical to hold sheep in the bath for a sufficient length of time. As footbathing—even when done under ideal conditions—is never anywhere near 100% effective, this method will not clear up all infections, nor will it prevent the transmission of infection from one paddock to another.

CHOICE OF FOOTBATH CHEMICALS   A most important aspect of footbathing is the choice of chemical. Copper sulphate is extremely toxic to sheep (and fish in nearby streams) and should never be used. Formalin probably remains the most commonly used chemical, but also has a number of disadvantages, including causing considerable pain to sheep with footrot, especially when in too strong a solution (e.g. more than 5%). It must not be used in enclosed spaces as the fumes are toxic, and it does not work in the presence of organic matter (dung or mud) and therefore must be replenished frequently. Otherwise formalin is an effective treatment even at dilutions of 2 to 3%.

Zinc sulphate as a 10% solution may be used straight, or with an added agent to aid penetration into the horn of the hoof, which, it is claimed, will not only kill the bacteria more effectively, but should also give some measure of protection for a number of weeks following treatment. Also, because of the superior penetration, much less paring of the feet should be necessary. However, these penetrating products require a long stand-in time of up to one hour and this necessitates the construction or purchase of a large bath to accommodate many sheep.

Zinc sulphate with a penetrant is much less effective when the horn of the hoof is hard. So where formalin has been used previously, it may take a couple of months for the feet to soften up sufficiently for the zinc

599

preparation to be fully effective. Zinc products are expensive to purchase initially but can be reused if the manufacturer's instructions are followed, since they remain effective even in the presence of organic matter such as mud or faeces. (There is no evidence that zinc sulphate given as an oral drench helps prevent footrot and, as it is a toxic chemical, this method should not be used.)

Different chemicals should never be mixed together in the footbath. As they are all toxic in concentrated form, they should be kept in a lockable store. After footbathing, the solution should be disposed of in a responsible manner well away from any watercourse. See Quick Reference Chart.

Antibiotic aerosols

A number of antibiotics are effective against the bacteria causing footrot and can be used both topically—by spraying the affected foot with an aerosol preparation—and by injection. The same rules apply when using an aerosol preparation as for footbathing. Namely, the foot should be adequately pared to allow penetration of the infected tissues, sprayed and then allowed to dry before turning the sheep onto dry pasture. These sprays are very useful when catching individually lame sheep in the field, but are often used ineffectively—for example, in wet weather when the antibiotic is immediately washed off the foot by the wet grass. Obviously, feet should not be sprayed prior to footbathing.

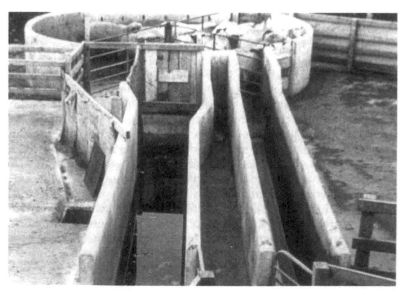

Plate 15.14 A walkthrough footbath with shedder at the end. Sheep must be made to stand in the solution for at least two or three minutes, longer if possible.

QUICK REFERENCE CHART
Footbathing chemicals

Chemical (symbol) (Concentration)	Safety	Comments & recommendations
Zinc sulphate (ZnSO$_4$) and zinc sulphate plus a detergent or penetrant (ZnSO$_4$+) (10%)	Toxic if drunk; eye irritation in dogs; non-corrosive.	Both products: No hardening of horn; work in presence of organic matter so can be re-used many times; non-irritant to sheep's feet.
		Penetrant: Prevents blood clotting, so avoid cuts when paring; long stand-in time (30 to 60 minutes) for full protective benefit, so large footbath required for many sheep. Expensive initially, but competitive long term. Foaming may inhibit sheep from entering footbath.
		Will probably replace formalin as first choice in time – kind to sheep and good penetration (ZnSO$_4$+), if long stand-in time observed; but change in shepherd's attitude necessary if benefits to be fully exploited.
Formalin (2 or 3%; never more than 5%)	Toxic fumes – cannot be used indoors (hazardous to humans) – concentrate is inflammable and corrosive.	Painful to damaged skin; strong solutions may cause scald or more severe cracking of skin; must be made up fresh; ineffective in presence of organic matter so cannot be re-used; concentrate needs special storage facilities.
		Probably outdated on welfare and safety grounds, but likely to continue in use. Effective where used correctly and where penetration is not essential (e.g. early or benign footrot and scald).
Copper sulphate (CuSO$_4$) (10%)	Very toxic to sheep if drunk. Poisonous to fish if it contaminates watercourses.	Stains fleece; corrosive to metal. Should **NOT** be used.

NOTE: Sheep should have a longer stand-in time than is usually allowed. All products present disposal problems.

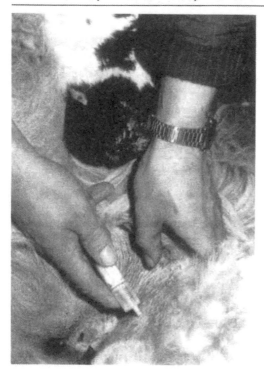

Plate 15.15 Antibiotics by injection are a most effective treatment for footrot—especially where more than one foot is infected or in particularly severe cases where paring would increase the animal's suffering.

Injectable antibiotics

Considering the high success rate and the rapid cure following the use of injectable antibiotics—in particular, penicillin with streptomycin—it is surprising that this treatment is not used more frequently, especially for valuable sheep, or on humanitarian grounds for severely lame or chronically affected animals. Where more than one foot is affected, an injection will treat all of them simultaneously and without the need for paring initially. The cost of the drugs is substantial, because a high dose is required, but a cure is often achieved after only one injection. Only a small proportion of sheep will need a second injection about a week later. The few which do not then respond should be culled. Sheep can be treated in any weather, but as for all other treatments, the results are more satisfactory when the disease is not spreading in the flock.

Heavily pregnant ewes with footrot should not be tipped up and extensively pared if avoidable; these are often ideal candidates for treatment by injection, but strictly under veterinary supervision. If rams with bad footrot have been neglected until very close to mating, but must be used to tup the flock, it is often preferable to inject penicillin and streptomycin rather than embark upon extensive paring of the feet, which may cause more pain initially and reduce willingness to work.

602

The best results are obtained where badly affected sheep are kept indoors on clean, dry bedding for 24 hours after injection. Animals should be kept under surveillance near the farm and re-inspected after a week.

If milking sheep are given antibiotics by injection, the milk should be withdrawn from human consumption for at least the period specified by the manufacturer for dairy cows. If in doubt, consult your veterinary surgeon.

Vaccination

Vaccination against footrot has been practised on some farms for many years, but for a variety of reasons the technique has augmented rather than superseded other control methods. Nonetheless, vaccination can play an important role in the control and prevention of this intractable disease on many farms.

Natural footrot infection does not produce a good immunity and a sheep may become reinfected on a number of occasions during its life. This means that producing a highly effective vaccine is a difficult task. The vaccines presently available are directed at protecting against *B. nodosus* only, which exists in many strains. It is only in recent years that multistrain vaccines containing all ten of the *B. nodosus* types have been available.

Vaccination is a technique aimed at protecting animals against infection expected sometime in the future, although modern vaccines also have some curative effect in sheep already suffering from the disease. Unfortunately, the level of protection from vaccines is modest and relatively short-lived. The results also vary considerably from farm to farm and from breed to breed. There are a number of possible reasons for this, such as incorrect vaccination technique, inappropriate timing, inadequate supportive treatment (paring and footbathing) or a very high level of infection on the farm.

TIMING AND FREQUENCY OF VACCINATIONS Because of the vagaries of the British climate, it is not possible to forecast with any degree of accuracy or precision when footrot is likely to spread within a flock. However, the weather conditions in late spring and early summer and again in autumn and early winter are usually suitable for spread. Therefore new vaccination programmes should be timetabled to allow a primary injection, followed by a secondary injection four to six weeks later, to be completed a few weeks before the expected period of risk.

If sheep have been vaccinated previously, the single booster vaccination required should precede the risk period. Because the protection is short-lived, repeated vaccination may be necessary in flocks where the normal measures have not given adequate control in previous years. These booster doses may be required twice or occasionally three times a year, depending upon the degree of protection required and the disease challenge in the flock.

VACCINATION IN HOUSED FLOCKS Housing sheep overwinter—or for even a short period during lambing—significantly increases the risk of an outbreak of footrot, the conditions underfoot being ideal for spread. The disease should therefore be reduced to as low a level as possible within the flock immediately before housing. If housing conditions are less than perfect, or problems have arisen in previous years, vaccination should be considered. If ewes are to be housed over the whole winter period, say from December onwards, then vaccination in early autumn with regular, effective footbathing up until housing may be sufficient. Where necessary, a further booster could be used a couple of weeks before housing.

For ewes housed only over lambing, for example in March, footrot is likely to take off once the ewes are put indoors, even though the level of infection in the flock at pasture may be low in late winter. A booster vaccination would therefore be useful shortly before housing. However there is a difficulty here, because this would mean vaccinating in late pregnancy, around the time booster clostridial and pasteurella vaccines are given. These are given not only to protect the ewe, but also the lambs via colostrum. In the case of footrot, the antibodies produced from vaccination are also concentrated in colostrum and what relatively little protection there is goes mostly to the lamb, often leaving the ewes inadequately protected. Therefore in these circumstances it may be better to vaccinate in autumn and to rely on footbathing in the period up to housing. Also a multiplicity of vaccinations and other treatments should be avoided in late pregnancy. Vaccination should not be carried out in milking flocks, nor in suckling ewes during early lactation, since it may cause a sharp fall in milk production. This could affect peak milk yield and therefore overall lactation performance. Growth rate may also be affected in sucking lambs, especially twins and triplets.

VACCINATION ABSCESSES The modern ten-strain vaccines are prepared

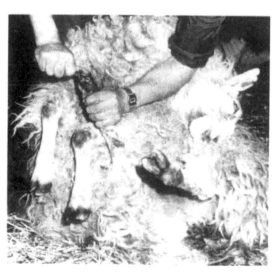

Plate 15.16 A heavily pregnant ewe with footrot in a sheep shed. Such animals must be handled with great care. It is essential not to over-pare and make the animal even more lame, as this could predispose to pregnancy toxaemia.

604

in an oily base as this helps to boost their effectiveness by increasing the amount of protective antibody the ewe produces in response to vaccination. However, there is a drawback, since the oily base produces an adverse reaction at the site of injection. In the majority of sheep this is only a slight swelling with some 'woolbreak' over the area surrounding the injection site. In a small percentage, however, there may be a severe reaction consisting of a large, painful and unsightly abscess, which may burst, soiling the surrounding fleece and presenting a fly strike risk in summer. Abscesses may take several weeks to heal and in a few cases may cause some loss of body condition.

The risk can be reduced, but not eliminated, by good vaccination technique. The recommended site is under the skin on the side of the neck, although this is not acceptable to all flockmasters. Do **not** vaccinate under the skin of the cheek, as is sometimes advocated, since, if there is a reaction at this site, it may be very painful and interfere with chewing. Sheep should not be vaccinated within two months of going to a show or sale, nor within two months of shearing in case the abscesses are cut by the machines. Lambs can be vaccinated from as early as a fortnight old, but only healthy, well-grown lambs should be injected. Lambs destined for marketing should not be vaccinated in the three months prior to slaughter.

The abscess risk can be substantially reduced by using the three-strain footrot vaccine (Clovax, Coopers Pitman-Moore), since the base used to carry the vaccine is much less irritant. However, the level of protection is also reduced. Nevertheless, many farmers have used this vaccine successfully for many years.

As the aim is to reduce substantially the proportion of sheep with footrot, all animals in the flock should be vaccinated. Unless and until more effective vaccines become available, 100% protection should not be expected and supportive control measures should continue to be applied.

Some strategies for control and eradication—with and without vaccination—are described below, but it should be appreciated that individual farms need a tailor-made footrot control programme to take account of particular needs and circumstances. Advice from your veterinary surgeon is therefore essential in helping to decide if and when to vaccinate and which vaccine to use and how best to use it.

Footrot in rams

Because footrot in rams can have such profound effects upon their working ability and therefore upon lambing results, there is usually a strong case for routine vaccination of the stud. A special effort should be made in late summer or during a suitable dry spell to clear up any infection. Vaccination should be carried out at least two months before mating is scheduled to begin. Because resistance or susceptibility to footrot appears to be an inherited characteristic (see below), it is probably unwise to breed from rams which have repeated attacks of footrot which do not respond to treatment, or which have deformed feet.

CONTROL AND ERADICATION OF FOOTROT

The measures for dealing with footrot in the flock are so laborious, tedious and costly that it makes sense to consider attempting to eradicate the disease from the flock once and for all, and so avoid having to repeat the procedures year in and year out. Eradication of a disease means the total elimination of the infection—in this case of B. *nodosus*—from the flock, so that not a single foot remains infected. Providing the infection is not reintroduced through purchased (or stray) sheep, goats or cattle, then the flock should remain footrot-free.

Planning

As stated already, footrot is an infectious disease and a flock problem rather than simply that of an occasional lame sheep. Control measures must therefore be planned rather than applied on an ad-hoc basis. The aim should be to reduce the level of footrot infection in the flock to such a low level—for example, to less than 1 or 2% infected sheep—that eradication becomes a more feasible and less daunting proposition. Shepherds today are being asked to look after more and more sheep; therefore any scheme which will reduce the need to upturn and examine many hundreds of sheep, on numerous occasions during the year, is surely worthy of consideration.

Whilst control measures are essential in all sheep flocks, eradication may not necessarily be attainable or sustainable on many farms. Flocks which regularly buy in sheep, for example, would need to set aside quarantine pastures for purchased sheep and to keep them separate from the main flock, often for long periods. This could impose difficult or impossible management problems on some farms. On the other hand, small and medium sized self-contained flocks, which purchase only an occasional ram each year, could, with vigilance, maintain footrot-free status. Other farms again may not have the adequate handling facilities crucial to the attainment of eradication status.

Feasibility of eradication

Shepherds must be trained to diagnose footrot, especially in its early stages and in its chronic or 'hidden' form. Identification is not always easy—even experts make mistakes—and nobody can identify infected feet during the incubation period of the disease, when no clinical symptoms are present.

Probably the best time of year to start in most flocks will be immediately after weaning, since lambs are being sold and total sheep numbers on the farm will be reducing week by week. Occasionally a spell of dry weather in late summer may slow or halt the spread of the disease. This helps considerably, since all control measures work better when the disease is not spreading. Also, there is a degree of self-cure during non-transmission periods.

The first step to take is to find out the level of infection present in the flock by examining every foot of every animal. If the number of cases is very low, say below 5%, then eradication may be feasible in many flocks. If the incidence is higher than this—and 50% or more may be encountered—it will be necessary to use control measures to reduce the level before even considering eradication. This will take some time, but in the meanwhile the success or failure of the treatments employed can be assessed and a judgement made on whether to proceed to eradication.

Blitz approach

Control must first focus on reducing the number of affected sheep by using a combination of the techniques already described, namely paring, footbathing and injectable antibiotics. Where antibiotics are used, treated sheep must be identified so that they can be re-examined to see if they have been cured. If not, then they must be culled immediately, before they contaminate the grazings further. Such non-responsive animals would wreck any chances of eradicating footrot from the flock. Where the incidence of footrot is high, vaccination may be used to augment these measures. Whilst vaccination and antibiotic injections are relatively expensive initially, neither should be necessary, of course, once footrot is successfully controlled or eradicated. Paring should also be reduced to a minimum, since footrot infection is probably the main reason for overgrowth and deformities of the feet.

Segregation

Separation of unaffected and affected sheep into temporary 'clean' and 'dirty' flocks respectively is a useful, although not a foolproof, way of attempting to keep clean sheep clean—a most important part of any control or eradication scheme. However, this can lead to management difficulties where footrot-clean grazings may be difficult to find, or where there are simply insufficient fields for the extra groups of sheep. When control measures are applied whilst footrot is spreading in the flock, such separation is essential. However, during non-transmission periods—which are difficult to predict in the UK and which may not last for long—there is no need to segregate. Remember that handling pens, farm tracks and similar areas will be infected if they have been used by sheep during the previous week to 10 days. If foot parings have been left lying around they will be contaminated for several weeks.

Cattle may harbour benign footrot infection and should therefore be kept apart from the sheep flock. Mixed grazing should not be practised and sheep should not move onto cattle ground until 10 days have elapsed. Goats can be run with sheep, but only provided they too are included in the eradication programme. Any animals which have away-wintered must also go into quarantine on their return, since they present a real risk to the home flock. Even one infected animal slipping through the net can undo months or years of hard work. So too can stray animals, so farms where footrot has been eradicated must be thoroughly stockproof. Escapes will still occur and precautionary measures such as immediate and careful footbathing followed by a check-up examination at least two weeks later will be necessary.

Inherited resistance or susceptibility to footrot

One of the most important control measures, which is worth stressing again, is the rigorous culling of all sheep which do not respond to treatment, are chronically infected or have deformed feet. Not only do these animals perform inefficiently but they continually contaminate the pastures and so increase the risk of infection for the rest of the flock. They are therefore very costly animals to retain.

There is also a longer term benefit to be gained from culling these animals, since work in New Zealand and the United States has shown that susceptibility or resistance to footrot is a heritable characteristic. That is to say, the offspring of susceptible animals are themselves likely to be more prone to the disease. Therefore, they should not be retained as breeding replacements, since they will merely perpetuate the disease in the flock.

There is also evidence to show that the skin between the cleats of sheep which do not get footrot, or which suffer less severely or less frequently from the disease, is more resistant to invasion by the bacteria responsible for footrot. These sheep also produce more protective antibodies following vaccination than do less resistant animals.

Some ewes and rams remain consistently free from footrot and these should be identified in some way, since the offspring from the matings of apparently resistant parents are likely to be more resistant. The New Zealand workers investigated other inherited traits, such as the number of lambs born and weight at weaning, and found that selecting for resistance to footrot did not prejudice these other important factors. In the long term, therefore, selecting for resistance and culling for susceptibility to footrot could be another useful technique in the control of this disease.

Summary of steps towards the eradication of footrot

- Examine every foot of every sheep in the flock to ascertain the extent of infection.
- If the incidence is low (e.g. below 5%), consider the pros and cons of going for eradication at the earliest opportunity.
- If the incidence is high, take veterinary advice on the measures and methods necessary to reduce the infection rate. (These will differ from flock to flock, depending on the level of infection, the commitment of staff, the availability of handling facilities and of footrot-free grazings, the time of year and the climatic conditions, etc.)
- Once the level of infection has been substantially reduced, and providing weather conditions are such that infection is not spreading, then all remaining infected sheep must be individually identified, and either cured—by treatment with injectable antibiotics (e.g. penicillin or lincomycin)—or culled immediately. Treated sheep must be marked and

re-examined after a week. All those which are not completely cured must be culled immediately.

- The flock can be said to be provisionally free from footrot after no infected feet can be found following an inspection of the whole flock.
- Full eradication status cannot be assumed until no cases can be detected following a period of risk.

Scald

Scald or scad is the name given to an inflammation of the skin between the digits which makes the skin swollen, moist, red and very painful. It may be due to any number of causes, including the bacterium *Fusobacterium necrophorum* (which is responsible for the early stage of footrot), the use of too strong a solution of formalin in the footbath, mild frostbite, sandy soils causing abrasion, clay soils 'balling' between the cleats and many others.

Scald may occur at any time of the year and in any age group, but is probably most familiar as a condition of lambs grazing lush spring or early summer grass, particularly in a wet season. This form is thought to be most commonly caused by *Fusobacterium necrophorum*, which is probably able to establish an infection because the skin of the foot has been denatured by the wet conditions. Sudden outbreaks occur, so that during the course of a few days it may appear that the whole flock is lame. Sometimes lambs may be affected in all four feet at once and are therefore very reluctant to move about, spending a lot of time lying down. If the other footrot bacterium, *Bacteroides nodosus*, is present on the pasture then scald may progress to true footrot if not treated promptly and effectively.

TREATMENT

The flock should be footbathed in 2 or 3% formalin or 10% zinc sulphate, allowing at least two minutes' stand-in time. They should then be stood on concrete for an hour to allow the feet to dry, before moving on to drier and less verdant pasture which has not been grazed for at least 10 days.

It should be noted that scald may be caused by using too strong a solution of formalin (e.g. 5% or greater), either through inaccurate dilution of the concentrate, or through deliberately increasing the strength with the idea that this will do more good. It is the **time** that sheep are allowed to stand in the footbath solution which is important. Weak solutions of formalin, given time, will kill the bacteria just as efficiently as stronger solutions and will not damage the skin so much in the process. As scald can be a particularly painful condition, a 10% zinc sulphate solution is a kinder treatment than formalin.

Severe cases of scald due to *F. necrophorum* infection respond well to local treatment with an antibiotic aerosol preparation. Animals must not be put through the footbath immediately after such treatment since it will wash off the antibiotic, but the rest of the flock should be footbathed. Response to treatment is often rapid. Scald due to other causes will have to be dealt with appropriately, which initially means removing them from the source of irritation.

Outbreaks may occur in adult ewes during winter—for example, shortly after they are housed. Providing virulent footrot is not the cause, this type of scald is often successfully cured by prompt footbathing and by the provision of generous clean bedding. Ewes fed from a silage face or from big-bale silage feeders may also become affected, especially where conditions underfoot are allowed to become dirty and wet. In this case it is necessary to tidy up the feeding area daily and to use the footbath routinely.

Foot Abscesses

These are quite a common, painful and serious condition. They may occur in any age group, but are most common in lambs and younger sheep, possibly because the horn of the sole is softer and therefore more vulnerable to bruising and penetration by sharp foreign bodies, such as flints, nails, glass, thorns and barbed wire left lying around. Even stubbles and kale and rape stalks may cause sufficient damage if the feet are softened due to tramping through mud in prolonged periods of wet weather.

Where a sharp object punctures the sole or other part of the foot, it is inevitable that bacteria will contaminate the wound. The outcome will depend upon how deep and into what structures the object penetrated, the type and degree of bacterial contamination and the speed and vigour of the treatment given. Examination of early cases may or may not reveal a puncture mark. Bruising or accumulation of pus under a darkly pigmented sole is not easy to spot. The absence of footrot or any other obvious infection may give a clue. Eventually the foot will become swollen, hot

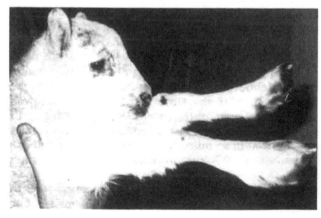

Plate 15.17 Lamb with a foot abscess due to a puncture wound.

and painful as pus accumulates. Neglected cases, or those which do not respond to treatment, may eventually develop sinuses, that is, tracks from the infected site within the foot to the exterior, often at the coronet, from which pus may ooze. This often gives some relief, since the pain from an abscess is mainly due to the pressure from the build-up of pus.

The diagnosis and treatment of foot abscesses is a veterinary job, often requiring a surgical approach to allow for drainage of pus and to clean up the area. Antibiotics by injection are likely to be prescribed for at least a week or longer. Painkillers may give the sheep some respite meanwhile. Where the foot has been operated upon surgically, it will require special dressings for several weeks. Even in cases which respond well to treatment, healing is a slow process.

Where infection has involved tendons, joints or bones, the outlook is less hopeful. In some cases, amputation of one digit may be performed, or the foot and fetlock joint may be encased in plaster of Paris and the joint allowed to 'seize-up', with antibiotic treatment to counteract the infection. Others may be incurable or may recur repeatedly, in which case the sheep should be destroyed on humane and economic grounds.

Fibromas

Fibromas are growths situated between the digits which frequently become infected or ulcerated and cause considerable pain. They are most common in younger sheep, but are especially common in rams, where they are found most often in the hind feet. They appear to be an inherited condition and therefore affected animals should be culled. Rams with the defect should not be purchased or bred from. The Suffolk breed appears to be particularly susceptible.

Fibromas must be treated surgically under local anaesthetic by a veterinary surgeon. As animals take some time to recover, fibromas in rams should be treated promptly so that they do not have to be operated on in the weeks leading up to mating, as they will probably be unable to mount and thrust, especially when the hind feet are affected. Cases have an annoying habit of recurring in future years.

Granulomas

Granulomas look very similar to fibromas but are excessive growths of tissue, caused either through the constant rubbing of horn on flesh—as in cases of neglected footrot—or damage to the delicate tissues by over-zealous use of the hoof knife when paring feet. Granulomas must be surgically removed by your veterinary surgeon and are often slow to heal.

611

Orf and *Dermatophilus congolensis*

These infections may affect the lower limbs of lambs, especially in the late summer or early autumn when sheep are grazing stubbles or kale stems. Damage to the skin, however slight, may allow entry of the orf virus with the formation of soft, spongy tissue, especially around the coronary band at the top of the hoof. The infection may spread to the lips and face as lambs nibble at their painful feet.

These lesions bleed easily as the lambs brush against the harsh herbage and their appearance gives the disease its common, though somewhat misleading, name of **strawberry footrot**. The worst cases may require individual treatment with injectable antibiotics and local soothing ointments, but the lesions are slow to heal.

The treatment and control of both infections are discussed in detail in Chapter 14. (See Colour plate 61.)

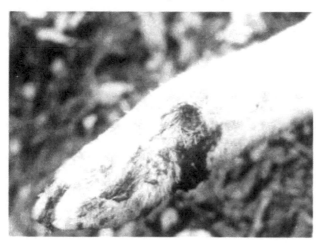

Plate 15.18   Strawberry footrot.

Laminitis

Laminitis is an inflammation of the laminae, which are the very sensitive structures within the hoof immediately below the outer horny layer. Because they are tightly confined within the rigid hoof, any swelling of the laminae causes intense pain. If laminitis is not treated promptly and effectively, the damage may cause permanent deformity.

Laminitis may occur in sheep under a number of different circumstances, most of which are concerned with diet. Animals on a high grain diet, such as those being prepared for show or sale, may succumb, as may housed ewes in the last third of pregnancy when suddenly introduced to a concentrate ration. Sudden unlimited access to lush pasture may also bring on cases. Ewes suffering from metritis—an inflammation of the uterus due to infection at lambing—may suffer from laminitis as a consequence. Laminitis is also involved in some cases of post-dipping lameness (see Chapter 13).

A number of animals may become affected at around the same time and often in all four feet simultaneously. Because of the severe pain, sheep are disinclined to move and spend long periods lying down and experience difficulty in rising. The feet are warm to the touch, the sheep resent being handled and they may run a high temperature.

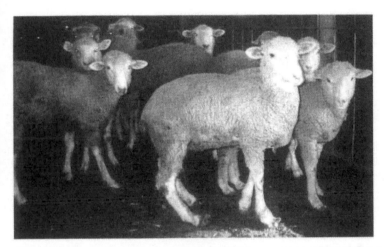

Plate 15.19 Almost every animal in this large group of fattening lambs was suffering from laminitis due to overfeeding on concentrates. (*Below*) Grossly deformed feet of the lamb in the foreground of the top plate. This unfortunate animal was in extreme pain and spent most of its time lying down.

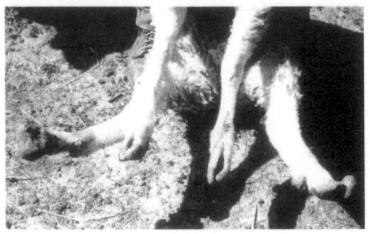

613

In cases where the diet is thought to be the cause, this should be remedied immediately by removing the concentrate portion of the ration or by transferring the flock from lush pasture onto more sparse grazing. Laxatives or purgatives may be suggested by your veterinary surgeon, who may also prescribe pain killers to help sheep over the acutely painful stages of the disease. Metritis and post-dipping lameness will require antibiotic treatment. Severely affected animals which do not respond to treatment or grossly deformed animals (see Plate 15.19) should be slaughtered or knackered, as appropriate, on humane grounds.

Redfoot

This is a rare and unusual condition which affects lambs of the Scottish Blackface breed or their crosses. It is encountered most frequently in central and southern Scotland and the north of England, particularly on heather hills. In flocks where redfoot occurs, roughly one in a hundred lambs will be affected. The cause of the condition is unknown, but it is most likely to be genetically inherited.

CLINICAL SIGNS

The condition affects very young lambs. The horn of the hoof becomes detached, leaving the delicate underlying structures of the foot exposed and bleeding—hence the name redfoot (see Colour plates 78 and 79). Sometimes all the feet are affected, but surprisingly, lambs are not usually very lame at this early stage. However, as they get older the affected areas become damaged and infected and very painful. Lambs then become very lame and lie down a lot, or crawl about on their knees. Often they are unable to keep up with their dams and die of starvation or from other diseases.

The condition also affects other parts of the body. The horns and the horn on the small accessory digits above the hoof may be shed. Blisters can form in the mouth, especially on the tongue, lips and gums and these burst, ulcerate and bleed. Blisters may also form on the ears and nostrils and on the coronary band at the top of the hoof. The surface of the eye—the cornea—may also become ulcerated which may cause blindness.

This is a most unpleasant condition for which there is no treatment. Lambs become very sick and miserable and are often in great pain before they finally die from some other condition such as pneumonia. They should therefore be destroyed on humanitarian grounds sooner rather than later.

Because rams are usually run in multi-sire groups with hill ewes, it is often difficult to identify the offending male, which should not be used for further breeding.

Foot and Mouth Disease

This very important disease should always be at the back of the mind when a number of sheep suddenly become lame. It is a **notifiable disease**, which means that any person in charge of or tending animals possibly suffering from this disease is required by law to inform the relevant authorities (see Appendix 5).

There is no cure for foot and mouth disease and vaccination is not allowed in the UK, the authorities considering a slaughter policy to be the most effective method of control should the disease be imported into the country. In many areas of the world—parts of Europe and South America, for instance—the disease is ever present (endemic).

The disease is caused by a virus—in fact, the most infectious agent known in either human or animal medicine. The virus may spread through direct contact, animal to animal, or via foodstuffs such as milk, meat, bones and offal. It may also be carried on air currents or by mechanical means—such as on Wellington boots or lorry tyres, or by birds or other wild animals. It is a disease affecting cloven-hoofed animals and in an outbreak it is most commonly seen first in cattle and pigs with subsequent spread to sheep.

The first indication of the disease in a flock would be sudden and acute lameness in a number of animals almost simultaneously, with rapid spread to the rest of the flock. If the disease is allowed to run its course, every animal in the flock will become infected. The feet are warm and painful and careful examination reveals small blisters, which often merge to form larger blisters around the coronary band and also on the skin in between the digits and at the back of the heels. The horn may start to separate from the underlying tissues as the disease progresses. Less commonly in sheep,

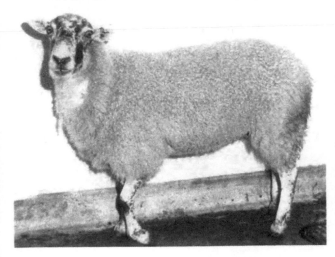

Plate 15.20 Foot and mouth disease in an adult ewe. This notifiable disease should always be considered as the possible cause of illness, especially when a number of sheep in a flock suddenly become lame. (See Colour plates 75 to 77.)

there may be blisters in the mouth and on the gums, lips and tongue. Profuse salivation does not occur in sheep as it does in cattle. Affected animals are obviously ill, lose their appetite and run a high temperature. (See Colour plates 75 to 77.)

Depending upon when the disease occurs in a flock, some pregnant ewes may abort and lactating ewes will go off their milk. There may be some sudden deaths in baby lambs due to the effect of the virus on the heart muscle.

The disease is less easy to diagnose in sheep than in other species, so **if in doubt, report the matter immediately**. Remember also that it is a legal requirement to keep an **up-to-date livestock movements book**, which is essential to the authorities in tracing the spread of this and other notifiable diseases.

16

POISONS AND RADIOACTIVITY

Poisoning

A diagnosis of poisoning probably occurs less frequently in sheep in the UK than it does in cattle, despite the much greater numbers of sheep. A large proportion of the national sheep flock graze extensively on hill and upland grazings and are therefore probably less likely to come into contact with poisonous chemicals or plants than animals kept more intensively and in enclosed fields. It is also possible that sheep may be more tolerant of certain poisonous substances than cattle, although this is difficult to substantiate. However, it is very likely that many cases of poisoning in sheep go unrecognised.

Detoxification

Most poisons, although not all, are taken in by mouth in the case of grazing animals. The toxic substance is then diluted to a degree in the large quantity of rumen contents and this may reduce the risk or delay the symptoms of poisoning. The poison may then be absorbed from the gut into the blood stream, in which case its first port of call will be the liver, which will attempt to detoxify the poison by changing it chemically. This is not always possible, however, and sometimes products are produced in the liver which are even more toxic than the original poison. Other poisons may simply accumulate in the organ, so that liver damage is a common sequel to many poisonings.

Diagnosis

Most poisons are excreted via the kidneys and in consequence this organ is also frequently damaged. Urine is commonly analysed in an attempt to confirm a suspected diagnosis. However, some poisons are deposited selectively in other parts of the body—for example, fluorine in the bones, or iodine in the thyroid gland. Therefore, if a particular poison is suspected, it is important to know which organs or tissues are required for laboratory analysis. Equally, it is essential that the laboratory staff be given as much information as possible, since in many types of poisoning there are no specific post-mortem signs to give a clue as to which chemical or plant poison may have been involved.

A full history of where the animals have been grazing over recent days and weeks or what they have been fed indoors is essential information. Details of any recent operations on the farm or adjoining land—such as crop spraying or basic slag application—may be highly relevant. Animals may occasionally have access to dangerous materials, such as discarded lead accumulators in dumps, or old lead paint in a building used as temporary lambing pens. Simply delivering a carcass at the laboratory with a message that poisoning is suspected is very unlikely to result in a diagnosis. The scientists would have to analyse every organ for a list of substances as long as your arm and at great expense, and this they are unlikely to do.

A celebrated veterinary story tells of the Australian who dug up his dead cat in the middle of the night after reading an Agatha Christie novel, chopped off its whiskers, placed them in an envelope and drove round to his local veterinarian in the small hours insisting that he analyse them for the presence of arsenic!

Toxicity

The degree of toxicity of poisonous chemicals and plants varies considerably. For example, sheep would have to eat considerable amounts of bracken over a prolonged period before its effects would be seen, whereas animals may fall dead whilst still eating leaves from a yew tree. Apart from notable exceptions such as yew, the amount of poison taken in is obviously important to the outcome, as is the frequency of intake. In poisonous plants the toxic substance may be more concentrated in one part of the plant than another—the seeds and roots are often most dangerous. In the case of oak, the unripe acorns are the most toxic part of the plant.

Palatability

Poisonous plants often have a very disagreeable taste and are normally avoided by stock, except where grazing is sparse or the plant is incorporated into hay or silage, when the animal has little or no choice. Some repulsive plants become more palatable after wilting and ragwort is an example. Occasionally animals develop a perverse liking for a poisonous plant, and even though it has already been unwell through eating the plant, it actively seeks it out. Some inorganic chemicals, including deadly ones such as lead and arsenic, have a sweet taste and many animals have a sweet tooth like humans.

Garden plants

Many cultivated garden shrubs and plants are very poisonous and this can pose a hazard to 'good-life' sheep kept in the back garden or orchard. It can also be a problem for farmers when gardeners deposit clippings and other garden refuse over the fence. The author can recall a case where six prime, heavily pregnant pedigree Friesian heifers were found dead after clippings from a yew hedge had been deposited in their field. One heifer still had a

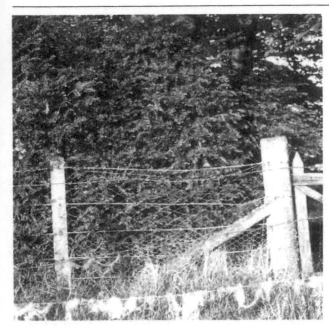

Plate 16.1   The yew hedge of a private garden adjacent to farmland. At the bottom of the photograph, note the wool on the barbed wire where sheep have gone under the secondary fence to have a nibble!

sprig in her mouth as she lay dead. (Diagnosis is easier when the evidence is left lying around so conveniently!)

Care of poisoned animals

How an animal fares after being poisoned will obviously depend upon what it has been poisoned with and how much it has taken or been exposed to. However, the animal's age, sex, body condition and general health may all influence the outcome. For example, a thin, pregnant ewe suffering from liver fluke disease is much more likely to succumb to ragwort poisoning from eating 'contaminated' hay in late pregnancy than a fit, healthy, dry ewe taking the same quantity of ragwort during a period of sparse grazing in a hot summer.

In the absence of a positive diagnosis there is often only circumstantial evidence or a strong suspicion to go on. Obviously, the first thing to do is to separate the animals at risk from the suspect or identified poison. This may mean moving the sheep where a poisonous plant is the culprit, or removing the poison (such as an old car battery) from the sheep's surroundings. Sick animals should be brought indoors and made comfortable, or at least near the farm steading where they can be closely observed. There are few poisons for which there is a specific antidote or cure, but your veterinary surgeon will be able to help with both specific and general treatment and about what to do with animals which have been exposed to a poison but are showing no clinical signs. Animals must be offered good-quality food and fresh, clean water.

The list set out below—which is selective—includes poisons which are potentially harmful to sheep, even if there are only a few, or even no, recorded cases. The list is divided into chemical and plant poisons and each is arranged alphabetically for ease of reference. If specific treatments are mentioned, this is on the assumption that a definite diagnosis has been made or that the circumstantial evidence is overwhelming.

Chemical Poisons

ARSENIC

Poisoning from arsenic used to be relatively common in the days when it was used in dips, in weed killers and as a defoliant on the potato crop. These uses are now banned and the emissions from smelting works which could contaminate pastures are now strictly controlled. Consequently arsenic poisoning is rare.

Animals die within a day or two of the ingestion of a large dose, but may suffer from diarrhoea and considerable abdominal pain for days before they die after a lesser dose. Sheep with mild symptoms may be treated with painkillers and given liquid paraffin by stomach tube if they are sufficiently conscious to swallow the tube, but few cases recover from arsenic poisoning. Very sick animals should be humanely destroyed.

BASIC SLAG

Slag—a by-product of the steel industry—is less commonly used as a source of phosphate than it used to be because it is less readily available and has increased in price in recent years. Nevertheless, it is still used and cases of poisoning may therefore arise from time to time. Slag is a severe irritant to the gut and causes a diarrhoea. Young lambs apparently find the taste appealing and will nose around where bulk slag has been dumped in the field. If substantial amounts are eaten, lambs may lose control of their hind legs and fall about in a manner reminiscent of delayed swayback, with which it may be confused. These severe cases usually die as there is no specific treatment. Sudden deaths may also occur in a flock grazing contaminated ground.

Sheep should on no account be allowed access to slagged pastures until heavy rain has thoroughly washed it into the soil. Bare pastures are more dangerous than those with a lush growth because animals are forced to graze closely and therefore will ingest more slag. Bulk slag should not be dumped in the field unless it is fenced off, and empty slag bags should be burned in a safe place.

CARBOLIC ACID (PHENOL)

Sheep may be poisoned by various dangerous phenolic compounds by mouth, inhalation or absorption through the skin. For example, they may graze pasture contaminated with industrial waste containing phenols or inhale them from the atmosphere. This is likely to be a local problem, but much more widespread is the use of phenols in wood preservatives such as creosote, in disinfectants such as Jeyes fluid and in 'bloom' dips for show sheep. On one occasion the author attended a badly blowfly-struck sheep which the shepherd had treated liberally with neat Jeyes fluid. The poor animal could not rise, was breathing only with great difficulty and had to be destroyed. It must have suffered terribly, not only from the results of the compound being absorbed through the skin, but also from the intense pain the chemical must have caused on the extensive wounds.

Animals may be poisoned if they lick wood recently treated with creosote or if compounds are left lying around or are spilt or poured away irresponsibly so that they contaminate watercourses. Bloom dips may cause poisoning if sheep accidentally drink some dip, but more commonly when the dip is incorrectly diluted in the dipper so that it is at too high a concentration. The sheep may look very pretty, but using extra strength phenolic dips is highly dangerous, since they are readily absorbed through the skin—not only of the sheep, but also of the operators if they are not properly protected.

Carbolics are very irritant to the gut and cause diarrhoea when they are ingested. If the animal receives a large dose, it is likely to convulse and die very quickly. Following bloom dip poisoning, sheep will stop eating and lie away from the rest of the flock, often breathing with great difficulty. These signs normally appear within a day or two of being dipped and once symptoms appear death follows within hours. Your veterinary surgeon may attempt to treat other animals which were dipped in the same bath but which have so far shown no untoward signs, but the prospects are poor for any animal which has received an overdose.

COPPER

This important potential poison of sheep is discussed fully in Chapter 11.

FLUORINE

Brick works and scores of other industrial processes may emit fluorine which can be deposited on downwind pastures if precautions are not taken. Animals usually have to graze contaminated herbage for many months before any symptoms develop. The mineral is selectively deposited in the hard tissues—namely teeth and bone. All ages can be affected, but young growing animals are usually afflicted worst. When poisoning coincides with the eruption of the permanent teeth these may wear down excessively fast

621

and bits may break off. This is due to defects of the enamel—the hard outer covering of the tooth. However, tooth defects are usually only noted when animals are examined because they appear unwell.

The most frequent symptom seen in fluoride poisoning is lameness. The bones tend to be softer and thicker than normal and are painful when handled. They are more liable to be fractured, in particular the 'coffin' bone (which lies within the hoof) and the ribs. If the poisoning is particularly severe, hard lumps may be felt when handling the jaw bones and long bones of the limbs. These lumps interfere with the movement of tendons and muscles and may be particularly painful when they affect the edges of joints. Affected animals have a poor appetite and fail to thrive in consequence.

The presence of clinical signs on farms within a few miles of a factory where fluorine is known to be a by-product of the industrial process used, would be grounds for an initial diagnosis of fluorosis. This would need to be confirmed by carrying out a post-mortem analysis of bones, when the fluoride levels would be elevated. Urine samples from sheep with clinical signs may also contain higher levels of fluorine than normal sheep. Pasture samples would also be analysed.

There is no specific treatment for fluorosis but where alternative grazing can be taken further afield, stock should be moved off the suspect pastures. Contamination levels are usually higher immediately downwind from factories, and depending upon the geography of a farm and the prevailing wind direction, some pastures may be less severely affected and may therefore be less risky for grazing animals. Symptoms will eventually subside if animals are moved to clean ground. Your veterinary surgeon may decide to treat animals which have to remain on contaminated ground but such animals are unlikely to be profitable and some may have to be destroyed.

INSECTICIDES AND ACARICIDES

See control of ectoparasites in Chapter 13.

LEAD

Sheep are less commonly affected by lead poisoning than cattle, who are generally more inquisitive and less fastidious feeders. However, the sources of lead are similar for both species and these include the soils and grazings around old lead mine workings, old lead-containing paint, discarded car and tractor batteries, tarpaulins, roofing felt, lead shot, putty and various lotions and liniments. Sheep grazing close to busy roads or eating hay made from the 'long meadow' (roadside verges) may take in lead from petrol. If any of the items mentioned above are burned, then the ashes will contain lead and animals—especially calves—will investigate such interesting places.

Acute lead poisoning (where large quantities are consumed over a short period) is not commonly met with in sheep, but may result in sudden death or in the animals becoming highly excitable and throwing fits before they collapse and die. If animals survive an acute attack they are frequently left blind. Chronic lead poisoning occurs where small amounts of lead are ingested over a long period and accumulate in the body. Such animals lose their appetite and hence body condition and pregnant ewes may abort on occasion. Young lambs may suffer from defects of the skeleton and may fracture bones easily. (This syndrome is sometimes seen in the old lead mining hill areas of northern England and southern Scotland.) Adult ewes may occasionally show symptoms of abdominal pain (colic) and the dung may be either loose or firm.

The majority of animals poisoned with lead die despite treatment. However, once a diagnosis has been confirmed in the laboratory, or if the circumstantial evidence is overwhelming, your veterinary surgeon may be able to save some cases if they are spotted quickly enough. He will probably use a preparation (calcium disodium versenate given directly into the bloodstream) which combines with the lead so that it can be excreted in the urine. Dosing with Epsom salts may also help, since it precipitates lead (as lead sulphate) so that it cannot be absorbed from the gut. It also causes the animal to purge, so ridding itself of lead remaining in the gut. This treatment will not help where large quantities of lead have already entered the bloodstream or are accumulated in body tissues through chronic poisoning. Affected animals must be brought indoors, made comfortable and offered wholesome food and fresh clean water.

MOLYBDENUM

See copper deficiency in Chapter 11.

Plant Poisons

ACORNS

Occasionally sheep (and cattle) will develop a craving for acorns, which are particularly poisonous in their green, unripe state because of their high tannin content. Animals lose their appetite and are constipated initially, although diarrhoea soon follows and there may be blood in the faeces in some cases. Animals may urinate frequently. Oak buds (unripe leaves) are also toxic, but sheep are less likely to be able to reach leaves than are cattle.

Poisoning is more likely to occur when grazing is sparse and the flock should be moved if they are seen eating acorns or if any animals develop suspicious symptoms. A mild purgative such as liquid paraffin may speed the removal of the acorns from the gut to prevent further absorption of the toxin, but otherwise there is no specific treatment.

BRACKEN

Bright blindness, or bracken blindness, is a slowly progressive poisoning, due to the ingestion of bracken (*Pteridium aquilinium*) over a long period of time. It is most commonly recognised in northern Britain, where there are vast tracts of this insidious plant, considered by botanists to be one of the most successful plant species on earth and one which is encroaching onto productive agricultural land at an alarming rate each year.

Where adequate grazing is available, sheep will normally ignore the plant, but in times of shortage they may nibble at bracken shoots. Once cut and dried the plant becomes more palatable and will be eaten readily in hay or ensiled material, although it remains toxic.

Since the poisoning takes some time to produce symptoms in sheep, due to its slowly accumulating effect, bright blindness is seen most frequently in mature animals. The toxin in bracken destroys the retina of the eyes, so that sheep eventually become totally blind.

Cases may not be immediately obvious, but when the flock is gathered, blind sheep become separated and show a degree of alarm and agitation. They hold their heads up as if listening carefully but are very difficult to catch despite their blindness, which may only be partial in the early stages of the condition. Affected sheep move with an unusual, high stepping style and stumble and bump into objects on unfamiliar territory. Hill ewes on their own heft may cope quite well until they are disturbed, but a number become casualties of road accidents or fall into rivers, or simply starve to death in some cases.

Close examination of the eyes reveals that there is no inflammation of the tissues surrounding the eye, as in pinkeye. Also there is no cloudiness of the cornea (the surface of the eye) or of the lens, deep inside the eye itself. The pupil—the dark central area of the eye—is abnormally large and round in shape, rather than rectangular, and in fading light the eyes shine excessively brightly, especially in torchlight—hence the name of the condition.

Bracken blindness can be distinguished from other forms of blindness by the history of access to bracken and the absence of any inflammation of, discharge from or damage to the eye. It may occasionally be confused with twin lamb disease, in which blindness may be a feature.

Affected sheep are untreatable and should be culled since they are unlikely to survive a winter on the hill.

Control of bright blindness depends on restricting access to bracken, but this, of course, is not always practical. Control of bracken by spraying is expensive and it is unlikely that bracken control will be a first priority on many hill and upland farms in the immediate future. Bracken should obviously never be included in hay or silage or used as bedding.

ERGOT

Ergot is a fungus (*Claviceps purpurea*) which affects certain grasses and cereals by replacing the seed or grain respectively with its own spores. The toxic substances are alkaloids which cause narrowing of the blood vessels in animals eating affected herbage with the result that the extremities, such as the feet, nose and ears, are deprived of their blood supply. They become cold and gangrenous and may eventually slough off (see Colour plates 80 and 81).

Animals must be moved from the offending pastures and on to safe grazings. Close grazing and topping of pastures will prevent grasses going to seed and thereby reduce the risk as well as encouraging grass growth.

FESCUE ENDOPHYTE

Much of the tall fescue which covers vast areas of the United States (and other parts of the world) is infected with the fungus *Acremonium coenophialum*. This fungus produces ergot alkaloids which cause a dry gangrene of the lower limbs of grazing sheep (see 'Ergot' above) for which there is no cure.

Control measures include the elimination or dilution of infected fescue swards, the avoidance of overstocking and overgrazing, the topping of pastures (to prevent heading), rotation with other crops and the avoidance, where feasible, of infected pastures during the hottest and coldest months when the risk is greatest.

HELLEBORES

Stinking green hellibore is common in the south of England, and the Christmas rose (black hellibore) is a common garden plant all over the country. This family of plants causes drastic purging and affects the heart and nervous system. Sheep are likely to eat them only when nothing else is available.

HEMLOCK WATER DROPWORT

The roots of this plant are particularly poisonous but are only likely to be unearthed during ditching operations. Sheep are more tolerant to the poison than cattle, but some may suffer from convulsions and die.

HORSETAILS

Stock are unlikely to eat these plants unless grazing is sparse. They may be included in hay, in which case they will be eaten and will poison. The symptoms are diarrhoea, dehydration, loss of condition and death. There is no specific treatment.

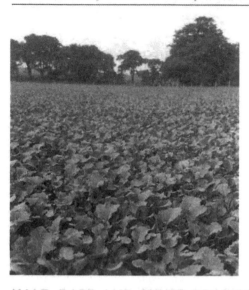

Plate 16.2 Brassica crops pose risks of anaemia and goitre.

KALE, RAPE AND OTHER BRASSICAS

A number of different types of poisoning can occur following the folding of sheep on these crops, but they all result from overfeeding.

Anaemia

If sheep are given unlimited access to kale without being rationed and are fenced back on pasture for part of the day, heavy intakes may cause a severe anaemia due to the destruction of red blood cells. Affected animals become very depressed and weak as a consequence. Jaundice develops and the yellow coloration can be seen in the eyes and mouth and if the fleece is parted even the skin is yellow. Some animals develop a diarrhoea, there may be blood in the urine and breathing may be more rapid than normal. There is often a high death rate with this acute poisoning.

Sheep, such as fattening lambs, which are grazed for prolonged periods on kale, rape or any brassica crop, may develop a temporary blindness from which they usually recover after several weeks.

Goitre

All brassica crops contain goitrogenic substances which interfere with the uptake of iodine by the thyroid gland. Occasionally sheep grazing these crops may develop goitre and if pregnant ewes are affected the goitrogen may cross the placenta and cause goitre in the unborn lamb. In consequence abortions and stillbirths may occur, whilst other lambs may be born weakly or deformed and may perish.

When any of the above syndromes occur, the flock should be removed from the crop immediately and put onto pasture. They should not be returned until all animals are completely recovered and only then if they can be strictly rationed. As a guide, these crops should not constitute more than about one-third of the total daily dry matter intake and a sheltered grass lay back should always be provided.

LABURNUM

All parts of this tree, especially the beautiful flowers and seeds, are very poisonous, but apparently somewhat less so to sheep than some other species. Animals become very excited, uncoordinated and eventually die in a convulsion.

LUPINS

When lupins are grown as cash crops for seed, sheep may break into the crop. Lupins vary in their toxicity, which is thought to be caused by a fungus which grows on the plant rather than the plant itself. Poisoned animals act stupidly, stop eating and become jaundiced because of liver damage. Death is common.

NITRATES AND NITRITES IN PLANTS

Under certain circumstances some plants may accumulate high concentrations of nitrates, which may be converted to nitrites in the sheep's rumen. These nitrites are absorbed into the bloodstream where they combine with

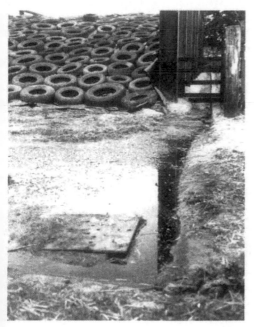

Plate 16.3 Silage effluent may be rich in nitrates.

627

the haemoglobin of red blood cells and so prevent them from taking up oxygen in the lungs. The result is that affected animals rapidly become very weak, fall about, gasp for breath, collapse and die—sometimes within only an hour or two of consuming high nitrate fodder.

In hot dry weather or in warm muggy 'growy' weather, heavily fertilised grasses such as ryegrass may accumulate high levels of nitrates. Certain weedkillers—such as 2,4-D—alter plant metabolism and may lead to the accumulation of nitrates. Silage itself does not pose a particular risk, but the effluent may be rich in nitrates. If hay is stacked when 'sappy' it may become dangerous because of an increase in nitrate content.

If sick animals are spotted early enough, your veterinary surgeon may be able to treat them effectively, but rapid or sudden death is a feature of nitrate poisoning. The flock should be moved onto safer, poorer grazing. Animals in poor condition which are put onto lush grazing or rapidly growing root crops are at special risk.

OAK

See acorns.

RAGWORT

Ragwort is a very common and persistent weed, especially in permanent pastures, and poisoning cases appear with depressing regularity. The plant has a bitter taste and stock will normally avoid it, but if grazing is short they may nibble at it and symptoms will develop after several weeks. When the weed is cut and left to wilt it loses much of its bitterness and stock are more likely to eat it. If it is ensiled or included in hay or grass nuts, stock will eat it unknowingly, and this is a common method of poisoning.

The toxin in ragwort causes permanent liver damage, so that animals gradually lose their appetite and therefore body condition. They are often constipated and may strain frequently, often to the point where they prolapse the rectum. Affected animals become very sick and as there is no treatment and the liver damage is permanent, they should be destroyed.

Sheep can graze affected pastures more safely than cattle, but they are just as likely to be poisoned by contaminated hay. Good pasture management should reduce the weed, but if it is cut, it must be gathered up and burned. Great care should be taken not to include it in hay or silage.

RHODODENDRONS AND AZALEAS

These beautiful shrubs, whose flowers are so attractive in late spring and early summer, grow particularly well on poor, acid soils. They often 'escape' from private gardens and may grow where stock are grazed. As with most poisonous plants they are usually ignored by stock, but may be

628

eaten in times of shortage, as for example, by sheep in a snow storm, or if stock have access to clippings which have wilted.

The leaves contain a toxin which causes very distressing symptoms of salivation, colicky pains, vomiting (very rare in ruminants), weakness, collapse and death. If animals survive, they need careful nursing and take a long time to recover from the damage to the nervous system.

SUGAR BEET TOPS

Wilted sugar beet tops are a safe and useful feed for sheep, but the fresh tops contain high levels of oxalates and are toxic, especially to sheep which have not been acclimatised to the crop. Oxalates are excreted by the kidneys into the urine and may crystalise out, causing blockages and urine retention.

YEW

The wood of the yew tree was used in times past to make the English longbow. As all parts of the tree are deadly poisonous in the fresh, wilted or dry state, it was planted in churchyards, which were one of the few places walled off from livestock.

The toxic substance is an alkaloid (taxine) which has a powerful slowing action on the heart, which eventually stops. There is no treatment. It takes very little yew to poison an animal, and since the action is so quick, it is rare to see any symptoms, sudden death being the rule. Sometimes the animal is still chewing the leaves or berries when it drops dead. It is hardly ever practical for your veterinary surgeon to operate and empty the rumen of an animal it is thought may have eaten the plant, because if it has, it will die very quickly even after only small amounts.

If a death occurs and yew is suspected, the flock should be removed from the source, but there may still be further deaths. A common source is wilted yew hedge clippings, or perhaps the broken limb of a tree blown down in a storm (see introduction to this chapter and Plate 16.1).

Colour plates 82 to 96 illustrate some poisonous plants.

Radioactivity

The atomic nucleus of a chemical element comprises particles called protons and neutrons. Elements may exist in a number of different forms depending upon the number of neutrons in the nucleus. These different forms are known as **isotopes**, some of which are unstable and liable to disintegrate at any time. These unstable forms are known as **radionuclides**. When the nuclei of these unstable forms disintegrate, they emit alpha or beta particles or gamma rays and this is called **radiation**. The **half-life** of a radionuclide is a measure of its stability and is the time taken for one-half of the nuclei of the element to disintegrate. Some have half-lives of only a fraction of a second whilst in others it may be measured in thousands or even millions of years.

SOURCES OF CONTAMINATION

It has long been known that heavy doses of radiation are harmful to the body but it is now known that there is an increased risk of cancer and of genetic defects from even very low doses of radiation. Humans and animals cannot avoid radiation because they are constantly bombarded from outer space and because there is a background of radiation from the earth's crust. Some rocks in Cornwall, the Lake District, the Scottish Highlands and other regions emit significant amounts of natural radiation. Added to this is a small, although significant, amount of man-made radiation, which comprises about one eighth of the total we are subjected to. This comes from controlled waste from nuclear power stations and reprocessing plants, from the testing of nuclear weapons and from nuclear accidents such as the Windscale fire of 1957 and the Chernobyl disaster of 1986.

NUCLEAR ACCIDENTS

In 1957 the author was a hill shepherd/assistant herdsman in Cumberland when the Windscale fire showered strontium-90 (^{90}Sr) and iodine-131 (^{131}I) abroad in the countryside. The milk from the Ayrshire herd had to be tipped down the drain for several weeks, along with the milk from producers from a wide area around Windscale (now Sellafield). The fortunate thing about this accident was that the iodine-131 (the main contaminant) had a short half-life of only eight days, so that it was cleared relatively quickly.

In the Chernobyl accident of April 26, 1986, the main contaminant of concern was caesium-137 (^{137}Cs), together with some of the 134 isotope, (^{134}Cs). Caesium-137 (radiocaesium) has a half-life of 30 years and so poses a long-term problem in areas which were heavily contaminated. In the UK the worst affected were north Wales, Cumbria, south-west Scotland and parts of the Scottish Highlands, all of which received heavy rain when the Chernobyl 'cloud' passed over between 2 and 5 May, 1986. Monitoring and analysis carried out at the time showed that the level of iodine-131 (of which there was some fallout) was low in cow's milk, probably because many cows in affected areas were still housed and therefore not grazing contaminated ground.

ROUGH GRAZINGS WORST AFFECTED

The situation in sheep was, unfortunately, much less satisfactory. Herbage analysis showed that the rough hill grazings and unimproved upland pastures were the worst affected. Contrary to early predictions, the level of radioactivity on these grazings remained high for a long period. Sheep were therefore accumulating considerable amounts of radiocaesium. Many more animals than expected had body counts of greater than 1,000 Becquerels per kilogram of fresh tissue weight. (A Becqueral represents one nuclear disintegration per second and is the unit of radioactivity.) Indeed, at the time of writing, more than three years after the event, there are farms in Cumbria that still have restrictions on the sale of lambs.

Rough hill and upland grazings may retain high levels of radiation for a number of reasons. There is much less plant growth than in the lowland situation and so less dilution of the contamination. Also, much more dead contaminated material remains on the rough herbage. Heather tends to retain more radioactivity than the hill grass species in the same area and the mosses apparently trapped more of the airborne contamination at the time of the incident. The acid peaty soils with a high organic content tend to hang on to the radiocaesium for very much longer than lowland clay soils, so that it continues to be taken up by plant roots. It is also probable that the original contamination was not easily washed off the rough herbage on the hills.

Removing sheep from contaminated grazings down onto uncontaminated lowland pastures will result in a rapid loss of radioactivity, but of course this is hardly a practical or economic proposition for many of the hard-pressed hill farmers who have found themselves in this most unfortunate situation. Certain clays, such as bentonite, are able to reduce the absorption of radiocaesium. However, there is the impracticality and the cost of spreading it, not to mention its unpalatability, which could lead to ewes refusing to graze dressed areas and thus losing body condition. Dosing sheep with potassium or caesium chloride will reduce their level of radiation by about one-fifth, but this again is not a practical or worthwhile option for most of the affected flocks.

APPENDIX 1

A HUSBANDRY AND HEALTH PROGRAMME FOR A SPRING LAMBING FLOCK

Key

H = Husbandry
V = Health
Italics = Items that will not apply to all farms

Suggestion: use a highlight pen to mark the items which will apply in your flock and enter the calendar dates in the empty left-hand column.

Weaning to mating

Ewes

H **Wean**, allowing sufficient time (at least 8 weeks) to recover from lactation before mating.

H **Dry-off** by removing to sparse pasture at a high stocking rate or yard on straw. (Do **not** deprive of water.)

    V *Dry-ewe therapy may be appropriate in some flocks.*

H **Select ewes for breeding and identify those for culling.**

H Divide ewe flock according to **condition score** (CS) and graze appropriately to achieve CS 2.5 for hill ewes and 3.5 for lowland ewes by mating time. (Some trough feeding may be necessary for very thin ewes or where grazing is scarce.)

    V Control **fly strike** and **headfly** worry as appropriate.

V **Control footrot** by 'blitz' treatment during dry (non-transmission) weather. Consider vaccination where incidence high.

V *Vaccinate against enzootic abortion (EAE) every 1 to 3 years in infected flocks or open flocks purchasing breeding females.*

V *Vaccinate against louping ill on affected farms where autumn tick rise is expected.*

V *Clostridial vaccination—extra booster on flukey farms with a high risk of black disease.*

V *Pasteurella vaccination—extra booster before mating on high risk farms.*

V Ewes may benefit from a pre-flushing worming dose, and where the fields are to carry lambs next season this dosing is essential.

H **Flush** ewes from around 3 weeks pre-mating on good-quality grazing. (Some trough feeding may be necessary where grazing is scarce.)

V **Check mineral and trace element status** by blood sampling a selection of ewes and take appropriate action on veterinary advice.

V **Control ectoparasites** as appropriate and observe **compulsory dipping regulations.**

Weaned lambs

H After weaning allow to settle for a few days and then simultaneously **worm and move to clean grazing** (such as a silage aftermath).

V If no worm-free grazing is available for lambs, they must be **dosed every 3 weeks** until slaughter.

V Where autumn nematodirus has occurred in previous years, lambs should be dosed at 3 week intervals during August and September if clean grazing is not available.

V Ewe lamb replacements must be brought into the **clostridial and pasteurella vaccination scheme,** with two doses initially, 4 to 6 weeks apart, starting no earlier than 2 or 3 months of age. Fattening lambs and store lambs which are to be kept on beyond 4 months of age must also be vaccinated.

Rams

H **Physical examination of whole ram stud**. Cull any unsatisfactory rams not disposed of at the end of last breeding season.

H Purchase replacement ram lambs or shearlings as early as possible and only after a **thorough physical examination**. Ensure there are **sufficient rams to serve the flock** satisfactorily. Always enquire about the health status of the vendor flocks. Blood test rams for Border disease and **isolate** new purchases for at least a month.

H **Flush** rams on good-quality grazing (with trough feeding where appropriate) for 6 to 8 weeks. Aim for CS4 by mating.

H **Teaser rams** should be prepared by your veterinary surgeon at least a month before they are required.

> *V* Vaccinate all rams against the **clostridial** diseases, **pasteurella** and **footrot**. Newly purchased rams should be assumed unvaccinated and given both primary and secondary doses at appropriate intervals.
>
> *V* *Vaccinate against **louping ill** on affected farms at least a month before grazing tick-infected pastures.*
>
> *V* **Footrot** and other lamenesses must be cured well before mating.
>
> *V* Rams may benefit from a pre-flushing worm dose, and where they are to graze pastures earmarked for grazing lambs next season this worming is essential.

Purchased breeding females (open flocks)

H Purchase only from flocks of a **high health status** (especially enzootic abortion-free) and **isolate** for at least a month and preferably until after lambing.

> *V* Bring into the **clostridial and pasteurella vaccination scheme** soon after arrival on the farm unless ewes are certified as being vaccinated, in which case give them a booster dose for safety.
>
> *V* Vaccinate against **enzootic abortion** before mating.
>
> *V* *Vaccinate against **louping ill** if home farm is tick-infected and autumn rise expected.*

Mating and early pregnancy

Ewes

H **Maintain CS** throughout this period on good grazing. (Supplementary concentrates may be required if grazing is in short supply.)

H To reduce early embryonic death, minimise stress by avoiding any unnecessary medications and gatherings.

H Analyse hays and silages.

> *V One or two **fluke treatments** (6 weeks apart) will be required during the October–November period on affected farms. Watch for media forecasts of degree of risk.*

Rams

H **Handfeed** throughout mating period and beyond to make up for inevitable loss of CS.

H Use **appropriate number of rams** to ewes for mating—this is especially crucial in teased or sponged flocks. **Observe closely** to ensure rams are working satisfactorily.

> *V **Fluke treatments**—as for ewes.*

Mid and late pregnancy

Ewes

H **Optimal growth of the placenta** is crucial to lamb survival and growth. Do not under- or over-feed during this period.

H **Ultrasound scanning** to determine foetal numbers will allow for more precise late pregnancy feeding.

H **Condition score** a representative selection of ewes whenever the opportunity arises. Pull out any **thin ewes** for preferential feeding or for treatment (e.g. liver fluke). Allow **adequate trough space**, especially for housed ewes in late pregnancy.

H Ewe **rations must be balanced** for energy, protein, minerals, trace elements and vitamins to minimise the risk of metabolic and deficiency diseases.

H **Do not feed spoiled silage (listeriosis risk) or mouldy hay (abortion risk).**

V Ask your veterinary surgeon to **blood sample a selection of ewes** and correct any discrepancies (e.g. copper deficiency) promptly, so as not to compromise the ewes or the unborn lambs.

V If ewes are to be housed over the whole winter period, **footrot must be effectively controlled before housing.** Consider vaccination if the prevalence in the flock is high.

V Control **lice** by treating ewes with a pour-on pyrethroid before housing.

V **Hill ewes can be dosed for worms** in the last third of pregnancy with a broad-spectrum anthelmintic, especially if food is scarce. They should respond by milking better. (A combined fluke and worm dose can be used, providing it contains the appropriate drugs.)

V *Housed ewes should be dosed with a broad-spectrum* **anthelmintic shortly after housing.**

V *On affected farms one or two* **fluke doses** *will be necessary during the January–February period.*

V *If ewes are to be vaccinated against* **orf** *(on infected farms only), this must be done at least 2 months before the start of lambing. (Ewes must* **not** *be vaccinated in the area where they are to lamb, as the scabs are infectious.) Vaccinating ewes does not provide protection for their lambs via colostrum.*

H **Feed concentrate rations in increasing amounts** from around 8 weeks prior to lambing. For more precise feeding, it is useful to have ewes grouped according to foetal numbers and lambing date.

V *If* **toxoplasma abortion** *is expected to be a problem,* **monensin sodium** *can be included in the ewe rations during the second half of pregnancy. Monensin will also reduce coccidial oocyst output and help protect lambs. Accurate mixing is vitally important, as monensin is toxic in excess.*

637

V Any **abortions** must be dealt with promptly by **isolating** and **identifying** the ewe and collecting up the foetus and placenta for **laboratory diagnosis.** Strict **personal hygiene** will reduce the risk of human infection from a number of sheep abortion agents.

V *E. coli vaccination of ewes to protect lambs against colibacillosis where appropriate.*

V *Where* **erysipelas joint-ill** *in lambs has been a flock problem in the past, ewes can be vaccinated pre-lambing.*

V **Clostridial and pasteurella vaccination boosters** should be given on manufacturer's advice before lambing begins. If lambing is prolonged, late lambing ewes should be vaccinated as a separate group to maximise colostral protection for lambs.

V **Warning:** Do not subject ewes to too many manipulations, vaccinations or medications at the same time during late pregnancy as this may precipitate deaths through pregnancy toxaemia or other causes. Always consult your veterinary surgeon before administering any combination of treatments. For similar reasons, any period of starvation, however short, should be avoided.

Lambing and lactation

Ewes and lambs

V **Note:** Please see separate detailed list on **'The husbandry measures aimed at reducing infectious disease in newborn lambs'** in Chapter 9.

V Record any ewe which has a problem around lambing time. Mark permanently for culling any ewes which prolapse, get mastitis or develop some other serious condition.

H Observe as many lambings as possible and interfere with as few lambings as possible.

H Observe **strict hygiene** when lambing ewes.

H Always inject assisted ewes with **antibiotic** on veterinary advice.

H Check ewes' **udders** hygienically for adequate milk or signs of mastitis.

H Ensure lambs suck sufficient **colostrum** early.

H Examine **suspect lambs** immediately, take their temperature and act promptly.

H Treat lambs' **navels** with tincture of iodine promptly.

H Feed ewes sufficiently on a well-balanced diet to **maximise peak milk yield.**

H Introduce **magnesium supplement** to ewe ration gradually to reduce the risk of grass staggers.

V **Worm ewes** before turn-out onto clean, worm-free grazing (unless they were wormed at housing). Ewes and lambs on clean grazings should not then require dosing until weaning.

V If only **contaminated grazing** is available, worm ewes at 3 weeks and 6 weeks after lambing and lambs at 6 weeks of age and every 3 weeks thereafter until weaning.

V **Hill ewes** can be wormed at the lamb marking.

V *Where* **nematodirus** *is a risk, lambs must be dosed every 3 weeks from the end of April through to June (watch out for forecasts).*

V *Where* **coccidiosis** *is a risk a coccidiostat can be provided in the creep feed where this is fed; otherwise lambs can be treated at 3 and 6 weeks of age with a long acting sulphonamide.*

V Be alert for the signs of **mastitis** in ewes (apparently lame ewes, starving lambs etc.) and treat cases promptly and effectively.

V If deaths from **pasteurellosis** have occurred in young lambs in previous years, they can be vaccinated at around a fortnight old and again 3 to 4 weeks later, but **not** with a vaccine containing a clostridial component.

V *Control* **ticks on lambs** *with spot-ons with or without tetracycline antibiotic injection and on ewes and hoggs by dipping.*

639

V On hill farms, ensure lambs are infected with **tickborne** *fever by returning them to the hill before the end of the tick rise.*

V *On affected farms, ewes will require a* **fluke dose** *around late April–early May.*

H Identify clean grazings for **next** year before weaning.

Dogs

V Sheepdogs and other farm dogs should be treated for roundworms and tapeworms at 2 month intervals. Consult your veterinary surgeon, who will prescribe effective drugs.

APPENDIX 2

FLOCK HUSBANDRY AND HEALTH PROGRAMMES

From just a glance at the husbandry and health programme in
Appendix 1, it will be obvious that a lot of planning and many important
and sometimes difficult decisions have to be made to keep a flock
healthy, productive and profitable. On most well-run sheep farms, disease
rarely limits productivity to the extent that stocking rates, inadequate
fertiliser usage or poor grazing management can do. Nevertheless, every
year in some flocks and some years in most flocks, disease may
seriously limit the output and compromise the welfare of animals.

Years ago farmers would complain—possibly with some
justification—that they could not find many veterinary surgeons who
were interested in sheep. The situation today is very different, as
evidenced by the large membership of the Sheep Veterinary Society.
Most veterinary practices with a significant amount of sheep work have
a member with a special interest in sheep, who will be able to assist you
in formulating a programme tailor-made for your particular flock and farm
circumstances, whether sheep are the main or a subsidiary enterprise, or
simply a hobby flock.

Many of these programmes have begun out of a request from the flock
owner for help to deal with a particular problem, such as an outbreak
of abortion. However, it is not necessary to begin in this way. Indeed,
it may be more satisfactory to begin simply from a desire to increase
the productivity and profitability of the flock by improving the standard
of husbandry and upgrading the health status of the flock. Whatever
the motive, these schemes almost always work best when initiated by
the farmer, because then the commitment is there to make it work.
Before entering into a contract of this kind, it is preferable that the
veterinary charges are fully discussed and agreed. Also, it is essential
that all parties involved—the veterinary surgeon, the flock owner and
the shepherd—are enthusiastic and committed to the project. This will
usually work best where everyone already knows and respects each other

and where the veterinary surgeon has experience of the implementation of such schemes.

There are many ways of initiating and running flock health programmes, and an example of how it might be done follows.

Initial farm visit

It is vital at the outset to clearly identify the aims of the flock owner and the way the sheep fit into the whole farm policy if there are other enterprises. A farm walk is helpful at this stage so that the veterinary surgeon can become familiar with the topography, the quality of land, the cropping, the stocking and any other enterprises. It is also helpful to arrange this initial visit when the flock is to be gathered for some reason, so that both ewes and rams can be examined to give the veterinary surgeon an overall appraisal of the condition and health of the flock and of its structure.

Records

Back at the farmhouse or office the flock records can be examined. If none are kept, it will be important to discuss what information is required and how it should be recorded. Keeping a record of the physical and gross margin data is essential in order to judge the success or failure of such a venture. Any health and husbandry programme already in place, however basic, should be reviewed. Records of particular disease problems which have occurred in the past should be collated, so that a picture of the current health status can be arrived at.

Priorities

Armed with this information, your veterinary surgeon can then identify the factors—be they husbandry or health—which are likely to be limiting flock performance. He or she can attempt to list these in order of importance and give priority to those which, if corrected, are likely to have the most initial impact on the profitability of the flock. It may be advantageous at this stage to bring in other specialists in areas such as nutrition or housing.

Implementation and monitoring

Once the priorities are agreed by all parties, a health and husbandry programme can be drawn up and implemented. At the same time, physical and financial targets can be set. These should be challenging, but realistic and achievable. The progress of the programme should be continuously monitored to ensure that it is being carried out as agreed, that it is working effectively and that it continues to make economic sense. The veterinary surgeon should provide written reports at agreed intervals—perhaps following flock visits at strategic times of year, such as pre-mating and mid pregnancy—in which the successes and failures are recorded. This report should then be fully discussed and any recommendations agreed and implemented.

Disease problems must be reported promptly, so that a thorough investigation—with laboratory support where necessary—can be carried out. If production targets are not reached, the reasons should be identified and corrected, and if the targets are unrealistic they should be adjusted. If the programme is successful after a year, in terms of the health and welfare of the sheep and the economic returns from the flock, then new targets and horizons can be set.

APPENDIX 3

HUMANE EUTHANASIA OF CASUALTY CASES

In any livestock enterprise, animals can be so severely injured or sick that the most appropriate action is to destroy them in as humane a manner as possible.

A decision must first be made on whether the animal is fit to travel. There is legislation in the UK—**The Transit of Animals (Road and Rail) Order 1975**—under which it is an offence to transport any animal if it is likely to cause unnecessary suffering through illness, injury or fatigue (see Appendix 4). If you are in doubt, the animal is probably unfit to travel, but you can consult your veterinary surgeon, who will in any case have to furnish you with a **Certificate of Casualty Slaughter** if the animal is to go to the abattoir, either alive or as an undressed carcass [**Slaughterhouse (Hygiene) Regulations 1977**]. The abattoir must also be alerted that you wish to send in a live animal or carcass for dressing.

If the animal is unfit to travel then it **must** be killed on the farm. If it is unfit for human consumption then it **should** be killed on the farm, even though it may be fit to travel. Killing an animal is an unpleasant and sometimes emotional task to perform and it is always preferable to employ a skilled person to do it, such as a veterinary surgeon or a licensed slaughterman or knackerman. If the carcass is likely to be fit for human consumption—for example, in the case of a recently acquired limb fracture—a captive bolt pistol or a firearm (free bullet) must be used. Your veterinary surgeon may use barbiturate drugs when the animal is unfit for human consumption, in which case it is important that the carcass does not go to the hunt kennels, since these drugs are toxic to the hounds. If the carcass is to remain on the farm it must be deeply buried or incinerated.

Firearms

In the event that you decide to destroy the animal yourself, it is always preferable to use a firearm. Many farms have a rifle, but only a few of the larger estates will be licensed to possess a captive bolt pistol. Firearms

644

are dangerous weapons at any time, particularly a rifle used in a confined space, where the bullet may ricochet. Extra care is necessary when other people are present or have to assist in handling the animal.

Aims

The aim of humane slaughter is to **render the animal dead in the shortest possible time and with the minimum of distress**. It is most important to keep calm and essential to know where to apply the firearm and in which direction to fire it, so that the animal will be killed efficiently at the first attempt. If the animal is down and cannot rise, it may not be necessary to have another person restrain it. A halter may be helpful if the animal can move about, or it may be set in a sheep cradle. The method of restraint should take account of any pain or panic which may be caused to the animal.

Method

The firearm should be held lightly against the head in the most appropriate site as shown in the figure overleaf. The animal should be allowed to settle down before the weapon is fired in the direction indicated. If the animal is not dispatched with the first shot, a second shot should be delivered as soon as possible, but taking care to position and aim it correctly.

Rams

Rams, like all adult male animals, are more difficult to destroy than ewes. In heavily horned breeds there is a formidable thickness of skull which may make the task considerably more difficult. Do not attempt the job unless you are confident and preferably experienced.

Lambs

Baby lambs in distress are a sad prospect. If it is obvious that a lamb is eventually going to die, or is in pain or distress, it should be destroyed without delay. If the farm is close to the veterinary surgery, it is best to take the lambs in for destruction. Your veterinary surgeon will most probably use an overdose of a barbiturate anaesthetic and in special circumstances may prescribe a single dose to a trusted client. These drugs quietly put the animal to sleep and the overdose halts respiration. Do not attempt to inject into the chest cavity as this can be most stressful if not done expertly. The site and technique used for intraperitoneal glucose injections for hypothermic lambs may be suitable and is considerably less traumatic (see Chapter 8).

Stunning lambs (concussion) is a most unpleasant method and should only be used by experienced people as a last resort.

Some alternative sites and directions of fire for captive bolt or firearm (free bullet).

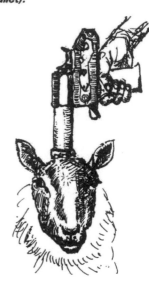

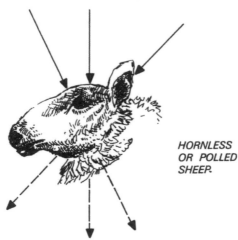

Some alternative sites and directions of fire for captive bolt or firearm (free bullet).

HORNLESS OR POLLED SHEEP.

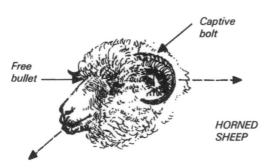

If the top of the head is unsuitable, place the captive bolt behind the poll and fire towards the throat.

Free bullet

Captive bolt

HORNED SHEEP

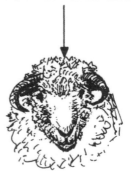

When using the captive bolt on the highest point of the head, fire towards the throat.

APPENDIX 4

TRANSPORT OF SHEEP

UK legislation in regard to the transport of animals is covered by the
Animal Health Act, 1981 and various **Transit of Animals Orders** and
these can be obtained from HM Stationery Office, 49 High Holborn,
London WC1V 6HB. There are hefty penalties for contravention of up to
£2,000 (or £400 per animal if more than ten animals are involved). Second
and subsequent offences attract up to a month's imprisonment. These
orders apply to anyone who loads, carries or unloads animals, or anyone
in charge of animals in transit.

The following notes summarise a number of the more important points
covered in the orders.

Loading and unloading

Sticks and electric goads must not be used excessively so as to
lead to injury or suffering, directly or indirectly, by causing animals
to damage themselves against the vehicle or its fittings. There are a
number of prescribed methods for loading and unloading animals and for
moving animals between decks. A ramp must be carried in the vehicle for
emergency unloading.

During the journey

Animals must not suffer unnecessarily from exposure to weather, from
inadequate ventilation, through escaping or from any other cause. Floors
must be anti-slip, or sand or other suitable material must be applied.

The driver of a vehicle may act as the attendant and in that
event is responsible for ensuring that animals are fed and watered
adequately (see later) and that they come to no harm during the
journey.

647

Overcrowding

Animals must not be overcrowded so as to cause injury or suffocation through lack of ventilation or trampling.

In large vehicles, pens of no more than 3.1 m (10' 2") in length must be constructed by means of partitions. Smaller pen divisions are permitted but not larger.

Feed and water

Animals must be offered wholesome and appropriate food in sufficient amount and fresh, clean water at intervals of not more than 12 hours. If the journey lasts 15 hours or less it is acceptable if the person who takes charge of them at unloading feeds and waters them immediately.

Unfit animals

If an animal is likely to suffer unnecessarily during transit—for example, through illness or injury—then it **must not be carried**. Nor must any animal which is likely to give birth during transit unless upon certification by a veterinary surgeon. If an animal becomes unfit during the journey it must be unloaded at the earliest opportunity in order to receive attention.

Dead animals

Carcasses of animals must not be carried on the same vehicle along with live animals. Any animals which die in transit must be removed at the first opportunity.

Cleaning and disinfection

This exercise must be completed as soon as possible after unloading the last animals and always before loading other animals.

The vehicle and accessories must be swept, washed and scrubbed with water, followed by a soaking in an approved disinfectant. The sweepings must be disposed of so that they cannot come into contact with other animals. Special requirements apply if the vehicle is carrying diseased animals or those suspected of being infected, or if it has carried carcasses or dung.

Construction of vehicles

Detailed requirements are specified in the orders.

NB Although there are certain exemptions in regard to the construction of vehicles to the provision of **The Transit of Animals (Road and Rail)**

Order, 1975, if you own and use a small vehicle, you must nevertheless comply with the general requirements. This includes the requirement to carry a ramp in the vehicle for loading or unloading if the vehicle floor is more than 31 cm from the ground.

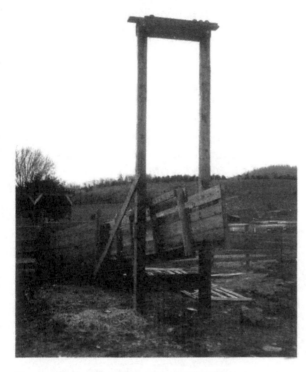

A shute for loading and unloading sheep on and off vehicles. The height can be adjusted by means of pulleys attached to the 'guillotine' (eastern United States).

Separation of animals in transit

Rules regarding the carrying of different species and classes of animals in the same vehicle are specified in Schedule 2.

Records

A **Form of record in respect of the carriage of animals by road** must be completed within 18 hours of carriage, except that the details relating to times of loading and unloading, feeding and watering, must be entered **immediately** these tasks are performed. Records must be available for inspection by the police, inspectors of MAFF and Animal Health Inspectors.

These records are over and above those which must be kept under the **Movement of Animals (Records) Order, 1960.** These latter are vital for tracing animal movements during outbreaks of notifiable diseases such as foot and mouth disease and sheep scab.

APPENDIX 5

NOTIFIABLE DISEASES

In the UK, by Act of Parliament (Diseases of Animals Act, 1950; Animal Health Act, 1981) a number of important diseases are notifiable—that is to say, the owner or person in charge of an animal suffering from a suspected notifiable disease must immediately report the suspicion to the police or to a veterinary officer of the Ministry of Agriculture in England and Wales or the Department of Agriculture in Scotland.

The acts give powers to the authorities to enable them to prevent certain diseases from entering the UK (e.g. foot and mouth), to eradicate diseases already present (e.g. sheep scab) or to control the spread of others (e.g. bovine spongiform encephalopathy, BSE). All the notifiable diseases are infectious and/or contagious and most are of considerable economic significance. A number are zoonoses—that is, they are transmissible to human beings (e.g. rabies and anthrax).

The methods used to deal with individual notifiable diseases have been developed to do so in the most efficient and cost-effective manner, but they need to be under constant review, since disease patterns change and new challenges arise. Although the present measures for dealing with sheep scab have failed to eradicate the disease to date, the costs to the taxpayer and to individual farmers for the current scheme are far less than if the disease were to be allowed to run its course unchecked.

Accounts of the most important notifiable diseases are given throughout the text at appropriate places. For example, foot and mouth disease is described in the chapter on lameness. Many notifiable diseases have been eradicated from the UK but remain on the list because the risk remains, even though it may be slight.

As of February, 1989, the law requires the existence, or suspected existence, of the following to be notified immediately to the police or a Ministry veterinary officer:

African horse sickness
African swine fever
Anthrax
Aujeszky's disease
Bovine spongiform encephalopathy
(BSE)
Brucella melitensis in cattle
Cattle plague in ruminants and
swine
Classical swine fever
Contagious equine metritis
Dourine in horses, asses, mules
and zebras
Enzootic bovine leukosis
Epizootic lymphangitis in horses,
asses and mules
Equine encephalomyelitis

Equine infectious anaemia
Foot and mouth disease in
ruminants and swine
Fowl pest (fowl plague, Newcastle
disease and paramyxovirus) in
poultry of all kinds
Glanders and farcy in horses,
asses and mules
Paramyxovirus in pigeons
Pleuro-pneumonia in cattle
Rabies
Sheep pox
Sheep scab
Swine vesicular disease (SVD)
Warble fly
Teschen disease of pigs
Tuberculosis in cattle (certain forms)

Further information can be obtained from Animal Health Division A, Hook Rise South, Tolworth, Surbiton, Surrey KT6 7NF.

Anthrax

Anthrax is a notifiable disease which is also transmissible to humans, in whom it can cause a dangerous and sometimes fatal disease. It is caused by the bacterium *Bacillus anthracis*, which is generally taken in by mouth from contaminated foodstuffs, usually of imported origin.

Anthrax is usually rapidly fatal, animals simply being found dead, although occasionally there may be a short illness where the animal runs a high fever of 107°C (41.5°F), becomes very dull and breathes rapidly before collapsing and dying. The blood of affected animals fails to clot and may run freely from the nose, mouth, rectum or vagina. This should make the owner even more suspicious and the authorities (police and state veterinary service) should be informed immediately. This blood will be teeming with anthrax bacteria which contaminate the area where the animal dies. As soon as the blood is exposed to the air the bacteria immediately form spores which are highly resistant and can survive for very many years—certainly for 50 years, but perhaps for a century or longer.

The author once diagnosed anthrax following the sudden death of a dairy cow in a herd which had been grazing in a field adjacent to a site where once a tannery had stood. Although the tannery had been closed down some 60 years previously, the suspicion was that material from contaminated hides could have polluted the stream running alongside the works. Recent heavy rain had caused erosion and flooding of the surrounding pastures. Cows may have become infected by grazing these pastures or by drinking from the stream. A number of other cows in the herd became ill with a fever, but recovered after treatment with penicillin.

Anthrax cases are much less common than they used to be, due to restrictions on the imports of certain types of meat products. Indeed, in 1988 there were only three recorded cases in the UK, whereas before the implementation of these restrictions there used to be several hundred cases annually. Cases in sheep are relatively rare because they eat fewer concentrate feeds than cows or pigs, but cases still occur occasionally. Any suspicion must be reported to the police or to Ministry veterinary officers. On no account should the carcass of any suspect animal be moved or cut open. Apart from the risk of contaminating the area further, there is also a risk to humans, particularly from the blood of infected animals. The greatest risk to humans, however, is from inhaling the bacterial spores which have dried on the hide or fleece of infected animals—so-called wool sorter's disease—a frequently fatal septicaemia unless treatment is applied early.

Ministry veterinary staff will confirm the diagnosis and place a movements order on the premises until the carcass has been burned, along with the turfs or bedding where the animal lay, and the area disinfected.

APPENDIX 6

ZOONOSES

A number of diseases are transmissible to humans and these are known as zoonoses. Some are merely inconvenient, whilst others are downright dangerous and even life-threatening.

Should anyone become ill whilst shepherding or assisting with the flock and it is known or suspected that a zoonotic disease is present on the farm, **medical advice should be sought without delay**. The doctor should be informed of the presence of the suspect disease in the flock and referred to your veterinary surgeon where appropriate for further information. Abortion in ewes and diarrhoea in lambs carry particular risks, and **pregnant women and young children should not assist at lambing time**.

Below is a list of zoonoses, some of which are rare, but cases of all of which are on record.

Disease	Risk to humans
abortion agents	foetus, placenta and birth fluids all pose a risk
brucella	rare in UK, common elsewhere in the world
campylobacter	severe diarrhoea but uncommon
chlamydia (enzootic abortion)	**life-threatening in pregnant women**
listeria	risk of abortion or still birth in women
Q fever (*Coxiella burnetii*)	mainly unapparent infection in man or flu-like disease; occasionally serious complications in compromised patients
salmonella	relatively uncommon but a real risk to humans when it does occur
toxoplasma	cat faeces and improperly cooked meat are the main sources of infection for

653

	man, but the products of abortion do pose a risk; **especially dangerous to pregnant women** in whom it may cause serious defects in the unborn child
anthrax	rare in the UK; potentially fatally septicaemia
brucella	see 'abortion'
cryptosporidia	from faeces of scouring lambs; unpleasant diarrhoea
contagious pustular dermatitis	see 'orf'
dermatophilus	see 'lumpy wool'
enzootic abortion	see 'abortion agents, chlamydia'
erysipelas	skin rash, usually from contaminated dip (see post-dipping lameness in text)
leptospirosis	variety of serious symptoms in man but rarely contracted from sheep
listeriosis	see 'abortion agents'
louping ill	from handling infected brain at post-mortem, so mostly in veterinary surgeons, laboratory workers or vaccine manufacturers; also, but rarely, from tick bites
lumpy wool (dermatophilus)	rare but recorded
orf (contagious pustular dermatitis)	painful lesions and occasionally fever and generalised symptoms
post-dipping lameness	see 'erysipelas'
salmonella	from diarrhoea in lambs; see also 'abortion agents'. Diarrhoea, vomiting or septicaemia in man
strawberry footrot	see 'lumpy wool' and 'orf', as both organisms may be involved
toxoplasma	see 'abortion agents'

APPENDIX 7

DIPPING TECHNIQUE

Dipping is a stressful procedure for sheep which is not without risk. Unfortunately, there is, at present, no alternative technique which is approved for the control of sheep scab. It is to be hoped that less traumatic measures will eventually become available. Meanwhile, it is important to carry out the task correctly and with the welfare of the sheep firmly in mind.

The following notes are reproduced with the permission of the Agricultural Training Board from their trainee guide, *Dipping Sheep*.

Preparing materials and equipment

First of all, clean out all grilles and channels to ensure that the draining pens have good drainage back into the bath.

Several days before dipping will begin, thoroughly clean the dip bath.

Clean the filter which excludes solid dung (if applicable).

If you do not know it, calculate the exact capacity of the dip bath and check the existing calibrations, or calibrate the bath by marking the side at 50 litre or 100 litre (10 gallon or 20 gallon) intervals.

Alternatively, paint marks or carve notches at intervals on a dip-stick to indicate the bath's capacity at varying depths. It is advisable to copy the stick markings on a permanent site, such as a door or wall, for making replacements.

Ensure that:

- sufficient dip concentrate/powder is available
- an adequate water supply is available
- the outlet tap or plug on the dip bath is working correctly and not leaking
- all the holding and draining pens are clean

Examine any wooden steps out of the dip bath for condition and secure fixing, making repairs where necessary.

**If dipping controls are in force, the local authority must be
notified of the date of dipping and given at least three days' clear
notice.**

Bringing the sheep into the yard

Do not dip newly sheared sheep—each animal must have at least three
weeks' wool growth.

Bring the sheep into the yard at least six hours before dipping
(preferably the evening before).

Do not crowd the sheep in holding pens.

Do not feed the sheep whilst they are yarded, but ensure that they have
ample drinking water.

Dag adult sheep if necessary.

Do not dip sheep which are due to be slaughtered fairly soon (see
the dip concentrate manufacturer's instructions for the length of the safe
period).

Making up the dip wash

Always make up the dip wash on the day it will be used.

If in a hard water area, either use rain water or soften the tap water with
washing soda.

When using washing soda to soften the water:
- soften the water an hour or two before mixing the dip
- calculate the quantity of soda and weigh out 2 to 5 grams of soda
  for every litre of water required in the dip (2 to 5 lb soda for every
  100 gallons of water)
- first, dissolve the soda in a small quantity of hot water and then stir this
  into the remaining quantity of water

Wear rubber gloves and a face-shield at all times when handling dip
concentrate.

Wear rubber boots and a waterproof bib-apron at all times when
handling diluted liquid and freshly dipped sheep.

If you are splashed in the face or eyes with concentrate, wash
thoroughly with plenty of water and obtain medical attention as soon as
possible.

When mixing the dip, read and follow the dip manufacturer's instructions
carefully.

Measure the quantities of concentrate and water carefully.

Do not increase the strength of the dip wash even when a badly
infested flock is to be dipped

Wash out the empty concentrate containers and add the washings to the dip bath.

Mix the diluted liquid well, stirring it right to the bottom of the bath, including vertical movements.

Moving the sheep into the holding pen

Move the sheep to the holding pen through a foot bath of plain water if possible. This will help to keep the dip wash clean and reduce the frequency of refilling.

Decide upon the order in which the sheep will be dipped. Points affecting the order chosen may include:

- if rams are dipped first, their size may cause the bath to overflow but
- it is easier to put heavy ewes and rams in the bath first, when the operators are not tired
- lambs, having more wool, tend to strip the dip wash, so may be best left till last

At regular intervals during the dipping operation, hose down the holding pen to keep dung and dirt in the pen from being transferred to the dip wash.

Dipping sheep

Do not dip sheep which are heated, wet, recently fed, tired or thirsty.

Wear rubber boots, rubber gloves and a waterproof bib-apron.

Stir the dip wash thoroughly from the bottom of the bath (along its entire length) before dipping any sheep, occasionally between sheep and also whenever there has been a break during dipping.

When dipping:

- do not dip sheep in dip wash which is becoming very dirty or fouled (replace with fresh dip wash)
- do not eat, drink or smoke without removing all protective clothing (except overall or rubber boots), washing your hands and face and leaving the dipping area

Finish a day's dipping in time to allow all the sheep to dry before evening.

When dipping sheep in cold weather, do not use a warm dip wash.

Do not dip sheep in wet weather or when they are wet or when the air temperature is falling.

Smear any wounds on the sheep with petroleum jelly before dipping.

(a) Simple dip baths (non-mechanical).

Move a sheep to the end of the bath and lower it tail first into the bath, at the same time pushing it forward.

When lifting a sheep, place one arm under its neck (low down towards its breast) and grip the loose skin of its opposite flank with the other hand.

Do not lift the animal by its fleece.

Do not put a sheep into the bath on its back.

(b) Semi-automatic baths (i.e. having a trap-door).

Do not overcrowd the sheep in the bath.

Ensure that each sheep:

- is in the bath for the correct period of time
- goes completely beneath the surface of the dip wash
- does not get into difficulties

(c) All dip baths.

After the initial shock of entry is over, use a brush or crutch to duck the sheep's head under once or twice, quickly enough to avoid the animal taking in any of the dip wash.

Ensure that each animal stays in the dip for at least one minute.

Do not overcrowd the sheep in the bath.

Skim off any scum from the surface of the dip wash as it forms (i.e. between batches).

Remove or change immediately any clothing which becomes heavily contaminated with dip wash.

Replenish the dip bath when necessary (see later).

Do not use any dip wash in the bath for more than one day.

Do not dip more than about three sheep for each 4.5 litres (1 gallon) of the original dip wash before completely renewing it.

Do not use a running water hose to keep up the dip wash level in the bath as this will weaken the solution.

Assist weak sheep or sheep in poor condition if they become exhausted during the swim and are in difficulties or are unable to climb out of the bath.

Hose down the holding pen regularly to avoid transferring any dung and dirt from the pen to the dip wash.

Releasing sheep into the draining pen

Do not overcrowd the sheep in the draining pen.

Ensure that there is good drainage of the dip wash back into the bath and that the filter does not become blocked with dung.

Do not herd the sheep into a closed shed after dipping.

Allow the sheep to rest in the shade for a few hours; do not drive them immediately after dipping.

Newly dipped sheep which are not fully dry **must** be given shelter from rain.

Brush out the draining pens regularly to prevent a build-up of dung. (Do not hose down these pens since this will dilute the dip wash in the bath.)

Replenishing the dip bath

The level in the bath must not be allowed to fall by more than one-fifth (i.e. by not more than 250 litres in a 1,250 litre bath or 50 gallons in a 250 gallon bath).

Make up the replenishing solution carefully in accordance with the dip manufacturer's instructions.

NB The replenishing dip wash is usually more concentrated than the original solution in the bath.

Returning the sheep to grazing

After dipping, do not carry out other stock tasks on the sheep on the same day.

After allowing the sheep to drain, turn them out into shady yards or a nearby paddock, where there is shelter.

Do not drive dipped sheep any distance until they are fairly dry.

If the sheep are to be housed after dipping, ensure that they are almost dry before putting them indoors.

Emptying the bath

Dispose of the used dip wash in a suitably safe manner (e.g. in a soakaway or by a waste disposal company).

Do not pour the used dip wash into a pond, stream or anywhere that it might be a hazard to people, livestock or natural life.

Avoid putting the used dip wash in a slurry system, where it might eventually be put back on the land.

Cleaning the equipment and disposing of rubbish

Hose down all the equipment and pens thoroughly.

Wash all protective clothing thoroughly.

Store all loose equipment and protective clothing away in their correct places.

Send returnable empty containers back to the supplier without delay.

Burn empty packages and cartons in an open space—but keep away from the fumes which may be toxic.

Puncture and flatten non-returnable drums and cans and bury them, or use the local authority waste disposal service.

Do not dump empty containers in situations where they might drain into ditches, drains or wells.

Store unused liquid or powder concentrate in sealed containers in a locked store inaccessible to children.

Thoroughly wash your hands and exposed skin before meals and after work.

APPENDIX 8

GLOSSARY

Definitions are given as used in the context of this book.

adhesion	the sticking together of internal organs during the healing process following inflammation, causing restriction of movement and pain.
adjuvant	substance added to a medicine to modify the action of the main ingredient (e.g. an oily substance added to a vaccine to slow the release of the antigen).
aftermath	a regrowth of grass after mowing.
anoestrus	period of suspended sexual activity in ewes, which in the UK occurs during spring and early summer when the days are long (lactation and poor nutrition may also influence).
attenuation	weakening the potency of a microorganism, toxin, or drug.
basic slag	a phosphorus-rich by-product of the steel industry used as a slow-release fertiliser (also contains trace elements).
bolus	a rounded mass of medicine.
cast ewe	older hill ewe sold to lowland farms for further breeding under kinder conditions.
carrier state	the harbouring of infection without displaying clinical illness.
clamp (silage)	method of storage of grass for conservation in a compact pile.
cleats (clays, claws, clees)	the two halves of the sheep's foot.
closed flock	one breeding its own female replacements and purchasing only rams.
comatose	in a state of profound unconsciousness from which the patient cannot be roused.

661

contagious disease	one transmissible by direct physical contact between animals.
crutch	remove wool around the genitalia.
cull	dispose of animals before the end of their productive life because of disease, injury or poor productivity.
degradable	dietary protein which is broken down into amino acids by the rumen microorganisms (see undegradable).
dehydration	loss of water from the body tissues.
devitalised	deprived of life.
dystocia	abnormal (difficult) labour.
ensile	to make crops into silage.
flushing	feeding of better-quality grazing (or occasionally concentrates) to ewes in the weeks prior to mating to improve ovulation rate (number of eggs shed).
gangrene	death and putrefaction of tissues due to loss of blood supply, often as a result of infection.
gimmers	female sheep between first and second shearing.
gross margin	the enterprise output less its variable costs.
heft	portion of a hirsel (there are normally about 5 or 6 hefts to the hirsel).
hirsel	large area of hill ground and the flock grazing it, usually tended by one shepherd.
hogg	male or female sheep between weaning and first shearing—e.g. wether hogg, ewe hogg.
implant	solid substance (such as a hormone or medicine) embedded in the tissues (usually under the skin) to ensure sustained action.
in-bye	fenced land between fields and open hill.
infectious disease	one transmissible by direct means.
lambing percentage	the number of lambs born, weaned, or sold (must define which applies) per 100 ewes run with the ram.
lay-back	area of pasture adjacent to (for example) a root crop.
lesion	any morbid change in the structure or function of the living tissues of the body.
ley	temporary grassland (e.g. three year ley).
open flock	one which purchases a significant proportion of animals—particularly breeding females.
parasite	an organism which lives on (or in) another living organism (host) at the expense of the latter.
parks	low ground fenced fields.
raddle	paint or crayon applied to a ram's chest to mark females he mates.

parturition	the process of giving birth.
rumen	a forestomach of a ruminant.
runty	small and undeveloped.
scour	diarrhoea
septicaemia	serious infection in which the bloodstream is invaded by large numbers of causal bacteria which multiply there.
shearling	male, female or castrated sheep from first to second shearing.
singleton	single lamb.
secondary infection	one superimposed on a primary infection by opportunist microorganisms.
steading	farmstead.
sub-fertile	less than acceptably fertile.
superovulation	use of natural or artificial methods of increasing the number of eggs shed at ovulation.
teaser	vasectomised ram.
toxaemia	generalised poisoning, due to soluble (usually bacterial) toxins entering bloodstream.
toxin	any poisonous substance of biological origin.
tup	ram.
tupped	(of ewes) mated.
tucked up	hunchbacked and empty bellied.
undegradable	dietary protein which escapes destruction by the rumen microorganisms and is digested later in the small intestine (see degradable).
unthrifty	poor-growing.
viraemia	viruses in the blood stream.
wintering (away)	practice of sending young stock to overwinter on grazings elsewhere.

APPENDIX 9

Some Metric Conversion Factors

British to Metric

Metric to British

LENGTH

inches to cm × 2.54	centimetres to in × 0.394
or mm × 25.4	millimetres to in × 0.0394
feet to m × 0.305	metres to ft × 3.29
yards to m × 0.914	metres to yd × 1.09
miles to km × 1.61	kilometres to miles × 0.621

AREA

sq feet to m^2 × 0.093	sq metres to ft^2 × 10.8
sq yards to m^2 × 0.836	sq metres to yd^2 × 1.20
acres to ha × 0.405	hectares to ac × 2.47

VOLUME (LIQUID)

pints to litres × 0.568	litres to pints × 1.76
gallons to litres × 4.55	litres to gallons × 0.22

WEIGHT

ounces to g × 28.3	grams to oz × 0.0353
pounds to g × 454	grams to lb × 0.0022
pounds to kg × 0.454	kilograms to lb × 2.20
hundredweights to kg × 50.8	kilograms to cwt × 0.020
hundredweights to t × 0.0508	tonnes to tons × 0.984
tons to kg × 1016	
tons to tonnes × 1.016	

TEMPERATURE

(°C × 1.8) + 32 = °F

SOME DOUBLE CONVERSIONS

fertiliser units/acre	× 1.25	= kg/hectare
cwt/acre	× 0.125	= t/ha
lb/acre	× 1.1	= kg/ha
pints/acre	× 1.4	= litres/ha

INDEX

MALE REPRODUCTIVE ORGANS

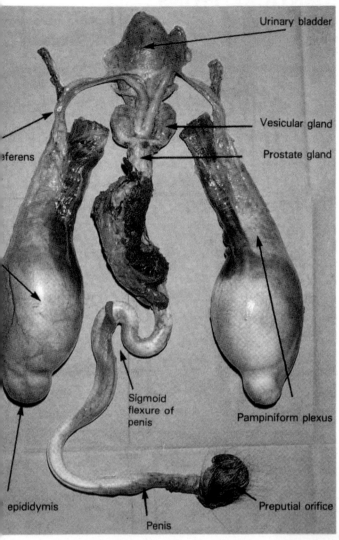

Urinary bladder

Vesicular gland

Prostate gland

eferens

Sigmoid flexure of penis

Pampiniform plexus

epididymis

Penis

Preputial orifice

1 Reproductive organs of the ram dissected out.

2 Testis and epididymis of the ram.

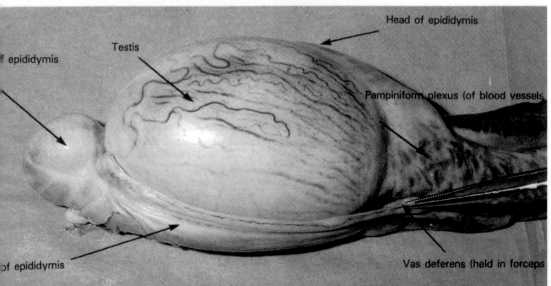

Head of epididymis

Testis

f epididymis

Pampiniform plexus (of blood vessels

of epididymis

Vas deferens (held in forceps

EMBRYO SPLITTING FOR THE PRODUCTION OF IDENTICAL TWINS

Photos taken down a light microscope. This technique is carried out using a micromanipulator. See Plate 3.22 on page 129, where the resulting lambs are also shown.

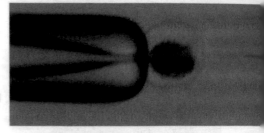

3   Sheep embryo of six days' development is held by suction to a pipette (left) whilst the eggshell is pierced by the glass knife.

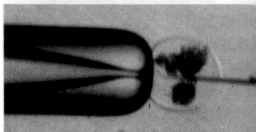

4   Knife pierces embryo.

5   Embryo transferred to top of pipette which acts as support whilst embryo is cut in half by sawing action of knife.

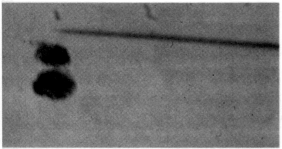

6   Two halves of embryo removed from eggs

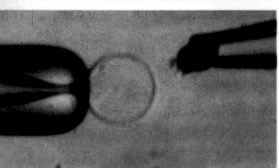

7   Empty eggshell (centre) held ready to acce half of divided embryo.

8   Other half of embryo transferred to spare eggshell.

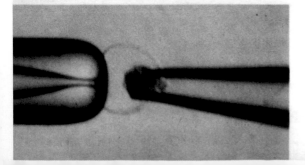

FOETAL DEATH

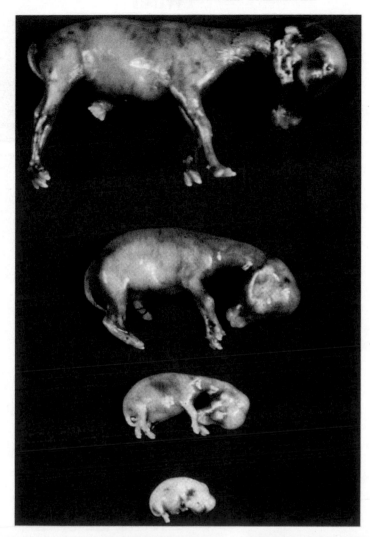

9 Sheep foetuses at 34, 41, 48 and 55 days' gestation (bottom to top).

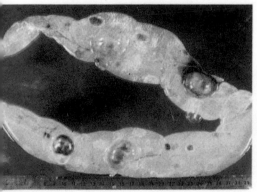

The contents of the uterus at 34 days pregnancy (trophoblast) containing four ?uses, one of which is dead (upper left). ?mbing the triplets born would only have ? the size of quads.

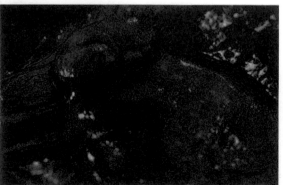

11 A dead foetus the size of a finger nail found in the afterbirth at a normal lambing. This foetus died at around one month of gestation and the twins born alive were approximately 30 per cent lighter than expected.

FOETAL LIFE

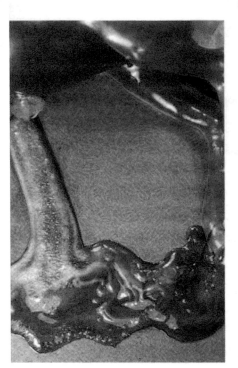

12 The lifeline of the foetal lamb—the umbilical cord.

13 Part of a normal placenta of a foetal lamb. Note the clean, fresh pink appearance.

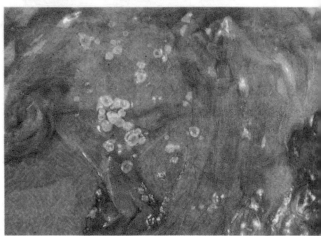

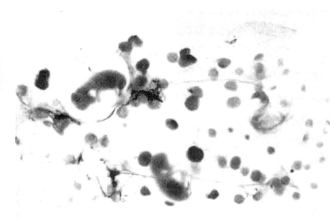

14 Early twin foetuses in their individual placental membranes. Note the early placentomes or 'buttons'.

15 Comparison of two foetuses and their placentae at 120 days' (top) and 70 days' gestation. Note the fluid-filled sacs (stained) which surround and protect the foetus.

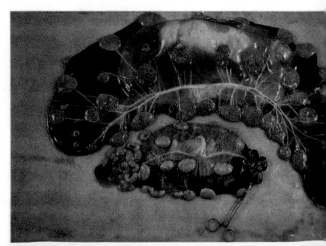

ABORTION

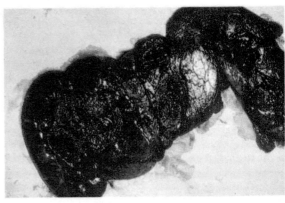

16 An infected placenta from a case of enzootic abortion of ewes. Note the abnormally thickened red tissues between the 'buttons'.

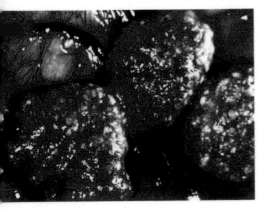

17 Toxoplasma abortion. Note the white spots (foci of infection) in the 'buttons'.

OTHER CONDITIONS OF PREGNANCY

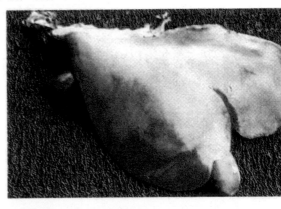

18 Liver from a ewe with pregnancy toxaemia. Note the pale, pasty appearance due to heavy fat deposits.

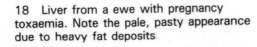
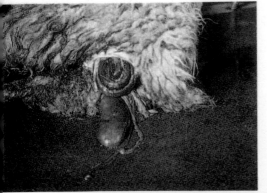

19 Prolapse of the intestines through a prolapsed vagina. This serious complication usually results in rapid death or the humane destruction of the ewe.

MASTITIS

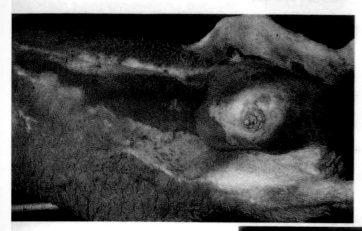

20 Acute fatal mastitis in a ewe. Note that the inflammation has spread along the belly.

21 Abscesses in the udder at post-mortem. Note the creamy pus and the inflamed appearance of the whole 'half' of the gland.

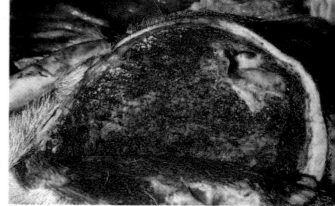

WELFARE OF LAMBS

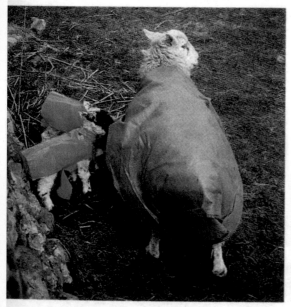

22 The latest designer plastic fashion macs for the whole family!

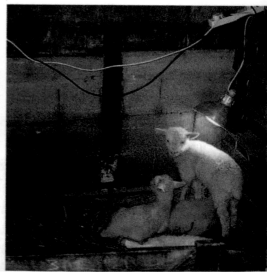

23 Lambs under a dangerously close infra-red lamp. Lambs have been barbecued in this way.

GUT CONDITIONS OF THE LAMB

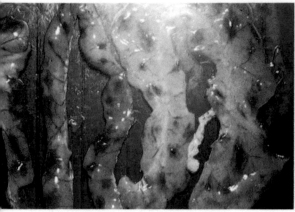

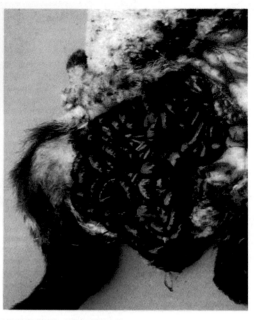

24 Intestine of a lamb with lamb dysentery. Note the raw bleeding areas where the gut lining has stripped off.

25 Redgut—there has been massive haemorrhage into the intestines from ruptured blood vessels.

CONDITIONS RESULTING FROM NAVEL OR WOUND INFECTIONS

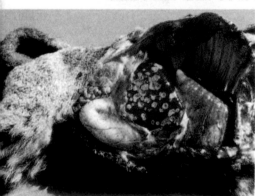

26 Numerous liver abscesses caused by one of the bacteria responsible for footrot (*Fusobacterium necrophorum*) which invaded the body via the navel cord.

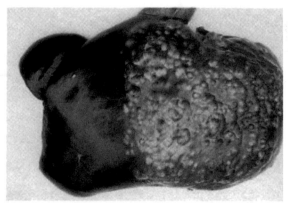

27 Tick pyaemia—numerous abscesses in the liver of a lamb at post-mortem.

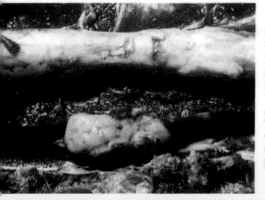

28 Spinal abscess in a shearling ram. The spinal cord has been lifted out of the spinal canal—note the narrower portion of the cord which was caused by pressure from the abscess which can be seen (pale yellow) bulging into the now empty spinal canal. The ram had difficulty walking initially and eventually went off its hind legs altogether. The bacteria responsible may have entered the body via the navel at birth or via some wound in later life and travelled in the bloodstream to the spinal canal.

PNEUMONIA

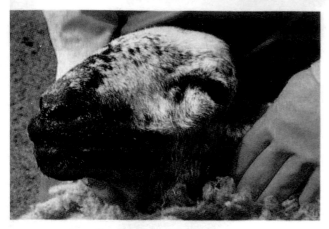

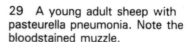

29 A young adult sheep with pasteurella pneumonia. Note the bloodstained muzzle.

30 Pasteurella pneumonia at post-mortem. Note the plum-coloured consolidated lungs which look like liver and the large amount of bloodstained fluid.

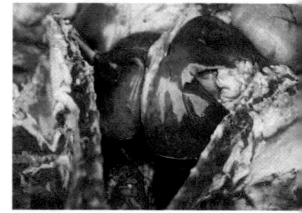

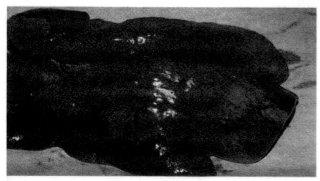

31 Lung from a case of atypical pneumonia. The darker liver-coloured areas (mainly around the bottom) are solid and functionless. Only the salmon-pink areas are capable of exchanging oxygen for carbon dioxide, and so this animal had only a half to two-thirds lung capacity. This would reduce feed conversion and slow weight gain very significantly.

32 The plucks of lambs with atypical pneumonia, which often goes undiagnosed until slaughter.

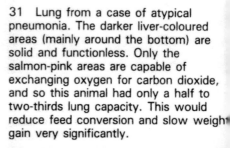

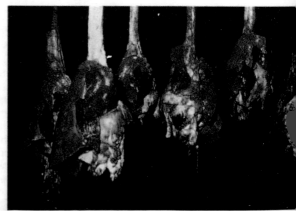

TRACE ELEMENTS

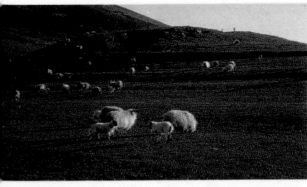

33 Scottish Blackface ewes and lambs on improved marginal land. Productive pastures such as these allow the stocking rate to be increased, but they may pose a risk to both ewes and lambs from mineral and trace element deficiencies.

34 Free-access minerals. The rich brown colour suggests a high iron content that may make copper unavailable and thereby induce copper deficiency.

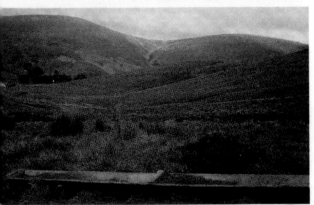

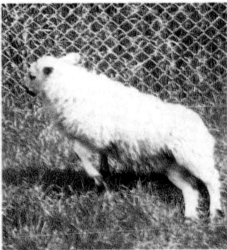

35 Swayback lamb.

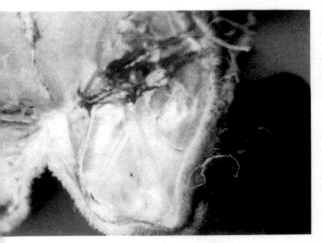

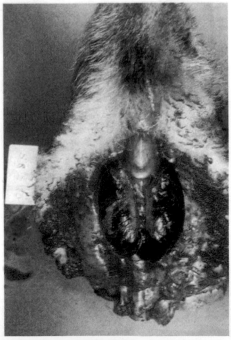

36 White muscle disease in a lamb at post-mortem. Note the extreme pallor of the muscles.

37 Lamb's head at post-mortem showing the enlarged thyroid gland (damson-coloured) in a case of goitre.

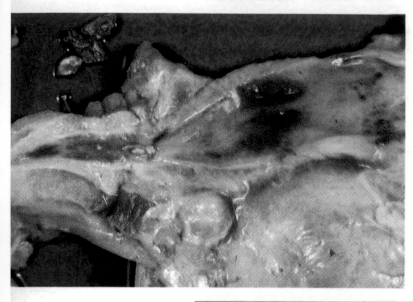

38 Male urinary tract opened up to show inflammation (red areas) caused by urinary calculi, some of which have been removed (on blue background).

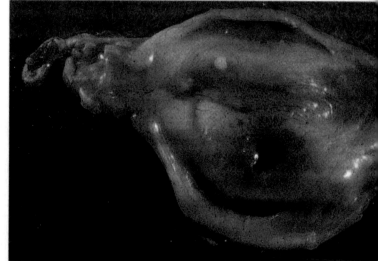

39 Bladder. Note severe bruising (deep red) due to damage by calculi.

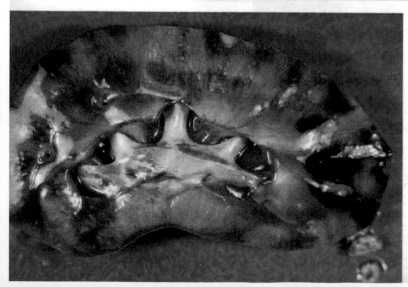

40 Kidney. Bruising (almost black areas) was due to calculi (removed, on blue background).

INTERNAL PARASITES

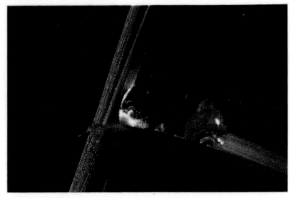

41　Third stage infective larvae of a parasitic worm in a dewdrop on a blade of grass.

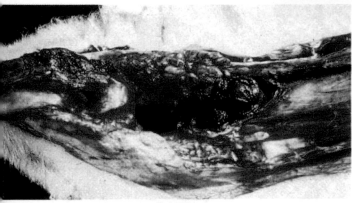

42　Dosing gun injury to the pharynx of a lamb. Animals will die or have to be destroyed as a consequence of this type of serious injury.

BLADDERWORMS

43　Bladderworm (*Coenurus cerebralis*) in the brain of a sheep. The pressure of such a large cyst in the brain causes the nervous symptoms associated with gid.

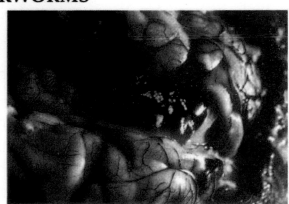

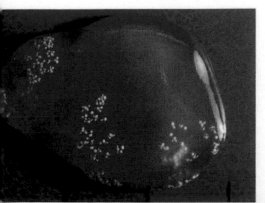

44　A very large bladderworm (3 inches or 7.6 cm long) removed from the brain of a sheep with gid. The small white circular spots (scolices) on the inner surface of the cyst develop into adult tapeworms (*Taenia multiceps*) when eaten by dogs.

PARASITIC CONDITIONS OF THE SHEEP'S LIVER

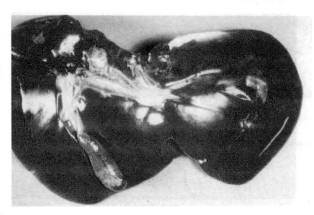

45 Normal sheep's liver. The dark green sausage-shaped object is the gall bladder.

46 Chronic liver fluke infection. Note the grossly thickened bile ducts (top) caused by the blood sucking activity of large numbers of adult liver flukes.

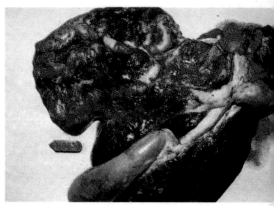

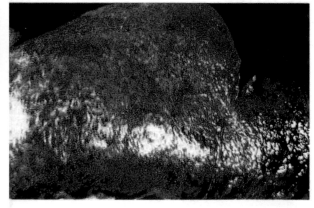

47 Liver of a lamb with acute liver fluke disease. Note how totally different it looks from a normal liver. The black areas are haemorrhaged blood caused by the burrowing of thousands of immature flukes.

48 Hydatid liver of a sheep. The lighter areas indicate the location of hydatid cysts. Dogs eating these become infected with the tapeworm *Echinococcus granulosus*, the eggs of which are passed out in faeces and constitute a source of infection for sheep and, more importantly, humans.

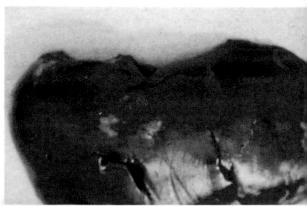

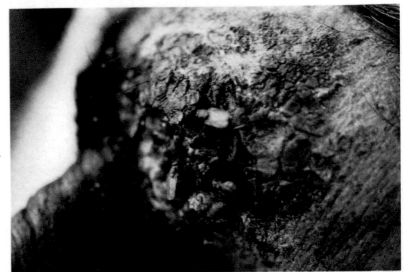

49 Headfly damage ('broken head') at the hornbase of a young Scottish Blackface sheep. A few flies remain feeding. The rasping action of their mouthparts initiates these lesions, and self-inflicted damage makes them worse.

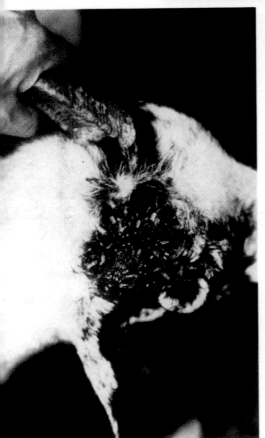

50 Headfly. In this distressing case, the lamb has broken off its horn in trying to rid itself of the headflies. Note the large number of flies feeding. This type of damage is also prone to blowfly strike.

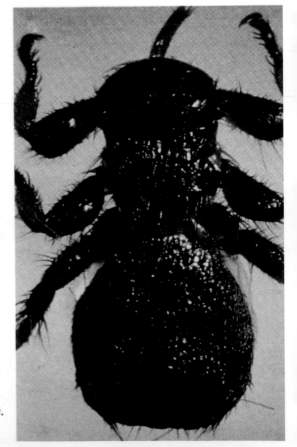

51 The sheep ked—*Melophagus ovinus*.

SOME SKIN CONDITIONS IN MAN CONTRACTED FROM SHEEP

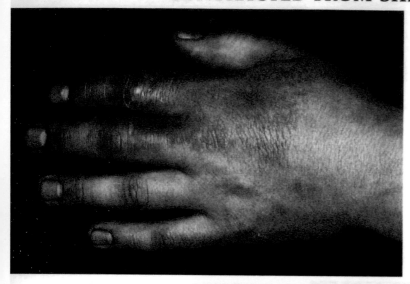

52 Erysipeloid in man from contaminated dip (see Colour plate 63).

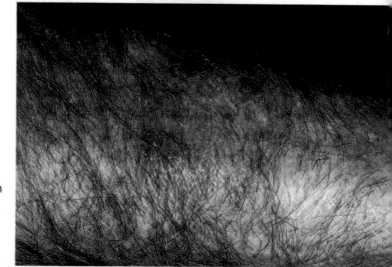

53 Ringworm—a human case on the forearm, contracted from an animal.

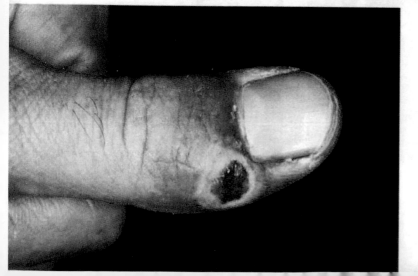

WOOL

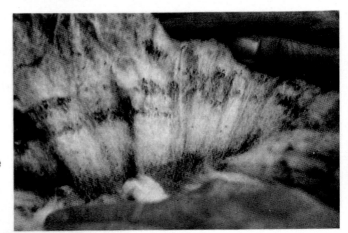

55 Lumpy wool or mycotic dermatitis. Note the brown colouration close to the skin and the crusty layer within the fleece which is evidence of an earlier episode.

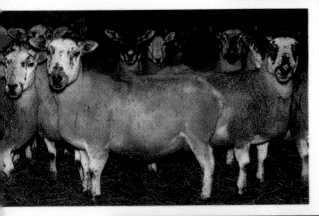

56 Wool slip in housed shorn Greyface ewes.

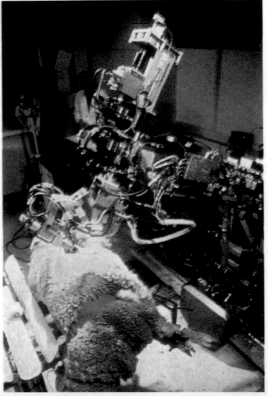

57 Sheep being sheared by a prototype robotic machine in Australia. We have a duty to consider very carefully the welfare aspects of any new husbandry procedures before they are widely used and accepted.

CONTAGIOUS PUSTULAR DERMATITIS—ORF

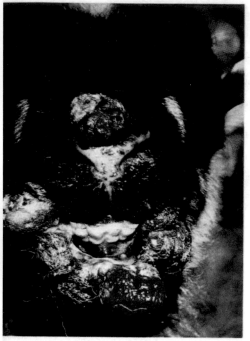

58 A severe case of orf on the muzzle of a Scottish Blackface lamb.

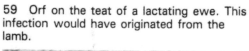

59 Orf on the teat of a lactating ewe. This infection would have originated from the lamb.

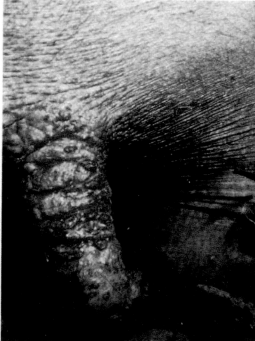

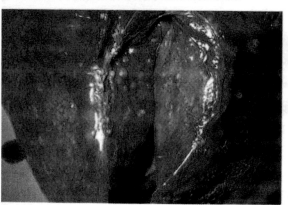

60 Orf infection in the lungs. The pea-sized lumps are the orf lesions. This is a most unusual case.

61 Strawberry footrot is an unsightly and unpleasant lameness, usually of older lambs. Both the orf virus and dermatophilus may be found in the lesions.

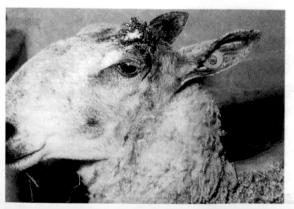

62 Crusty orf lesions on the poll of a Blueface Leicester ram. Lesions of this type tend to come and go and may be one way that the virus persists in a flock.

SOME SKIN CONDITIONS

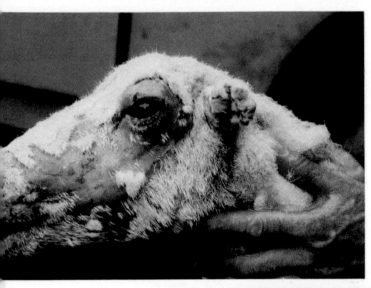

63 Erysipelas infection of the head from contaminated dip (see Colour plate 52).

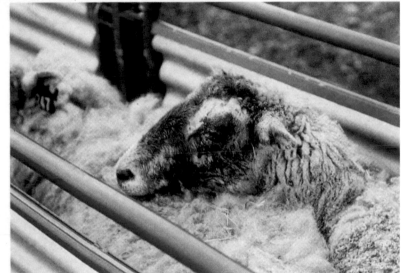

64 Facial dermatitis or peri-orbital eczema.

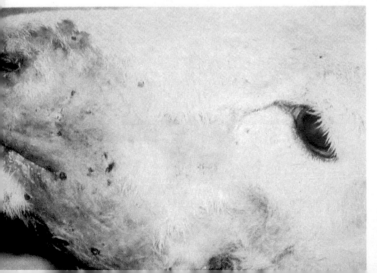

65 'Cruels' or actinobacillosis. Abscesses may discharge thick green pus onto the skin surface.

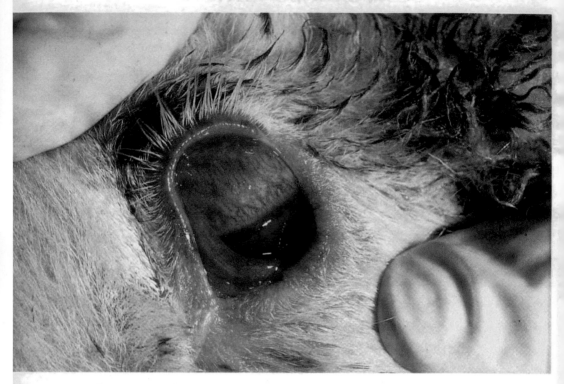

66 Pinkeye due to *Mycoplasma conjunctivae* — a highly infectious and contagious disease.

67 Pinkeye in an adult animal which has progressed to cause serious damage to the cornea and temporary blindness in that eye.

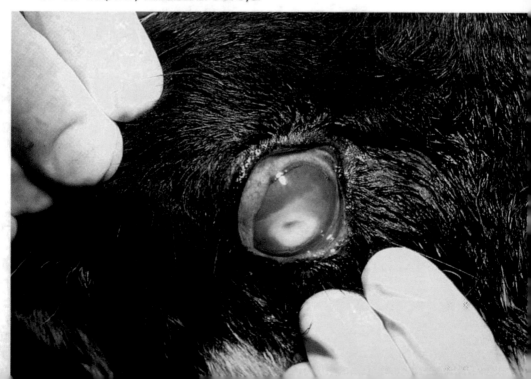

INCISOR TEETH

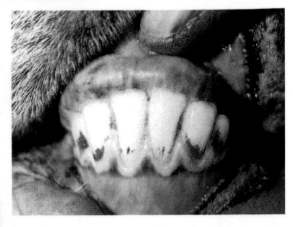

68 A good mouth of teeth in an adult ewe. The incisors are held firmly in healthy gums and also meet the upper dental pad snugly. (The slight brown discolouration is of no consequence.)

69 An early stage in the development of broken mouth—erosion of the gums. Note how the crowns of the teeth (the bits you can see) are longer than normal and how the gums are swollen, inflamed and bleeding.

70 Broken mouth in a ewe. One pair of incisors have been lost and those remaining have sharp front edges. The central incisors have very long crowns due to receding gums and lack of wear against the dental pad and are likely to be the next to be lost.

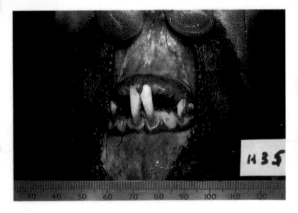

CHEEK TEETH

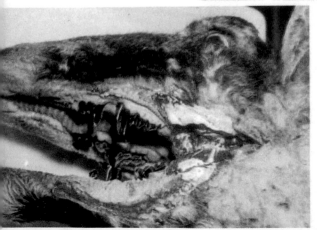

71 Disease of the cheek teeth in a ewe at post-mortem. A number of teeth are missing, and their opposite numbers in the other jaw have grown long sharp crowns due to lack of wear. The sharp edges can lacerate the gums, cheeks and tongue. Sheep with loose or overgrown cheek teeth as shown here cannot grind their food adequately. In consequence they may develop digestive upsets and frequently lose body condition.

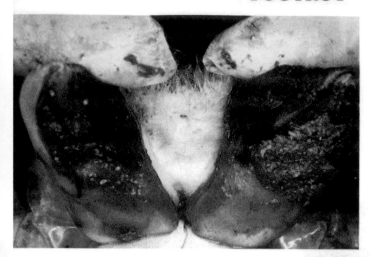

72 Normal foot (washed). Note the pale pink colour of normal interdigital skin and the undamaged horn.

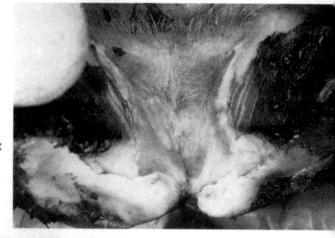

73 Footrot (washed). Note how the skin between the cleats is inflamed and how the soft horn at the bulbs of the heels has been eaten away by the bacterial infection.

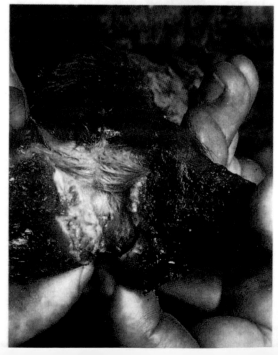

74 Footrot (unwashed). Note how wet and angry the tissues are — this virulent form of footrot is very painful.

FOOT AND MOUTH DISEASE

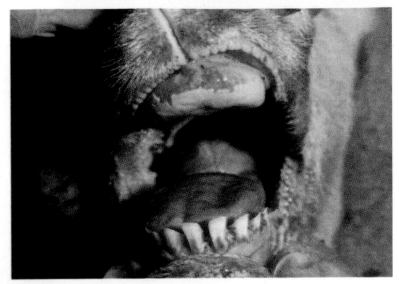

75 Ulcers on the dental pad and gums (two days after infection).

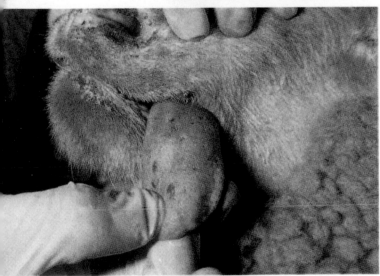

76 Ulcers on the tongue (two days after infection).

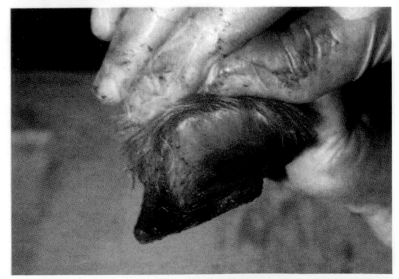

77 Unruptured vesicle on the coronary band (24 hours after infection).

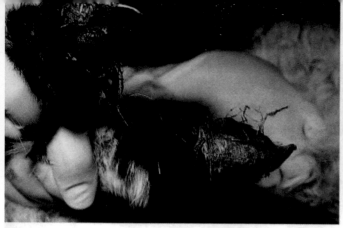

78 Redfoot—the whole horny shell of one cleat of each foot has been lost, exposing the bleeding, sensitive tissues underneath.

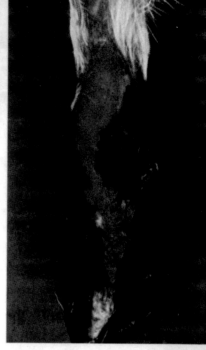

79 Redfoot—the skin of the leg is splitting and peeling and the hoof horn has split and is about to be shed.

80 Ergot poisoning.

81 Ergot poisoning.

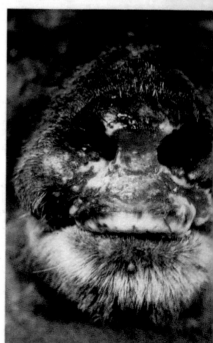

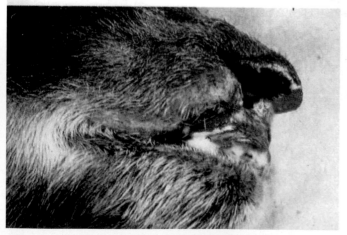

SOME POISONOUS PLANTS

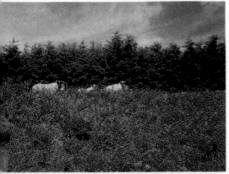

82　Bracken.

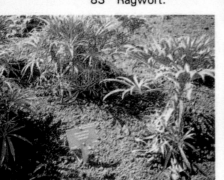

83　Ragwort.

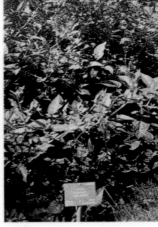

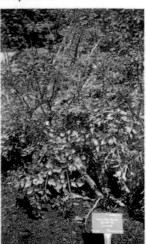

86　Deadly nightshade.

87　Woody nightshade.

88　Foxglove.

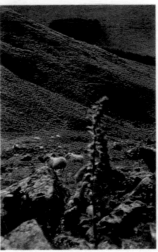

89　Hemlock water dropwort.

84　Stinking hellebore.

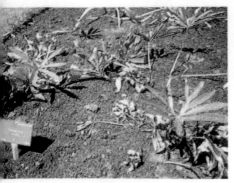

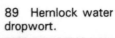

85　Green hellebore.

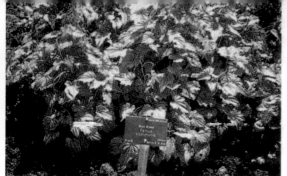

90 Black bryony.

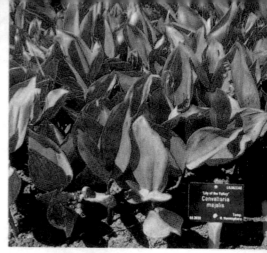

91 Lily of the valley.

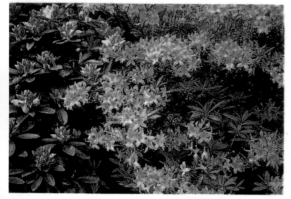

92 Rhododendron (left of photo) and azalea (yellow).

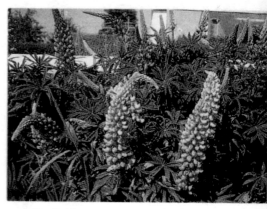

93 Lupins.

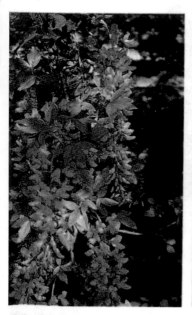

94 Laburnum.

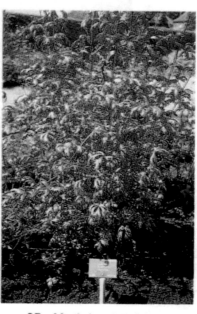

95 Monkshood (foliage only).

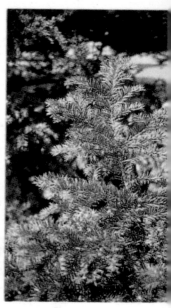

96 Yew.